Postgraduate Review Series
MCQs in Hematology

Postgraduate Review Series
MCQs in Hematology

Third Edition

Editors

Sanjeev Kumar Sharma
MD (Medicine, UCMS and GTBH) DM (Clinical Hematology, AIIMS, New Delhi)
Senior Consultant and Head
Department of Hemato-oncology and
Bone Marrow Transplantation
Venkateshwar Hospital, Sector 18A, Dwarka, New Delhi, India

Pawan Kumar Singh
MD (Medicine, KGMC) DM (Clinical Hematology, AIIMS, New Delhi)
Senior Consultant and Head
Department of Hematology and
Bone Marrow Transplantation
Artemis Hospital
Gurugram, Haryana, India

Foreword

Nitin Gupta

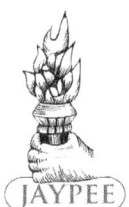

JAYPEE BROTHERS MEDICAL PUBLISHERS
The Health Sciences Publisher
New Delhi | London

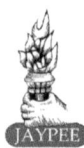
Jaypee Brothers Medical Publishers (P) Ltd

Headquarters
Jaypee Brothers Medical Publishers (P) Ltd
EMCA House, 23/23-B
Ansari Road, Daryaganj
New Delhi 110 002, India
Landline: +91-11-23272143, +91-11-23272703
+91-11-23282021, +91-11-23245672
Email: jaypee@jaypeebrothers.com

Corporate Office
Jaypee Brothers Medical Publishers (P) Ltd 4838/24,
Ansari Road, Daryaganj
New Delhi 110 002, India
Phone: +91-11-43574357
Fax: +91-11-43574314
Email: jaypee@jaypeebrothers.com

Overseas Office
J.P. Medical Ltd
83 Victoria Street, London
SW1H 0HW (UK)
Phone: +44 20 3170 8910
Fax: +44 (0)20 3008 6180
Email: info@jpmedpub.com

Website: www.jaypeebrothers.com
Website: www.jaypeedigital.com

© 2022, Jaypee Brothers Medical Publishers

The views and opinions expressed in this book are solely those of the original contributor(s)/author(s) and do not necessarily represent those of editor(s) of the book.

All rights reserved. No part of this publication may be reproduced, stored or transmitted in any form or by any means, electronic, mechanical, photocopying, recording or otherwise, without the prior permission in writing of the publishers.

All brand names and product names used in this book are trade names, service marks, trademarks or registered trademarks of their respective owners. The publisher is not associated with any product or vendor mentioned in this book.

Medical knowledge and practice change constantly. This book is designed to provide accurate, authoritative information about the subject matter in question. However, readers are advised to check the most current information available on procedures included and check information from the manufacturer of each product to be administered, to verify the recommended dose, formula, method and duration of administration, adverse effects and contraindications. It is the responsibility of the practitioner to take all appropriate safety precautions. Neither the publisher nor the author(s)/editor(s) assume any liability for any injury and/or damage to persons or property arising from or related to use of material in this book.

This book is sold on the understanding that the publisher is not engaged in providing professional medical services. If such advice or services are required, the services of a competent medical professional should be sought.

Every effort has been made where necessary to contact holders of copyright to obtain permission to reproduce copyright material. If any have been inadvertently overlooked, the publisher will be pleased to make the necessary arrangements at the first opportunity. The **CD/DVD-ROM** (if any) provided in the sealed envelope with this book is complimentary and free of cost. **Not meant for sale.**

Inquiries for bulk sales may be solicited at: jaypee@jaypeebrothers.com

Postgraduate Review Series: MCQs in Hematology

First Edition: 2015
Second Edition: 2020
Third Edition: **2022**

ISBN: 978-93-5465-065-9

Dedicated to

My beloved father late Shri Subhash Sharma for his simplicity, never-ending encouragement and passion for life.
—**Sanjeev Kumar Sharma**

My wife who is always supporting in my career.
—**Pawan Kumar Singh**

Contributors

Aditi Mittal MD (Pathology)
Attending Consultant
Department of Hematology
BLK-MAX Super Speciality Hospital
New Delhi, India

Amee Patel MD DNB (Clinical Hematology)
Consultant Hemato-oncologist and
BMT physician,
Shashwat Superspeciality Center
Surat, Gujarat

Anamika Bakliwal MD DM
(Trainee, Clinical Hematology, 3rd year)
Senior Resident
All India Institute of Medical Sciences
Rishikesh, Uttarakhand, India

Avinash Kumar Singh
MD DM (Clinical Hematology)
Consultant Hematologist
Paras HMRI Hospital
Patna, Bihar, India

Bhawna Sahay MD DNB
(Trainee, Clinical Hematology, 2nd year)
Department of
Hemato-oncology and BMT
BLK-MAX Superspeciality Hospital
New Delhi, India

Deepankar Bhattacharya MD FNB
(Hemato-oncology)
Consultant Hematologist
Medanta Hospital, Lucknow
Uttar Pradesh, India

Divya Doval MD
Attending Consultant
Department of Hemato-oncology and
Bone Marrow Transplantation
BLK MAX Super Speciality Hospital
New Delhi, India

Esha Kaul MD
Board Certified in
Internal Medicine and Hematology
(American Board of Internal Medicine)
Executive Consultant
Department of Hemato-oncology and
Bone Marrow Transplantation
Jaypee Hospital
Noida, Uttar Pradesh, India

Gopila Gupta MD, DM (Clinical Hematology)
Consultant
Clinical Hematology and
Bone Marrow Transplant Unit
Fortis Hospital, Shalimar Bagh
New Delhi, India

Gurmeet Singh MD DM
(Hematopathology)
Specialist Hematopathologist and
Hematologist
Consultant
JLN Hospital and Research Centre
Bhilai, Chhattisgarh, India

Isha Gambhir MD
Registrar
Department of Hematology and
Bone Marrow Transplantation
Artemis Hospital
Gurugram, Haryana, India

Jitendra Mohan Khunger MD DM
(Hematopathology)
Senior Consultant Hematologist
Department of Hematology
Vardhman Mahavir Medical College
and Safdarjung Hospital
New Delhi, India

Kostubh Sekhar MD
DNB (Trainee, Clinical Hematology, 3rd year)
Department of
Hemato-oncology and BMT
BLK-MAX Superspeciality Hospital
New Delhi, India

Manisha Jain MD DM (Hematology)
Associate Consultant
Department of Hematology & BMT
Artemis Hospital, Gurugram
Haryana, India

Meena Verma MD DNB
(Trainee, Clinical Hematology, 1st year)
Department of
Hemato-oncology and BMT
BLK-MAX Superspeciality Hospital
New Delhi, India

Meet Kumar MD DM (Clinical Hematology)
Consultant
Department of Hemato-oncology and
Bone Marrow Transplantation
Fortis Hospital (FMRI)
Gurugram, Haryana, India

Narendra Agrawal MD DM
(Clinical Hematology)
Senior Consultant
Department of Hemato-oncology and
Bone Marrow Transplantation
Rajiv Gandhi Cancer Institute
New Delhi, India

Neha Bhanot Sharma MD DNB
(Trainee, Clinical Hematology, 1st year)
Department of
Hemato-oncology and BMT
BLK-MAX Superspeciality Hospital
New Delhi, India

Nisarg Thakkar MD DNB
(Trainee, Clinical Hematology, 3rd year)
Senior Resident
Department of Clinical Hematology
and Bone Marrow Transplantation
Sahyadri Super Speciality Hospital
Pune, Maharashtra, India

Nishit Gupta MD PDCC (Hematopathology)
Fellow AACC, Washington
(Flow Cytometry Division)
Visiting Fellow, Kings College London
(Hematological Malignancy Division)
Attending Consultant
Department of Hematology
BLK-MAX Super Speciality Hospital
New Delhi, India

(Col) Rajiv Kumar
MD DM (Clinical Hematology)
Senior Advisor (Medicine) and
Clinical Hematologist
Professor of Medicine
INHS Asvini
Mumbai, Maharashtra, India

Rakhi Maiwall DM (Gastroenterology)
Additional Professor
Institute of Liver and Biliary Sciences
New Delhi, India

Rasika Setia DNB (Pathology) MNAMS
Associate Director and Head
Department of Hematology and
Transfusion Medicine
BLK-MAX Super Speciality Hospital
New Delhi, India

Rohan Halder DM (Clinical Hematology)
Associate Consultant
Department of Hematology and
Bone Marrow Transplantation
Artemis Hospital
Gurugram, Haryana, India

Saroj Bala MD DNB
(Trainee, Clinical Hematology 3rd year)
Department of
Hemato-oncology and BMT
BLK-MAX Superspeciality Hospital
New Delhi, India

Satyam Arora MD (Transfusion Medicine)
Assistant Professor
Department of Transfusion Medicine
Super Speciality Pediatric Hospital and
Post Graduate Teaching Institute
Noida, Uttar Pradesh, India

Sonal Jain MD DNB DM (Hematopathology)
Head, Department of Hematology
Dr Dang's Lab LLP
New Delhi, India

Sudhir Kumar Atri MD DM
(Clinical Hematology)
Senior Professor, Medicine and Incharge
Department of Clinical Hematology
Post Graduate Institute of
Medical Sciences
Rohtak, Haryana, India

Suhail Qureshi DNB (Medicine)
DNB (Medical Oncology)
Consultant
Department of Medical Oncology
Fortis Hospital, Shalimar Bagh
New Delhi, India

(Col) Suman Kumar
MD DM (Clinical Hematology)
Consultant Hematologist
Department of Clinical Hematology
Army Hospital (Research and Referral)
New Delhi, India

Sunil Debadwar MD DNB
(Trainee, Clinical Hematology, 2nd year)
Department of
Hemato-oncology and BMT
BLK-MAX Superspeciality Hospital
New Delhi, India

Tina Dadu DNB (Pathology) MNAMS
ASH Fellow (Flowcytometry)
Principal Consultant and Head
Department of Hematology
BLK-MAX Super Speciality Hospital
New Delhi, India

Vikrant Singh Bhar DM
(Hematopathology)
Consultant
Department of Hematology and
Bone Marrow Transplantation
Artemis Hospital
Gurugram, Haryana, India

Vipin Khandelwal MD FNB
(Pediatric Hematology and BMT)
Consultant and Incharge
(Pediatric Hemato-oncology)
Department of Hemato-oncology and
Bone Marrow Transplantation
BLK-MAX Super Speciality Hospital
New Delhi, India

Foreword

The previous two editions of MCQs in Hematology were highly successful and a new edition was very much needed. As we know Hematology and Oncology fields are rapidly advancing with the innovations in diagnostic and therapeutic medicine occurring at a lightening speed. For the students preparing for competitive examinations, there is a need to stay abreast of advances happening in the field to be successful.

This book on MCQs in Hematology is highly recommended and directed for students dreaming of a career in hematology, medical-oncology, hemato-pathology and bone marrow transplantation. It is well adept for postgraduate students pursuing MD (Medicine), MD (Pathology), MD (Pediatrics), MD (Biochemistry) and for students preparing for superspeciality training course in hematology, including United States Medical Licensing Examination (USMLE), Professional and Linguistic Assessments Board (PLAB), National Eligibility cum Entrance Test (NEET) and various other entrance examinations based on multiple choice questions. Written and contributed by highly trained and experienced faculties, it also gives immense clarity of concepts on various aspects of both benign and malignant hematological diseases for students undergoing superspeciality training in hematology and junior faculty in their early years of hematology.

The new edition incorporates new and updated MCQs, keeping in mind the progress made in this field in last few years. To the students it will provide competitive edge as in previous editions and to the professionals it will help in updating their knowledge.

Nitin Gupta MD DM
Department of Hematology and
Bone Marrow Transplantation
Sir Ganga Ram Hospital
New Delhi, India

Preface to the Third Edition

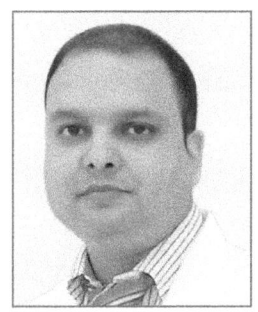

Sanjeev Kumar Sharma

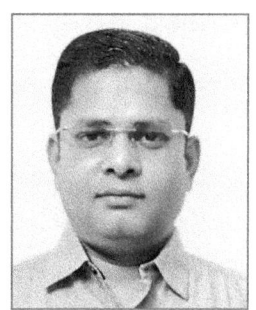

Pawan Kumar Singh

In order to keep up with the progress in hematology and the ever increasing demand of clinical hematologist, hemato-oncologist and bone marrow transplant physicians, we have come up with the third edition of the "*MCQs in Hematology*" book. This edition has many new features added to it including the addition of multiple chapters on hemato-pathology, recent advances and image-based questions. The chapters on pathology, novel therapies, stem cell transplantation and self-assessment have been expanded.

The questions have been collected and provided by the contributors who are the experts in their respective field. The explanations and references have been collected from the standard textbooks and various recent guidelines in hematology and oncology.

This book will help not only those preparing for specialization in clinical hematology and hemato-oncology but also those who want to study and prepare for various competitive examinations in hemato-pathology, medical oncology, laboratory medicine, clinical pathology, consultative hematology, transplant biology and immunohematology.

Preface to the First Edition

Hematology is an upcoming branch in the field of medicine, with lots of prospects in the near future. Multiple choice questions in hematology are compulsory in nearly all MD entrance exams though this subject still lags much behind other subjects like cardiology, gastroenterology, neurology, etc. when it comes to teaching during graduation and postgraduation. There is no MCQs book in hematology and the students keep on searching various medicine MCQs books to get questions related to hematology. Hematology is also one of the favored subjects in USMLE and PLAB entrance exams. Moreover, there were hardly 3 institutes in India where DM hematology was taught about 3 years back but now the number of seats in hematology and number of institutes offering DM hematology have increased.

Hematology not only covers clinical but also a major part of lab oriented topics and includes benign and malignant hematology which covers most of the oncology as well.

We hope that this book which will be first of such kind in *MCQs in Hematology* will be liked by many students preparing for various entrance exams as well as for others interested in hematology. The answers and references have been taken from standard textbooks of hematology, and NCCN, BCSH and other guidelines. We have tried to cover almost all the aspects of hematology, however, still some topics may have been missed. We will definitely appreciate the comments, suggestions and any other queries. If anybody wants to get answer to any doubtful or difficult question they are welcome and the doubts can be e-mailed to us. We will try to improve this book further.

Sanjeev Kumar Sharma
Pawan Kumar Singh

Acknowledgments

I would like to thank my teachers, seniors and colleagues for providing guidance and inspiration in completing the third edition of this book. I am grateful to all the contributors for their hard work and dedication in making this book a reality.

I am also indebted to my parents, my wife, brother and sister who have been an inspiration and guide to me, without whose support this work would have not been completed.

Last but not the least, I am also thankful to Jaypee Brothers Medical Publishers(P) Ltd, New Delhi, India for their support and help in publishing this book.

Only you know your dreams and only you can chase them.

—Sanjeev Kumar Sharma

I would like to thank my teachers, friends and colleagues who have inspired me to authorize this book. I would also like to thank all the contributors for providing important inputs in this third edition of the book.

—Pawan Kumar Singh

Contents

Section 1: Basic Sciences

1. Cell Biology 3
2. Basic Sciences 8
3. Hematopoiesis 11
4. Red Blood Cells 16
5. Lymphocytes 24

Section 2: Benign Hematology

6. Iron Deficiency Anemia and Anemia of Chronic Diseases 31
7. Megaloblastic Anemia 38
8. Platelets and Hemostatic Disorders 42
9. Thrombosis 53
10. Red Blood Cell Membrane Disorders 59
11. Disorders of Red Cell Enzymes 65
12. Sickle Cell Anemia 69
13. Methemoglobinemia 73
14. Immune Hemolytic Anemia 75
15. Primary Immunodeficiency Diseases 79
16. Thalassemia Syndromes 83
17. Eosinophilic Disorders 89
18. Neutrophilic Disorders 91
19. Hemophilia and Other Coagulation Factor Defects 94
20. Inherited Bone Marrow Failure Syndromes and Aplastic Anemia 103
21. Mast Cells/Basophilic Disorders 110
22. Monocyte/Macrophage Disorders 112
23. Paroxysmal Nocturnal Hemoglobinuria 114
24. von Willebrand Disease 117

Section 3: Malignant Hematology

25. Acute Lymphoblastic Leukemia 125
26. Acute Myeloid Leukemia 135
27. Acute Promyelocytic Leukemia 148
28. Chronic Lymphocytic Leukemia 153
29. Chronic Myeloid Leukemia 161
30. Hodgkin Lymphoma 171

31. Non-Hodgkin Lymphoma 181
32. Multiple Myeloma and Amyloidosis 203
33. Hairy Cell Leukemia 216
34. Myeloproliferative Neoplasms 219
35. Myelodysplastic Syndrome 223
36. Tumor Lysis Syndrome 229

Section 4: Hematopoietic Stem Cell Transplantation and GVHD

37. Stem Cell Transplantation 235
38. Graft versus Host Disease 251

Section 5: Consultative Hematology

39. Consultative Hematology 259

Section 6: Hematopathology

40. Hematopathology 271

Section 7: Transfusion Medicine

41. Blood Banking and Transfusion 305

Section 8: Immunohematology

42. Immunohematology 319

Section 9: Case-based Questions

43. Case-based Questions 325

Section 10: Novel Therapies

44. Novel Therapies 345

Section 11: Drugs and Miscellaneous

45. Drugs 357
46. Miscellaneous 365

Section 12: Self-Assessment

47. Self-Assessment 379

Section 13: Tables

48. Tables 427

Index 437

SECTION 1

Basic Sciences

1. Cell Biology
2. Basic Sciences
3. Hematopoiesis
4. Red Blood Cells
5. Lymphocytes

CHAPTER 1

Cell Biology

1. **Which is not true regarding normal cell cycle?**
   a. DNA replication occurs in G1 phase
   b. The normal cell cycle is G1 – S – G2 – M
   c. Cyclin-dependent kinase phosphorylates the protein targets
   d. Cyclin proteins are formed during specific phases

2. **Which is true regarding apoptosis?**
   a. Caspases are the ultimate effectors of apoptosis
   b. Fas and tumor necrosis factor (TNF)-R have an extracellular death domain
   c. Bcl-2 is a proapoptotic protein
   d. Entry of cytochrome C into mitochondria is a critical step

3. **All of the following are proapoptotic proteins, *except*:**
   a. Bax
   b. Bid
   c. Bcl-2
   d. Bak

4. **All of the following are antiapoptotic proteins, *except*:**
   a. Bcl-Xl
   b. Bcl-2
   c. Bcl-6
   d. None of the above

5. **Which of the following statements is not true regarding transcription factors?**
   a. Contains DNA binding and activation domain
   b. Helix-loop-helix is a DNA-binding domain (DBD)
   c. c-Abl gene translocation in chronic myeloid leukemia (CML) is an example
   d. They regulate gene expression by regulating the transcription of specific genes

6. **Which one of these statements is not true regarding cell adhesion molecules?**
   a. Chemokines are a major family
   b. They include the immunoglobulin super family
   c. They are important in the spread and localization of tumor cells
   d. Integrins can bind cells to extracellular matrix

7. **Which one of these molecules does not have a role in the transduction pathway of growth factors?**
   a. p 53
   b. Ras
   c. Signal transducer and activator of transcription (STAT)
   d. Janus kinase (JAK)

8. **Which of the following statement is not true regarding clonal abnormality in cytogenetic analysis?**
   a. Two cells with translocation, deletions or inversions signifies abnormal chromosome
   b. Single cell showing loss of chromosome
   c. Single cell with recurring structural abnormality
   d. Two cells with gain of same chromosome

9. **All of the following are major cell cycle check points, *except*:**
   a. DNA damage check point
   b. The spindle check point
   c. The spindle pole body duplication check point
   d. RNA damage check point

10. **The most abundant protein found in the red cell membrane is:**
    a. Glycoprotein
    b. Lipoprotein
    c. Mucoprotein
    d. Nucleoprotein

11. **The shape of any cell is maintained by:**
    a. Microtubules
    b. Spindle fibers
    c. Endoplasmic reticulum
    d. Membrane proteins

12. **Accumulations of cerebral gangliosides occurs due to deficiency of:**
    a. Beta-glucocerebrosidase
    b. Beta-galactosidase
    c. Hexosaminidase A
    d. Sphingomyelinase

13. **Enzyme deficient in Hunter disease is:**
    a. L-iduronidase
    b. Iduronate sulfatase
    c. Heparan sulfamidase
    d. Hyaluronidase

14. **If a chromosome divides in an axis perpendicular to usual axis of division it is going to form:**
    a. Ring chromosome
    b. Isochromosome
    c. Telocentric chromosome
    d. Mosaicism

15. Genomic imprinting includes:
a. DNA methylation
b. Histone deacetylation
c. Histone methylation
d. All of the above

16. Preferential expression of the gene depending upon the parent of origin is called:
a. Genomic imprinting
b. Anticipation
c. Mosaicism
d. Pleotropism

17. All are true for gonadal mosaicism, *except*:
a. Mutation occurs post-zygotically
b. Phenotypically normal parents
c. Can transmit the mutation to offsprings, if gametes are mutated
d. Only one child of gonadal mosaic parent would be affected

18. No change of genetic material occurs in which of the following cytogenetic abnormalities?
a. Deletion
b. Insertion
c. Translocation
d. Inversion

19. Isochromosomes are:
a. Duplication of one arm, when the other arm is lost
b. Rearrangement within chromosome involving two breaks
c. Loss of a portion of arm of chromosome
d. Transfer of a segment of one chromosome to another

ANSWERS WITH EXPLANATIONS

1. Ans. a. DNA replication occurs in G1 phase
Ref: Hoffman 7/e

Interphase is the phase of cell cycle in which the cell spends majority of its time and performs the majority of its purposes including preparation for cell division. There are three stages of interphase:
1. *G1 (gap 1)* in which the cell grows and functions normally. During this time, protein synthesis occurs and the cell grows, and organelles are produced. If the cell has not to divide again, it will remain in this phase.
2. *S (synthesis) phase*, in which the cell duplicates its DNA (via semiconservative replication).
3. *G2 (gap 2)*, in which the cell resumes its growth in preparation for cell division. Some cells do not divide often or ever, enter a *G0 (gap zero) stage*, which is either a stage separate from interphase or an extended G1 phase, which follows the restriction point (a cell cycle check point at the end of G1). Examples are terminally differentiated cells viz., neuron, myocyte, neutrophils, etc.

M (mitotic phase) has four stages—prophase, metaphase, anaphase, and telophase.

Resting lymphocytes are in G0 phase until antigen and cytokine stimulation induces them to proliferate.

Cell cycle is regulated by the phosphorylation of various cyclin-dependent kinases and these cyclins appear and disappear at different phases of cell cycle.

2. Ans. a. Caspases are the ultimate effectors of apoptosis
Ref: William's 8/e p161-3

Activation of caspases constitutes an irreversible event and the caspases are the ultimate effectors of apoptotic cell destruction. A key role is played by mitochondria in the regulation of apoptosis and cytochrome from inner mitochondrial membrane (electron transport chain) and is released into the cytosol. Where it may participate in caspase activation.

There are multiple pathways through which activation of caspases may occur but two are marked out in detail:
1. *Receptor mediated:* Fas or TNF-α receptor. Binding of these receptors by their respective ligands cause recruitment of systolic adapter molecule called Fas-associated death domain (FADD) or TNFR-associated activates the effective caspase 3.
2. *Activation of caspase 9:* Through interaction of apoptotic protease activating factor-1 (Apaf-1) which binds to cytochrome c and d ATR (ataxia telangiectasia and Rad3-related) or adenosine triphosphate (ATP) and this complex has caspase activation and recruitment domain (CARD).

The participation of mitochondria in these apoptotic events is regulated by Bcl-2. Bcl-2 is an antiapoptotic protein and it does so by preventing the release of cytochrome C into the cytosol. Release of cytochrome C to cytosol is promoted by proapoptotic factors.

3. Ans. c. Bcl-2
Ref: William's 8/e p161-162

Bcl-2 is an antiapoptotic protein.

Proapoptotic	Antiapoptotic
Bax	Bcl-X1
Bid	Bcl-2
Bad	
Bak	

4. Ans. c. Bcl-6 *Ref: William 8/e p161-2*

Bcl-6 is a sequence-specific repressor of transcription and it modulates the STAT-dependent IL-4 response of B cells. It interacts with several corepressor complexes to inhibit transcription. It is also involved in pathogenesis of various lymphoma, e.g., diffuse large B-cell lymphoma (DLBCL), Burkitt lymphoma, follicular lymphoma, and nodular lymphocyte predominant Hodgkin lymphoma (NLPHL).

5. Ans. c. c-Abl gene translocation in CML is an example *Ref: Hoffman 7/e*

c-Abl gene translocation results in the formation of abnormal protein kinase B involved in leukemogenesis.

Transcription factors regulate gene function by upregulating or downregulating its transcription. They have a sequence specific DBD and the activation domain. There are other proteins which also regulate gene function but due to the lack of DBD, they are not classified as transcription factors and examples are histone acetylases, deacetylases, kinase methylases, and chromatin remodelers (also called epigenetic factors).

Transcription factors have following domains:
- DNA-binding domain and corresponding DNA sequence are called response elements.
- Trans-activating domain (TAD) which contains binding sites for other proteins such as corregulators (also called activation functions).
- Optional signal sensing domain (SSD) which senses external signals.

The various DBD families are:
- Basic helix-loop-helix
- Basic leucine zipper (b-ZIP)
- Helix-turn-helix
- Homeodomain protein—bind to homeobox on DNA
- SRF like (serum response factor)
- Zinc fingers
- Winged helix.

Three groups of transcription factors are important in human cancers:
1. NF-Kappa B and AP-1 families
2. STAT family
3. Steroid receptors.

6. Ans. a. Chemokines are a major family *Hoffman 7/e*

Adhesion molecules are macromolecules present on cell surface which adhere through noncovalent bond with macromolecules on other cell surface and extracellular matrix (ECM). These macromolecules can be grouped into families:
- *ECM proteins:* These are adhesive proteins and proteoglycans and examples are von Willebrand factor (VWF), thrombospondin, collagen, fibronectin, laminin, and vitronectin.
- *Integrins* contain α and β submits—generally mediate cell—matrix adhesion.
- *Immunoglobulin-like receptors*—examples are intercellular adhesion molecule (ICAM), vascular cell adhesion molecule (VCAM), platelet endothelial cell adhesion molecule (PECAM), CD 2, CD 4, CD 8, and CD 3.
- *Selectins.*
- *Lectin adhesion receptors*—CD44.
- *Others*, DC—SIGN, GP—1b/1x, CD36, and cadherins.

Functional value of these cell adhesion molecules:
- Platelet adhesion and aggregation through fibrinogen, collagen, VWF, GP 1B/IX, and GP IIb/IIIa.
- Neutrophil rolling, adhesion, and migration through selectins, ICAM, and VCAM.
- Adhesion of T-cells to antigen-presenting cells (APCs) through CD 3, MHC, CD 4, and CD 8.
- Deficiency can lead to various diseases, e.g., leukocyte adhesion deficiency (LAD) type 1, LAD type 2, Glanzmann thrombasthenia, and Bernard-Soulier syndrome.
- Inappropriate expression of adhesion is implicated in thrombosis, inflammation, and tumor metastasis.

7. Ans. a. p 53 *Ref: William's 7/e p184-7*

There are two stages included in signal transduction:
1. Signaling molecule activates specific receptor protein on cell membrane.
2. A second messenger transmits the signal into the cell, eliciting a physiological response.

In either stage, the signal can be amplified.

First messengers are the intracellular chemical messenger (hormones, neurotransmitters, and paracrine/autocrine agents) which reach the cell from ECF and bind to their specific receptors. Second messengers enter the cytoplasm and act within cell to trigger a response.

The major signaling pathways are:
- Mitogen-activated protein kinase/extracellular signal-regulated kinase (MAPK/ERK) pathway for hematopoietic growth factors.
- Cyclic adenosine monophosphate (cAMP)-dependent pathway.
- Inositol trisphosphate/diacylglycerol (IP_3/DAG) pathway—involved in taste, manic depression, and tumor progression.
- JAK/STAT pathway—also involved in growth factors.
- AKT pathway—involved in cell survival and/or cell cycling (tumor).

- Ras pathway—turn on genes involved in cell growth, differentiation and survival (mutation in Ras family of proto-oncogene (H-Ras, N-Ras, and K-Ras).

p53 is a tumor suppressor protein encoded by TP53 gene. It has many mechanism of anticancer function and plays a role in apoptosis, genomic stability, and inhibition of angiogenesis. It can activate DNA repair proteins, induce growth arrest by holding the cell cycle at G1/S regulation point, and can initiate apoptosis if DNA damage proves to be irreparable.

8. Ans. b. Single cell showing loss of chromosome
Ref: William's 8/e p146

The observation of at least two cells with the same structural rearrangements (e.g., translocation, deletions, inversions and gain of same chromosome, or three cells showing loss of same chromosome) is considered evidence for the presence of an abnormal clone. However, one cell with a normal karyotype is considered evidence for the presence of a normal cell line. Patients whose cells show no alteration or nonclonal (single cell) abnormalities are considered to be normal. However, a single cell characterized by a recurring structural abnormality is an exception to this.

9. Ans. d. RNA damage check point
Ref: William's 8/e p169

A number of surveillance systems (check points) control the cell cycle and interrupt its progression when DNA damage occurs or when the cells have failed to complete a necessary event. There are three major cell cycle checkpoints. These are DNA damage checkpoints, the spindle checkpoints, and the spindle pole body duplication checkpoints. Cancer cells usually fail one or more checkpoints, which facilities a malignant transformation.

10. Ans. a. Glycoprotein *Ref: William's 7/e p573*

Glycophorins are the most abundant integral membrane glycoproteins in red blood cells (RBCs).

11. Ans. a. Microtubules *Ref: William's 7/e p1588*

The circumferential band of microtubules present below the plasma membrane plays an important role in platelet formation from megakaryocytes and contributes to platelet's discoid shape.

12. Ans. b. Beta- galactosidase *Ref: Robbins 9/e chapter 5 Genetic disorders p151*

GM1 gangliosidosis is caused by deficiency of lysosomal acid β-galactosidase; It has autosomal recessive inheritance. It leads to neurodenegerative disorder with progressive brain dysfunction due to accumulation of cerebral gangliosides.

13. Ans. b. Iduronate sulfatase *Ref: Robbins 9/e chapter 5 Genetic disorders, p151*

Mucopolysaccharidosis type II (MPS II; Hunter syndrome) is a rare X-linked recessive disease caused by deficiency of the lysosomal enzyme iduronate-2-sulphatase, leading to progressive accumulation of glycosaminoglycans in nearly all cell types, tissues and organs. Clinical manifestations include severe airway obstruction, skeletal deformities, cardiomyopathy and, in most patients, neurological decline. Death usually occurs in the second decade of life, although some patients with less severe disease have survived into their fifth or sixth decade.

14. Ans. b. Isochromosome *Ref: Robbins 9/e chapter 5 Genetic disorders*

Isochromosomes result when the centromere divides horizontally rather than vertically. One of the two arms of the chromosome is then lost, and the remaining arm is duplicated, resulting in a chromosome with only two short arms or two long arms. The most common isochromosome present in live births involves the long arm of the X chromosome and is designated i (Xq). When fertilization occurs by a gamete that contains a normal X chromosome, the result is monosomy for genes on Xp and trisomy for genes on Xq.

15. Ans. d. All of the above *Ref: Robbins 9/e chapter 5 Genetic disorders, p172*

Genomic imprinting is the inheritance out of Mendelian borders. Many of inherited diseases and human development violates Mendelian law of inheritance, this way of inheriting is studied by epigenetics. Epigenetics shows that gene expression undergoes changes more complex than modifications in the DNA sequence; it includes the environmental influence on the gametes before conception. Genomic imprinting is a process of silencing genes through DNA methylation. The repressed allele is methylated, while the active allele is unmethylated. Genomic imprinting is a reversible form of gene inactivation and is not considered a mutation.

16. Ans. a. Genomic imprinting *Ref: Robbins 9/e chapter 5 Genetic disorders, p172*

Imprinted genes are genes whose expression is determined by the parent that contributed them. Imprinted genes violate the usual rule of inheritance that both alleles in a heterozygote are equally expressed. We all inherit two copies of every autosomal gene, one copy from our mother and one from our father. Both copies are functional for the majority of these genes; however, in a small subset one copy is turned off in a parent-of-origin dependent manner. These genes are called 'imprinted' because one copy of the gene was epigenetically marked or imprinted in either the egg or the sperm. Thus, the allelic expression of an imprinted gene depends upon whether it resided in a male, in a female in the previous generation.

17. **Ans. d. Only one child of gonadal mosaic parent would be affected**   *Ref: Robbins 9/e chapter 5 Genetic disorders, p174*

Gonadal mosaicism results from a mutation that occurs post zygotically during early development. If mutation affects only cells destined to form the gonads, the gametes carry the mutation but the somatic cells of the individual are completely normal. A phenotypically normal parent who has germ-line mosaicism can transmit disease causing mutation to the offsprings through mutant gamete. Since the progenitor cells of the gametes carry the mutation, there is definite possibility that more than one child of such parent would be affected. It is seen with osteogenesis imperfecta and tuberous sclerosis.

18. **Ans. d. Inversion**   *Ref: Robbins 9/e chapter 5 Genetic disorders, p160*

Inversion refers to rearrangement that involves two breaks within a single chromosome with reincorporation of the inverted, intervening segment. It is not associated with any change in genetic material.

19. **Ans. a. Duplication of one arm, when the other arm is lost**   *Ref: Robbins 9/e chapter 5 Genetic disorders, p160*

Isochromosome results when the centromere divides horizontally rather than vertically. One of the two arms of the chromosome is then lost, and the remaining arm is duplicated, resulting in a chromosome with only two short arms or two long arms.

CHAPTER 2

Basic Sciences

1. **Intracellular destruction of proteins can occur by all of the following, *except*:**
   a. Lysosome
   b. Proteasome
   c. Spliceosome
   d. Aggresome

2. **Intron splicing occurs in:**
   a. Nucleus
   b. Cytoplasm
   c. Both
   d. Golgi body

3. **Ubiquitinated proteins are destroyed by:**
   a. Proteasome
   b. Endosome
   c. Aggresome
   d. Microsome

4. **Stem cell markers are all, *except*:**
   a. CD34
   b. CD33
   c. Thy1
   d. AC133
   e. c-Kit

5. **True about umbilical cord stem cells compared to bone marrow stem cells are all, *except*:**
   a. Contain more stem cells
   b. Causes less graft-versus-host disease (GvHD)
   c. Contains less T cells
   d. All of the above

6. **The most important mediator for physiological changes to hypoxia is:**
   a. Activation of the erythropoietin-receptor pathway
   b. Stimulation of new blood vessels
   c. Transferrin receptor (TfR) upregulation
   d. Hypoxia inducible factor (HIF) activation

7. **False regarding hemosiderin is:**
   a. Water soluble
   b. Higher iron/protein ratio than ferritin
   c. Formed by the partial digestion of ferritin
   d. All are true

8. **True regarding hepcidin is:**
   a. Predominantly expressed by the kidney
   b. Increases iron absorption
   c. Levels are increased in iron deficiency
   d. Produced by HAMP gene

9. **Mutations of matriptase-2 gene cause:**
   a. Congenital erythropoietic porphyria
   b. Porphyria cutanea tarda
   c. Iron refractory iron deficiency anemia
   d. Hepcidin deficiency

10. **True about transferrin deficiency are all, *except*:**
    a. Microcytic hypochromic anemia
    b. Tissue iron overload
    c. Treatment is with intravenous iron
    d. Fresh frozen plasma may be given

11. **Which of the following statements are false about adhesion molecules?**
    a. Chemokines are major family
    b. Involved in metastasis of tumor cells
    c. Integrins bind cells to extracellular matrix (ECM)
    d. Immunoglobulins are a superfamily
    e. Directs stem cells to bone marrow during hematopoietic stem cell transplantation (HSCT)

12. **GATA2 deficiency is not characterized by which of the following?**
    a. MONOMAC syndrome
    b. Emberger syndrome
    c. Familial MDS/AML
    d. DCML
    e. ATR-X syndrome

13. **Which of the following is genomic editing technology?**
    a. CRISPR
    b. Meganucleases
    c. TALENS
    d. ZINC FINGER NUCLEASES
    e. All of the above

ANSWERS WITH EXPLANATIONS

1. **Ans. c. Spliceosome**
   Ref: Will CL. Spliceosome structure and function. Cold Spr Harb Pers Biol. 2011;3(7):a003707.

   Lysosomes are the cytoplasmic organelles, where the intracellular destruction of endogenous or exogenous proteins occurs. The other pathway of intracellular destruction of proteins occurs through the usual ubiquitin-proteasome system. An aggresome is a proteinaceous inclusion body of abnormal or mutant protein in the cytoplasm, which fails to be eliminated by the proteasome pathway. Aggresome forms around the microtubule organizing center in eukaryotic cells. Substrates are targeted to the aggresome by an ubiquitin-independent pathway mediated by stress induced co-chaperon BAG 3 (Bcl-2 associated athanogene 3). The aggresome is eventually targeted for autophagic clearance for the cell. Some pathological proteins cannot be degraded and cause the aggresome to form inclusion bodies, e.g., Lewy bodies and Mallory's hyaline.

A spliceosome is a complex of small nuclear RNA (snRNA) and protein subunits that remove introns from a transcribed pre-mRNA (hnRNA) segment. This process is called intron splicing. The snRNAs that make up nuclear spliceosomes are named V1, V2, V4, V5, and V6. The RNA component of snRNA (small nuclear ribonucleoprotein) is rich in uridine.

A group of less abundant snRNAs, V11, V12, V4 atac, and V6 atac, together with V5 are subunits of so-called minor spliceosome. These snRNAs form the V12 spliceosome and are located in cytosol. Spliceosome is actually a ribozyme (RNA with enzyme like activity).

2. Ans. c. Both

Refer to explanation for Q. No 1.

3. Ans. a. Proteasome

Refer to explanation for Q. No 1.

4. Ans. b. CD33   *Ref: William's 8/e p234*

Human HSCs are negative for expression of mature hematopoietic lineage cell surface markers, such as those found on B-lymphoid cells (CD19), T-lymphoid cells (CD4, CD8, and CD3), macrophages (CD15 and Mac-1), and granulocytes (Gr-1). Positive selection for human HSCs is based on expression of CD34, c-kit, IL-6R, Thy-1, AC133, and CD45RA markers.

5. Ans. a. Contain more stem cells
Ref: William's 8/e p316; Hoffman 6/e p1544

Umbilical cord blood (UCB) appears to offer an advantageous source of HSCs for several reasons—UCB HSCs are young, being harvested at the neonatal stage of development, thus circumventing concerns about the ageing of HSCs. UCB contains many fewer activated T cells than adult bone marrow, therefore UCB transplantation induces less frequent, delayed engraftment, and less severe GvHD. Also, UCB HSCs are highly proliferative. However, only relatively small numbers of stem cells are harvested (approximately 10-fold lower than those in adult bone marrow) which limits their use to pediatric patients.

6. Ans. d. Hypoxia-inducible factor HIF activation
Ref: William's 8/e p824-31

In addition to activation of the erythropoietin (Epo), EpoR receptor (EpoR) pathway tissue hypoxia induces a variety of physiological responses. Parallel responses include the stimulation of new blood vessels by vascular endothelial growth factor (VEGF) and metabolic changes (e.g., in glycolytic pathway enzymes) that enable continued energy production despite inadequate oxygen availability. Also, the expression of TfR is upregulated. The most important mediator of this cellular response is a transcription factor called HIF. It activates the genes that influence the adaptive responses to hypoxia including those encoding Epo, glycolytic pathway enzymes, TfR, and VEGF.

7. Ans. a. Water soluble

Hemosiderin, unlike ferritin, is a water-insoluble, crystalline, protein-iron complex that is visible by light microscopy when stained by the Prussian blue (Perls') reaction. It has an amorphous structure, with a higher iron/protein ratio than ferritin, and is probably formed by the partial digestion of ferritin aggregates by lysosomal enzymes.

8. Ans. d. Produced by HAMP gene
Ref: Hoffman 6/e p433-4

Hepcidin plays a central role in the regulation of iron metabolism. It is a product of the HAMP gene. It is predominantly expressed in the liver. It regulates iron homeostasis by binding to cell-surface ferroportin, causing its tyrosine phosphorylation, internalization, ubiquitination, and degradation in lysosomes. It therefore acts to inhibit iron absorption, iron release from macrophages, and iron transport across the placenta. The major route of clearance is the kidney. ELISA or mass spectrometry-based techniques can be used to measure hepcidin in serum or urine. These have shown low or undetectable levels in iron deficiency and extremely high levels in inflammatory conditions, with inappropriately low levels in hemochromatosis and iron-loading anemias. Rise in serum iron, iron overload, and inflammation increases hepcidin expression, and iron deficiency, hypoxia, and increased erythropoietic activity suppress it.

9. Ans. c. Iron refractory iron deficiency anemia
Ref: Hoffman 6/e p434, 440

Homozygous or doubly heterozygous germline frameshift, splice junction, or missense mutations of matriptase-2 (TMPRSS6) are a cause of iron refractory iron deficiency anemia. The patients show a microcytic hypochromic anemia with normal or raised serum and urine hepcidin levels and low serum iron and percentage saturation of iron-binding capacity. The patients absorb iron poorly and are refractory to oral iron therapy but are partially responsive to parenteral iron. Congenital erythropoietic porphyria is due to mutations in the uroporphyrinogen III synthase gene. Either the homozygous or heterozygous presence of the C282Y and H63D mutations in the HFE gene may predispose to the development of porphyria cutanea tarda.

10. Ans. c. Treatment is with intravenous iron

Ref: Hoffman 6/e p440-2

Deficiency of serum transferrin due to mutations of the transferrin gene causes a hypochromic microcytic anemia with tissue iron overload, caused by increased plasma nontransferrin bound iron and low hepcidin levels. Treatment has been with infusions of fresh frozen plasma or apotransferrin.

11. Ans. a. Chemokines are major family

Ref: Hoffman's 6/e p97-107

Cells adhere through noncovalent bond formation between macromolecules on cell surfaces with macromolecules on other cell surfaces or in the ECM. These interactions involve either protein-protein or protein-carbohydrate recognition. ECM constitutes proteins and proteoglycans. The major proteins are collagen, von Willebrand factor (vWF), thrombospondin, elastin, fibronectin, laminin, and vitronectin. Integrins are a broadly distributed group of cell-surface adhesion receptors that consist of noncovalently associated α and β subunits. All blood cells have several different integrins for example glycoprotein IIb-IIIa (GpIIb-IIIa) on platelets and 4 β2 integrins each paired with a unique α subunit are expressed only on leukocytes. Multidomain adhesive proteins of the ECM are ligands for integrins. So options c is correct that integrins bind cells to ECM. Immunoglobulin-like receptors are present on cells, are responsible for cell-cell adhesion. The immunoglobulin-like molecules, intercellular adhesion molecule (ICAM)-1 and 2 and vascular cell adhesion molecule 1 (VACM-1), expressed on endothelial cells, as well as ICAM-3, expressed on leukocytes, mediate cell-cell contact through recognition of specific integrins on leukocytes. Immunoglobulin-like molecules like CD8 and CD4 expressed on T cells bind to the class I and class II, respectively, the T-cell receptor (TCR) (CD3) binds to the polymorphic antigen presenting domain. So option d is also correct that immunoglobulin-like molecules are a superfamily of cell adhesion molecules.

Other adhesion receptors that mediate protein-protein interactions are cadherins. Cadherins bind to homotypic binding to other cadherins on the different cell. GPIb-IX-V is other type of adhesion molecules present on platelets which bind to vWF on exposed endothelium. Selectins are other group of adhesion molecules. P-selectins cause leukocyte adhesion to activated endothelial cells and platelets. E-selectins cause leukocyte adhesion to activated endothelial cells. L-selectins cause leukocyte adhesion to other leukocytes; lymphocyte homing to lymph node; activated endothelial cells and platelets.

12. Ans. e. ATR-X syndrome

Ref: GATA2 deficiency and related myeloid neoplasms. Seminars in Hematology

Previously established clinical entities known to be caused by GATA2 mutations include monocytopenia and Mycobacterium avium complex (MONOMAC)/ dendritic cell, monocyte, B and NK lymphoid deficiency (DCML), Emberger syndrome, and familial MDS/ acute myeloid leukemia (AML). Additional recurrent manifestations include primary pediatric MDS and chronic neutropenia.

13. Ans. e. All of the above

Ref: Gai T. Genome-editing technologies: Principles and applications. Cold Spring Harb Perspect Biol 2016

The core technologies now most commonly used to facilitate genome editing, are (1) clustered regularly interspaced short palindromic repeats (CRISPR)-CRISPR-associated protein 9 (Cas9), (2) transcription activator-like effector nucleases (TALENs), (3) zinc-finger nucleases (ZFNs), and (4) homing endonucleases or meganucleases.

CHAPTER 3

Hematopoiesis

1. Which of the following is the primary site of hematopoiesis in a fetus at 20 weeks of gestation?
   a. Spleen
   b. Liver
   c. Bone marrow
   d. Yolk sac

2. Which of the following interleukin (IL) is implicated in early hematopoiesis?
   a. IL-1
   b. IL-2
   c. IL-3
   d. IL-4

3. Very high reticulocyte count is seen in:
   a. Acute hemorrhage
   b. Pure red cell aplasia (PRCA)
   c. β-thalassemia
   d. Hemoglobin E (HbE) disease

4. Which of the following stains are used for manual reticulocyte count, *except*?
   a. New methylene blue
   b. Azure B
   c. Brilliant cresyl blue
   d. Methylene blue

5. Bone marrow biopsy is indicated in:
   a. Non-Hodgkin lymphoma
   b. Acute lymphoblastic leukemia
   c. Megaloblastic anemia
   d. Disseminated intravascular coagulation

6. Bone marrow aspiration is not indicated in:
   a. Myelofibrosis
   b. Acute myeloid leukemia (AML)
   c. Multiple myeloma
   d. Leishmaniasis

7. CD 34 is a marker of:
   a. Angiogenesis
   b. T-Lymphocytes
   c. B-Lymphocytes
   d. Myeloblasts

8. Corrected reticulocyte count corrects for:
   a. Differences in blood volume
   b. Differences in hematocrit
   c. Differences in Hb
   d. Differences in red cell number

9. Hematopoiesis in the fetus starts in the:
   a. Liver at 12 weeks
   b. Liver at 6 weeks
   c. Bone marrow at 8 weeks
   d. Yolk sac at 4 weeks

10. Definitive hematopoiesis begins in embryo proper in:
   a. Liver
   b. Yolk sac
   c. Aorta-gonad-mesonephros (AGM) region
   d. Spleen

11. Which of the following growth factors/cytokines are not of potential clinical value to stimulate hematopoiesis?
   a. Thrombopoietin
   b. Erythropoietin
   c. Granulocyte macrophage colony-stimulating factor (GM–CSF)
   d. Interleukins
   e. Gamma interferon (IFN-γ)

12. Earliest hemoglobin to appear is:
   a. Portland
   b. Gower-1
   c. Gower-2
   d. HbF

13. Division occurs up to which stage of erythroid development?
   a. Proerythroblast
   b. Early normoblast
   c. Intermediate normoblast
   d. Late normoblast

14. Erythropoietin (EPO) levels are low in:
   a. Polycythemia vera
   b. Hydronephrosis
   c. Chronic obstructive airway disease
   d. Cerebellar hemangioblastoma

15. What is true regarding normal adult bone marrow?
   a. It is composed of 90% hematopoietic cells, 10% fat
   b. It has a M:E ratio of 1:2
   c. It is present in adults in the skull
   d. It secrets erythropoietin

16. Which of the following is not true about hematopoietic stem cell (HSC)?
   a. Stem cell constitute 1% of bone marrow cells
   b. Has an immunophenotype of CD 34$^+$ CD38$^-$
   c. Morphologically, it resembles small to medium sized lymphocyte
   d. Can form full hematopoietic system upon transplantation

SECTION 1 | Basic Sciences

17. Which is not a normal component of bone marrow?
   a. Endothelial cells
   b. Adipocytes
   c. Epithelial cells
   d. Fibroblasts

18. Granulocyte colony-stimulating factor (G-CSF) increases the neutrophil production by all of the following mechanism, *except*:
   a. Increased differentiation from stem cells
   b. Increased rate of proliferation of immature myeloid cells
   c. Suppression of apoptosis of myeloid cells
   d. Reduction in the self-renewal of hematopoietic stem cells

19. Which of the following statements is not true regarding extramedullary hematopoiesis?
   a. Occurs in severe hemolytic anemia
   b. May rarely be seen in megaloblastic anemia
   c. Occurs in fetus
   d. Occurs in secondary polycythemia

20. Which statement is not correct about hypersplenism?
   a. Commonly seen in chronic liver disease
   b. Peripheral blood counts are increased
   c. Splenectomy may be indicated in case the symptoms are severe
   d. May develop in patients with chronic blood transfusion

21. Which of the following is not a cause of hypersplenism in a patient who is on chronic transfusion therapy?
   a. Stimulation of immune system by allogeneic red cells
   b. Increased work of splenic macrophages
   c. Iron overload in liver and spleen with portal hypertension
   d. Pooling of blood cells in spleen

22. During final stages of red cell maturation the nucleus:
   a. More condensed
   b. Less condensed
   c. More acidophilic
   d. Increase in size

23. Metarubricyte is also known as:
   a. Pronormoblast
   b. Orthochromatic normoblast
   c. Basophilic normoblast
   d. Polychromatophil

24. All are false statements regarding normal adult marrow, *except*:
   a. Hematopoietic element constitute 90% of it
   b. M:E ratio is 1:2
   c. It is the major source of thrombopoietin
   d. Sternum and pelvis are the major site of hematopoiesis
   e. It is the major source of erythropoietin

25. All are true about HSCs, *except*:
   a. Has immunophenotype of $CD34^+/CD38^-$
   b. Morphologically looks like small to medium sized lymphocytes [mononuclear cells (MNCs)]
   c. Constitute 1% of marrow cells
   d. Can be mobilized to peripheral blood with G-CSF

26. All of these cells are normally seen in marrow, *except*:
   a. Adipose cells
   b. Osteoblasts
   c. Endothelial cells
   d. Fibroblasts
   e. Epithelial cells

27. All of the following can be used for stem cell mobilization, *except*:
   a. G-CSF
   b. GM-CSF
   c. Plerixafor
   d. Steel factor
   e. M-CSF

28. In the bone marrow, red cell precursors are located:
   a. In the center of hematopoietic cords
   b. Along the megakaryocytes
   c. Surrounding fat cells
   d. Surrounding macrophages near the sinus membrane

29. Which of the following is a multilineage cytokine?
   a. Interleukin 1
   b. Interleukin 2
   c. Interleukin 3
   d. Interleukin 4

ANSWERS WITH EXPLANATIONS

1. Ans. b. Liver Ref: *Newborn Infant Nursing Review.* United Kingdom: WB Saunders; 2004.

2. Ans. c. IL-3 Ref: *Hoffman 5/e p259 Table 24.1*

IL-3 stimulates the proliferation of multipotential progenitors and enhances the survival of early hematopoietic progenitors. It is also called multi-GSF. Other early acting cytokines are stem cell factor (SCF), flat 3 ligand (FL), TPO, IL-6, and G-CSF.

3. Ans. a. Acute hemorrhage Ref: *Dacie and Lewis 10/e p52*

Reticulocyte count can be measured using manual or automated methods. Various degrees of reticulocyte maturation can be measured using fully automated instruments. The most immature reticulocyte fraction (IRF) is produced when EPO levels are high, has more RNA and fluorescence more strongly than the mature reticulocyte normally present in peripheral blood. Presence of IRF may be an early sign of engraftment in bone marrow transplantation (BMT) patients and responsiveness to immunosuppressive therapy in severe aplastic anemia.

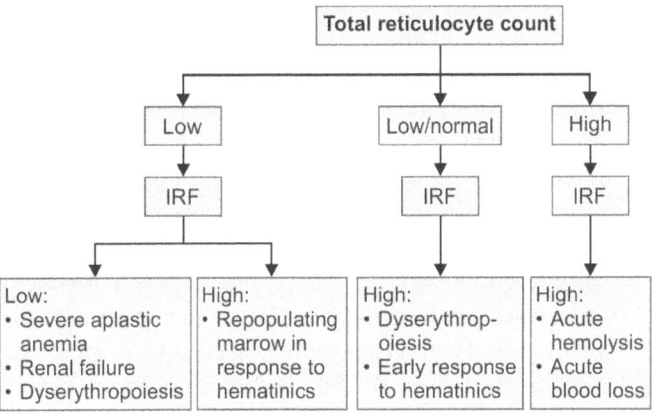

(IRF: immature reticulocyte fraction)

In PRCA, there is reticulocytopenia and in β-thalassemia and HbE disease there is ineffective erythropoiesis so reticulocyte count does not increase.

4. Ans. d. Methylene blue *Ref: Dacie and Lewis 10/e p36*

New Methylene blue is chemically different form methylene blue, which is a poor reticulocyte stain.

Stains used in automated reticulocyte counters are fluorescent dye, e.g., auramine O, thiazole orange, CD4K 530 and nonfluorescent dyes oxazine 750 and new methylene blue (Beckman Coulter).

5. Ans. a. Non-Hodgkin lymphoma
Ref: Dacie and Lewis 10/e p124-7

Bone marrow trephine biopsy is indicated in dry tap (myelofibrosis), lymphoma, AML with fibrosis (especially AML-M7), MDS (for reticulin stain), granuloma, metastasis, cellularity (aplastic anemia), and marrow infiltration.

6. Ans. a. Myelofibrosis
Ref: Dacie and Lewis 10/e p124-7

Myelofibrosis is usually diagnosed with the characteristic leukoerythroblastic blood picture and reticulin fibrosis in bone marrow biopsy. Aspirate is not helpful in the diagnosis and usually is dry tap. Rest all other requires aspirate for diagnosis.

7. Ans. a. Angiogenesis *Ref: Hoffman 6/e p124*

Circulating $CD34^+$ EPCs (endothelial progenitor cell) from human cord blood participate in new vessel formation and these angioblast-like precursor cells form new vessels via postnatal vasculogenesis. This statement also supports the first option "Although no single unique cell surface molecule serves to define an EPC, in human subjects, CD34 expression serves as fundamental marker." Capillaries of most tissues are CD34 positive, but not the endothelium of most large vessels.

8. Ans. b. Differences in hematocrit
Ref: William's 8/e p443

Absolute reticulocyte count = % reticulocyte × red cell count/100

Corrected reticulocyte % = Reticulocyte % × actual hematocrit/normal hematocrit

Reticulocyte index = absolute reticulocyte count/correction factor (usually 2)

The elevated reticulocyte count may give an erroneous impression of the actual rate of daily red cell production. Dividing the absolute reticulocyte count by a factor may provide a more accurate estimate of red cell production in case of anemia. And this factor depends on the degree of anemia—1.5 in mild, 2.5 in moderate cases, and 3.0 in severe case.

9. Ans. b. Liver at 6 weeks *Ref: Hoffman's 6/e p271*

Hematopoiesis is believed to start in two anatomic sites in developing embryo—extraembryonic (primary yolk sac) and intraembryonic (AGM), and from here the hematopoietic precursors migrate and get implanted in liver which occurs at 10 days postconception.

First erythropoiesis starts in blood islands of yolk sac (here they are immature). Before their maturation, they begin to migrate to vascular spaces of rudimentary liver by week 5. At about the same time, foci of immature erythroid cells emerge within fetal liver as the fetal (or hepatic) phase of erythropoiesis commences. From week 7 onward, liver becomes the dominant site of erythropoiesis until gestational week 30. There afterward the cavities of long bone start producing erythroid cells. Shortly after birth, all bone cavities are engaged in erythroid production, and the hepatic phase of erythropoiesis comes to an end, as the final (adult) phase of erythropoiesis unfolds exclusively within bone marrow.

10. Ans. c. Aorta-gonad-mesonephros (AGM) region
Ref: Hoffman 6/e p271/273

Throughout human development, waves of hematopoiesis are initiated sequentially in newly recruited sites. The first wave of erythropoiesis is seen in yolk sac (extraembryonic site) between 15 and 18 weeks postconception. In addition to yolk sac, foci of hematopoietic activity have been detected within the embryo proper (intraembryonic) around the developing aorta [in para aortic-splanchnopleura (P-Sp) and AGM area].

11. Ans. e. Gamma interferon (IFN-γ)
Ref: Hoffman 6/e p136

Types I or class-I cytokines (also called hematopoietins) regulate, development, differentiation, and activation of hematopoietic and immune cells. These include:
- CSFs, e.g., G-CSF and GM-CSF
- Interleukins:

- Erythropoietin
- Thrombopoietin
• Growth hormone
• Leptin.

12. **Ans. a. Portland** *Ref: Hoffman 6/e p416; Protein Science. 2007;16:1641-58.*

α-Like chains are→α and ζ(Zeta); β-like chains are ε, γ, β and δ. Hb Portland-1 is ζ2γ2, Hb Portland-2 is ζ2β2, Hb Gower-1 is ζ2ε2, and Hb Gower – 2 is α2ε2. The order of expression of globin submits is determined by their relative gene positions, i.e. ζ→α (2 copies) on chromosome 16 and ε→γ (2 copies) →δ→β on chromosome 11. Hence, the combination of ζ and ε will occur first and thus the first form of Hb produced during embryonic period will be Hb Gower-1.

13. **Ans. c. Intermediate normoblast**
Ref: William's 8/e p411-3

Early erythroblast, intermediate erythroblast, and late normoblast are also called basophilic erythroblast, polychromatophilic erythroblast, and orthochromatic erythroblast, respectively. Mitotic divisions occur till the intermediate erythroblast stage and Hb also starts appearing at this stage.

14. **Ans. a. Polycythemia vera** *Ref: William's 8/e*

A low EPO level is among the minor diagnostic criterion for polycythemia vera.

15. **Ans. c. It is present in adults in the skull**

At birth, hematopoietic activity is distributed throughout the human skeleton but it gradually recedes with time, so that in normal adult life hematopoiesis is found mainly in sternum and pelvis, with small amounts in other bones like the ribs, skull, and vertebrae. An average fragment cellularity is normally between 25 and 75%, except at extremes of age. 90% hematopoietic cells compose only during infancy. It has been shown by various studies that normal M:E ratio is of 2.2:2.4. Kidney secretes EPO but not the bone marrow.

16. **Ans. a. Stem cell constitutes 1% of bone marrow cells**
Ref: Hoffman 6/e p79-80, 1477; William's 8/e p231-2

Hematopoietic stem cells are rare, occurring at a frequency of 1 stem cell per 10,000–100,000 bone marrow cells. HSCs are capable of rescuing lethally irradiated hosts by reconstituting the entire repertoire of hematopoietic cells in the host.

17. **Ans. c. Epithelial cells**
Ref: Bone Marrow Pathology. Barbara Bain 3/e p4

The bone marrow stroma is composed of fat cells and a meshwork of blood vessels, branching fibroblasts, macrophages, some myelinated and nonmyelinated nerve fibers, and a small amount of reticulin. Besides this, osteoblasts and osteoclasts are also found.

18. **Ans. d. Reduction in the self-renewal of HSCs**
Ref: Hoffman 6/e p282-283; van Raam BT, et al. Blood. 2008;112(5):2046-54

Early progenitor cells express receptors for multiple cytokines but expression becomes more restricted as the cell becomes committed to a specific lineage. Early progenitor cells have capabilities of dividing and one daughter cell can produce new HSC and other can differentiate or undergo apoptosis. The "early acting cytokines include IL-1, IL-6, SCF, FLT-3 ligand, and G-CSF. IL-63 drives the stem cells toward myelomonocytic lineage, subsequently leading to commitment and lineage restricted differentiation. The major cytokines mediating neutrophil maturation are G-CSF and GM-CSF. G-CSF supports the survival and proliferation of developing myeloid cells at all stages of differentiation and increases the functional activity of mature neutrophils. Studies have shown that the mature neutrophils are more susceptible to apoptosis. Self-renewal capacity of HSC is actually increased rather than decreased.

19. **Ans. d. Occurs in secondary polycythemia**
Ref: Hoffman 5/e p510, 1065

A recognized cause of extramedullary hematopoiesis is severe chronic hemolytic anemia which is particularly seen in thalassemia syndromes. Nontender hepatomegaly, but more often mild splenomegaly, may rarely be caused by extramedullary hematopoiesis in severe anemia. In secondary polycythemia, marrow is hyperplastic because of increased EPO production in response to hypoxia or other factors.

20. **Ans. b. Peripheral blood counts are increased**
Ref: Hoffman 6/e p2261

A common feature of chronic liver disease with portal hypertension is hypersplenism. The bone marrow is hyperplastic and the peripheral blood cell counts are decreased due to destruction of mature formed elements. Any cell line can be affected, alone or in combination. Splenectomy should be performed for clinical indications rather than for specific diagnosis. In some cases, it improves the condition, e.g. erythrocyte disorder due to membrane (HS) or enzyme disorders, storage disorder, portal hypertension, immune thrombocytopenia (ITP), and in thalassemia when the requirement of blood transfusion is high [>200 mL/kg/day of packed red blood cell (RBC)].

21. **Ans. d. Pooling of blood cells in spleen**
Ref: Hoffman 6/e p2261

Hypersplenism develops in patients who receive chronic transfusion. The possible reasons are:
• Antigenic load of allogeneic transfused cells stimulates the immune system.
• Transfused cells have shorter survival than normal red cells, which increases the work of splenic macrophages.
• Iron overload causes hemosiderosis of both the spleen and liver and portal hypertension thus developed further increases splenic pathology.

22. Ans. a. More condensed *Ref: Hoffman's 6/e p261*

As the red cell matures and after final mitotic division, the nucleus becomes more condensed and is smaller in size. Nucleus is mostly basophilic and not acidophilic.

23. Ans. b. Orthochromatic normoblast

The various stages of RBC development are rubriblast (proerythroblast) then prorubricyte then rubricyte then metarubricyte (orthochromatic normoblast-last nucleated cell) then polychromatic erythrocyte (reticulocyte) and then finally the mature erythrocyte.

24. Ans. d. Sternum and pelvis are the major sites of hematopoiesis

Ref: Hoffman 5/e p296; Hoffbrand 5/e p2; Barbara Bain. BM Pathology 3/e p10, 37

At birth, hematopoiesis occurs throughout the skeleton, but gradually as the child becomes adult it is mainly confined to sternum and pelvis, with small amounts in ribs, skull, and vertebrae. An average fragment cellularity is normally between 25 and 75%, except at extremes of ages. 90% hematopoietic cells compose during infancy only. The normal M:E ratio is 2.2:2.4. Thrombopoietin is mainly produced by liver and kidney and EPO is mainly produced by JG cells of kidney. Inducible expression of thrombopoietin has been detected by more sensitive methods in bone marrow and spleen in the setting or thrombocytopenia, although this likely accounts for only a minor fraction of thrombopoietin production. Low level expression has also been reported in the amygdala and hippocampus of brain.

25. Ans. c. Constitute 1% of marrow cells

Ref: William's 7/e p302; Hoffman 5/e p190, 200, 202

HSCs are rare, occurring at a frequency of 1 stem cell per 10,000–100,000 bone marrow cells. Human HSCs are CD34$^+$CD38$^-$ and are negative for other lineage specific markers. The HSCs morphologically look like MNCs that are why in peripheral blood stem cell (PBSC) collection product MNC count is done; however, in bone marrow stem cell collection, TNC is done which means all nucleated cell count. The HSCs can be mobilized from bone marrow to peripheral blood with the help of G-CSF and GM-CSF.

26. Ans. e. Epithelial cells *Ref: William's 7/e p38-42*

The normal cells in bone marrow are endothelial cells, adipocytes, osteoclasts, osteoblasts, stromal cells (derived from fibroblasts), macrophages and lymphocytes, and obviously the hematopoietic cells.

27. Ans. e. M-CSF *Ref: Hoffman's 6/e p1477-1479*

The ability of recombinant hematopoietic cytokines to increase the level of myeloid progenitor cell in blood was reported in 1988 by different groups for both G-CSF (recombinant methionyl human G-CSF, FILGRASTIM; recombinant human G-CSF, LENOGRASTIM) and GM-CSF. Recognition of mobilization potential of G-CSF led many investigators to study other cytokines, including erythropoietin, M-CSF, IL-3, PIXY 321 (a fusion molecule), and SCF (steel factor) for their capacity to mobilize HSCs to peripheral blood. Only SCF is approved for human use (in Europe), and none of these cytokines are widely used in clinical HSC transplantation. Plerixafor is a small molecule inhibitor of CXCR4 which used for HSC mobilization in myeloma and lymphoma case where patients had received multiple chemotherapies or have daily G-CSF mobilization (poor mobilizers). Usually, it is given in combination with G-CSF.

28. Ans. d. Surrounding macrophages near the sinus membrane *Ref: William's 5/e p369*

The anatomical unit of erythropoiesis in the normal adult is the erythroblastic island, which consists of 1 or 2 centrally located macrophages surrounded by maturing erythroid cells. When the erythroblast is sufficiently mature for nuclear expulsion, it makes contact with an endothelial cell, passes through a pore in the cytoplasm of the endothelial cell, and enters the circulation. The erythroblastic island is a fragile structure and is disrupted during the process of bone marrow aspiration.

29. Ans. a. Interleukin 1 *Ref: William's 7/e p207*

IL-1 induces production of other cytokines from many cells, works in synergy with other cytokines on primitive cells. IL-2 is T cell growth factor, IL-3 stimulates the growth of multiple myeloid cell types, involved in delayed hypersensitivity reactions and IL-4 stimulates B cell growth and modulates the immune response by affecting immunoglobulin class switching.

CHAPTER 4

Red Blood Cells

1. Mature red blood cells (RBCs) produce energy by:
   a. Glycolytic pathway
   b. Oxidative phosphorylation
   c. Hexose monophosphate (HMP) shunt
   d. Cori cycle

2. Blood for complete blood count (CBC) should normally be anticoagulated with:
   a. Heparin
   b. Citrate
   c. Ethylenediaminetetraacetic acid (EDTA)
   d. Fluoride

3. Which order for taking blood samples is recommended?
   1. Serum sample
   2. EDTA sample
   3. Heparin sample
   4. Fluoride sample
   5. Blood culture sample
   a. 1 → 2 → 3 → 4 → 5
   b. 5 → 1 → 3 → 2 → 5
   c. 5 → 4 → 3 → 2 → 1
   d. 5 → 3 → 2 → 4 → 1

4. The measurement most likely to correlate with hypochromia observed on a blood film is:
   a. Red cell distribution width
   b. Packed cell volume (PCV)
   c. Mean corpuscular hemoglobin (MCH)
   d. Mean corpuscular hemoglobin concentration (MCHC)
   e. Mean corpuscular volume (MCV)

5. Erroneous measurement of hemoglobin (Hb) concentration by cyanmethemoglobin method may result from the presence of significant proportion of:
   a. Oxyhemoglobin
   b. Carboxyhemoglobin
   c. Deoxyhemoglobin
   d. Methemoglobin

6. An automated differential white cell count may be inaccurate because of all, *except*:
   a. The presence of nucleated RBC (nRBC)
   b. Inherited peroxide deficiency
   c. An increased reticulocyte count
   d. Nonlysis of RBCs

7. All of the following will lead to shift of dissociation of curve toward right, *except*:
   a. Decreased pH
   b. Increased 2,3-bisphosphoglyceric acid (2,3-BPG) level
   c. Increased CO_2
   d. Decreased CO_2

8. Major histocompatibility complex (MHC) class I antigens are present on all, *except*:
   a. T-lymphocyte
   b. Macrophages
   c. Platelet
   d. RBC

9. Basophilic stippling is seen in all, *except*:
   a. Iron deficiency anemia (IDA)
   b. Megaloblastic anemia
   c. Thalassemia
   d. Liver disease

10. Bedside test to distinguish between hemoglobinuria and myoglobinuria:
    a. Color of serum
    b. RBC in urine
    c. Urine for hemosiderin
    d. Benzidine test

11. A 60-year-old patient is a known case of carcinoma prostate has become more sick with development of anemia. The most likely finding in his CBC would be:
    a. Microcytic hypochromic anemia
    b. Myelophthisic anemia
    c. Presence of schistocytes
    d. Normocytic normochromic anemia

12. Which statement is true regarding hemoglobin (Hb)?
    a. One Hb molecule carries 1 iron atom
    b. Catabolized in macrophages
    c. Type of Hb varies in children and adult
    d. Hb level is low at birth as compared to adult life

13. Which statement is true about reticulocytes?
    a. Contains DNA but no RNA
    b. Count is increased in megaloblastic anemia
    c. Raised after chemotherapy
    d. Raised after hemorrhage

14. Which one of the following is not true regarding erythropoietin (EPO)?
   a. Its gene has hypoxia response elements
   b. High altitude dwellers have more EPO levels
   c. About 90% of hormone is made in liver
   d. Levels are high in polycythemia secondary to tumor secreting EPO but are low in severe renal disease and polycythemia vera

15. Which one of the following is true regarding erythropoietin?
   a. Hypotension can be a side effect
   b. Mainly indicated for treatment of anemia associated with leukemia
   c. Can be given orally
   d. Oral or parental iron is often needed for good response

16. Which of these statements is not true about the hemoglobin (Hb)?
   a. Hb is 70% saturated in arterial blood
   b. When O_2 is released, the β-chain is pulled apart and thus entry of 2,3-BPG is allowed and resulting in lower affinity of the O_2 molecule
   c. P50 of normal blood is 26.6 mm Hg
   d. As the Hb molecule loads and unloads O_2, the globin genes move on each other

17. Which one of these is not true regarding RBCs?
   a. Each cell traverses ≥ 1,500 km in its life
   b. Generates adenosine triphosphate (ATP) by Embden-Meyerhof-Parnas (EMP) pathway
   c. Generates reducing equivalents as nicotinamide adenine dinucleotide (NADH) by EMP pathway and as reduced nicotinamide adenine dinucleotide phosphate (NADPH) by HMP shunt
   d. Has a maximum diameter of 3.5 μm

18. In individuals living at high altitudes, the hemoglobin:
   a. Higher   b. Lower
   c. Same   d. No change

19. The types of hemoglobins seen in a normal adult are:
   a. A, A_2, F   b. S, A, F
   c. A, C, A_2 d. A, F

20. The heme part of normal adult Hb consists of:
   a. Porphyrin ring with a Fe molecule in center
   b. Pyrrole ring with four Fe molecule in the center
   c. Polypeptide chain with single Fe molecule
   d. Four porphyrin ring containing Fe molecule in center

21. The polypeptide chains found in normal adult Hb:
   a. 1 alpha and 3 beta chains
   b. 2 alpha and 2 beta chains
   c. 1 alpha, 2 beta, and 1 delta chains
   d. 2 alpha

22. Normally bilirubin is metabolized by:
   a. Reused in RBCs
   b. Excreted as it is
   c. Converted to biliverdin
   d. Taken up by macrophages in liver

23. Stain used for reticulocyte is:
   a. Supravital stain   b. Counter stain
   c. Nonvital   d. Ultravital

24. In the reticulocyte, after staining with new methylene blue the reticulum is:
   a. DNA   b. RNA
   c. Ribosome   d. Organelle

25. When reticulocytes are stained with supravital stain like new methylene blue, they may be confused with:
   a. Döhle bodies
   b. Heinz body
   c. HbH inclusions
   d. Pappenheimer bodies

26. A red cell which is not biconcave disc is called:
   a. Anisocyte   b. Microcyte
   c. Spherocyte   d. Poikilocyte

27. A red cell with slit-like central pallor is called:
   a. Stomatocyte   b. Drepanocyte
   c. Schistocyte   d. Echinocyte

28. Fragmented red cells are called:
   a. Schistocyte   b. Drepanocyte
   c. Acanthocyte   d. Echinocyte

29. Round, purple staining nuclear fragments in the red cells are called:
   a. Basophilic stippling
   b. Pappenheimer bodies
   c. Howell-Jolly bodies
   d. Polychromatophilic granules

30. Small, peripheral, basophilic punctate iron laden granules in a red cell are called:
   a. Basophilic stippling
   b. Pappenheimer bodies
   c. Howell-Jolly bodies
   d. Polychromatophilic granules

31. Cyanmethemoglobin measures all types of Hb, *except*:
   a. Deoxyhemoglobin   b. Sulfhemoglobin
   c. Carboxyhemoglobin   d. Methemoglobin

32. The principle of cyanmethemoglobin method for determination of Hb concentration is:
   a. Potassium ferricyanide converts Hb iron from the ferrous to the ferric state to form methemoglobin, which combines with potassium cyanide to produce cyanmethemoglobin
   b. Ferricyanide converts Hb from the ferric state to the ferrous state to form methemoglobin, which combines with potassium cyanide to produce cyanmethemoglobin

c. Potassium cyanide converts Hb from the ferrous to the ferric state to form methemoglobin, which combines with ferricyanide to produce cyanmethemoglobin
d. Potassium ferricyanide converts Hb iron from the ferric to the ferrous state to form methemoglobin, which combines with ferricyanide to produce cyanmethemoglobin

33. In cyanmethemoglobin method, the concentration of hemoglobin level is measured by:
a. Light scatter
b. Nephelometry
c. Electrical impedance
d. Spectrophotometry

34. The hematocrit is the:
a. Volume of packed red cell
b. Volume of total red cell
c. Volume of average red cell
d. Weight of average red cell

35. The special stain for sideroblast, siderocyte, iron stores, and siderotic granules:
a. Nitroblue tetrazolium
b. Periodic acid-Schiff (PAS)
c. Prussian blue
d. Sodium metabisulfite

36. In Hb electrophoresis, with alkaline buffer (pH 8.4), the normal or abnormal Hb moves toward:
a. Anode
b. Cathode
c. Both directions
d. Does not move

37. The red cell indices of a patient were—MCV of 65 fL, MCH 22 picogram and MCHC of 24%, then the most likely finding on peripheral blood smear would be:
a. Microcytic and hypochromic
b. Microcytic and normochromic
c. Macrocytic and normochromic
d. Normocytic and hypochromic

38. In megaloblastic anemia, the defect in red cell lies in the:
a. Nucleus
b. Cytoplasm
c. Hb
d. Iron metabolism

39. Which of the following statement is FALSE regarding Hb?
a. It has quaternary protein structure
b. It is metabolized in macrophages of spleen
c. At birth, the level is high
d. One molecule has only 1 iron atom

40. Which of the following features of RBCs is responsible for limiting their life span?
a. Loss of nucleus
b. Loss of mitochondria
c. Increased red cell membrane fragility
d. Reduction of Hb

41. Which of the following molecule of Hb has the least affinity for oxygen?
a. Tense state
b. Relaxed state
c. Arterial
d. Venous

42. The HMP shunt pathway in RBCs provides:
a. Glucose and lactic acid
b. 2,3-BPG and methemoglobin
c. NADPH and glutathione
d. ATP

43. A 65-year-old man presented with abdominal pain, heaviness in left hypochondrium with 1 episode of small hematemesis. On examination, he was found to be having, moderate ascites, hepatomegaly, and very big spleen. His blood investigations reveal Hb—7 g/dL, total Leukocyte Count (TLC)—2,700, platelet count of 90,000/cumm and leukoerythroblastic blood picture. He is diagnosed to be having primary myelofibrosis. Which is the type cell seen in peripheral blood of this patient?
a. Schistocytes
b. Sickle cells
c. Dacryocytes
d. Spherocytes
e. Target cells

44. A 40-year-old male, nonsmoker presented with heaviness in head, and flushing of face. On evaluation, he was found to be having plethora and redness in hand and feet. There is also hepatosplenomegaly. He is suspected of having polycythemia vera. Which of the following will be seen in this patient?
a. Low EPO level and low red cell mass
b. Raised EPO level and low red cell mass
c. Raised EPO level and raised red cell mass
d. Normal EPO level and normal red cell mass
e. Low EPO level and raised red cell mass

45. Which of the following are coeluting Hb with HbA1c in same window?
a. Hb Hope
b. Hb N-Baltimore
c. Hb New York
d. Hb Fannin-Lubbock

ANSWERS WITH EXPLANATIONS

1. Ans. a. Glycolytic pathway

Mature RBCs produce energy by only glycolytic pathway because they do not have mitochondria for oxidative phosphorylation. HMP shunt is present in RBC but it produces reducing equivalents (NADH, NADPH).

2. Ans. c. Ethylenediaminetetraacetic acid (EDTA)

3. Ans. b. 5 → 1 → 3 → 2 → 5   *Ref: Barbara Bain 4/e p5*

Recommended order for taking blood samples:
- Blood culture
- Serum samples in plain glass tube
- Sodium citrate tubes
- Gel separator tubes/plain plastic tubes for serum
- Heparin tubes
- EDTA tubes
- Fluoride tubes.

4. Ans. d. Mean corpuscular hemoglobin concentration (MCHC)   *Ref: Barbara Bain 4/e p40*

5. Ans. b. Carboxyhemoglobin

Ref: Barbara Bain 4/e p22-3

In cyanmethemoglobin method Hb, methemoglobin (MetHb)_ and carboxyhemoglobin are all converted to cyanmethemoglobin and are thus included in measurement of Hb. Sulfhemoglobin is not at all converted to cyanmethemoglobin which can lead to slight under estimation of Hb. Carboxyhemoglobin is slowly converted to cyanmethemoglobin which can lead to over estimation of Hb, if the test is read at 3 minutes because carboxyhemoglobin absorbs more light at 540 mm than does cyanmethemoglobin.

6. Ans. c. An increased reticulocyte count

Ref: Barbara Bain 4/e p47

White blood cell (WBC) measured by automated counter based on impedance principle is falsely elevated due to presence of nRBCs. WBC in the optical channel excludes nRBC by means of a moving threshold. However, optical channel employs less potent lytic agent so WBC may be falsely elevate in the presence of osmotically resistant red cells (neonatal RBC).

7. Ans. d. Decreased CO_2

Shift to left	Shift to right
Increased pH	Decreased pH
Decreased CO_2	2,3-bisphosphoglyceric acid
CO	Increased CO_2
Methemoglobinemia	Increased temperature Sulfhemoglobinemia

As the O_2 affinity of Hb increases, curve is shifted toward left and vice versa.

8. Ans. d. RBC   *Ref: William's 8/e p2269-70*

Major histocompatibility complex (MHC) class I	MHC class II
Present on all nucleated cells and platelets	B cells, dendritic cells, monocytes, macrophages, and endothelial cells
Bind to peptides that are derived from proteins synthesized in cytosol (e.g., viral-encoded proteins) and usually are of 8–10 amino acids	Bind to peptides derived from endogenous proteins degraded in intracellular vesicles usually > 13 amino acids long
Human leukocyte antigen (HLA)–A, HLA–B, and HLA–C	HLA–D (DP, DQ, and DR)

9. Ans. a. Iron deficiency anemia (IDA)
Ref: Dacie and Lewis 10/e p84-85

Basophilic stippling (or punctate basophilia) indicates disturbed erythropoiesis and is seen in thalassemia, megaloblastic anemia, infections, liver disease, lead poisoning, unstable Hbs, and pyrimidine 5' nucleotidase deficiency.

10. Ans. a. Color of serum

After centrifuging, the serum of myoglobinuria is clear, whereas the serum of hemoglobinuria after centrifugation is pink.

11. Ans. b. Myelophthisic anemia

Ref: William's 8/e p614-15

The most likely cause of anemia in this patient is myelophthisic anemia; however, he can have microcytic hypochromic anemia due to iron deficiency or microangiopathic hemolytic anemia (MAHA) with presence of schistocytes, but these possibilities are less likely. Almost all cancers can metastasize to the marrow, but the most common are lung, breast, and prostate. Ca prostate is less likely to cause MAHA.

12. Ans. b. Catabolized in macrophages

Ref: William's 8/e p13, 89, 452

After the first week of extrauterine life, Hb level falls from 17 g/dL to 11 g/dL by 2 months age. Normal adult levels of HbA_2 are achieved by 2 months of age so type of Hb in a normal person is mostly HbA_2 at all ages. Intravascular Hb is taken by haptoglobin and each molecule can combine 2 molecules of Hb. This complex is carried to liver parenchyma where macrophages take it up and heme is separated from globin. Globin goes for proteolytic destruction in lysosome and heme is converted to biliverdin and CO by heme oxygenase. Biliverdin is further catabolized to bilirubin by biliverdin reductase. Heme-hemopexin is taken up by a low-density lipoprotein related receptor, CD91. Haptoglobin-Hb is taken up by CD163.

13. Ans. d. Raised after hemorrhage
Ref: William's 8/e p414-15

The reticulocyte, as it enters circulation, retains mitochondria, small numbers of ribosome, the centriole and remnants of Golgi body, and does not contain nucleus (or DNA). Maturation of reticulocyte requires 24-48 hours. Reticulocyte count is not increased in megaloblastic anemia due to ineffective erythropoiesis. After acute hemorrhage reticulocyte is markedly raised.

14. Ans. c. About 90% of hormone is made in liver
Ref: William's 8/e p828, 830

HIF-1 (hypoxia inducible factor-1) is the transcriptional factor responsible for activation of EPO gene and its production is increased by hypoxia. High-altitude dwellers have usually more EPO levels due to chronic hypoxia but there is no correlation between the level and altitude. EPO is mainly produced by kidneys. In severe renal failure and polycythemia vera, EPO levels are characteristically low. Polycythemia secondary to tumors is due to inappropriate secretion of EPO and thus levels are high in blood.

15. Ans. d. Oral or parental iron is often needed for good response
Ref: William's 8/e p500-01

Hypertension is the side effect of EPO therapy and not hypotension. EPO therapy is mainly required for treatment of anemia of chronic renal failure or chronic inflammation. Anemia of chronic malignancy, myeloma, or anemia of leukemia does not respond to EPO therapy. This is a recombinant protein and can be given only by parenteral route. Coadministration of iron by oral or parenteral route with EPO is required for optimal response to EPO therapy.

16. Ans. a. Hb is 70% saturated in arterial blood
Ref: Harper's Biochemistry 23/e p50-6

P50 is the partial pressure of oxygen that half saturates a Hb. For Hb A, P50 is 26 mm of Hg; for Hb F, P50 is 20 mm Hg.

On oxygenation, the iron atoms of deoxyhemoglobin move into the plane of the heme ring. Fully deoxygenated molecule lies in the T-structure (Taught) and fully oxygenated molecule lies in R structure (Relaxed), but these structures are too unstable to exist in significant numbers.

One molecule of BPG is bound per Hb tetramer in the central cavity formed by all four submits. This cavity is of sufficient size for BPG only when the Hb is in T-form (deoxygenated form). Thus BPG stabilizes the T or deoxygenated form of Hb.

Arterial oxygen saturation is 95% and not 70%.

17. Ans. d. Has a maximum diameter of 3.5 μm
Ref: William's 8/e p649, 650

Glucose is metabolized in RBC through EMP pathway or HMP shunt. Glycolytic pathway leads to formation of pyruvate and lactate. In glycolysis, ADP is phosphorylated to ATP and NAD^+ is reduced to NADH. 2,3-BPG is also formed by glycolysis. HMP shunt oxidizes glucose 6-phosphate, reducing $NADP^+$ to NADPH. The normal diameter of RBC is 6-8 microns; however, it is flexible so that it can pass through vessels of diameter 3-5 microns. A single RBC travels about 1,500 km in its brief 4-month lifetime.

18. Ans. a. Higher
Ref: Hoffman's 6/e p1003

High-altitude results in hyperventilation, alkalosis, and shift of oxygen dissociation curve to the left, leading to the impaired release of oxygen from Hb and ultimately tissue hypoxia. Healthy highlanders develop pulmonary hypertension, right ventricular hypertrophy (RVH) leading to increased pulmonary vascular resistance, and pulmonary arterial pressure as compared with individuals at sea level. These pulmonary pressures are normalized after living for 2 years at sea level. Despite these changes high landers are able to perform their normal or even strenuous activities.

19. Ans. a. HbA, HbA2 and HbF
Ref: Hoffman's 6/e p414

In adult the types of Hb seen are HbA ($\alpha_2\beta_2$—97%), HbA_2 ($\alpha_2\delta_2$—2.5%), and HbF ($\alpha_2\gamma_2$—1%).

20. Ans. a. Porphyrin ring with a Fe molecule in center

A heme group consists of an iron (Fe) ion held in a heterocyclic ring, known as porphyrin. This porphyrin ring consists of four pyrrole molecules cyclically linked together. So in a Hb there are four heme molecule linked to four different globin molecule.

21. Ans. b. 2 alpha and 2 beta chains
Ref: Hoffman's 6/e p408-09

Normal Hb has 2 alpha and 2 nonalpha chains (which is beta in case of adult Hb).

22. Ans. b. Excreted as it is

In the macrophage heme is converted to Biliverdin (by heme oxygenase) and then this biliverdin is converted to bilirubin (by biliverdin reductase). Then this bilirubin is excreted as it is in intestine through bile duct, where it is converted to stercobilin by intestinal bacteria or transported back to liver by enterohepatic circulation.

23. Ans. a. Supravital stain
Ref: Hoffman's 6/e p1003

Reticulocytes are visualized by supravital staining such as new methylene blue, brilliant cresyl blue, crystal violet, or pure azure blue that precipitates the RNA and organelles, forming a filamentous reticulum.

24. Ans. c. Ribosome
Ref: William's 7/e p373-4

Supravital staining with brilliant cresyl blue or new methylene blue produces aggregates of ribosomes, mitochondria, and other cytoplasmic organelles. These artifactual aggregates stain deep blue and arranged in reticular strands, give the reticulocyte its name. Option c is preferred over d (organelle) because it is more specific.

25. Ans. c. HbH inclusions *Ref: William's 7/e p374*

Hemoglobin H is composed of β_4 tetramers, indicating that β chains are present in excess as a result of impaired α chain production. These supravital stains cause the formation of a large number of small membrane bound inclusions, giving the cell the characteristic golf-ball like appearance. Color looks like reticular inclusions of reticulocytes.

26. Ans. d. Poikilocyte *Ref: Hoffman's 6/e p609*

In poikilocytosis means variation in cell shape. Poikilocyte may be oval, tear-drop shaped, sickle shaped, irregularly contracted, spherical, or any other shape. Normal red cells are biconcave disks. A poikilocyte is an abnormal shaped cell.

27. Ans. a. Stomatocyte *Ref: Dacie and Lewis 10/e p95-6*

Stomatocytes are red cells in which the central biconcave appears slit-like in dried films. In wet preparations, the stomatocyte is a cup-shaped cell. They are seen in hereditary stomatocytosis and South-East Asian ovalocytosis.

28. Ans. a. Schistocyte *Ref: Hoffman's 6/e p609*

Schistocytes (schizocyte) are the fragmented red cells and are seen in disseminated intravascular coagulation (DIC), thrombotic thrombocytopenic purpura-hemolytic uremic syndrome (TTP-HUS). They can be of various shapes like helmet cells, etc.

29. Ans. c. Howell-Jolly bodies

Ref: Dacie and Lewis 10/e p97

Howell-Jolly bodies are nuclear remnants and (usually single) may be seen in a small percentage of red cells in pernicious anemia. Cells containing them are regularly present after splenectomy and splenic atrophy. Usually, only a few such cells are present, but they may be numerous in case of coeliac disease in which there is splenic atrophy and coexisting folate deficiency.

30. Ans. b. Pappenheimer bodies

Ref: Dacie and Lewis 10/e p39, 84, 97-8

Pappenheimer bodies are small peripherally located basophilic (almost black) erythrocyte inclusions. Usually, small numbers are present in a cell. They are composed of hemosiderin, and their presence is related to iron overload and hyposplenism. It should be differentiated from punctate basophilia (basophilic stippling), which means the presence of numerous basophilic granules distributed throughout the cells. In contrast to pappenheimer bodies, they do not give a positive Perl's reaction for ionized iron. Basophilic stippling is indicative of disturbed erythropoiesis for example thalassemia, megaloblastic anemia, infections, liver disease, lead or other heavy metal poisoning, unstable Hb, and pyrimidine 5'-nucleotidase deficiency.

The reticulofilamentous material of reticulocyte is less bluish than Pappenheimer bodies. Phase contrast microscope can differentiate between these two.

HbH undergoes denaturation in the presence of brilliant cresyl blue or new methylene blue, resulting in round inclusion bodies that stain greenish-blue. These can be easily differentiated from reticulofilamentous material.

Heinz bodies are also stained by new methylene blue, but they stain lighter shade of blue than the reticulofilamentous material of reticulocytes and stain well with methyl violet.

31. Ans. b. Sulfhemoglobin

Ref: Dacie and Lewis 10/e p26-7

There are two methods commonly used for measurement of Hb: cyanmethemoglobin and oxyhemoglobin. In cyanmethemoglobin, the blood is diluted with a solution containing potassium cyanide and potassium ferricyanide. When blood is mixed with a solution of potassium ferricyanide, potassium cyanide, and Drabkin's solution, the red cells are lysed by producing evenly disturbed solution. Potassium ferricyanide transforms Hb to methemoglobin, and methemoglobin combines with potassium cyanide to produce cyanmethemoglobin. Hb, methemoglobin, and carboxyhemoglobin are converted to cyan-methemoglobin but not sulfhemoglobin.

The other method is Sahli's method (acid-hematin method), but it is less accurate, because the color develops slowly, is unstable, and begins to fade immediately after it reaches its peak. The alkaline-hematin method gives true estimate of total Hb even if carboxyhemoglobin, sulfhemoglobin, or methemoglobin is present. Plasma proteins and lipid proteins have little effect on color.

32. Ans. a. Potassium ferricyanide converts Hb iron from the ferrous to the ferric state to form methemoglobin, which combines with potassium cyanide to produce cyanmethemoglobin

Ref: Dacie and Lewis 10/e p26-7

33. Ans. d. Spectrophotometry

Ref: Dacie and Lewis 10/e p26-7

Once the Hb is converted to cyanmethemoglobin, the absorbance of solution is measured in a spectrometer at a wavelength of 540 nm or a photoelectric colorimeter with a yellow-green filter.

34. Ans. a. Volume of packed red cell

Ref: Dacie and Lewis 10/e p108

The hematocrit measures the volume percentage of RBCs in blood. The measurement depends on the number and size of RBCs. The hematocrit is slightly more accurate as the PCV includes small amounts of plasma trapped between the red cells. The PCV can be determined by centrifuging heparinized blood in a capillary tube at 10,000 rpm for 5 minutes. With modern laboratory equipment, the hematocrit is calculated by automated analyzer and is not directly measured. Another way of measuring is optical methods such spectrophotometry.

35. Ans. c. Prussian blue

Ref: Dacie and Lewis 10/e p292, 323; Hoffman's 6/e p662

Siderocytes contain one or two (rarely many) small unevenly, distributed iron-containing granules that stain a Prussian-blue color (Perl's reaction). Nitroblue tetrazolium is the dye use to detect the NADPH oxidase activity. If less than 50%, cells neutrophils show change in color of granules, then the test is considered positive. The other test is flow cytometry based in which the oxidase activity is measured by conversion of dihydroxyrhodamine 123 to rhodamine 123. Sodium metabisulfite is the reagent used as sickling agent in diagnosing sickle cell anemia, but nowadays sodium dithionite is used.

36. Ans. a. Anode *Ref: Dacie and Lewis 10/e p282-6*

At alkaline pH, Hb is negatively charged protein and when subjected to electrophoresis will migrate toward the anode (+). At alkaline pH of 8.5 on cellulose acetate, satisfactory separation of Hb C, S, F, A, and J, in general Hb S, D, and G migrate closely together as do Hb C, E, and O. Differentiation between these HbS can be obtained by using acid agarose gels, citrate agar electrophoresis, high-performance liquid chromatography (HPLC), or isoelectric focusing. HbC migrates slightly cathodal.

37. Ans. a. Microcytic and hypochromic

Ref: William's 7/e p12

This patient is having low MCV, MCH and MCHC. The normal range of MCV, MCH, and MCHC is 80-100 fL, 27.5-33.2 pg/red cell and 33.4-35.5 g/dL RBC, respectively. An MCHC greater than 35 g/dL is associated with hereditary spherocytosis and a low MCHC is typical of iron deficiency, but its diagnostic value is limited. Low MCHC means hypochromia.

38. Ans. a. Nucleus *Ref: Hoffman's 6/e p473*

The common feature of megaloblastic anemias is defect in DNA synthesis, with lesser alterations in RNA and protein synthesis, leading to a state of unbalanced cell growth with impaired cell division.

39. Ans. d. One molecule has only 1 iron atom

Ref: William's 7/e p1192; Hoffman's 6/e p420

Hemoglobin has a quaternary protein structure. The liganded (oxygen bound) is in relaxed state (R-state) and has high affinity for oxygen, while the unliganded (reduced, deoxygenated) is intense state (T-state) and has low affinity for oxygen. Carbon monoxide binds to Hb with 400 times more affinity than oxygen, as a result of which it shifts the oxygen dissociation curve toward left. Quaternary structure of Hb contains four globin chains and attached to it are four heme parts with four iron atoms attached to it in ferrous state. Hb at birth is usually high as compared to adults. RBCs are removed from the circulation by splenic macrophages, probably by several mechanisms. SHPS-1, a surface glycoprotein and a member of immunoglobulin like superfamily that interacts with RBC membrane protein CD47, abundant in macrophages.

40. Ans. a. Loss of nucleus *Ref: Hoffman's 6/e p407*

The most remarkable feature of RBC is its durability, given that it is enucleated cell devoid of organelles that appear to be critical for the survival and function of most other cell types. The RBC has no mitochondria for oxidative metabolism; no ribosomes for regeneration of damaged or lost proteins; a very limited metabolic repertoire that largely precludes de-novo synthesis of lipids; and no nucleus to direct regenerative processes, adaption to circulatory stresses, or cell division to replenish itself. Thus the most important part responsible for limiting the red cell lifespan is the loss of nucleus.

41. Ans. b. Relaxed state *Ref: William's 7/e p1192*

The liganded or oxygen bound (relaxed—R state) has the highest affinity for oxygen. As 1 oxygen atom binds to Hb, it makes oxygen molecule in relaxed state and causes other oxygen molecules to bind to it.

42. Ans. c. NADPH and glutathione

Ref: Hoffman 5/e p581-3

Maintenance of RBC reducing power: The red cells have the remarkable ability to absorb extreme oxidative stress by virtue of the enzymes involved in glutathione metabolism and generation of NADPH. These enzymes provide RBCs the reducing equivalents to reduce Hb, lipoprotein, and other intracellular proteins damaged by oxidative stress.

Generation of ATP: In RBCs, ATP is required for pumps, membrane transport mechanisms and for the production of reduced form of NADH. In RBCs, ATP is produced by EMP pathway as they do not have mitochondria.

Maintenance of Hb in its functional state: NADH and NADPH play a critical role in maintaining Hb in its reduced state by supplying Cb5R (the major Hb reductase) and the alternative methemoglobin reductase with its cofactors. The enzymes that catalyze the formation of 2,3-BPG via the Rapoport-Luebering pathway also plays an important role in Hb function, because it binds to beta-globin chain and facilitates the off-loading of oxygen from Hb to the tissues.

Degradation of ribosomal proteins: RBCs must modify its membrane and volume accordingly and expel ribosomal proteins, which could otherwise prove deleterious. Pyrimidine 5'-nucleotidase is effective in degrading ribosomal contents into smaller components that can pass through the membrane.

The function of HMP shunt (pentose pathway) is to provide NADPH. The glutathione is produced by the glutathione pathway. This NADPH is responsible for reducing the oxidized form of glutathione to reduced form. The Rappaport-Luebering pathway is responsible for the production of 2,3-BPG. The EMP pathway is responsible for production of ATP and lactic acid.

43. Ans. c. Dacryocytes
Ref: William's 7/e p1059

The leukoerythroblastic picture is characterized by the presence of nRBCs and immature myeloid elements in 96% of case. Megathrombocytes and megakaryocyte fragments are frequent findings. The number of tear drop erythrocytes (dacryocytes) decreases after splenectomy or institution of chemotherapy.

44. Ans. e. Low EPO levels and raised red cell mass
Ref: Hoffman's 6/e p1019-21

In PV, the red cell mass is high and serum EPO levels are low in two-thirds of patients even after normalization of hematocrit.

45. Ans. a. Hb Hope

HbA1c which is increased in diabetes elutes in the P2 window. Only one variant, Hb Hope with a percentage of >40% elutes in this window.

CHAPTER 5

Lymphocytes

1. **Which of the following are not the methods for cell separation?**
   a. Fluorescence-activated cell sorting (FACS)
   b. Panning
   c. Density gradient centrifugation
   d. High-performance liquid chromatograph (HPLC)

2. **Which of the following infections can cause lymphocytosis in young children?**
   a. Typhoid fever
   b. Tuberculosis
   c. *Bordetella pertussis*
   d. *Haemophilus influenzae*

3. **Which one of these statements is correct about T-lymphocytes?**
   a. Express CD5
   b. Produce immunoglobulins (Igs)
   c. Recognize soluble free antigens
   d. Activate complements

4. **Which statement is true about B-lymphocytes?**
   a. Are short lived
   b. Are of two types helper and cytotoxic cells
   c. They become atypical lymphocytes in infectious mononucleosis
   d. Secrete surface immunoglobulins

5. **Which of the following is primary lymphoid organ?**
   a. Thymus
   b. Peyer's patches
   c. Lymph node
   d. Spleen

6. **Which of the following statements is not true about Igs?**
   a. IgM is the largest class
   b. IgG is the most common type of antibody in human plasma
   c. Each Ig has one Kappa and one lambda light chain
   d. IgM fixes complement more early than other classes

7. **Which statement is not true regarding generation of heavy chain in B cell development?**
   a. There are multiple functional heavy chain variable region genes
   b. B cells have only 1 in-frame copy of Ig heavy chain
   c. Somatic hypermutation occurs in RNA transcript
   d. Endonuclease enzymes encoded by recombination activating gene (RAG)-1/RAG-2 genes produce diversity between V, D, and J segments

8. **Which of the following is not true regarding complement system?**
   a. Macrophages and neutrophils have C3b receptors
   b. Alternate pathway is activated by complement fixing immune complex attached to cells
   c. C5-9 produces holes in cell membrane of target cell
   d. Most abundant is C3

9. **Which of the following statements is not true about human leukocyte antigen (HLA)?**
   a. HLA genes are located on chromosome no 6 and are highly polymorphic
   b. HLA molecules on antigen presenting cells (APCs) present peptide antigens to T-lymphocyte
   c. HLA class II molecules contains alpha- and beta-chains
   d. HLA class I molecules are heterodimers consisting of covalently bound alpha-chain and beta-microglobulin

10. **Which of the following is not true about Epstein-Barr virus (EBV) mononucleosis?**
    a. It occurs after the primary infection with EBV
    b. Corticosteroids are required in all cases
    c. Patients treated with penicillin group of antibodies typically develop rashes
    d. Monospot test detects IgM antibodies that agglutinate sheep red cells

11. **Which of the following does not causes generalized lymphadenopathy?**
    a. Sarcoidosis
    b. Myeloma
    c. HIV infection
    d. Non-Hodgkin lymphoma

12. **Which of the following vaccine is not recommended prior to splenectomy?**
    a. *Neisseria meningitides*
    b. *Streptococcus pneumoniae*
    c. *Haemophilus influenzae b*
    d. *Neisseria gonorrhoeae*

13. Which of the following is the important function of spleen?
a. Enucleation of red cells released from bone marrow
b. Production of antibody for limiting infection by encapsulated bacteria
c. Storage of blood cells which can be released at the time of stress
d. None of the above

14. An increase in leukocytes is called:
a. Leukemoid reaction
b. Leukocytosis
c. Leukemia
d. Leukopenia

15. In a normal differential count, the smallest percentage of cell is:
a. Metamyelocyte
b. Basophil
c. Monocyte
d. Eosinophil

16. In a 1-year-old child there is relatively increased percentage of which cell:
a. Lymphocyte
b. Neutrophil
c. Monocyte
d. Eosinophil

17. Majority of cell types in peripheral blood lymphocyte are:
a. T cells
b. B cells
c. NK cells
d. Large granular lymphocytes

18. Atypical or reactive lymphocyte was first described by:
a. Downey cells
b. Sabin
c. Lancefield
d. Landsteiner

19. The cells that synthesize normal Igs are:
a. Lymphocyte
b. Plasma cells
c. Monocyte
d. Turk cell

20. May-Hegglin-like inclusions containing rough endoplasmic reticulum (RNA) are:
a. Döhle bodies
b. Auer rods
c. Barr body
d. Y tag

21. Inclusion body found only in white cell:
a. Heinz body
b. Howell-Jolly body
c. Auer rods
d. Pappenheimer body

22. The periodic acid-Schiff (PAS) stain is positive due to the presence of:
a. Lipids
b. Abnormal proteins
c. Mucoproteins and polysaccharides
d. Glucose

23. All of these types of white blood cells (WBCs) are effective in destroying bacteria with the help of digestive enzymes (phagocytosis), *except*:
a. Lymphocyte
b. Monocyte
c. Neutrophil
d. Dendritic cells

24. Basket cell in peripheral blood smear is also called:
a. Smudge cell
b. Turk cell
c. Mott cell
d. Target cell

25. Which of the following may develop in sites other than marrow?
a. Monocyte
b. Lymphocytes
c. Neutrophil
d. Megakaryocyte

ANSWERS WITH EXPLANATIONS

1. Ans. d. High-performance liquid chromatograph (HPLC)

The various methods of cell separation or sorting are:
- *Separation according to density (and size):*
  - Gradient centrifugation (simple or with Ficoll-hypaque).
- *Separation according to adhesion:*
  - Adhesion to surfaces
  - *Adhesion to sheep erythrocytes:* E-rosette formation.
- *Separation according to surface markers:*
  - Panning
  - Dynal beads/magnetic-activated cell sorting (MACS)
  - Fluorescence-activated cell sorting.

2. Ans. c. *Bordetella pertussis*
Ref: Harrison 18/e p1244

In pertussis lymphocytosis, an absolute lymphocyte count of > 10^8–10^9/L is common among young children (in whom it is unusual with other infections) but not among young adolescents and in adults.

3. Ans. a. Express CD5
Ref: William's 7/e p1083-4

CD 5 is found on all T cells and appears to be a signal transducer. It appears early in T cell ontogeny.

Immunoglobulins are produced by plasma cells and not by T cells. T cells generally recognize peptide antigens that are bound to a molecule of major histocompatibility complex (MHC) on APCs. T cells do not activate complements; in fact classical pathway is activated by complement fixing immune complexes (IgG and IgM). Alternative pathway is triggered by IgA aggregates, endotoxin, cobra venom factor, and the polysaccharide components of some bacterial and fungal cell walls and the 3rd pathway, the Mannan-binding lectin (MBL) pathway, is activated when MBL binds to carbohydrate-coated microbes.

4. Ans. d. Secrete surface immunoglobulins
Ref: William's 8/e p1116, 1201

B cells secrete surface Igs. A normal adult has preexisting B lymphocytes that can interact with almost any foreign antigen. In the presence of accessory T lymphocytes and macrophages, an antigen binding clone of B lymphocytes may transform into antibody-secreting plasma cells or memory B cells, which can be readily reactivated during an immune response to antigen. In infectious mononucleosis, massive T-lymphocyte response to the neoantigens in infected B cells is evident by the lymphocytosis with reactive blood T lymphocytes and other disease manifestations.

5. Ans. a. Thymus
Ref: William's 8/e p75

Primary lymphoid tissues are sites where lymphocytes develop from progenitor cells into functional and mature lymphocytes. The major primary lymphoid tissue is bone marrow and other is thymus where T cell development occurs.

Secondary lymphoid tissues are sites where lymphocytes interact with each other and nonlymphoid cells to generate immune responses to antigens. These include spleen, lymph node, and mucosa-associated lymphoid tissue (MALT).

6. Ans. c. Each Ig has one Kappa and one lambda light chain

IgM represents the predominant Ig class formed during primary immune response and pentavalent IgM antibodies fix complement more efficiently.

	IgG	IgA	IgM	IgD	IgE
Heavy chain subclass	γ1, γ2, γ3, and γ4	α1, α2	mu	delta	epsilon
Secretory form	Monomer	Monomer/Dimer	Pentamer	Monomer	Monomer
Serum concentration (mg/mL)	8–16	1.4–4.0	0.5–2.0	0–0.4	17–450 mg/mL
Percentage of total Ig	80	13	6	1	0.002
Complement fixation:					
• Classical	Yes	No	Yes	No	No
• Alternate	No	Yes	No	No	No
Antibody-dependent cell mediated cytotoxicity	Yes	No	No	No	No
Serum half-life (days)	21	5.8	10	2.8	2.3

IgG1 and IgG3 fix complement more efficiently than other subclasses of Igs.

7. Ans. c. Somatic hypermutation occurs in RNA transcript
Ref: William's 8/e p1110-4

There are three unlinked gene complexes—1 for heavy chain, 1 for κ-light chain, and 1 for λ-light chains. Heavy chain gene complex is composed of 39 functional heavy chain variable region (VH) genes, >120 nonfunctional VH pseudogenes, 25 functional diversity (D) segments, six functional JH minigenes, and exons encoding the constant region for each heavy chain isotypes. Each germline V gene, D element, and J segment are flanked by recognition sequences that direct site specific recombination. This sequence is called heptamer-spacer-monomer sequence (also called recombination signal sequence—RSS), is the targets of lymphocyte-specific endonuclease enzymes encoded by RAG-1 and RAG-2. Mutation in RAG-1 and RAG-2 genes can result in combined immune deficiency called Omenn syndrome. VDJ recombination occurs mostly in G0 and/or G1 stage of cell cycle. Somatic hypermutation is also called class switching, which occurs in DNA and not in RNA transcript. During differentiation, a single B cell can synthesize chains with different constant regions coupled to the same variable region. The switch from IgM to IgG, IgA or IgE requires active transcription of the downstream constant regions exons encoding future Ig isotype. This process requires interaction of B cell with antigens and ligation of CD 40 via ligand for CD 40 (CD 154) and inherited defects of either is called hyper-IgM syndrome type I. Ig class switch recombination (CSR) occurs in the intron between rearranged VDJH sequences the gene. CSR requires DNA replication which is helped by expression of activation-induced deaminase (AID) present in activated B cells and deficiency of it results in hyper-IgM syndrome type II.

8. Ans. b. Alternate pathway is activated by complement fixing immune complex attached to cells
Ref: William's 8/e p258-260, 996

Actually classical pathway is activated by complement fixing immune complexes attached to cells. The most important activation products of complement appear to be C5a, the major chemotactic factor, and the anaphylatoxins (C3a, C4a, and C5a) of which C3 is most abundant. C5b–9 is the major cytotoxic product forming the membrane attack complex and produces holes in target cell. Neutrophils express receptors for complement components, including CD1 qr, CR 1 (CD 35), CR 3(CD11/CD18), and CR4. CR1 binds C3b, C4b, and C3bi. CR3 recognizes C3bi. Macrophages have CD11b through which they bind to C3bi. Through these receptors macrophages and neutrophils phagocytose C3b-coated cells.

9. Ans. d. HLA class I molecules are heterodimers consisting of covalently bound alpha-chain and beta-microglobulin
Ref: William's 7/e p2269-73

HLAs are highly polymorphic glycoproteins encoded by a cluster of genes on the short arm of chromosome 6. The biologic function of HLA molecules is the presentation of antigenic peptides to T-cells. Class I molecule is a hetero dimer of noncovalently bound α-heavy chain (consists of α-1, 2, and 3 domains) and β-light chain (β-2 microglobulin—nonpolymorphic globular protein) and it stabilizes class I molecule on cell surface. Class II molecules formed by two noncovalently brand protein chains—an α-heavy chain (α1 and 2) domain and β-light chain (β-1 and β-2 domains). In HLA-DR, α-chain is constant and β-chain is polymorphic whereas in HLA-DQ and HLA-DR both α- and β-chains are polymorphic.

Class I	*Class II*
• Present on all nucleated cells	• Present in B cell, monocyte, macrophages, dendritic cells, and endothelial cells
• Binds to peptides derived from proteins synthesized in cytosol (e.g. viral encoded proteins)	• Binds to peptides derived from exogenes proteins degraded in intracellular vesicles
• Usually peptides are 8–10 amino acid	• Usually peptides are > 13 amino acid
• Human leukocyte antigen (HLA)–A, HLA-B, and HLA-C	• HLA-D (DP, DQ, and DR)

10. Ans. b. Corticosteroids are required in all cases

Primary infection in infants and young children either is asymptomatic or accompanied by mild nonspecific symptoms and signs such as fever, upper respiratory tract infection (URTI), pharyngitis, tonsillitis, and cervical lymphadenopathy. But 50% of adolescents and young adults present with the clinical picture of infectious mononucleosis. Most patients with primary EBV infection have symptoms for 2–4 weeks and recover without significant complication or sequelae. Corticosteroids are needed in only severe condition associated with marked tonsillar inflammation and hypertrophy with impending airway obstruction. Acyclovir reduces EBV shedding into oral secretions with no clinical benefits. Heterophile antibodies are present in 90–95% of EBV infections at some point of illness. Infants and children younger than 4 years may have negative monospot test. Heterophile antibodies are IgM antibodies, which agglutinate erythrocytes of bovine, camel, horse, goat, and sheep. VCAs–IgM (viral capsid antigens) are good markers for an acute infection because they rapidly disappear in 4–8 weeks. VCA-IgG persists for life. IgG antibodies against EA are present at the onset of clinical illness in approximately 70% of patients. IgG antibodies to EBMA appear late in the course of almost all patients and presence early in a suspected case of primary infection rules out diagnosis.

Latency pattern in EBV infection:

Latency/ malignancy	*Latent gene expression*	*Viral membrane*	*Immunogenicity*
Type III LPD after solid organ or stem cell transplant (PTLD) HIV associated immunoblastic lymphoma	EBNAs-1, 2, 3A, 3B, 3C, EBNA leader protein (LP)	LMP–1 and LMP–2	+++
Type II Hodgkin lymphoma nasopharyngeal carcinoma T/NK cell lymphoma	EBNA–1	LMP–1 and LMP–2	++
Type I Burkitt lymphoma Gastric adenocarcinoma	EBNA	-	+

Humans are the only source of EBV.

11. Ans. b. Myeloma *Ref: Harrison 18/e p465*

12. Ans. d. *Neisseria gonorrhoeae*
Ref: Hoffman 6/e p2262-4

The major risk of postsplenectomy sepsis is with encapsulated organisms such as *Streptococcus pneumoniae*, *Neisseria meningitidis* and *Haemophilus influenzae type b*, which require opsonization for effective phagocytosis.

13. Ans. b. Production of antibody for limiting infection by encapsulated bacteria *Ref: Hoffman 6/e p2257*

Normal adult spleen contains 20–40 mL (5%) of blood and it is not the reservoir for blood or erythrocytes. It is not the normal site of hematopoiesis in postnatal life. The white pulp of the spleen is the largest mass of lymphoid tissue in the body. Antibody producing B cells predominate in the germinal centers and mantle zones of spleen. These areas increase in size and activity with immunization or infection. The complex interaction between the cells of the spleen contributes to the extraordinary repertoire of innate and adaptive immunity. In hypersplenism, the red cell pool can increase to 40% of total body pool.

14. Ans. b. Leukocytosis *Ref: Hoffman's 6/e p640-1*

Leukemoid reaction is a reactive (nonclonal) neutrophilic leukocytosis with WBC count above 50,000/cumm. Leukopenia is decrease in number of WBCs below the normal range. Leukemia is a hematological malignant process in which the WBCs can be low or high. Blasts are usually seen in peripheral blood, but may be absent rarely (aleukemic leukemia).

15. Ans. a. Metamyelocyte

In fact in a normal differential white cell count, the metamyelocytes are not seen, they are seen in peripheral blood only in case of stress myelopoiesis, chronic myeloid leukemia (CML), or marrow infiltrative diseases.

16. Ans. a. Lymphocyte *Ref: Hoffman's 6/e p647*

Infants have total lymphocyte count between 5,500 and 7,000/cumm, but this number declines beginning at about 1 year of age to reach 2,000–2,400/cumm in adults.

17. Ans. a. T cells *Ref: Hoffman's 6/e p647-8*

Circulating T cells exceeds B cells by a ratio of approximately four to one with ration exceeding slightly with age.

18. Ans. a. Downey cells *Ref: Hoffman's 6/e p640-641*

Reactive or variant lymphocyte is cytotoxic (CD8$^+$) lymphocytes that become large after antigenic stimulation. The nucleus can be round, elliptic, indented, cleft, or folded. The cytoplasm is often abundant and can be basophilic. Vacuoles and/or azurophilic granules can also be present. It was first described Hal Downey in case of EBV or cytomegalovirus (CMV) infection and are also called Downey cell.

19. Ans. b. Plasma cells *Ref: Dacie and Lewis 10/e p108*

The normal function of plasma cells is to produce normal antibodies or Igs. In infections, both bacterial and viral, transforming lymphocytes may be present. These immunoblasts or Turk cells are 10–15 microns in diameter, with a round nucleus and abundant, basophilic cytoplasm. They may develop into plasmacytoid lymphocytes and plasma cells, and these are occasionally seen in blood in severe infections.

20. Ans. a. Döhle bodies
Ref: Dacie and Lewis 10/e p39, 84, 97-8

The May-Hegglin anomaly (MHA) is a rare autosomal dominant disease due to MYH9 gene mutation characterized by neutrophils with abnormal cytoplasmic inclusions, large platelets, and variable thrombocytopenia. It is part of myosin heavy chain (MHC) single gene defect group that also includes Fechtner syndrome, Sebastian syndrome, and Epstein syndrome. All of these entities represent hereditary forms of macrothrombocytopenia associated with leukocyte inclusions (Dohle-like bodies), and variable clinical features of sensorineural hearing loss, presenile (early) cataracts, and renal failure.

21. Ans. c. Auer rods *Ref: Dacie and Lewis 10/e p330*

Auer rods are characteristically seen in acute myeloid leukemia (AML) blasts. Rest all inclusions are seen in red blood cells.

22. Ans. c. Mucoproteins and polysaccharides
Ref: Dacie and Lewis 10/e p323

Periodic acid specifically oxidizes 1-2 glycol groups to produce stable dialdehydes. Positive reactions occur with carbohydrates, principally glycogen, but also monosaccharides, polysaccharides, glycoproteins, mucoproteins, phosphorylated sugars, inositol derivatives, and cerebrosides.

23. Ans. a. Lymphocyte *Ref: Hoffman's 6/e p175-6*

Phagosome is a vesicle formed around a particle engulfed by a phagocyte via phagocytosis. Phagosomes have membrane bound proteins to recruit and fuse with lysosomes to form phagolysosomes. The lysosomes have hydrolytic enzymes and reactive oxygen species which kill and digest pathogens. Professional phagocytes include macrophages and dendritic cells. Neutrophils have multiple functions, including the direct killing of foreign organisms via phagocytosis or release of hydroxylases or oxidative enzymes from primary and secondary granules, release or pattern recognition receptors (PRRs), and the formation of neutrophil extracellular nets. Neutrophils are at first attracted to a site, where they proliferate, before they are phagocytized by macrophages.

24. Ans. a. Smudge cell
Ref: William's 7/e p12; Dacie and Lewis 10/e p94-5

During the process of preparing the film, leukocytes may be damaged, with consequent appearance and staining. They are specifically seen in chronic lymphocytic leukemia (CLL), because the cells are fragile. They are also called crushed cells or basket cells. In infections, both bacterial and viral, transforming lymphocytes may be present. These immunoblasts or Turk cells are 10–15 microns in diameter, with a round nucleus and abundant, basophilic cytoplasm. They may develop into plasmacytoid lymphocytes and plasma cells, and these are occasionally seen in blood in severe infections.

Target cells refers to a cell in which there is central round stained area and a peripheral rim of hemoglobinized cytoplasm separated by nonstaining or more lightly staining cytoplasm. They are bell shaped and also called codocytes. Seen in liver disease, hemoglobinopathies especially HbC, E, and S.

25. Ans. b. Lymphocytes *Ref: Hoffman's 6/e p173, 175*

Lymphocytes initially arise in the bone marrow and subsequently undergo maturation in peripheral lymphoid organ (thymus for T cells and lymph nodes, spleen or other lymphoid tissues for B cells). Monocytes develop in the bone marrow and then circulate through the blood and lymphatics with an average half-life of 1–3 days before migrating into the tissues and maturing into macrophages. Neutrophils mature in the bone marrow, where 80–90% of the body's store of mature neutrophils reside. Megakaryocyte production and maturation occurs in bone marrow only.

SECTION 2

Benign Hematology

6. Iron Deficiency Anemia and Anemia of Chronic Diseases
7. Megaloblastic Anemia
8. Platelets and Hemostatic Disorders
9. Thrombosis
10. Red Blood Cell Membrane Disorders
11. Disorders of Red Cell Enzymes
12. Sickle Cell Anemia
13. Methemoglobinemia
14. Immune Hemolytic Anemia
15. Primary Immunodeficiency Diseases
16. Thalassemia Syndromes
17. Eosinophilic Disorders
18. Neutrophilic Disorders
19. Hemophilia and Other Coagulation Factor Defects
20. Inherited Bone Marrow Failure Syndromes and Aplastic Anemia
21. Mast Cell/Basophilic Disorders
22. Monocyte/Macrophage Disorders
23. Paroxysmal Nocturnal Hemoglobinuria
24. von Willebrand Disease

CHAPTER 6

Iron Deficiency Anemia and Anemia of Chronic Diseases

1. A 29-year-old woman was found to have a Hb of 7.8 g/dL with reticulocyte count of 0.8%. Peripheral smear showed microcytic hypochromic anemia. Hb A2 and Hb F levels were 2.4% and 1.3%, respectively. Serum iron and TIBC were 15 mcg/dL and 420 mcg/dL, respectively. The likely diagnosis is:
   a. Iron deficiency anemia (IDA)
   b. β-thalassemia minor
   c. Sideroblastic anemia
   d. Anemia of chronic inflammation

2. A child presented with microcytic hypochromic anemia with normal levels of RBC protoporphyrin. Most likely, the diagnosis is:
   a. Lead toxicity
   b. Iron deficiency anemia
   c. Thalassemia
   d. Anemia of chronic inflammation

3. Which of the following test is best suited for community-based screening program for identifying iron deficiency?
   a. Serum ferritin
   b. Red cell protoporphyrin level
   c. Serum iron
   d. Total iron binding capacity

4. Which of the following test is best in differentiating between anemia of chronic inflammation and IDA?
   a. Serum ferritin
   b. Serum transferrin receptor
   c. TIBC
   d. Transferrin saturation

5. Elevated serum ferritin, serum iron, and transferrin saturation percentage are most consistent with diagnosis of:
   a. IDA
   b. Hemochromatosis
   c. Anemia of chronic inflammation
   d. Lead poisoning

6. Which of the following is earliest recognizable change in RBC morphology in case of iron deficiency?
   a. Hypochromia
   b. Anisocytosis
   c. Target cells
   d. Poikilocytosis

7. All of the following are causes of iron deficiency anemia, *except*:
   a. Chronic renal failure
   b. Celiac sprue
   c. Hookworm
   d. Carcinoma colon

8. Iron absorption is increased in all, *except*:
   a. Iron deficiency
   b. Pregnancy
   c. Hypoxia
   d. Alkaline pH of stomach
   e. Ferrous iron salts

9. All of the following in the diet lead to decreased iron absorption, *except*:
   a. Oxalates
   b. Ascorbate
   c. Phytates
   d. Phosphates

10. The earliest sign of iron deficiency anemia is:
    a. Increased TIBC
    b. Decreased serum iron
    c. Decreased serum ferritin
    d. Decreased percentage saturation

11. Which of the following is true about oral therapy for iron deficiency anemia?
    a. Of 300 mg elemental iron given, only 100 mg gets absorbed
    b. Reticulocytosis appears in 1–2 weeks and then peaks in 3–4 weeks
    c. Hemoglobin levels are usually corrected in 6 weeks after starting therapy
    d. Stop the treatment after normalizing Hb
    e. Decrease in absorption of iron with improvement of Hb

12. A patient presents with increased serum iron, decreased TIBC, increased percentage saturation, and increased serum ferritin. Most likely, the diagnosis is:
    a. Anemia of chronic disease (ACD)
    b. Sideroblastic anemia
    c. IDA
    d. Thalassemia major

13. Features of Paterson-Kelly/Plummer-Vinson syndrome includes all of the following, *except*:
    a. Esophageal web in postcricoid region
    b. Iron deficiency
    c. Koilonychia
    d. Gum hypertrophy

14. Macrocytic anemia may be seen with all of the following conditions, *except*:
    a. Liver disease
    b. Copper deficiency
    c. Thiamine deficiency
    d. Orotic aciduria

15. Anemia of chronic renal failure can be attributable to all of the following, *except*:
    a. Low erythropoietin (EPO) level
    b. Decreased RBC renewal
    c. Decreased RBC supply
    d. Decreased plasma volume
    e. Bleeding due to platelet dysfunction

16. Erythropoietin levels will be low in all, *except*:
    a. Polycythemia vera
    b. Renal failure
    c. Autoimmune hemolytic anemia
    d. Anemia of chronic disease

17. Which is the first stage of iron deficiency?
    a. Negative iron balance
    b. Decreased iron stores
    c. Decreased mean corpuscular volume (MCV)
    d. Decrease in hemoglobin

18. Which statement is true regarding oral iron therapy?
    a. Treatment should be given along with vitamin C
    b. Enteric-coated and prolonged-release preparations should be given
    c. Best given after meals
    d. Maximum dose is 200 mg of elemental iron per day
    e. Carbonyl iron is usually not tolerated in high dose

19. In which of the following conditions iron absorption will be increased?
    a. Pregnancy
    b. Chronic inflammation
    c. Iron overload
    d. Phosphates

20. Which of the following is not true about serum iron concentration?
    a. It is low in ACD
    b. Raised in hemochromatosis
    c. Transported by ferritin
    d. Shows a diurnal variation

21. The ferritin complex which combines with phosphate and hydroxide:
    a. Hemopexin
    b. Hemosiderin
    c. Haptoglobin
    d. Oxyhemoglobin

22. A 45-year-old lady who is a known case of rheumatoid arthritis for the past 5 years and is on disease-modifying antirheumatic drug (DMARD) therapy, but she still has clinical features suggestive of active disease. On evaluation, she was found to be having anemia with Hb 8.5 g/dL, MCV 83 fL and ESR 76. Which of the following combinations of tests are consistent with this patient?
    a. Elevated hepcidin, elevated ferritin, low TIBC, and decreased serum iron
    b. Elevated hepcidin, decreased ferritin, elevated TIBC, and elevated iron
    c. Elevated hepcidin, elevated ferritin, elevated TIBC, and elevated iron
    d. Decreased hepcidin, elevated ferritin, elevated TIBC, and elevated iron
    e. Decreased hepcidin, decreased ferritin, elevated TIBC, and elevated iron

23. In the iron metabolism, transferrin receptor carries:
    a. Iron out of duodenal cells from the intestinal lumen
    b. Iron out of duodenal cells into the plasma
    c. Transferrin bound iron in the plasma
    d. Transferrin bound iron into the red blood cells

24. A 45-year-old lady generalized weakness and effort intolerance for the past 3 months. There is no history of bleeding from anywhere and on examination only, positive finding is pallor. The CBC showed Hb 8 g/dL, MCV 75 fL, RDW 18.5 and reticulocyte count 0.5%. What is the most likely diagnosis?
    a. Iron deficiency anemia
    b. Sideroblastic anemia
    c. Thalassemia
    d. Anemia of chronic disease

25. A 55-year-old man presented with 2 months history of generalized weakness and easy fatigability with significant weight loss. Blood investigations showed Hb 10 g/dL, MCV 90 fL, platelet count 175,000/cmm, TLC 11,500/cmm, serum iron 10 µg/dL, serum ferritin 160 ng/mL, and TIBC 40 µg/dL. The most likely diagnosis for him would be:
    a. IDA
    b. Sideroblastic anemia
    c. Thalassemia
    d. ACD
    e. Megaloblastic anemia

26. The response to iron administration would be seen earliest by:
    a. Increased TIBC
    b. Increase in hemoglobin
    c. Increased hematocrit
    d. Reticulocytosis

27. Which of the following is not true about sideroblastic anemia?
    a. May be inherited
    b. It may respond to pyridoxine
    c. May be caused by folate deficiency
    d. Most frequently caused by myelodysplasia

CHAPTER 6 | Iron Deficiency Anemia and Anemia of Chronic Diseases

28. All of the following are associated with vacuolated erythroblast with ring sideroblast in bone marrow, *except*:
a. Chronic alcoholism
b. Chloramphenicol toxicity
c. Pearson marrow-pancreas syndrome
d. Copper deficiency
e. Lead poisoning

29. Which of the following statement is not correct?
a. A unit of blood contains 200–250 mg iron
b. 1 mg of dietary iron is absorbed daily
c. One molecule of transferrin carries 4 atoms of iron
d. None of the above

30. Which of the following may be used to treat iron deficiency in general population?
a. Ferric carboxymaltose   b. Desferrioxamine
c. Ferric gluconate   d. Erythropoietin

31. What is true about hemochromatosis?
a. Has autosomal dominant inheritance
b. Usually caused by mutation in *HFE* gene
c. Patients have low percentage transferrin saturation
d. More common in females

32. Which of the following organ is not damaged by transfusional iron overload?
a. Kidneys   b. Parathyroid
c. Heart   d. Liver
e. Pituitary

33. Which one of the following is seen in iron deficiency?
a. High serum transferrin
b. Low protoporphyrin level
c. High MCV
d. Raised serum hepcidin levels

34. Regarding erythroferrone true statement is:
a. It is a steroid hormone encoded in humans by *ERFE* gene
b. It is produced by erythroblasts
c. It increases the production of hepcidin
d. Its level is decreased in thalassemia

ANSWERS WITH EXPLANATIONS

1. Ans. a. Iron deficiency anemia (IDA)
Ref: Harrison 18/e p846-8

Such a high level of TIBC with microcytic hypochromic blood picture is very much suggestive of IDA. Anemia of chronic inflammation usually have normocytic normochromic red cells. Serum ferritin is very important in diagnosing IDA and is usually <15 ng/mL. Differential diagnosis of microcytic hypochromic anemia are given in the tables here.

Parameter	IDA	ACD	Thalassemia	Sideroblastic anemia
Smear	MCHC	Normal/MCHC	MCHC with targeting	Variable
Serum iron	<30	<50	Normal to high	Normal to high
TIBC	>360	<300	Normal	Normal
% Saturation	<10	10–20	30–80	30–80
Ferritin	<15	30–200	50–300	50–300
Hb pattern electrophoresis	Normal	Normal	Abnormal with β-thalassemia; it can be normal in α-thalassemia	Normal

(ACD: anemia of chronic disease; IDA: iron deficiency anemia; Hb: hemoglobin; MCHC: mean corpuscular hemoglobin concentration; TIBC: total iron binding capacity).

	Normal	Negative iron balance	Iron-deficient erythropoiesis	IDA
Marrow iron stores	1–3+	0–1+	0	0
Serum ferritin (ng/mL)	50–200	<20	<15	<15
TIBC (mcg/dL)	300–360	>360	>380	>400
Serum iron (µg/dL)	50–150	N	<50	<30
% Saturation	30–50	N	<20	<10
RBC protoporphyrin (µg/dL)	30–50	N	>100	>200

(IDA: iron deficiency anemia; RBC: red blood cell; TIBC: total iron binding capacity).

2. Ans. c. Thalassemia   *Ref: William's 8/e p582*

Both lead toxicity and IDA have microcytic hypochromic blood pictures and the red cell protoporphyrin levels are elevated in both conditions.

3. Ans. b. Red cell protoporphyrin level

Erythrocyte protoporphyrin is a more sensitive but less specific test than ferritin, and it can be used as a first-line diagnostic test in the evaluation of iron deficiency and in diagnosing IDA in infants. The measurement of erythrocyte protoporphyrin levels as an indicator of iron deficiency has particular advantages in pediatric hematology and in large-scale surveys in which the small sample size and simplicity of the test are important.

4. Ans. b. Serum transferrin receptor
Ref: William's 8/e p581-2

Serum transferrin receptor is elevated in IDA but not in ACD. Serum ferritin is an acute phase reactant which can be falsely elevated. It has been shown by many studies that transferrin receptor/log of ferritin is more accurate in differentiating between IDA and ACD. The gold standard for IDA is absent stainable iron in bone marrow (BM) aspirate but it has drawbacks, e.g., it is invasive procedure and difficulty in differentiating from artefacts within macrophages. Iron in BM aspirate (stained with Prussian blue) can be found as storage iron in cytoplasm of macrophages or as functional iron (siderosome) in nucleated red cells (sideroblasts). Approximately, one third of nucleated red cells contain 1-4 fine blue inclusion bodies (siderosome). Both sideroblast and macrophage iron are increased in ACD.

5. Ans. b. Hemochromatosis
Ref: William's 8/e p583, 594

Hemochromatosis is the increase in tissue iron with associated tissue damage with evidence of bronzing of skin, cirrhosis, and diabetes. Hemosiderosis is increase in tissue iron without tissue damage. Primary hemochromatosis is most commonly due to *HFE* gene mutation. It is associated with increased percentage saturation, serum iron, and serum ferritin. ACD will have low serum iron, and IDA will have all three parameters low.

6. Ans. b. Anisocytosis *Ref: William's 8/e p579*

Variation in the size of red cells (anisocytosis) can be quantified and expressed as red cell distribution width (RDW) or as red cell morphology index. In iron deficiency, anisocytosis (increased RDW) may be the first laboratory abnormality, even before anemia and microcytosis are seen.

7. Ans. a. Chronic renal failure
Ref: William's 8/e p573-5

Iron deficiency anemia usually occurs due to blood loss, poor absorption, increased requirement, or dietary deficiency. The most common cause of IDA all over the world is in fact dietary deficiency, while others are:
- *Blood loss*:
  - GI blood loss
  - Menstrual blood loss
  - Frequent blood donations
  - *Urinary blood loss*: Ca urinary bladder
  - *Hemoglobinuria*: Paroxysmal nocturnal hemoglobinuria (PNH), prosthetic valve.
- *Malabsorption*:
  - Achlorhydria
  - Chronic gastritis
  - Celiac sprue
  - Tropical sprue.
- *Increased iron requirement*:
  - Pregnancy and lactation
  - Growth.

8. Ans. d. Alkaline pH of stomach
Ref: William's 8/e p567; Harrison 18/e p843

Factors that increase iron absorption from gastro-intestinal (GI) tracts are:
- *Dietary factors*:
  - Increased heme iron (particularly in meat)
  - Ferrous iron salts.
- *GI factors*: Acid pH.
- *Increased requirement*:
  - Iron deficiency
  - Increased erythropoiesis
  - Pregnancy
  - Hypoxia.

Factors that decrease iron absorption are:
- Ferric iron salts
- Malabsorption
- Proximal bowel resection
- Presence of oxalates, phytates, and phosphates in diet
- Inflammatory disorders (due to increased hepcidin level).

9. Ans b. Ascorbate *Ref: William's 8/e p567*

Reducing substances in diet which will lead to increased iron absorption are: Hydroquinone, lactate, ascorbate, pyruvate, succinate, fructose, cysteine, and sorbitol.

10. Ans. c. Decreased serum ferritin
Ref: Harrison 18/e p846

11. Ans. e. Decrease in absorption of iron with improvement of Hb *Ref: Harrison 18/e p848-9*

A dose of 200-300 mg of elemental iron result in absorption of 20-50 mg/d. As the Hb level rises, EPO stimulation decreases and the amount of iron absorbed is reduced. Typically, the reticulocyte increment begins within 4-7 days and peaks at 1-1½ weeks after initiation of therapy. Hb level usually normalizes in 1 month of therapy. Minimum treatment of 4-6 months should be given for building iron stores.

12. Ans. b. Sideroblastic anemia

Anemia of chronic disease can be differentiated from sideroblastic anemia by the presence of low serum iron and low percentage saturation.

13. Ans. d. Gum hypertrophy *Ref: William's 8/e p578*

14. Ans. b. Copper deficiency
Ref: William's 8/e p609, 554, 556, 545; Harrison 18/e p867-9

Microcytic hypochromic anemia is caused due to copper deficiency. Rest other conditions are associated with macrocytic anemia. Copper deficiency is unresponsive to iron therapy and is associated with hypoferritinemia, neutropenia, and usually the presence of vacuolated erythroid precursors in the BM.

15. Ans. d. Decreased plasma volume
Ref: William's 8/e p495-7

The pathogenesis of anemia in renal failure can be multifactorial:
- Low EPO level (main cause)
- Shortening of RBC life span
- Marrow suppression
- Blood loss
- Mechanical red cell destruction.

16. Ans. c. Autoimmune hemolytic anemia (AIHA)
Ref: William's 8/e p457, 495, 504, 833

- In renal failure, the main cause of anemia is decreased production of EPO by failing kidneys.
- In polycythemia vera, EPO levels are almost always low but is not pathognomonic of polycythemia vera.
- EPO production is low in ACD, but is not the major mechanism.
- EPO concentration can increase from approximately 10 mU/mL at normal hemoglobin concentrations to 10,000 mU/mL in severe anemia.

17. Ans. a. Negative iron balance
Ref: Harrison 18/e p867-9

18. Ans. d. Maximum dose is 200 mg of elemental iron per day
Ref: William's 8/e p586, 587

Although vitamin C increases oral absorption, it is not routinely recommended with iron therapy. Iron should be readily released in acidic or neutral gastric or duodenal juice, because maximal iron absorption occur in duodenum. Enteric-coated and prolonged-release preparations dissolve slowly in any of these fluids. It should be given 1 hour before meals. A common generic approach for iron deficiency in adults consists of a daily dose of 150–200 mg of elemental iron. This approach entails prescribing one ferrous sulfate tablet 3 times daily since each tablet contains approximately 60 mg of elemental iron.

19. Ans. a. Pregnancy

Factors that increase iron absorption from GI tracts are the factors that increase the demand of iron requirement. Since pregnancy is associated with increased iron demand, the absorption of iron is also increased.

20. Ans. c. Transported by ferritin
Ref: William's 8/e p581

Physiologically, the serum iron concentration has a diurnal rhythm; it decreases in late afternoon and evening, reaching a nadir near 9:00 pm and increases to its maximum between 7:00 am and 10:00 pm. Iron is transported by transferrin in Fe^{3+} form and not by ferritin (storage protein for iron).

21. Ans. b. Hemosiderin
Ref: William's 7/e p370, 807

Hemosiderin is largely composed of dense clusters of ferritin, most of which are membrane enclosed. Ferritin is converted into hemosiderin upon partial degradation of its protein shell by lysosomal enzymes. Heme is readily oxidized in vitro to hemin, i.e., ferric protoporphyrin IX. Hemin has one residual positive charge and usually is isolated as a halide, most commonly as chloride. In hematin, halide is replaced by a hydroxyl ion. Heme can further form hexacoordinated complexes with nitrogenous bases called hemochrome or hemochromogen. Iron is stored, mostly in the liver, as ferritin or hemosiderin. Ferritin is a protein with a capacity of about 4,500 iron (III) ions per protein molecule. This is the major form of iron storage. If the capacity for storage of iron in ferritin is exceeded, a complex of iron with phosphate and hydroxide forms. This is called hemosiderin; it is physiologically available. As the body burden of iron increases beyond normal levels, excess hemosiderin is deposited in the liver and heart. This can reach the point that the function of these organs is impaired, and death ensues.

Hemopexin binds heme with the highest affinity of any known protein. Its main function is scavenging the heme released or lost by the turnover of heme proteins such as hemoglobin. Haptoglobin bind to the hemoglobin molecule which is released outside the red blood cells.

22. Ans. a. Elevated hepcidin, elevated ferritin, low TIBC, and decreased serum iron
Ref: Hoffman 5/e p450-4

This patient is definitely having ACD. The diagnosis of ACD is made on the basis of elevated bone marrow iron stores (usually assessed by serum ferritin) and low serum iron level, low transferrin level, and low TIBC. Usually, there is normocytic normochromic anemia but can be microcytic as well, in which case it may difficult to differentiate from IDA. Moreover, in acute inflammation with iron deficiency, the ferritin would not be a reliable marker as it is falsely elevated. Algorithms that integrate serum ferritin, soluble transferrin receptor (sTfr) concentration (or ratio of sTfr to log ferritin, known as sTfr index), and other markers of inflammation (ESR and CRP) have been derived to know concomitant iron deficiency. A sTfr index above 0.8 may discern iron deficiency in subjects with inflammation, and an index above 1.5 may do likewise in subjects without inflammation. Hepcidin is elevated in ACD, but commercial tests are not available at the moment. Hepcidin causes degradation and internalization of ferroportin which decreases its absorption from duodenum epithelium and also block iron release from ferroportin-expressing macrophages.

23. **Ans. d. Transferrin bound iron into the red blood cells**
Ref: Hoffman's 6/e p427-8

Not only the red blood cells, but each cell needs iron for growth development and function. Each cell contains its share of transferrin-bound iron by expressing transferrin receptor 1, a glycoprotein on cell membrane that binds the transferrin-iron complex and is internalized in the endocytic vesicle, where iron is released and then returns to the cell membrane, liberating apotransferrin into the plasma. Transferrin receptor 1 has little affinity for apotransferrin, intermediate affinity for monoferric transferrin, and highest affinity for diferric transferrin.

24. **Ans. a. Iron deficiency anemia**
Ref: Hoffman's 5/e p440-1

This patient is most likely having IDA as the red cell indices are showing to be microcytic hypochromic. The RDW is high with reticulocytopenia.

25. **Ans. d. ACD**
Ref: Hoffman's 5/e p453

This patient is having normocytic anemia with low serum iron, low TIBC, and slightly elevated ferritin, so the most likely diagnosis is ACD. The diagnosis of ACD is made on the basis of low serum iron, low transferrin levels, low TIBC, and elevated ferritin levels. There is also reticulocytopenia as it is hypoproliferative anemia.

26. **Ans. d. Reticulocytosis**
Ref: William's 7/e p378-9

Mild reticulocytosis begins within 3-5 days, is maximal by days 8-10, and then declines. The hemoglobin begins to increase after 1st week and usually returns to normal in 6 weeks. Complete recovery from microcytosis may take up to 4 months.

27. **Ans. c. May be caused by folate deficiency**
Ref: Hoffman 5/e p469-72

Sideroblastic anemia is characterized by anemia of varying severity and presence of ring sideroblasts (presence of siderotic granules arranged in perinuclear distribution around one third or more of the nucleus). Marrow shows erythroid hyperplasia and there is ineffective erythropoiesis leading to iron overload. Most sideroblastic anemias are acquired as a clonal disorder of erythropoiesis with varying degrees of myelodysplasia. Inherited forms are uncommon and occur in males with X-linked inheritance and are due to the defect in ALAS (aminolevulinic acid synthase) which is corrected by pyridoxine (cofactor for ALAS). Inherited deficiency of flavin monooxygenase is a rare cause of sideroblastic anemia. It typically manifests in infancy or childhood. MCV correlates with the degree of anemia. They have high serum iron, transferrin saturation, and serum ferritin levels. Sideroblastic anemia can be differentiated from idiopathic by the presence of anemia and low MCV.

A trial of pyridoxine (100–200 mg/d) orally for 3 weeks should be given to each patient. Response rate is 25–50% in hereditary sideroblastic anemia and less in acquired form. After response, dose should be titrated as it can lead to peripheral neuropathy. Unresponsive patient require regular blood transfusion with iron chelation. Folate deficiency does not cause sideroblastic anemia.

28. **Ans. e. Lead poisoning**
Ref: Hoffman 5/e p469-70

Ring sideroblasts (RS) may be found in bone marrow of malnourished anemic alcoholics. Alcohol has direct toxic effect on hematopoiesis. Usually have increased MCV and vacuolation of red cell precursors with RS. RS disappear over 4–12 days when alcohol is withdrawn.

Chloramphenicol causes reversible suppression of erythropoiesis after several days of therapy (this effect is different from idiosyncratic aplastic anemia occurring in 1 in 20,000 exposed persons). Nearly all patients develop vacuolated erythroid RS. It occurs due to inhibition of mitochondrial protein synthesis and reduced cytochrome c3 and b levels.

Pearson marrow-pancreas syndrome also has associated mitochondrial myopathy and sideroblastic anemia. It has normocytic normochromic anemia with varying degrees of neutropenia and thrombocytopenia. Bone marrow shows vacuolation and sideroblasts.

Copper deficiency also presents with microcytic hypochromic red cells with RS and vacuolated erythroid and myeloid precursors in marrow. Zinc toxicity can also cause copper deficiency (Zn interferes with copper absorption).

In iron deficiency, Zn complex of protoporphyrins is produced because ferrochelatase uses Zn^{2+} during iron-deficient erythropoiesis.

Erythrocyte protoporphyrin levels are raised before changes appear in peripheral blood and may be helpful in diagnosing iron deficiency when serum iron and ferritin levels are rising as a result of iron therapy.

29. **Ans. c. One molecule of transferrin carries 4 atoms of iron**

Ref: William's 8/e p567; Taher A, Musallam K, Cappellini. Guidelines for the management of Nontransfusion dependent Thalassaemia (NTDT), 2nd edition. Cyprus: Thalassaemia International Federation; 2017. p33

In a rough estimate, 1 unit of blood, irrespective of its hematocrit contains 200 mg of iron. Normal intestinal iron absorption is about 1–2 mg/day. In patients with thalassemia who do not receive any transfusion, iron absorption increases several folds.

One molecule of transferrin has two binding sites for Fe^{3+}. One ferritin complex can store about 4,500 iron (Fe^{3+}) ions in crystals together with phosphate and hydroxide ions.

30. **Ans. c. Ferric gluconate**
Ref: William's 8/e p586-8

Oral supplement: From GI tract, iron is absorbed in the ferrous form, so only ferrous salt should be used.

Oral preparation should be nonenteric coated and should be taken 3-4 times a day at least 1 hour before meal. Adult dose is 150-200 mg elemental iron/day. Children may be given 6 mg/kg/day.

Other preparation is carbonyl iron which is actually metallic iron powder with a particle size < 5 μm. The bioavailability is about 70% of that of an equivalent amount of ferrous sulfate. Oral dose of 1-3 g/day may be required for optimal therapy and does not produce toxic effects.

Parenteral therapy: Indications are malabsorption, intolerance to oral therapy, large doses required which cannot be given orally and noncompliance of patient.

Iron sucrose is a complex of polynuclear iron ferric hydroxide in sucrose. It is taken up by macrophages.

Iron dextran is a complex of iron and dextran. Ferric carboxymaltose is given intravenously.

Iron ferric gluconate complex in sucrose injection is a stable macromolecular complex of innate and ferric ion.

31. Ans. b. Usually caused by mutation in *HFE* gene

Ref: William's 8/e p589-91

The most common cause of hereditary hemochromatosis is mutation in *HFE* gene and the mode of inheritance is autosomal recessive. These patients have high serum iron percentage transferrin saturation and serum ferritin. Actually the male to female ration is 18:1 (more common in males).

32. Ans. a. Kidneys

Ref: William's 8/e p691

Iron accumulates in the endocrine glands, particularly in the parathyroids, pituitary, pancreas, liver and most important, in the myocardium.

33. Ans. a. High serum transferrin

Ref: William's 8/e p580-1

The iron binding capacity is a measure of the amount of transferrin in circulating blood. Normally transferrin is about one third saturated with iron. The sum of serum iron and UIBC represents TIBC. In the iron deficiency, TIBC and UIBC are increased and the transferrin saturation is decreased to <15%. Red cell protophyrin levels are increased in iron deficiency. Hepcidin levels are raised in anemia of chronic disease and are decreased in iron deficiency. IL-6 is a potent inducer of hepcidin and hypoferremia develops within hours of onset of inflammation. Hepcidin inhibits release of iron from macrophages (and probably from hepatocyte) leading to hypoferremia. Hepcidin does this by ferroportin internalization and degradation which is the mediator of release of iron into plasma from macrophages, hepatocyte, and also enterocytes.

34. Ans. b. It is produced by erythroblasts

Ref: Hoffman 7/e p475

It is a peptide hormone encoded in humans by *ERFE* gene. It is produced by erythroblasts in response to erythropoetin. It decreases the production of hepcidin. Its level is increased in thalassemia.

CHAPTER 7

Megaloblastic Anemia

1. Megaloblastic anemia may be caused by all of the following, *except*:
   a. Phenytoin
   b. Methotrexate
   c. Pyrimethamine
   d. Amoxicillin

2. A 1-year-old child presented with severe macrocytic anemia with subnephrotic range proteinuria. His vitamin B_{12} levels are low. The diagnosis is:
   a. Imerslund-Gräsbeck disease
   b. Thiamine deficiency
   c. Roger syndrome
   d. Pearson syndrome

3. Which of the following is not true about tropical sprue?
   a. Not corrected by folate treatment
   b. Corrected by antibiotics treatment
   c. More severely affect the distal ileum
   d. Have both folate and cobalamin deficiency

4. The earliest specific indicator of folate deficiency is:
   a. Serum folate level
   b. Red cell folate level
   c. Anemia
   d. Elevated homocysteine level

5. A 30-year-old lady presented with severe generalized weakness and CBC shows Hb 6.0 g/dL, mean corpuscular volume (MCV–123fL), total leukocyte count (TLC–3000/cmm), and platelet count of 40,000/cmm. There is no hepatosplenomegaly or lymphadenopathy. Reticulocyte of 1% and peripheral smear is showing macrocytic blood picture. Which of the following is most likely diagnosis?
   a. Aplastic anemia
   b. Liver disease
   c. Megaloblastic anemia
   d. Hypothyroidism

6. Megaloblastic anemia should be treated with both folic acid and vitamin B_{12}, because:
   a. It is a cofactor
   b. It is enzyme
   c. Folic acid alone causes improvement of hematologic symptoms but worsening of neurological symptoms
   d. None of the above

7. The earliest neurological sign of megaloblastic anemia is:
   a. Loss of position sense
   b. Loss of vibration sense
   c. Dysdiadochokinesia
   d. Romberg's sign positive

8. Which of the following is true about megaloblastic anemia?
   a. Reticulocytosis begins on day 3–5 and peaks on day 4–10 after treatment.
   b. Marrow change from megaloblastic to normoblastic starts at 12 hours and completed in 2–3 days of therapy
   c. Nuclear hypersegmentation persists for 4–7 days of therapy
   d. Decrease in serum potassium

9. Cobalamin deficiency is characterized by all of the following, *except*:
   a. Angular cheilitis
   b. Glossitis
   c. Cognitive impairment
   d. Jaundice

10. A 60-year-old female patient presented with anemia requiring blood transfusion. There is also associated mild thrombocytosis. The most likely diagnosis could be:
   a. Gastrointestinal bleed
   b. Myelodysplastic syndrome 5q–
   c. Both of the above
   d. None of the above

11. Macrocytic anemia is seen in all, *except*:
   a. Acute blood loss
   b. Hemolytic anemia
   c. Vitamin B_{12} deficiency
   d. Folate deficiency

12. Which of the following form is used in the treatment of megaloblastic anemia?
   a. Methylcobalamin
   b. Folate polyglutamate
   c. Hydroxycobalamin
   d. Methyltetrahydrofolate

13. Which of the following may be associated with pernicious anemia?
   a. Ileal resection
   b. Anti-thyroid antibodies
   c. Rheumatoid arthritis
   d. Malabsorption

14. What is true regarding reduction of folate?
   a. Needs cobalamin
   b. Inhibited by methotrexate

c. Inhibited by sulfonamide
d. It occurs during thymidylate synthesis

15. What is not true about megaloblastic anemia?
a. Due to defective DNA synthesis
b. May be caused by nitrous oxide inhalation
c. Patient may have jaundice
d. Bone marrow changes are identical in vitamin B_{12} and folic acid deficiency
e. Always caused by vitamin B_{12} or folate deficiency

16. Folate deficiency during pregnancy can cause:
a. Hemolytic anemia
b. Neural tube defect
c. Phocomelia
d. Duodenal atresia

17. A 70-year-old man presents with history of malaise, weakness and effort intolerance for the past 6 months. He is having pallor and heart rate of 118/min. Schilling test is positive and there is macrocytic anemia with low reticulocyte count. The most likely diagnosis in his case would be:
a. Hemorrhage
b. Iron deficiency anemia
c. Pernicious anemia
d. Autoimmune hemolytic anemia
e. Anemia of chronic disease

18. A 75-year-old male presented with generalized weakness, tingling and numbness in feet and hands, and soreness in tongue. Schilling test showed impaired vitamin B_{12} absorption and peripheral blood smear showed macrocytic anemia. He is diagnosed to have pernicious anemia. Which of the following antibodies is most closely associated with it?
a. Anti-intrinsic factor antibodies
b. Anti-mitochondrial antibodies
c. Anti-tissue transglutaminase antibodies
d. Anti-gliadin antibodies
e. Anti-smooth muscle antibodies

19. All of the following are causes of falsely low serum cobalamin in the absence of true cobalamin deficiency, *except*:
a. Active liver disease
b. Multiple myeloma
c. Transcobalamin I deficiency
d. Megadose vitamin C therapy

ANSWERS WITH EXPLANATIONS

1. Ans. d. Amoxicillin *Ref: Williams 8/e p584*

2. Ans. a. Imerslund–Gräsbeck disease
Ref: Williams 8/e p540, 555

It is an autosomal recessive megaloblastic anemia associated with proteinuria, due to inherited failure of transport of intrinsic factor-cobalamin complex by ileum. Usually occurs in less than 2 years old children. Endogenous intrinsic factor and hydrochloric acid (HCl) secretion, transcobalamin/haptocorrin levels and gastric and interstitial histology are all normal. It is treated with intramuscular cobalamin but proteinuria persists.

3. Ans. a. Not corrected by folate treatment
Ref: William 8/e p546

Tropical sprue is endemic in West Indies, Southern India, parts of South Africa and Southeast Asia. It is rapidly corrected by folate therapy. Etiology is not known, although, response to antibiotics suggests infection. It is more severe in distal small intestine. Megaloblastic anemia is very common in these patients and may result from both folate and cobalamin deficiency. Celiac disease (Nontropical sprue) is related to ingestion of wheat gluten. It affects more severely the proximal small intestine. It is associated with weight loss, glossitis, diarrhea and passage of light-colored bulky stools with unusually foul odor. Iron deficiency, hypocalcemia, osteoporosis and osteomalacia may occur. Folate levels are low which may lead to megaloblastic anemia.

4. Ans. a. Serum folate level *Ref: Williams 8/e p547*

The earliest specific indicator of folate deficiency is low serum or plasma folate. Raised homocysteine level may precede decline in plasma folate level but it can be elevated in other conditions also, so it is not specific for folate deficiency. A better indicator of the tissue folate status is red cell folate, which remains unchanged while red cell is circulating and reflects better status in past 2–3 months. But again, it is also low in 50% of cobalamin-deficient megaloblastic anemia patients.

5. Ans. c. Megaloblastic anemia *Ref: Williams 8/e p547*

Hypothyroidism does not cause pancytopenia. All other conditions can cause macrocytic anemia but MCV usually rarely exceeds 110 fL. So, most likely diagnosis is megaloblastic anemia.

6. Ans. c. Folic acid alone causes improvement of hematologic symptoms but worsening of neurological symptoms *Ref: Williams 8/e p547*

Folic acid is not an enzyme or cofactor for cobalamin.

7. Ans. a. Loss of position sense *Ref: Williams 8/e p551*

Loss of position sense in second toe is the earliest neurological sign of megaloblastic anemia.

8. Ans. c. Nuclear hypersegmentation persists for 4–7 days of therapy *Ref: Williams 8/e p552*

Nuclear hypersegmentation persists for 10-14 days after starting of therapy.

9. Ans. a. Angular cheilitis *Ref: Williams 7/e p494, 524*

All the features can be seen in cobalamin deficiency except Angular cheilitis. Physical features of iron deficiency anemia (IDA) are pallor, glossitis (smooth, red tongue), stomatitis and angular cheilitis and koilonychia (rarely found nowadays).

Physical features of cobalamin deficiency are pallor, slight jaundice, smooth tongue (glossitis), knuckle hyperpigmentation, peripheral neuropathy, dementia, cognitive impairment, loss of position and vibration sense.

10. Ans. c. Both of the above *Ref: Williams 7/e p1162, 1785*

In gastrointestinal bleed because of IDA reactive thrombocytosis can be found. In myelodysplastic syndrome 5q-patients usually have anemia with macrocytic red cells and normal or elevated platelet.

11. Ans. a. Acute blood loss *Ref: Williams 7/e p767-9*

In vitamin B_{12} and folate deficiency, the anemia is macrocytic. In hemolytic anemia because of chronic nature, the marrow is depleted of folate so the anemia is macrocytic (megaloblastic crisis) in hemolytic anemia. In blood loss, the anemia is usually normocytic normochronic and hemoglobin is low because of increase in plasma volume.

12. Ans. c. Hydroxycobalamin *Ref: Hoffman 5/e p491, 493, 494; Williams 8/e p536*

Four types of cobalamins are seen in animal cell metabolism. Two are cyanocobalamin (Cn Cbl; vitamin B_{12}) and hydroxycobalamin (OH Cbl). Others are alkyl derivatives that are synthesized form of OH Cbl and serve as coenzymes. In one, adenosylcobalamin (AdoCbl)-deoxyadenosyl replaces OH as the cobalt ligand and in the other, methylcobalamin (MeCbl) OH is replaced by methyl group. MeCbl is the major form of cobalamin in human blood plasma and exists always in bound form with transcobalamin-I (accounts for 70–90% of total serum cobalamin).

Cobalamin in food is usually in coenzyme form AdoCbl or MeCbl, nonspecifically bound to protcins. On exposure to light, cyanide moiety (CN) is gradually lost with production of hydroxycobalamin. In vivo 5-methyl tetrahydrofolate readily donates its methyl group to cobalamin to form MeCbl catalyzed by methionine synthase.

Cyanocobalamin does not occur in nature and is prepared for pharmacological use for supplement because of its stability and lower cost. Hydroxycobalamin, MeCbl and AdoCbl can also be found inexpensive pharmacological products. Otherwise, MeCbl and AdoCbl are unstable forms ex vivo. Food and Drug Administration (FDA) recommends OHCbl for the treatment of cyanide poisoning. OHCbl is produced by many bacteria which are used to produce this form commercially.

Folate polyglutamate is the conjugated form of folate present intracellularly (75% of intracellular folate is conjugated). This form cannot move out of cell. This form is not commercially available and cannot be used for treatment of folate or vitamin B_{12} deficiency.

13. Ans. b. Anti-thyroid antibodies *Ref: Williams 8/e p548*

Antiparietal cell antibodies and pernicious anemia are unexpectedly frequent in patients with other autoimmune diseases including autoimmune thyroid disorders (thyrotoxicosis, Hashimoto thyroiditis and hypothyroidism), type I diabetes mellitus, Addison disease, hypoparathyroidism, postpartum, hypophysitis, vitiligo, acquired agammaglobulinemia, infertility in female and hypospermia and infertility in males (due to defective DNA synthesis rather than to autoimmune mechanism).

14. Ans. b. Inhibited by methotrexate *Ref: Williams 8/e p535, 536, 538, 539*

In folate metabolism, 1 carbon transfer occurs and M5, M10-methylene FH4 serve as hydrogen donor for reduction. So, thymidylate synthase oxidizes folate. In case of folate deficiency, uracil is incorporated into DNA instead of thymidine which leads to defective DNA synthesis.

Dihydrofolate reductase (DHFR) reduces FH2 back to FH4 form and this enzyme is inhibited by methotrexate and antibiotic trimethoprim. Bacteria are unable to take up folic acid from environment so they have to depend on de novo synthesis which eukaryotic cell can directly take up.

Cobalamin metabolism: It catalyzes two reactions:

Methylmalonyl-CoA and Succinyl-CoA

Adenosylcobalamin is a cofactor for methymalonyl CoA mutase.

Actually, this reaction has a complex of enzymes involving S-adenosyl methionine (SAM) and methionine synthase reductase.

This reaction is also important in converting the N5-methyl FH4 to FH4 and this demethylated form is a prerequisite for attachment of polyglutamate chain which prevents leakage of M5-methyl FH4. In cobalamin deficiency, M5 methyl FH4 level is increased and it cannot be converted to FH4 (required for polyglutamate), so tissue levels of other forms of folate decreases and that is why folate supplement corrects megaloblastic anemia in cobalamin deficiency. Conversely, anemia in folate deficiency is not corrected by cobalamin supplement. Reduction of folate is done by DHFR which does not require cobalamin.

15. **Ans. e. Always caused by B$_{12}$ or folate deficiency**
Ref: Williams 8/e p542, 538, 543, 544, 534

Megaloblastic anemias are disorders caused by impaired DNA synthesis. Nitrous oxide impairs methyltransferase by oxidizing cob(I)alamin (a catalytic intermediate in methyltransferase reaction) to cob(II)alamin and it depletes MeCbl and produces cobalamin deficiency like state. Slight jaundice can be seen in megaloblastic anemia. All megaloblastic anemias share certain general clinical features and bone marrow changes. Other causes of megaloblastic anemia include drugs (hydroxyurea, nucleoside analogues), hemolytic anemia causing folate deficiency and certain inborn errors of metabolism.

16. **Ans. b. Neural tube defect** *Ref: Hoffman 6/e p494*

Neural tube defects are the most common congenital malformation. Other defects could be decreased placental weight and premature, low birth-weight babies.

17. **Ans. c. Pernicious anemia** *Ref: Williams 7/e p489*

This patient is having macrocytic anemia and positive Schilling test means vitamin B$_{12}$ malabsorption. A common cause of cobalamin malabsorption is pernicious anemia, an autoimmune disease in which the fundamental defect is atrophy of gastric (parietal cell) oxyntic mucosa that eventually leads to the complete absence of intrinsic factor (IF) and HCl secretion. The autoimmune gastritis associated with pernicious anemia involves body and fundus of stomach. Although, the average of onset is about 60 years, pernicious anemia is no respecter of age, race or ethnic origin. Anti-IF antibodies are highly specific and confirmatory of pernicious anemia, but their absence does not rule out the condition. Despite the high incidence anti-parietal cell in 90% of patients with pernicious anemia, this test is not specific.

18. **Ans. a. Anti-intrinsic factor antibodies**
Ref: Williams 7/e p489

Pernicious anemia is characteristically diagnosed by the presence of anti-intrinsic factor antibodies. All patients with anemia, neuropathy or glossitis, and suspected of having pernicious anemia, should be tested for anti-intrinsic factor antibodies regardless of cobalamin levels. It identifies those patients with a need for lifelong cobalamin replacement therapy.

19. **Ans. a. Active liver disease** *Ref. Hoffmann 6/e p528*

All of these cause falsely low serum cobalamin in the absence of true cobalamin deficiency
- Folate deficiency (one-third of patients)
- Multiple myeloma
- Transcobalamin I (TCI) deficiency
- Megadose vitamin C therapy

All of these cause falsely raised cobalamin levels in the presence of a true deficiency
- Increased cobalamin binders (TCI and II) (e.g., myeloproliferative states, hepatomas, and fibrolamellar hepatic tumors)
- Activated macrophages producing TCII (e.g., autoimmune diseases, monoblastic leukemias and lymphomas)
- Release of cobalamin from hepatocytes (e.g., active liver disease)
- High serum anti-IF antibody titer

CHAPTER 8

Platelets and Hemostatic Disorders

1. All of the following are the normal hemostasis responses to vascular injury, *except*:
   a. Endothelium
   b. Stasis of blood flow
   c. Platelets
   d. Coagulation factors

2. Which of these statements is not true regarding platelets?
   a. During maturation megakaryocytes undergoes endomitotic nuclear division
   b. Thrombopoietin is mainly produced by liver
   c. Lifespan of platelets is 7–10 days
   d. They extrude their nucleus before forming mature platelets

3. Palpable purpura is seen in all, *except*:
   a. Immune thrombocytopenia
   b. Henoch-Schönlein purpura (HSP)
   c. Acute meningococcemia
   d. Polyarteritis nodosa (PAN)

4. One unit of random donor platelet ideally increases the platelet count in an adult by:
   a. $5,000/mm^3$
   b. $10,000/mm^3$
   c. $15,000/mm^3$
   d. $20,000/mm^3$

5. Most specific test in diagnosing heparin-induced thrombocytopenia (HIT):
   a. Enzyme-linked immunosorbent assay (ELISA)
   b. Serotonin release assay
   c. Prolonged prothrombin time/partial thromboplastin time (PT/APTT)
   d. Prothrombin fragment 1.2 level

6. Most common cause of thrombocytopenia in children is:
   a. Aplastic anemia
   b. Immune thrombocytopenia
   c. Thrombotic thrombocytopenic purpura (TTP)
   d. Drug induced

7. In TTP, which of the following is true?
   a. PT is prolonged
   b. APTT is prolonged
   c. Both PT and APTT are prolonged
   d. Both PT and APTT are normal

8. Falsely low platelets (pseudothrombocytopenia) are seen in all, *except*:
   a. Ethylenediaminetetraacetic acid (EDTA)
   b. Presence of giant platelets
   c. Multiple myeloma
   d. Heparin

9. Which of the following is not a first-line therapy in immune thrombocytopenia?
   a. Intravenous immunoglobulin (IVIg)
   b. Anti-D
   c. Rituximab
   d. Steroids

10. Which of the following is not true regarding post-transfusion purpura?
   a. It is most commonly due to anti-human platelet antigen-1a (anti-HPA-1a) antibodies
   b. Usually develops after 3 weeks of blood transfusion
   c. The treatment of choice is IVIg
   d. Even HLA matched platelets are not useful

11. Bernard-Soulier syndrome is characterized by all, *except*:
   a. Low platelet count
   b. Giant platelets
   c. Aggregation with ristocetin
   d. Has defect in GPIb/IX

12. In TTP, anemia is due to:
   a. Autoimmunity
   b. Hypersplenism
   c. Bleeding
   d. Platelet aggregates (microangiopathy)

13. Which of the following is true about von Willebrand factor (VWF)?
   a. It crosses links platelet to each other
   b. It is functional in large multimeric form
   c. Plasma VWF is derived from platelets
   d. It carries factor IX

14. Which of the following does not inhibit platelet activation?
   a. Ecto-ADPase
   b. Prostacyclins
   c. Nitric oxide
   d. Adenosine diphosphate (ADP)

15. Which of the following is the strongest activator of platelet?
   a. Thrombin
   b. Serotonin
   c. Thromboxane A2
   d. Epinephrine

16. Which of the following is not true?
   a. Coagulation is started by the interaction of tissue factor (TF) with factor VIIa
   b. Factor VIIa/TF complex activates IX and X
   c. TF is expressed on endothelial cell
   d. Small amount of factor VII circulates in activated form but is inactive unless bound to TF

17. Which of the following is not a risk factor for disseminated intravascular coagulation (DIC)?
   a. Amniotic fluid embolism
   b. Snake bite
   c. Abruptio placentae
   d. Major orthopedic surgery

18. Which of the following is not seen in DIC?
   a. Prolonged PT/APTT
   b. Thrombocytopenia with schistocytes in peripheral blood
   c. High levels of fibrin degradation product (FDP/D-dimer)
   d. Increased fibrinogen levels

19. A falsely low platelet count can be seen in all of the following, *except*:
   a. Platelet aggregation
   b. Platelet satellitism
   c. Presence of giant platelets
   d. Hypergammaglobulinemia

20. Macrothrombocytopenia is characteristically seen in all, *except*:
   a. Bernard-Soulier syndrome (BSS)
   b. Gray-platelet syndrome
   c. May-Hegglin anomaly
   d. Wiskott-Aldrich syndrome (WAS)

21. Which of the following is not true about WAS?
   a. Thrombocytopenia
   b. Autosomal recessive
   c. Small platelets
   d. Eczema
   e. Platelet dysfunction to various agonists

22. Thrombocytopenia is seen in all, *except*:
   a. Henoch-Schönlein purpura
   b. Disseminated intravascular coagulation
   c. Thrombotic thrombocytopenic purpura
   d. Leukemia

23. Immune destruction of platelets is seen in all, *except*:
   a. Chronic lymphocytic leukemia
   b. Human immunodeficiency virus (HIV)
   c. Systemic lupus erythematosus
   d. All of the above

24. All of the following can be seen in TTP, *except*:
   a. Microangiopathic hemolytic anemia
   b. Thrombocytopenia
   c. Prolongation of both PT and APTT
   d. Presence of fever

25. A 25 years old girl is brought to the emergency department in the state of altered sensorium with high-grade fever. Investigation revealed anemia, thrombocytopenia with fragmented red cells on peripheral blood smear examination. CT-brain is normal and a serum creatinine is 3.0 mg/dL. PT/APTT/thrombin time (TT) are normal. Which of the following is the most effective treatment?
   a. Plasma exchange therapy
   b. Steroids with IVIG
   c. Platelet transfusion
   d. Broad-spectrum IV antibiotics

26. All of the following are used in the treatment of TTP, *except*:
   a. Corticosteriods
   b. Plasma exchange therapy
   c. Cryosupernatant transfusion
   d. Platelet transfusion
   e. Vincristine

27. A 25-year-old healthy woman has delivered a baby who after birth, is drowsy and found to have a cerebral hemorrhage. Her platelet count is 21,000/mm^3 and the maternal platelet count is 130,000/mm^3. Maternal serum will most likely show:
   a. Antibodies to HIV
   b. Anti-HPA-1a antibodies
   c. Platelet autoantibodies
   d. Anti-HLA antibodies

28. A young pregnant lady is registered in ante-natal clinic and found to be having blood group B RhD positive. In previous pregnancy she was grouped as B positive RhD negative (B-) and has documenting evidence of her blood group:
   a. Laboratory error
   b. Weak/partial RhD group
   c. Rh null phenotype
   d. Presence of anti-D in her serum

29. A neonate is found to have petechial spots all over body with gum bleeding and hematuria after a full term normal vaginal delivery. CBC showing normal Hb and WBC with platelet count of 10,000/mm^3. Peripheral smear examination is normal. Mother did not have any major problem during pregnancy and has no h/o any autoimmune thrombocytopenia or other autoimmune disease and having a platelet count of 170,000/mm^3. What needs to be done urgently?

a. Platelet administration (random)
b. Administer mother's platelet
c. Steroids
d. High-dose IVIg
e. HPA matched platelet transfusion

30. An elderly gentleman develops purpura all over body 7 days after anterior resection for carcinoma colon. He was found to have platelet count of 10,000/mm^3 with normal WBC and Hb. Coagulation was normal. He was given 4 units of packed RBCs during surgery and was on low molecular weight heparin (LMWH) prophylaxis for deep vein thrombosis (DVT). What is to be done?
a. Platelet transfusion
b. Corticosteroids
c. High-dose IVIg
d. Stop heparin and start on warfarin/fondaparinux

31. A young lady presented with microangiopathic hemolytic anemia, thrombocytopenia and reduced level of consciousness. Her ADAMTS-13 level was low and was diagnosed as TTP. She was given plasma exchange to which she responded and then relapsed after 1 year. What is the treatment option now?
a. Plasma exchange
b. Plasma exchange plus rituximab
c. Plasma exchange plus splenectomy
d. High-dose steroids

32. A young lady presented with purpura all over body with gum bleeding and having platelet count of 15,000/mm^3. She was given steroid to which she responded and again the platelets dropped to 40,000/mm^3 after tapering of steroids was done. At this time she was found to be HIV positive. What treatment should be given to this patient?
a. Anti-D
b. High-dose IVIg
c. Highly active antiretroviral therapy (HAART)
d. No treatment

33. Which of the following is NOT a characteristic of platelet?
a. Absence of nucleus
b. Size of 2–4 microns
c. As a biconvex discoid shape in inactive form
d. Cytoplasm is a light blue with red purple granules
e. Has mitochondria

34. Platelets are direct fragments of:
a. Cytoplasm of megakaryoblast
b. Cytoplasm of megakaryocyte
c. Nucleus of megakaryoblast
d. Nucleus of megakaryocyte

35. Largest cell found in human bone marrow is:
a. Megakaryocyte   b. Osteoblast
c. Megakaryoblast   d. Monocyte

36. Platelet count is done best by:
a. Electron microscopy
b. Dark-field microscopy
c. Bright-field microscopy
d. Phase-contrast microscopy

37. A young lady presented to emergency room after an episode generalized tonic clonic seizure. She is still in confusional state and on examination there was no focal neurological deficit but she was febrile. Her laboratory evaluation showed Hb-7 g/dL, TLC-12000/mm^3, Platelet-30,000/mm^3, Creatinine-2.5 mg/dL and LDH-1500 U/l. What should be done next?
a. Intravenous immunoglobulin therapy
b. Immediately plan for therapeutic plasma exchange
c. Platelet transfusion
d. Pulse methylprednisolone

38. New drug approved for treatment of TTP is:
a. Concizumab   b. Caplacizumab
c. Fitusiran   d. Crizanlizumab

39. A 63-year-old lady underwent right total hip replacement therapy and 5 days later she developed swelling of right leg and on Doppler she was confirmed to have DVT. She is on unfractionated heparin (UFH) for DVT prophylaxis. On further evaluation her CBC showed Hb-11 g/dL, TLC-12500/mm^3 and platelet count of 55,000/mm^3. UFH was immediately stopped. What other intervention would be needed?
a. Start therapeutic dose of UFH
b. Start direct thrombin inhibitor
c. Start LMWH
d. Start fondaparinux

40. Anfibatide is used for:
a. Immune thrombocytopenia
b. Febrile neutropenia
c. Sickle cell disease
d. TTP

41. Which of the following is not a component of PLASMIC score?
a. Platelet count < 30,000/mm^3
b. Creatinine > 2 mg/dL
c. No active malignancy
d. Mean corpuscular volume (MCV) < 90 fL

42. Percentage of TTP cases presenting with classic pentad is:
a. 40–80%   b. 20%
c. 15%   d. 7%

43. Components of pentad in TTP include all, *except*:
a. Microangiopathic hemolytic anemia (MAHA)
b. Thrombocytopenia
c. Hypothermia
d. Neurological abnormalities

44. Which of the following is cause of fever in TTP?
 a. Hypothalamic infarcts
 b. Pontine infarcts
 c. Pituitary infarcts
 d. Medulla oblongata infarcts

45. Poor prognostic factors in TTP are following, *except*:
 a. Glasgow Coma Score (GCS) < 14
 b. Elevated troponin levels
 c. Autoimmune TTP
 d. Gastrointestinal involvement

46. Congenital TTP is also known as:
 a. Upshaw-Schulman syndrome
 b. Stiff person syndrome
 c. Weber's syndrome
 d. Moebius syndrome

47. Which of the following are long-term complications of TTP, *except*:
 a. Depression
 b. Chronic kidney disease
 c. Cognitive dysfunction
 d. Malabsorption syndrome

48. A 30-year-old woman who is 35 weeks pregnant with ITP and her current platelet count is 30,000/cumm. She is planned for delivery, so what is correct about the management of this patient?
 a. Minimum 50,000/cumm platelet count is needed for labour
 b. Type of delivery should be based on obstetric indication
 c. Dexamethasone can be given to increase the platelet count
 d. Elective caesarean (LSCS) can be done if platelet count is above 50,000/cumm
 e. Spinal anesthesia can be given if platelet count is above 80,000/cumm

49. The mother of a 3-year-old boy noticed small petechial hemorrhages on the skin. On examination besides petechiae, there were no other significant signs. CBC showed Hb of 13 g/dL, MCV 90 fL, WBC count of 7000/cumm and Platelet count of 15,000/cumm. These lesions resolved over next 2 weeks and the platelet counts also improved over next 1 month without any treatment. What is the most likely cause of this condition?
 a. Congenital HIV infection
 b. Vitamin B_{12} deficiency
 c. Respiratory syncytial virus infection
 d. Pain killer induced

50. All of the following are drugs for ITP, *except*:
 a. Fostamiatinib
 b. Rozanolixizumab
 c. Avathrombopag
 d. Efgartigimod
 e. None of the above

51. Which of the following is true about PFA-100?
 a. PFA-100 is a system for analyzing platelet function
 b. The PFA-200 is very similar but includes an additional cartridge
 c. Relatively insensitive to clotting factor deficiencies
 d. It has a high negative predictive value
 e. All of the above

52. Which of the following variable affect the result obtained with PFA 100?
 a. Citrate concentration
 b. Platelet count
 c. Blood group and VWF levels
 d. Drugs (Aspirin, NSAIDS)
 e. All of the above

53. A 10-year-old girl with newly diagnosed ITP is on tapering steroids. After 21 days platelet counts fall to 60000/micl. What is the next step?
 a. Advise splenectomy
 b. Add eltrombopag
 c. Increase dose of steroids
 d. Decrease dose and observe

54. True about thrombopoietin receptors agonist (TPO-RA) in Immune thrombocytopenia patient is:
 a. Eltrombopag cannot be used in splenectomised patients
 b. Romiplostim is administered at a dose of 10 mcg/kg/week
 c. TPO-RA should be discontinued if platelet count does not increase sufficiently after 4 weeks treatment at maximum doses
 d. Eltrombopag can be administered with meals

ANSWERS WITH EXPLANATIONS

1. Ans. b. Stasis of blood flow *Ref: Hoffbrand 7/e*

The hemostatic system is a complex mosaic of activating or inhibitory feedback or feed-forward pathways, integrating its five major components.

Activating	Inhibitory
Blood vessels (Endothelium)	Endothelium
Blood platelets	Coagulation inhibitors
Coagulation factors	Fibrinolytic elements

2. Ans. d. They extrude their nucleus before forming mature platelets *Ref: Williams 8/e p238, 1721-6*

The characteristic feature of megakaryocyte development is endomitosis in which the DNA is repeatedly replicated in absence of nuclear or cytoplasmic division. Endomitosis begins in megakaryocyte. Thrombopoietin is the primary regulator of megakarocyte maturation and is mainly produced by liver, though some amount is also produced by kidney, marrow stroma and skeletal muscle. The circulatory life span of platelet is approximately 10 days with normal platelet count, but shorter in patients with moderate (7 days) to severe (5 days) thrombocytopenia. Mature platelets are formed as proplatelet from megakaryocytes. Nucleus is not extruded from megakaryocyte.

3. **Ans. a. Immune thrombocytopenia** *Ref: Harrison 17/e*

Purpura can be of two types:

Palpable	Nonpalpable
Vasculitis (leukocytoclastic vasculitis)	Steroid purpura
• Drugs (antibiotics)	• ITP
• Infections (Hepatitis C)	• Vascular fragility
• Autoimmune connective tissue diseases (RA, lupus, Sjogren syndrome)	(Amyloidosis, Ehlers–Danlos syndrome)
• HSP	• Thrombi
• PAN	• DIC
Embolic type	• TTP
• Meningococcemia	• Warfarin reaction
• Disseminated gonococcal infection	• Cryoglobulinemia
• RMSF	• Thrombocytosis
• Erythema gangrenosum	• Fat emboli

(DIC: disseminated intravascular coagulation; HSP: Henoch-Schönlein purpura; ITP: immune thrombocytopenia purpura; PAN: polyarteritis nodosa; RMSF: Rocky Mountain spotted fever; TTP: thrombotic thrombocytopenic purpura).

4. **Ans. a. 5,000/mm³** *Ref: Williams 8/e p2306*

The increment in platelet count depends on many factors but if all other factors are absent then 1 unit of whole blood derived random platelet increases the platelet count by $5,000/mm^3/m^2$. So, in a person of BSA $2\ m^2$, it should raise by $10,000/mm^3$ and of $1.5\ m^2$ by $7,500/mm^3$, respectively.

5. **Ans. b. Serotonin release assay**

Ref: Williams 8/e p2176

Thrombocytopenia is the key laboratory finding in HIT and ranges from $20-100,000/mm^3$ or 50–70% decline from baseline. Two assay prototypes for confirming diagnosis are available. One is ELISA based for detection of immunoglobulin antibodies to heparin-PF4 complexes and the other measure heparin-dependent antibodies that activate platelets. Activation assays are not available commercially because specific platelet donors are needed each time and donor platelets vary greatly in their sensitivity to activation by HIT sera. The best-established activation assay is 14C-serotonin release assay. Activation assays have greater specificity than antigen assay. The risk status for HIT can be assessed by 4Ts.

	Points per category		
Clinical sign	0	1	2
Thrombocytopenia	<10,000/mm³ or <30% fall	10–20,000/mm³ or 30–50% fall	20–100,000/mm³ or >50% fall
Timing of Thrombocytopenia or Thrombosis	<4 days (unless prior heparin in last 3 weeks)	5–10 days (but not well documented) or <1 day with prior exposure in last 3 weeks	Documented occurrence in 5–10 days or <1 day with recent prior exposure
Thrombotic related event	None	Common thrombosis (DVT or line thrombus) or recurrent thrombosis	Major vessel thrombus or skin necrosis or skin lesion at the site of heparin infusion
Thrombocytopenia (Other Causes)	Definite	Possible	No other strong explanation for thrombocytopenia

Interpretation: 6–8 high risk, 4–5 intermediate risk, 0–3 low risk

6. **Ans. b. Immune thrombocytopenia**

Ref: Hoffman 7/e p1955-57

Immune thrombocytopenic purpura (ITP) is the most common cause of acquired severe thrombocytopenia and 50% of ITP cases are children, i.e., <10 years of age.

7. **Ans. d. Both PT and APTT are normal**

Ref: Hoffman 7/e p1985-88

In TTP, PT/APTT and fibrinogen levels are usually normal or only mild perturbed. Mild elevations in fibrin degradation products occur in 50% of patients.

8. **Ans. d. Heparin** *Ref: Williams 8/e p1892*

Pseudothrombocytopenia has been reported in association with the use of EDTA as an anticoagulant, with platelet cold agglutinins associated with multiple myeloma, platelet satellitism, giant platelets and platelet agglutination. Other anticoagulants such as sodium citrate, oxalate, acid citrate dextrose and heparin can also cause platelet agglutination but is less frequent.

9. **Ans. c. Rituximab** *Ref: Williams 8/e p1906-08*

Intravenous immunoglobulin, anti-D and steroids are the first-line treatment options given in ITP. Rituximab is usually given in cases of chronic ITP who fail to steroids.

10. **Ans. b. Usually develops after 3 weeks of blood transfusion** *Ref: Hoffman 7/e p2095-96*

The typical patient is a multiparous, middle aged or elderly female who presents with the acute onset of bleeding due to severe thrombocytopenia, a mean of 6–8 days (range 1–14 days) after receiving a blood product containing platelet material. Sera of more than

90% of patients contain antibodies to HPA-1a which is expressed on 97–98% of Caucasians. Bleeding usually lasts for 10 days, but can persists for 60–120 days with fatality rates of 10%. The treatment of choice is IVIg 1 g/kg/day × 2 days. More than 90% of patients respond within 2–3 days. HLA matched platelets are generally not useful.

11. Ans. c. Aggregation with ristocetin
Ref: Williams 8/e p1944-45

Thrombocytopenia is present in nearly all patients and ranges from 20,000/mm^3 to near-normal levels. Platelets can be large or small. The hallmark of BSS is the failure of platelets to aggregate in response to ristocetin or botrocetin. BSS platelets are deficient in GPIb, GPIX and GPV.

12. Ans. d. Platelet aggregates (Microangiopathy)
Ref: Williams 8/e p2166-7

Approximately one-third of patients have symptoms of hemolytic anemia (due to MAHA). Hemolysis is indicated by an elevated reticulocyte count, serum lactate dehydrogenase (LDH) and decreased serum haptoglobin. Direct Coombs' test (DCT) is almost always negative.

13. Ans. b. It is functional in largest multimeric form
Ref: Hoffman 7/e p2052-5

von Willebrand factor attaches platelets to the endothelium and vessel walls and not the platelets to each other. The biologically most potent form of VWF is the large multimeric form. VWF is secreted from the endothelium by one of the two pathways. The constitutive pathway–directly coupled to VWF synthesis and occurs without stimulation and the regulated pathway–involving VWF stored in Weibel-Palade bodies, is initiated by the action of secretagogues. VWF secreted by the constitutive pathway is in the largest multimeric form. Plasma VWF level is maintained by the constitutive secretion of VWF from endothelium. During activation after tissue injury, it is released from the Weibel–Palade bodies of endothelium and α-granules of platelet. VWF carries factor VIII and not IX.

14. Ans. d. Adenosine diphosphate
Ref: Williams 8/e p1788-9

The inhibitory pathways in platelets are CD39 (Ecto-ADPase), Nitric oxide and PGE2 (at high concentrations) and PGI2 also called prostacyclins (at low concentrations).

15. Ans. a. Thrombin

Activators of platelets are:

Strong	Weak
	Epinephrine
Thrombin	Thromboxane A2/Prostaglandin H2

Contd...

Contd...

Collagen	Serotonin
ADP	Platelet-activating factor
	Vasopressin
	Thrombospondin-1
Others-Shear	Thrombolytic agents

16. Ans. c. TF is expressed on endothelial cells
Ref: Williams 8/e p1830, 1835; Hoffman 5/e p1826

The major initiating event in hemostasis in vivo is the formation of a factor VIIa/TF complex at the site of injury. The factor VIIa/TF complex can activate both factor IX and X. TF is normally expressed on pericytes surrounding blood vessel and by epidermal, stromal and glial cells. In Contrast to other proenzymes, factor VII circulates in the blood in two forms: (1) the inactive zymogen factor VII and (2) the enzymatically active form VIIa. The concentration of factor VIIa is low but sufficient to generate significant factor X–activating activity when the factor VIIa forms a complex with newly exposed TF.

17. Ans. d. Major orthopedic surgery
Ref: Williams 8/e p2108-13

The risk factor for DIC are infections, purpura fulminans, solid tumors, leukemias, trauma, brain injury, burns, liver disease, heat stroke, snake bites, hemangiomas, aortic aneurysm, transfusion reaction, abruptio placentae, amniotic fluid embolism, preeclampsia and eclampsia, HELLP syndrome, dead fetus syndrome, and acute fatty liver of pregnancy.

18. Ans. d. Increased fibrinogen levels
Ref: Williams 8/e p2107-08

Fibrinogen levels are actually decreased and not increased in DIC.

19. Ans. d. Hypergammaglobulinemia
Ref: Dacie and Lewis 10/e p111-12

Pseudothrombocytopenia is seen with giant platelets (macrothrombocytopenia). In about 1% of individuals, EDTA causes platelet clumping, resulting in pseudothrombocytopenia. Occasionally platelets may be seen adhering to neutrophils (platelet satellitism). Presence of platelet cold agglutinins is seen with multiple myeloma. GP IIb/IIIa antagonists (e.g., abciximab) is associated with both pseudothrombocytopenia and true thrombocytopenia. Antiphospholipid antibodies (APLAs) are also associated with pseudothrombocytopenia.

20. Ans. d. Wiskott-Aldrich syndrome
Ref: Williams 8/e p1894, 1896, 1948, 1944

May-Hegglin anomaly, Fechtner syndrome, Sebastian syndrome and Epstein syndrome are autosomal dominant macrothrombocytopenia with mutations in the *MYH9* gene. WAS is a rare X-linked immunodeficiency disorder characterized by microthrombocytopenia, eczema, recurrent infections, T-cell deficiency and increased risk for autoimmune and lymphoproliferative disorders. Platelets appear larger than normal, pale, ghost-like, oval forms on blood smear in gray platelet syndrome. Thrombocytopenia is common and can be moderately severe. In BSS, thrombocytopenia is present in nearly all patients, but is variable in its severity, ranging from approximately 20,000/mm³ to normal levels.

21. Ans. b. Autosomal recessive

Ref: Williams 8/e p9 1954-5

Wiskott-Aldrich syndrome is a rare X-linked immunodeficiency disorder characterized by microthrombocytopenia, eczema, recurrent infections, T-cell deficiency and increased risk for autoimmune and lymphoproliferative disorders. Microthrombocytopenia is the most consistent feature. The bleeding time is usually prolonged. Platelet aggregation and release of dense body contents are variably abnormal.

22. Ans. a. Henoch-Schönlein purpura

Ref: Williams 8/e p1999-2000

Henoch-Schönlein purpura is a pediatric vasculitic syndrome characterized by the acute onset of abdominal pain and lower extremity eruption of diffuse urticarial plaques and palpable purpura. It affects patients of 2–20 years of age. Several environmental triggers are present, e.g. viral (Hepatitis B, hepatitis C, HIV, parvovirus B19) and bacterial (*Streptococcus* sp., *Staphylococcus aureus* and *Salmonella* sp.). Adult disease is precipitated by nonsteroidal anti-inflammatory drugs (NSAIDs), angiotensin-converting enzyme (ACE) inhibitors and antibiotics, food allergies and insect bites. In spite of its chronic relapsing pattern, the long-term evolution is benign in majority of patients. Glucocorticoids are reserved for cases with renal involvement.

23. Ans. d. All of the above *Ref: Williams 8/e p1902*

Secondary cause of immune destruction of platelets is seen in:
- *Autoimmune diseases*: Systemic lupus erythematosus (SLE), APLA, autoimmune hepatitis, autoimmune thyroiditis.
- *Lymphoproliferative disorders*: CLL, Hodgkin lymphoma, large granular lymphocytic leukemia.
- *Infections*: HIV, hepatitis C, *Helicobacter pylori* myelodysplastic syndrome (MDS).
- Agammaglobulinemia, hypogammaglobulinemia, immunoglobulin A deficiency.
- *Drugs*: Quinidine, gold, heparin, penicillin, procainamide.

24. Ans. c. Prolongation of both PT and APTT

Ref: Williams 8/e p2165-66

TTP has manifestations of MAHA and thrombocytopenia. Many patients have fever. Thrombocytopenia typically is severe. Almost all patients have normal fibrinogen levels, PT and APTT.

25. Ans. a. Plasma exchange therapy

Ref: Williams 8/e p2171

The mainstay of therapy for TTP is plasma exchange with the exception of factor H deficiency and possibly APS syndrome and quinine-induced disease. No compelling evidence indicates that plasma therapy is effective for thrombotic microangiopathy caused by a mechanism other than ADAMTS13 deficiency.

26. Ans. d. Platelet transfusion

Ref: Williams 8/e p2171, 2172

The treatment options for TTP are:
- Glucocorticoids (2 mg/kg/day)
- Plasma exchange therapy
- Plasma therapy
- Antiplatelet agents once platelet count exceeds 50,000/mm³
- Vincristine, rituximab, cyclosporine, cyclophosphamide, azathioprine, CHOP, autologous stem cell transplantation—usually all these used as second-line therapy
- Splenectomy.

27. Ans. b. Anti-HPA-1a antibodies

Ref: Williams 8/e p1912; BJH-152, p460-8

This patient is a case of neonatal alloimmune thrombocytopenia (NAIT) so maternal serum will show antiplatelet antibodies which are most commonly against anti-HPA-1a antigen (78%) in whites. However, in Asians most common is HPA-4a (80%). It is very important to differentiate between maternal ITP and NAIT and the features are:

Maternal ITP	NAIT
Rarely have severe thrombocytopenia or bleeding manifestation in fetus	Thrombocytopenia is severe and intracranial hemorrhage rate is higher (10–20%)
Maternal platelet count is low	Maternal platelet count is normal

Neonatal alloimmune thrombocytopenia is like Rh hemolytic disease of newborn but the first-born child is affected in 40–60% of cases (which is spared in Rh hemolytic disease of newborn). Platelet count recovers to normal in 1–2 weeks. The diagnosis is usually confirmed by tests for circulating maternal alloantibodies against fetal antigens (usually by MAIPA) or by platelet typing of the parents and neonate by genotyping or ELISA.

Postnatal management: Options are IVIg, glucocorticoids and platelet transfusions. In severe bleeding, platelets can be transfused and should be ABO and (Rh) D compatible and HPA-1a negative.

Prenatal management: In high-risk NAIT, weekly IVIg administration is indicated with or without glucocorticoids. In severe thrombocytopenia early delivery with cesarean section may reduce intracranial hemorrhage (ICH) in newborn.

28. Ans. b. Weak/partial Rh D group

Ref: Williams 8/e p2266

This pregnant lady is most likely to have weak Rh D expression and should be labeled as Rh (D) positive which was missed in previous testing. Blood donors and pregnant women who type D negative using standard typing sera should be tested further for weak expression using more sensitive methods, such as an ICT. Donors with weak D antigen are considered positive. Testing for weak D is optional for transfusion recipients.

29. Ans. d. High-dose IVIg

Ref: Williams 8/e p1912

The alternatives are IVIg, steroids and platelet transfusion. IVIg and/or glucocorticoids therapy may increase platelet count rapidly. Platelet transfusion will not increase the platelet count rapidly in cases of NAIT unless it is HPA-1a negative which may not be available on urgent basis. IVIg acts faster than steroids so the best answer would be IVIg.

Transfusion of washed and irradiated maternal platelets is an alternative but may not be appropriate for several reasons. Washing (to eliminate alloantibodies) and irradiation (to prevent GVHD) may damage the platelets.

30. Ans. c. High-dose IVIg

The differential diagnoses in this case are:

Diagnosis	In favor	In against
Immune thrombocytopenia	Very low platelet count with normal WBC and Hb	
Disseminated intravascular coagulation		Normal coagulation screen, no fever, sepsis
TTP/HUS/ malignancy associated microangiopathy	Low platelet count normal coagulation profile very low platelet count	No hemolysis/anemia, schistocytes
Post-transfusion purpura		Male patient, no transfusion of platelet, no history of previous transfusion
Heparin-induced thrombocytopenia	Patient has received LMWH	4Ts score is 3 (low-risk)

Intravenous immunoglobulin is the most effective treatment for ITP and has also been found effective in HIT.

31. Ans. a. Plasma exchange

Ref: Williams 8/e p2172

Complete response occurs after an average of 9–16 days of plasma exchange. Within 2 weeks following complete response, 25–50% of patients have an acute exacerbation that requires further treatment with plasma exchange. Relapses are defined as recurrence occurring 30 days after a complete response occur, which is usually seen in up to 1/3rd of patients. Most relapses occur during first year. Relapsing patients typically respond to plasma exchange therapy. Relapses in TTP are associated with severe ADAMTS13 deficiency and detectable ADAMTS13 autoantibody inhibitors. Immunosuppressive therapies are used only when the disease is refractory to plasma exchange therapy. Splenectomy can result in lasting remissions or reduce the frequency of relapses for some patients with TTP who are refractory to plasma exchange or immunesuppressive therapy, presumably by removing a major site of anti-ADAMTS13 antibody production.

32. Ans. c. Highly active antiretroviral therapy (HAART)

Ref: Williams 8/e p2174-77; Hoffman 7/e p2096

What was previously described as HIV-associated ITP is changed to primary HIV-associated thrombocytopenia (PHAT). PHAT is the most common cause of thrombocytopenia in persons with HIV. Differentiating features of PHAT from de novo ITP are:

- Higher rate of splenomegaly
- Less severe thrombocytopenia
- 20% spontaneous remission rate.

Multifactorial etiology—both decreased production and increased destruction.

Treatment options for PHAT are HAART, IVIg, interferon-γ anti-D, and splenectomy and glucocorticoids. HAART is an important treatment modality in patients with PHAT and should be the initial treatment of choice. There is no history of any drug exposure besides LMWH and compared to UFH, there is less risk of HIT. The most likely cause of thrombocytopenia in this case is ITP, so the treatment of choice is high dose IVIg if the patient is bleeding. As the patient has relapsed and not on HAART, so it needs to be started. Obviously, the LMWH needs to be stopped but no anticoagulation should be given in view of low platelet count.

33. Ans. e. Has mitochondria

Ref: Williams 7/e p1587

Blood films made from EDTA and stained with Wright stain, platelets appear as small bluish-gray, oval to round bodies with several purple-red granules. The mean diameter varies among individuals, ranging from approximately 1.5–3 microns, approximately one-third to one-fourth of diameter or red blood cells. They do not have nucleus or mitochondria.

34. Ans. b. Cytoplasm of megakaryocyte

Ref: Hoffman's 6/e p295

Each megakaryocyte produces between a few hundred to several thousand platelets. Platelets are released from dynamic megakaryocyte pseudopod extensions called proplatelets. This model was proposed by Becker and De Bruyn in 1976.

35. Ans. a. Megakaryocyte   *Ref: Hoffman's 6/e p292-3*

The largest cell in the bone marrow is the megakaryocyte. The normal development of platelet is—proliferating megakaryocytic progenitors (normal DNA content, 2N-4N), nonproliferating immature megakaryocytes (4N-8N) and nonproliferating immature megakaryocytes (8N-128N). Morphologically recognizable megakaryocytes exist in four distinct maturation stages. The megakaryoblast (stage I) is characterized by high NC ratio and scanty basophilic cytoplasm. The promegakaryocyte (stage II) is the cell in which the cytoplasm volume and number of platelet-specific granules increase. The granular or platelet-shedding megakaryocyte (stages III and IV) is the most mature cell.

36. Ans. c. Bright-field microscopy
Ref: Hoffman's 6/e p1896-9

Whenever platelet count is low, smear should be made and seen in bright-field microscope (simple optical microscope). Dark-field (in both light and electron beam) microscopy exclude the unscattered beam from the image. As a result, the field around the specimen is generally dark. Phase-contrast microscopy is an optical microscopy technique that coverts phase shift in light passing through the transparent specimen. It reveals many cellular structures that are not visible through simple optical microscopy. Electron microscopy technique is utilized to see cellular structures at high resolution.

37. Ans. b. Immediately plan for therapeutic plasma exchange   *Ref: Hoffman's 6/e p1936-7*

The clinical profile of this patient is consistent with TTP. The mortality rate of TTP exceeds 90% without therapy. With plasma-based therapy, the long-term outcome may now exceed 90%. Rituximab is being used with increasing frequency, primarily as salvage therapy for patients refractory to plasma exchange. Corticosteroids are often used as a part of initial therapy for patients who fail to show brisk response to plasma-based therapy. These drugs are of little benefit on their own. Currently, splenectomy is generally reserved for patient's refractory to plasma exchange and rituximab.

38. Ans. b. Caplacizumab

Caplacizumab is an anti-VWF humanized, bivalent variable-domain-only immunoglobulin fragment (nanobody), inhibits the interaction between VWF multimers and platelets. Its use in TTP has shown to shorten the time to platelet count increment, lower recurrence of TTP, shorter ICU stay, lesser number of plasma exchanges. Commonest adverse effect of the drug was mucocutaneous bleeding.

39. Ans. b. Start direct thrombin inhibitor
Ref: Hoffman 5/e p1918-20

This patient has developed DVT of lower limb while she was on prophylactic UFH for hip surgery and 2 days after starting UFH her platelet count dropped to 55,000/mm^3 which means she has developed heparin-induced thrombocytopenia and thrombosis (HITT). So, she definitely needs anticoagulation, but in case of HITT all forms of heparin, whether UFH or LMWH are contraindicated. Fondaparinux can be given but this also carries some risk so ideally be avoided. Direct thrombin inhibitors are absolutely safe, but as they are oral drugs and take some time to act so not good option for life threatening thrombosis like PE, etc. in this patient, as it is only DVT of lower limb, DTIs are best option to start which should immediately be done. We can do testing for HITT simultaneously.

40. Ans. d. TTP

Anfibatide is a potent platelet GP1b receptor antagonist derived from snake venom, which inhibits platelet aggregation by inhibiting its interaction with VWF. In a microfluidic shear model, anfibatide inhibited platelet adhesion, aggregation, and thrombosis formation under static and shear conditions and resulted in resolution of spontaneous thrombocytopenia in a Shiga toxin-induced murine TTP model.

41. Ans. b. Creatinine > 2 mg/dL

PLASMIC score is a robust, cost-effective prediction method for ADAMTS13 levels in TTP. Components of the score are:

Platelet count < 30 × 10^9/L-1 point

hemo*L*ysis; Reticulocyte >2.5%/Haptoglobin undetectable/indirect bilirubin >2 mg/dL-1 point

No *A*ctive cancer- 1 point

No history of *S*olid-organ or hematopoietic *S*tem cell transplant-1 point

*M*CV < 90 fL-1 point

*I*NR < 1.5-1 point

*C*reatinine level < 2 mg/dL-1 point

Interpretation:

Score	Risk category	Risk of severe ADAMTS13 deficiency (< 10%)
0–4	Low	4.3%
5–6	Intermediate	56.8%
7	High	96.2%

42. Ans. d. 7%

Clinical presentation in TTP:

MAHA with thrombocytopenia–100%

Neurological abnormalities: 39–80% Major-20–50%; Minor-25–40%

Fever: 10–70%

GI symptoms: 35–40%

Renal involvement: 10–15%

Classic pentad: 7%

43. **Ans. c. Hypothermia** *Ref: Williams 7/e p2034*

Classic pentad is seen in TTP in 7–10% cases. This includes MAHA, thrombocytopenia, neurological abnormalities, fever and renal dysfunction.

44. **Ans. a. Hypothalamic infarcts**

TTP is a condition that is associated with propensity for microthrombi formation in vasculature due to ADAMTS13 deficiency. Microthrombi can form in any of the vascular beds like central nervous system (CNS), renal, GI and cardiac. Hypothalamic infarcts are the cause for fever in TTP.

45. **Ans. d. Gastrointestinal involvement**
Ref: Alwan et al. Blood. 2017.

Poor prognostic factors in TTP are GCS < 14 which is associated with nine fold increase in mortality, elevated troponin levels in 68% patients and poor prognosis due to risk of myocardial infarction, autoimmune diseases are associated increased risk of relapse of TTP. Mortality was highest (27.3%) in patients with ADAMTS13 antibody levels in the highest quartile and ADAMTS13 antigen levels in lowest quartile. A GCS of < 14 was associated with a significant increase in mortality rate (20% versus 2.2%). Patients with anti-ADAMTS13 antibody levels in the higher versus lower quartile were more likely to have a raised troponin level, a reduced GCS, and a longer period of plasma exchange to achieve normal platelet count.

46. **Ans. a. Upshaw-Schulman syndrome**
Ref: Hoffman's 6/e p1925

Hereditary thrombotic thrombocytopenic purpura (Upshaw-Schulman syndrome) is a rare disorder characterized by thrombocytopenia as a result of platelet consumption, MAHA, occlusion of microvasculature with VWF-platelet-thrombic and ischemic end organ damage. It has autosomal recessive inheritance due to deficiency of ADAMTS13.

47. **Ans. d. Malabsorption syndrome**

Depression (most common), cognitive impairment, SLE and other autoimmune disorder manifestations and CKD with new onset hypertension are some of the long-term complications seen in patients with TTP.

48. **Ans. c. Dexamethasone can be given to increase the platelet count** *Ref: Gernsheimer T et al. How I treat thrombocytopenia in pregnancy. Blood. 2013;121(1):38-47*

A minimum platelet count of 30,000/cumm is generally needed for vaginal delivery. For LSCS, a platelet count of 50,000/cumm is needed. The mode of delivery, whether Vaginal or LSCS, is not based on platelet count rather based on obstetric indication. Dexamethasone is a long-acting steroid which crosses the placental barrier; prednisolone is shorter-acting and does not penetrate through the placenta. Therefore, prednisolone is preferred due to lower risk of complications (e.g., fetal orofacial clefts and adrenal insufficiency). Spinal anesthesia is generally considered to be safe with a platelet count of >80–100 × 10^9/L and should be done by experienced person. This is high-risk pregnancy should be managed in coordination with gynecologist and hematologist together.

49. **Ans. c. Respiratory syncytial virus infection**
Ref: Hoffman's 6/e p1883-7

This child is having acute ITP and in most cases it is self-limiting, so only observation is needed. So the patients who do not have any significant bleeding can safely be put on observation. 80% of childhood ITP resolve within 6 months without any treatment. However, if child is presenting with epistaxis or mucosal bleeding, treatment is required. In most cases there is no etiology, but infection (esp. viral infections) can be stimulus for formation of anti-platelet antibodies. Cross-reactive antibodies (molecular mimicry) have been described with H. pylori, HIV or HCV.

50. **Ans. e. None of the above**

Fostamatinib is an orally available small molecule inhibitor of spleen tyrosine kinase that is used to treat chronic immune thrombocytopenia. Rozanolixizumab, a subcutaneously infused humanized monoclonal antibody, specifically targets the IgG-binding region of FcRn. By blocking binding of IgG to FcRn, rozanolixizumab reduces IgG recycling, accelerates its lysosomal degradation, and lowers IgG levels. Avatrombopag is an orally available platelet thrombopoietin receptor (TPOR; MPL) agonist, with potential megakaryopoiesis stimulating activity was approved for thrombocytopenia (low platelets) in adults with chronic liver disease who are scheduled to undergo a procedure. Efgartigimod is designed as a first-in-class investigational antibody fragment to target the neonatal Fc receptor (FcRn).

51. **Ans. e. All of the above**
Ref: Emmanuel F. Clinical application of the PFA-100. Current Opinion in Hematology 2002

The PFA-100 is a system for analysing platelet function in which citrated whole blood is aspirated at high shear rates through disposable cartridges containing an aperture within a membrane coated with either Collagen and Epinephrine (CEPI) or Collagen and ADP (CADP). These agonists together with the high shear stress, induce platelet adhesion, activation and aggregation leading to rapid occlusion of the aperture and cessation of blood flow termed the closure time (CT). The PFA-200 is very similar but includes an additional cartridge – the INNOVANCE PFA P2Y cartridge, that detects platelet P2Y12-receptor blockade in patients on therapy with a P2Y12-receptor antagonist. The membrane of INNOVANCE PFA P2Y is coated with ADP, PGE1 (Prostaglandin E) and calcium chloride. The PFA-100 was designed as a screen to detect problems with primary hemostasis and in part to replace the bleeding time and in this respect it is better standardized. It is relatively insensitive to clotting factor deficiencies. It has high negative predictive value – i.e. if the PFA-100 gives a normal result then with some exceptions primary hemostasis is intact [Exceptions: Storage Pool Disorder (SPD), Primary Secretion Defects, mild Type 1 VWD]. If the PFA-100 is abnormal then formal platelet aggregation testing, platelet nucleotide assays and mutational analysis may be required to establish the underlying cause. The greatest strengths of the PFA-100 are its simplicity of use and excellent sensitivity to particular hemostatic disturbances such as VWD, platelet disorders, and platelet-affecting medication (asprin).

52. Ans. e. All of the above *Ref: Favaloro EJ. Clinical utility of closure times using the platelet function analyzer-100/200. Am J Hematol. 2017;92:398-404*

The PFA test may be performed up to 4 h after the blood collection. Platelet count of > 150×10^9/L is recommended for the PFA test. Platelet counts of less than 100,000/μL affect the closure time, as does a hematocrit of less than 15–20%. Closure times increase progressively as the platelet counts falls below 100×10^9/L. Heparin and oral anticoagulants do not affect the closure me, but antiplatelet drugs do. Incomplete fill of a 3.2% citrate blood tube is likely to affect results. Closure times correlate inversely with plasma VWF activity levels and may be increased in blood group O patients for the same reason (Blood group O individuals have lower VWF levels).

53. Ans. d. Decrease dose and observe *Ref: Provan D. Updated international consensus report on the investigation and management of primary immune thrombocytopenia, 2019*

Most children with newly diagnosed ITP do not have significant bleeding and can be managed without treatment. Hospital admission and medical treatment should be reserved for those with significant mucosal bleeding. If a response is there with medical treatment (platelet count >50×10^9/L), steroids should be tapered and stopped by 3 weeks, even if platelet count falls during dose tapering.

54. Ans. b. Romiplostim is administered at a dose of 10 mcg/kg/week

TPO-RAs (eltrombopag, avatrombopag, romiplostim) have provided excellent responses (60%) in splenectomized and non-splenectomized patients. Romiplostim is administered at an initial dose of 1 mcg/kg/week subcutaneously (dose up to 10 mcg/kg/week according to platelet response). Eltrombopag is administered at an initial dose of 25 or 50 mg/day, depending on patient age, Asian ancestry, and presence of hepatic dysfunction, up to a maximum of 75 mg/d. Eltrombopag is a chelator drug, it is administered orally 2 hours before or 4 hours after calcium-containing dairy products, etc. Avatrombopag has recently been approved by the FDA for adult patients with chronic ITP who have had an insufficient response to previous therapy. It is administered initially as 20-mg pill daily with dose increases up to 40 mg/d.

CHAPTER 9

Thrombosis

1. Which of the following can be given safely in pregnancy?
   a. Imatinib
   b. Heparin
   c. Warfarin
   d. Thalidomide

2. Five days after starting warfarin therapy in a patient of atrial fibrillation this 60-year-old man returns to his physician complaining of large patches of discolored stain over his gluteal region and legs. This complication is most likely the result of:
   a. Antithrombin III deficiency
   b. Protein C deficiency
   c. Drug allergy
   d. Very high international normalized ratio (INR)

3. All of the following can cause both arterial and venous thrombosis, *except*:
   a. Antiphospholipid antibody (APLA) syndrome
   b. Hyperhomocysteinemia
   c. Protein C deficiency
   d. Polycythemia vera

4. Most common inherited cause of thrombosis in Caucasians is:
   a. Protein S deficiency
   b. Factor V Leiden mutation
   c. Antithrombin III deficiency
   d. Protein C deficiency

5. Which of the following is a major risk factor for venous thrombosis?
   a. Smoking
   b. High cholesterol
   c. Hypertension (HTN)
   d. Diabetes mellitus (DM)
   e. Cancer

6. Which of the following is not a risk factor for arterial thrombosis?
   a. Diabetes mellitus
   b. Gout
   c. Male sex
   d. Smoking
   e. Hypohomocysteinemia

7. Which one of the following statement is TRUE regarding factor V Leiden gene mutation?
   a. In Caucasians, the incidence of factor V Leiden is 5%
   b. Individuals have an increased risk of bleeding
   c. Homozygous or heterozygous state carries the same risk
   d. Factor V Leiden mutation is the most common cause of activated protein C resistance (APCR) resistance

8. Which of the following statement is not true?
   a. Antithrombin III deficiency is sex linked
   b. Mucinous adenocarcinomas are more prone for disseminated intravascular coagulation (DIC)
   c. Protein C deficiency can develop Coumadin-induced skin necrosis when started without heparin
   d. Obesity is a risk factor for thrombosis in postoperative patient

9. Which one of the following test is not done in the evaluation of thrombophilia?
   a. Prothrombin time (PT) and activated partial thromboplastin time (APTT)
   b. Anticardiolipin and anti-B2GPI antibodies
   c. Serum cholesterol
   d. Protein C and S assay

10. Which one of these is not an advantage of low-molecular-weight heparin (LMWH) over unfractionated heparin (UFH)?
   a. There is a reduced risk of osteoporosis
   b. Has a half-life of 30 minutes so the effect can be easily reversed
   c. Dosing does not require monitoring by blood test
   d. Does not require continuous infusion

11. Antiphospholipid antibody syndrome is associated with all of the following, *except*:
   a. Pancytopenia
   b. Recurrent abortions
   c. Venous thrombosis
   d. Pulmonary HTN

12. Which of the following treatment is required in pregnant women with APLA?
   a. Aspirin + LMWH + Warfarin
   b. Aspirin + LMWH + Steroid
   c. Aspirin + LMWH
   d. No treatment

13. All of the following statements are true about hemolytic uremic syndrome (HUS), *except*:
   a. Uremia
   b. Thrombocytopenia

c. Positive direct Coombs test (DCT)
d. Fibrinogen normal

14. D negative HUS is due to the inherited deficiency of:
a. Factor I and H
b. Complement C3, C4
c. ADAMTS13
d. Large von Willebrand factor (vWF) multimers

15. A 30-year-old lady presented with pulmonary thromboembolism and is found to have APLA. She was given fondaparinux and warfarin and then maintained on warfarin. The appropriate target INR is:
a. 2.0
b. 2.5
c. 3.0
d. 3.5

16. A 30-year-old lady underwent prosthetic valve replacement surgery done for rheumatic heart disease and she is started on UFH by continuous infusion plus warfarin. 6 days after she developed deep vein thrombosis (DVT) of right lower limb. Her complete blood count (CBC) was normal preoperatively and now she has dropped her platelet count to 50,000/mm^3. Her INR is 2.3 and APTT is 90 (Control 35). The best therapeutic option would be:
a. IV immunoglobulin (IVIg) followed by steroids
b. Fondaparinux
c. Stop heparin and add aspirin to warfarin
d. Change to LMWH

17. A young patient developed unprovoked DVT for which he was started on LMWH and acitrom. LMWH should be continued:
a. For 5 days
b. For 5 days or until INR is between 2 and 3 for at least 24 hours, whichever is longer
c. Until the INR is between 2 and 3
d. For 7 days

18. A young male developed spontaneous DVT of right lower limb and he is having a sister who had DVT 5 years back and having protein C deficiency. He was started on warfarin and the INR came to 2–3 after which he had started following at local hospital where his warfarin dose was steadily increased as his INR never went higher than 1.5 and is currently on warfarin dose of 20 mg/day. He was referred back to hospital and was evaluated and found to be having warfarin level of 2.385 mg/L (therapeutic range 0.7–2.3 mg/L), protein induced by vitamin K absence (PIVKA) is >10 (Ref. range < 0.2). What is the most likely explanation for the subtherapeutic INR?
a. Cytochrome p450 mutation
b. VKORC 1 mutation
c. Not taking warfarin
d. Local hospital INR testing quality control is not good

19. All of the following are seen in a patient of APLA, *except*:
a. Preeclampsia
b. Infertility
c. Placental abruption
d. Intrauterine growth restriction (IUGR)
e. Preterm labor

20. All of the above following pathogens are associated with HUS, *except*:
a. *Escherichia coli* 0157:H7 strain
b. *Shigella dysenteriae* serotype I
c. *Citrobacter freundii*
d. *Yersinia enterocolitica*

21. What is the duration of anticoagulation in patients with antiphospholipid syndrome presented with DVT of lower limb?
a. 3 months
b. 6 months
c. Long-term
d. 6 weeks

22. A 65 years old man is on dabigatran for chronic atrial fibrillation and is planned for cholecystectomy. His preoperative evaluation showed normal hemogram and liver and kidney functions. For how much time the dabigatran be discontinued before surgery?
a. 3 days
b. 24 hours
c. 48 hours
d. No need to stop
e. 7 days

23. A young lady presented with acute DVT of right lower limb. She is also giving past history of DVT in same limb. Her grandmother died of pulmonary embolism and also having history of similar illness in family. The most likely diagnosis is:
a. Antithrombin III deficiency
b. APLA syndrome
c. Protein C deficiency
d. Protein S deficiency
e. Factor V Leiden mutation.

24. Constans clinical decision score is used in which of the following conditions?
a. Upper limb DVT
b. Lower limb DVT
c. Splanchnic system DVT
d. Cancer associated DVT

25. Which of the following is approved reversal agent for DOACs?
a. Idarucizumab
b. Andexanet alfa
c. Both of the above
d. None of the above

ANSWERS WITH EXPLANATIONS

1. Ans. b. Heparin

Ref: Essential of Medical Pharmacology 5/e p66

Human	Teratogenic Drugs
Thalidomide	Phocomelia, multiple defects
All anticancer drugs	Multiple defects, fetal death
Androgens	Virilization, limb, esophageal, cardiac defects
Progestins	Virilization of female fetus
Tetracycline	Discolored and deformed teeth, retarded bone growth
Warfarin	Nose, eye and hand defects, growth retardation
Phenytoin	Hypoplastic phalanges, cleft lip/palate, microcephaly
Phenobarbitone	Various malformations
Chlorpromazine	Neural tube defects
Valproate sodium	Spina bifida and other normal tube defects
Lithium	Fetal goiter, cardiac and other abnormalities
Isotretinoin	Craniofacial, heart
Imatinib	Multiple defects exomphalos, kidney abnormalities

2. Ans. b. Protein C deficiency

Ref: Williams 8/e p355-6

This is a case of warfarin-induced skin necrosis, a rare complication of warfarin therapy, which occurs early in the case of anticoagulation. Typical complaints are burning and tingling at the affected site, which usually involves a region with a large amount of subcutaneous tissue, such as breast, buttock or thigh. Painful hemorrhagic full thickness skin infarction develops and frequently required skin grafting. Thrombosis in dermal and subdermal venules is the underlying cause and this may be caused by disproportionately rapid reduction in protein C and S, in concert with relatively preserved levels of Factor II and X that are seen early in warfarin treatment. Also, heparin should have been started along with warfarin.

3. Ans. c. Protein C deficiency

Both arterial and venous:
- Cancer
- Oral hormone replacement therapy (HRT)
- APLA syndrome
- Polycythemia
- Hyperhomocysteinemia
- Factor V Leiden and prothrombin gene mutation G20210A.

Only venous:
- Protein C and S deficiency
- Antithrombin III deficiency
- Elevated factor VIII level
- Dysfibrinogenemia.

Only arterial:
- DM–HTN
- Obesity–hypercholesterolemia
- Smoking.

4. Ans. b. Factor V Leiden mutation

Ref: Williams 8/e p2122

Factor V Leiden (G1691A or Arg 506 Glu substitution) and prothrombin (G20210A) are rare in African and Orientals but they have prevalence in whites, highest prevalence of heterozygotes (11–14%) is reported in Sweden and Arabs.

5. Ans. e. Cancer

Cancer-associated thrombosis is a major cause of mortality in cancer patients, the most common type being venous thromboembolism. Armand Trousseau first reported on the relationship between thrombosis and cancer in 1865. Direct activation of coagulation and platelets can occur through several factors expressed on or released from cancer cells. These include the expression of tissue factor (TF), the key initiator of the coagulation cascade, which can also be released by TF-positive microparticles. Plasminogen activation inhibitor-1 (PAI-1), a key inhibitor of fibrinolysis, is highly expressed in cancer cells. Cancer cells also secrete platelet agonists such as adenosine diphosphate (ADP) and thrombin, thus further promoting platelet activation through P2Y12 and protease-activated receptors 1 and 4 (PAR1/4), respectively.

6. Ans. e. Hypohomocysteinemia

Ref: Hume M. Venous thrombosis and pulmonary embolism. J Clin Invert. p76; Williams 8/e p2122

Thrombosis and embolism has also been implicated as secondary to DM, gout, smoking, administration of adrenocorticotropic hormone (ACTH), but these cannot yet be substantiated as predisposing causes. Male sex has also been implicated as predisposing risk factor which may be related to differences in the way they secrete growth hormone and its effect on liver gene expression. Men secrete growth hormone not in pulses and women secrete it in pulses. Production of coagulation protein by liver is controlled by growth hormone; the differences in secretion may be related to differences in clotting and thrombosis risk. Hypohomocysteinemia, definitely is not a risk factor for thrombosis. However, hyperhomocysteinemia is a risk factor for thrombosis.

7. Ans. b. Individuals have an increased risk of bleeding
Ref: Williams 8/e p2122-2123; Hoffman 7/e p2030

Both factor V Leiden and prothrombin gene mutation G20210A are common in white population with prevalence of heterozygosity for these mutations are 5% and 2.7%, respectively. Homozygotes for factor V Leiden are at higher thrombotic risk than that noted for heterozygotes. Factor V Leiden is the most common cause of APCR resistance (>90%).

8. Ans. a. Antithrombin III deficiency is sex linked
Ref: Williams 8/e p2109; Hoffman 5/e p2025

Antithrombin III deficiency is inherited in an autosomal dominant fashion and thus affects both sexes equally. Microangiopathic hemolytic anemia frequently is induced by DIC in patients with malignancy and is particularly severe in patients with widespread intravascular metastases of mucin secreting adenocarcinoma. Obesity is definitely a risk factor for venous thrombosis, particularly in postoperative phase due to prolonged immobilization.

9. Ans. c. Serum cholesterol
Ref: Williams 5/e p2153, 2126, 2127

High serum cholesterol levels can be associated with risk of atherosclerotic arterial disease. All other investigations are routinely done for evaluation of both heritable and acquired risk factors for thrombophilia. PT/APTT is done to look for APLA syndrome screening. Anticardiolipin and B2 GP-I are helpful in diagnosis of APLA syndrome. Protein C and S deficiency are inherited cause of thrombophilia.

10. Ans. b. Has a half-life of 30 minutes so the effect can be easily reversed
Ref: Williams 8/e p357-358

LMWHs have a longer half-life than UFH, allowing once or twice daily subcutaneous administration. LMWHs exhibit less binding to plasma proteins and cells resulting in more predictable blood levels and anticoagulant effect. LMWHs have renal clearance so dose has to be adjusted in renal insufficiency. Protamine sulfate does not completely reverse the anticoagulant effect of LMWH but is partially effective. Animal and small clinical studies have shown that osteoporosis may be less common with LMWH. Normally dosing does not require monitoring by blood test. Monitoring by anti Xa level is done in obesity, renal failure, trauma, ischemic stroke, or history of gastrointestinal bleeding, and also in pregnancy and in children. There is smaller risk of heparin induced thrombocytopenia with LMWH compared to fractionated heparin.

11. Ans. a. Pancytopenia
Ref: Williams 8/e p2150 (Table)

Clinical manifestations associated with APS are:
- Venous and arterial thromboembolism
- Pregnancy complications
- Thrombocytopenia
- Cerebral venous thrombosis
- Coronary artery disease
- Kidney disease
- Pulmonary hypertension
- Acute respiratory distress syndrome (ARDS)
- Peripheral arterial disease
- Hemorrhagic adrenal infarction
- Budd–Chiari syndrome
- Sensorineural hearing loss
- Catastrophic APLA.

12. Ans. c. Aspirin + LMWH
Ref: Williams 8/e p2157

Women with a history of three or more spontaneous pregnancy losses and evidence of APL antibodies should be treated with a combination of low-dose aspirin (75-81 mg) and prophylactic doses of LMWH. However, UFH (i.e. 5000 units every 12 hours subcutaneously) can also be used. Treatment should be started as soon as the pregnancy is documented and continued until delivery.

13. Ans. c. Positive direct Coombs test (DCT)
Ref: Hoffman 7/e p1984-7

Hemolytic uremic syndrome is of two types, D+HUS and D–HUS; D+HUS is due to verotoxin *E. coli*-associated (VTEC) and Shiga-like toxin-related HUS. (0157:H7 strain of *E. coli*). *Shigella dysenteriae* serotype 1 is also associated with HUS in developing countries. *C. freundii* is also been implicated. D negative HUS is due to the congenital deficiency of complement regulatory proteins I and H.

The features of HUS/thrombotic thrombocytopenic purpura (TTP) are:
- Fever is typically absent or mild
- Uremia
- Microangiopathic hemolytic anemia with DAT being negative
- Thrombocytopenia
- Presence of neurological manifestation (~30%) usually irritability, somnolescence and less commonly confusion, paresis and seizure
- PT, APTT and fibrinogen levels are usually normal or only mildly perturbed
- Mild elevations in fibrinogen degradation products (FDPs) occur in 50% patients
- Moderate leukocytosis
- Elevated free plasma hemoglobin (Hb), low Haptoglobin, high LDH
- D+HUS is treated with plasma exchange, cryo-supernatant infusion (contains of ADAMTS13) steroids, etc.
- D–HUS-fresh frozen plasma (FFP) is indicated to replace factor I and H, which is the cause of pathogenesis.

14. Ans. a. Factor I and H

Refer to explanation for above question.

15. Ans. b. 2.5
Ref: Hoffman 5/e p1988

Treatment indications in APLA: Presence of lupus anticoagulant (LA), increased levels of anticardiolipin antibody (ACLA) or anti-B2 GPI antibodies are found in a patient with underlying autoimmune disease, treatment of underlying disease with immunosuppressive therapy is indicated.

When LA is found in association with severe prothrombin deficiency or thrombocytopenia (<20,000) treatment with steroids is indicated and if actively bleeding with severe hypoprothrombinemia. IVIg should be added and if patient is actively bleeding with severe thrombocytopenia, anti-D or IVIg can be given.

When LA, ACLA or anti-B2 GPI are found without any evidence of thrombosis or fetal loss treatment is not indicated. However, prophylactic low dose aspirin and or hydroxychloroquine plus aggressive treatment of comorbid conditions such as smoking, DM, hypertension, dyslipidemia is indicated.

For recurrent pregnancy losses prophylactic aspirin 75–81 mg/day plus LMWH (once a day) or UFH (5,000 units BD). If fetal loss recurs on this regimen then therapeutic LMWH (BD dose) or UFH 5,000 units s/c TID) should be given. Oral anticoagulants can be resumed in postpartum period for 4–6 weeks.

For catastrophic APS, UFH should be given at 80 units/kg IV bolus and then at 18 units kg/hour and continuous infusion or therapeutic dose of LMWH. Simultaneously, pulse injectable methylprednisolone 1 g IV once daily for 3 days should be given. If patient stabilizes in 24 hours, rituximab (375 mg/m^2) should then be administered. IVIg and plasmapheresis should be used as second-line therapy.

16. Ans. b. Fondaparinux
Ref: Hoffman 7/e p1973-6

The clinical profile of patient suggests heparin-induced thrombocytopenia (HIT). Features of HIT are:

Features	Details
Thrombocytopenia	Platelet count of 100,000/mm^3 or less or a 50% or more decrease
Timing	5–10 days after starting heparin
Type of heparin	More common with UFH than LMWH
Type of patient	More common in surgical than medical patients and more common in women than in men
Thrombosis	Venous thrombosis more common than arterial

Because it is HIT, so options A and D are excluded. Once HIT has developed, any type of heparin is contraindicated. Alternative anticoagulation should be given with lepirudin, argatroban, bivalirudin, danaparoid or fondaparinux. Platelet transfusion and warfarin are contraindicated. Patients with HIT, particularly with thrombosis have increased thrombin generation that can lead to consumption of protein C and thus warfarin alone can cause skin necrosis. If warfarin was administered, give vitamin K to restore the INR to normal.

17. Ans. b. For 5 days or until INR is between 2 and 3 for at least 24 hours, whichever is longer
Ref: ACCP guidelines, 2016

Recommendation in acute DVT is initial treatment with LMWH, UFH or fondaparinux for at least 5 days and until the INR is between 2 and 3 for 24 hours and VKA should be started together with LMWH, UFH or fondaparinux.

18. Ans. d. Local hospital INR testing quality control is not good

Proteins induced by vitamin K absence/antagonists is the test to detect inactive under-carboxylated forms of vitamin K dependent clotting factors which are formed in Vitamin K deficiency (particularly in neonates) and in the presence of antagonist. Its normal range is <0.2 mAV/mL. The form of PIVKA assessed is Des-P-carboxy prothrombin. As her serum warfarin levels are well in therapeutic range, so the option C, not taking warfarin, is wrong. Now her PIVKA levels are elevated so that means the option of warfarin resistance is also ruled out so option A and B are also wrong. It means that the INR tested locally is not correct which may be explained by different type of PT reagent being used.

19. Ans. b. Infertility
Ref: Williams 8/e p2150

Infertility is not associated with APLA syndrome.

20. Ans. d. *Yersinia enterocolitica*
Ref: Hoffman 7/e

E. coli 0157:H7 strain, *Shigella dysenteriae* type I and *C. freundii* (rare) have been associated with HUS.

21. Ans. c. Long-term
Ref: Hoffman's 6/e p2023

Patients with APLA syndrome with a persistent ACL or LA are also at high risk of recurrence and require long-term anticoagulation treatment.

22. Ans. c. 48 hours

Dabigatran should be discontinued for 1–2 days (CrCl ≥ 50 mL/min) or 3–5 days (CrCl < 50 mL/min) before invasive or surgical procedures because of increased risk of bleeding.

23. Ans. e. Factor V Leiden mutation
Ref: Williams 7/e p1981-7

This patient is having recurrent DVT with positive family history of venous thromboembolism so, there is high likelihood of inherited thrombophilic risk factor to be present. The common causes of inherited thrombophilic risk factors include Factor V Leiden mutation, Prothrombin gene mutation, increased Factor VIII levels, and homozygous *MTHFR* gene mutation. The rare causes are protein C and S deficiency, antithrombin deficiency. The very rare causes are dysfibrinogenemia and homozygous homocystinuria.

Ans a. Upper limb DVT

Ref: Constans J. A clinical prediction score for upper extremity deep venous thrombosis. Thrombs Hemostat, 2008

Constans Clinical Decision Score uses 4 variables to risk stratify patients with a suspected upper extremity DVT

Components

Central venous catheter or pacemaker thread: +1

Localized pain: yes +1

Unilateral edema: +1

Other diagnosis as plausible: (-1)

Maximum score: 3

Low probability: 12% (-1 to 0)

Moderate probability: 20% (1)

High probability: 70% (2-3)

25. Ans. c. Both of the above

Idarucizumab is a humanized monoclonal antibody against Dabigatran. It binds dabigatran noncompetitively. Total dose is 5 g. Andexanet alfa is human recombinant factor X a variant that lacks catalytic and membrane binding activity. It targets both direct and indirect factor X a inhibitors competitively.

CHAPTER 10

Red Blood Cell Membrane Disorders

1. Which of the following has decreased osmotic fragility?
   a. Hereditary spherocytosis (HS)
   b. Hereditary elliptocytosis (HE)
   c. Hereditary xerocytosis
   d. Hereditary stomatocytosis/hydrocytosis

2. Typical dominant hereditary spherocytosis is most commonly caused by deficiency of:
   a. Ankyrin
   b. Band 3
   c. Spectrin
   d. Protein 4.2

3. In what percentage of hereditary spherocytosis patients are spherocytes seen in peripheral smear?
   a. 30–40%
   b. 50–60%
   c. 70–80%
   d. 85–95%

4. Increased osmotic fragility is seen in all, *except*:
   a. Iron deficiency anemia (IDA)
   b. Hereditary spherocytosis
   c. Hereditary elliptocytosis
   d. Autoimmune hemolytic anemia

5. Which of the following is true about hereditary elliptocytosis/pyropoikilocytosis?
   a. Autosomal dominant inheritance
   b. Caused by defect in spectrin heterodimer self-association site
   c. Can be caused by defect in protein 4.1
   d. Degree of hemolysis correlates with the number of elliptocytes

6. A condition with an X-linked mode of inheritance, often associated with chronic granulomatous disease (CGD), hemolytic anemia, and characteristic red cell acanthocytosis is:
   a. Bruton's agammaglobulinemia
   b. Rh null phenotype
   c. McLeod phenotype
   d. Gerbich-negative phenotype

7. The characteristic red cell indices in HS are:
   a. Low mean cell volume (MCV), increased mean corpuscular hemoglobin concentration (MCHC), increased red cell distribution width (RDW)
   b. Low MCV, increased MCHC, decreased RDW
   c. High MCV, increased MCHC, increased RDW
   d. High MCV, increased MCHC, decreased RDW

8. Incubation increases the sensitivity of osmotic fragility test by:
   a. Overhydration of the cell
   b. Dehydration of the cell
   c. Increasing the loss of surface area
   d. Increasing the MCV

9. Membrane rigidity and fragility can be measured by:
   a. Osmocytometer
   b. Spherocytometer
   c. Ektacytometer
   d. Viscometer

10. Which of the following matching options is correct?
    1. Pincered red cell   A. Myelofibrosis
    2. Acanthocytic red cell B. Band 3 defect—HS
    3. Prickle cell   C. βXSpectrin defect—HS
    4. Dacryocyte   D. Pyruvate kinase deficiency

    Options
    a. 1-A, 2-C, 3-B, 4-D
    b. 1-B, 2-C, 3-D, 4-A
    c. 1-A, 2-C, 3-D, 4-B
    d. 1-D, 2-B, 3-A, 4-C

11. Southeast Asian ovalocytosis is due to a defect in:
    a. Band 3
    b. Ankyrin
    c. Protein 4.2
    d. Protein 4.1

12. Target cells are formed due to:
    a. Increase in surface area due to lipid gain
    b. Decrease in surface area due to lipid loss
    c. Weakening of skeletal protein
    d. All of the above

13. In HS, there is loss of connections between the membrane skeletal proteins. Which type of connections are lost?
    a. Horizontal
    b. Vertical
    c. Both
    d. Variable connections

14. Which of the following occurs in postsplenectomy?
    a. Neutropenia
    b. Thrombocytopenia
    c. Toxic cells
    d. Target cells

15. Target cells have:
    a. Decreased osmotic fragility
    b. Increased osmotic fragility
    c. Normal osmotic fragility
    d. None of the above

16. Pappenheimer bodies contain:
   a. Iron
   b. Deoxyribonucleic acid (DNA)
   c. Ribonucleic acid (RNA)
   d. Ribosomal proteins

17. Howell-Jolly bodies contain:
   a. Iron
   b. DNA
   c. RNA
   d. Protein

18. Which statement is true about red blood cell (RBC) membrane?
   a. Spectrin and ankyrin combined defect is the most common finding in HS
   b. Glycophorin is the most abundant integral protein followed by band 3
   c. Lipid compose 30% of red cell membrane mass
   d. Alteration in serum lipid concentration influences the red cell membrane

19. Which of the following is true about Inab phenotype?
   a. Inherited deficiency of CD55
   b. Inherited deficiency of CD59
   c. Inherited deficiency of both CD55 and CD59
   d. Acquired deficiency of CD55
   e. Acquired deficiency of CD59

20. Spherocytes in peripheral blood film are seen in:
   a. Thalassemia major
   b. Autoimmune hemolytic anemia
   c. Reticulocytosis
   d. Glucose-6-phosphate dehydrogenase (G6PD) deficiency

21. Which is true about chronic extravascular hemolytic anemia?
   a. Raised serum conjugated bilirubin
   b. Low reticulocyte count
   c. Hypocellular bone marrow
   d. Gallstones

22. Which of the following is not a cause of intravascular hemolysis?
   a. Rhesus incompatibility
   b. ABO incompatibility
   c. G6PD deficiency
   d. Red cell fragmentation syndrome

23. Which is not a feature of intravascular hemolysis?
   a. Jaundice
   b. Hemosiderinuria
   c. Low haptoglobin
   d. Hemoglobinuria

24. True about hereditary spherocytosis is:
   a. Defect of hemoglobin
   b. Commonly seen in males
   c. Splenectomy is the treatment
   d. Fresh frozen plasma may be given

25. Reagent used in osmotic fragility test is:
   a. Isotonic saline
   b. Hypotonic saline
   c. Hypertonic saline
   d. Varying concentrations of saline

26. A young boy is admitted in the surgery department for elective cholecystectomy, and hematology referral was called in view of anemia during preoperative evaluation. On further evaluation, he was found to be having mild icterus and splenomegaly. Complete blood count (CBC) showed Hb 10 g/dL, MCV 88 fL, reticulocyte count of 5%, and MCHC 37. The most likely diagnosis for this patient is:
   a. Hereditary spherocytosis (HS)
   b. Hereditary elliptocytosis (HE)
   c. Autoimmune hemolytic anemia (AIHA)
   d. Hereditary xerocytosis

27. The most common cause of nonspherocytic hemolytic anemia because of which there is enzyme deficiency in the hexose monophosphate (HMP) shunt pathway is:
   a. Pyruvate kinase deficiency
   b. Hexokinase
   c. G6PD
   d. Phosphofructokinase

28. A 14-years-old boy presented with the history of jaundice off and on for 6 years and heaviness and occasional pain in left upper abdomen for 4 years. Family history was positive for anemia and jaundice. On evaluation his Hb was 7.5 g/dL, white cell count 9000/micl and platelets 166,000/micl with spherocytes in the peripheral blood film. His ultrasonogram abdomen showed cholelithiasis and spleen size of 18 cms. His hemolytic workup was ordered and osmotic fragility test is reported below.

Osmotic Fragility Test (Room Temperature)

Tube no.	Reference interval NaCl (g/L)	Lysis (%)	Percentage lysis Test	Control
1	0	100	100	100
2	1	100	97.8	97.4
3	2	100	97.1	95.9
4	3	97 to 100	96.1	94.1
5	3.5	90 to 99	95.3	92.2
6	4	50 to 95	91.8	69.0
7	4.5	5 to 45	91.4	5.76
8	5	0 to 6	60.7	4.77
9	5.5	0	5.06	1.19
10	6	0	4.34	0.59
11	6.5	0	0.60	00
12	7.5	0	0.30	00

Contd...

Contd...

Tube no.	Reference interval		Percentage lysis	
	NaCl (g/L)	Lysis (%)	Test	Control
13	9	0	00	00
	Ref. interval		Test	Control
	(Grams per liter NaCl)			
MCF (50% lysis)	4 to 4.45		5.2	4.3

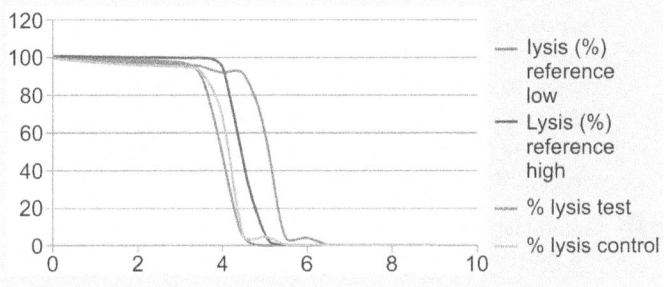

Courtesy: Dr Tina Dadu, MD, and Dr Nishit Gupta, MD, DM

The following statement is true:
a. The osmotic fragility test is positive
b. The patients should undergo splenectomy based on this report
c. He should not be evaluated for G6PD deficiency and Coombs (immune-mediated) hemolytic anemia
d. All of the above

29. Which of the following infections is not associated with cold agglutinin disease?
a. M. pneumoniae
b. Epstein Barr virus
c. HIV
d. Hepatitis A

30. In which of the RBC defects should splenectomy be avoided?
a. Hereditary spherocytosis
b. Hereditary elliptocytosis
c. Hereditary xerocytosis (Somatocytosis)
d. None of the above

ANSWERS WITH EXPLANATIONS

1. **Ans. c. Hereditary xerocytosis**
Ref: Williams 8/e p594-6

Osmotic fragility is typically increased in HS and HE. There are two types of hereditary stomatocytosis: Hereditary xerocytosis (complex permeability defect due to increased membrane lipids) and hereditary hydrocytosis (due to deficiency of band 7.2b or stomatin). Both have autosomal dominant inheritance. Osmotic fragility is decreased in xerocytosis and increased in hydrocytosis. Xerocytosis may result in recurrent fetal loss, hydrops fetalis, neonatal hepatitis, and familial pseudohyperkalemia.

2. **Ans. a. Ankyrin** Ref: William's 8/e p580-3

The most common cause of typical dominant HS (two-third of cases) is ankyrin defect, followed by band 3 defect and isolated spectrin deficiency. The degree of spectrin deficiency correlates with spheroidicity, ability of red cells to withstand shear stress, degree of hemolysis, and response to splenectomy. Protein 4.2 deficiency is inherited as autosomal recessive trait. Severe HS almost always have recessive inheritance and most have severe spectrin deficiency (<40%) which may be due to defect in β-spectrin.

3. **Ans. d. 85–95%**

4. **Ans. a. Iron deficiency anemia (IDA)**

Increased OFT	Decreased OFT
Hereditary spherocytosis	Iron deficiency anemia
Hereditary stomatocytosis	Southeast Asian ovalocytosis (SAO)

Contd...

Contd...

Increased OFT	Decreased OFT
Hereditary elliptocytosis	Thalassemia
AIHA–tail of fragile cells proportional to spherocytes	Hereditary xerocytosis

(AIHA: autoimmune hemolytic anemia; OFT: osmotic fragility test).

5. **Ans. d. Degree of hemolysis correlates with the number of elliptocytes** Ref: William's 8/e p598

The degree of hemolysis does not correlate with the number of elliptocytes in peripheral blood smear. Since there are several common features between HE and pyropoikilocytosis, they are considered together e.g. peripheral smear findings, thermal instability of erythrocytes. Elliptocytes appear in blood after 4–6 months of age.

6. **Ans. c. McLeod phenotype** Ref: William's 8/e p594

The McLeod phenotype is a recessive mutation of the Kell blood group system. The McLeod gene encodes the XK protein, which is located on the X chromosome, and has the structural characteristics of a membrane transport protein but an unknown function. It is an X-linked anomaly of the Kell blood group system manifested by mild hemolytic anemia not requiring blood support with variable acanthocytosis, late-onset myopathy, or chorea. It may be associated with CGD, retinitis pigmentosa, and Duchenne muscular dystrophy. McLeod phenotype has no XK antigen characterized by marked deficiency of 93-kDa protein that carries Kell antigen. In contrast, K null (Ko) red cells have a normal shape and they have twice the amount of XK antigen but only the Kell antigen carrying 93-kDa protein is absent.

7. Ans a. Low mean cell volume (MCV), increased mean corpuscular hemoglobin concentration (MCHC), increased red cell distribution width (RDW)
Ref: William's 8/e p586

The increased MCHC is an effective screening test to identify children with HS. An elevated erythrocyte distribution width adds additional specificity and is itself a powerful screening tool. The combination of the two tests is an excellent predictor for the diagnosis of HS. The MCV in HS is low to normal.

8. Ans. c. Increasing the loss of surface area
Ref: William's 8/e p586

After incubation at 37°C for 24 hours, HS red cells lose membrane surface area more readily because their membranes are leaky and unstable. Basically, incubation accentuates the defect in HS.

9. Ans. c. Ektacytometer
Ref: William's 8/e p586

The ektacytometer measures the deformation of a population of red cells or red cell membranes in response to shear. New-generation osmotic gradient ektacytometry has become a powerful procedure for measuring RBC deformability and therefore for the diagnosis of RBC membrane disorders like HS.

10. Ans. b. 1–B, 2–C, 3–D, 4–A

Type of red cell	Association
Drepanocyte (sickle cell)	Sickle cell disease/trait
Dacryocyte (tear drop cell)	Myelofibrosis, thalassemia, myelophthisic anemia
Spur cell (Acanthocyte)	• Alcoholic liver disease • Postsplenectomy • Abetalipoproteinemia
Burr cell (Echinocyte)	Uremia
Schizocyte (schistocyte)	Microangiopathic hemolytic anemia (TTP/HUS, DIC), Severe burn, March hemoglobinuria
Elliptocyte (oval)	Hereditary elliptocytosis Megaloblastic anemia IDA, thalassemia
Codocyte (target cell) (bell)	• Hemoglobinopathy (S, C) • Obstructive liver disease • Postsplenectomy • Thalassemia, IDA
Prickle cell	Pyruvate kinase deficiency
Pincered red cell	Band 3 deficiency
Bite cell	G6PD deficiency
Pencil cell (ovalocyte)	IDA

(DIC: disseminated intravascular coagulation; HUS: hemolytic uremic syndrome; IDA: iron deficiency anemia; TTP: thrombotic thrombocytopenic purpura).

11. Ans. a. Band 3

12. Ans. a. Increase in surface area due to lipid gain
Ref: William's 8/e p380

Target cell is characterized by relative membrane excess due to either increase in red cell surface area due to lipid gain (increased cholesterol-to-phospholipid ratio in obstructive liver disease) or decreased intracellular hemoglobin concentration (e.g., in IDA and thalassemia).

13. Ans. b. Vertical
Ref: William's 8/e p576

Hereditary spherocytosis is characterized by defects of vertical connections which lead to uncoupling of lipid bilayer from the skeleton and a release of membrane microvesicles. In contrast, a horizontal defect between the membrane proteins is seen in HE and hereditary pyropoikilocytosis (HPP).

14. Ans. d. Target cells
Ref: Dacie and Lewis 10/e p97, 98, 100

Postsplenectomy changes:
- Target cells
- Howell-Jolly bodies (nuclear remnants, single large inclusion)
- Acanthocytes
- Pappenheimer bodies (peripherally present, composed of hemosiderin)
- Neutrophilia (early after splenectomy)
- Lymphocytosis
- Thrombocytosis
- Giant platelets.

15. Ans. a. Decreased osmotic fragility
Ref: Dacie and Lewis 10/e p210

Seen specially in IDA and thalassemia, leptocytes are flattened cells (decreased volume-to-surface area ratio) which have decreased osmotic fragility. Similarly, target cells seen in liver disease also have decreased osmotic fragility owing to passive accumulation of lipids.

16. Ans. a. Iron

Refer to explanation for Q. No. 14.

17. Ans. b. DNA

Refer to explanation for Q. No. 14.

18. Ans. c. Lipids compose 30% of red cell membrane mass.
Ref: William's 8/e p617, 619, 627, 637, 638

Lipids compose 50–60% of red cell membrane. Mass alterations in the serum lipid concentrations can make changes in the RBC membrane and lead to alteration in the RBC shape, e.g., in dyslipidemia and in alcoholic liver disease (altered/loss of lipoproteins).

19. Ans. a. Inherited deficiency of CD55
Ref: Dacie and Lewis 10/e p266

The Inab phenotype of RBC is the congenital deficiency of CD55 (decay accelerating factor) on RBCs; therefore, to diagnose paroxysmal nocturnal hemoglobinuria (PNH) it is always recommended to test for at least two glycosyl-phosphatidylinositol (GPI) anchor proteins together (namely CD55 and CD59). In contrast with the situation in PNH, membranes from peripheral blood cells of the Inab phenotype individual lack decay accelerating factor (DAF), but retain the other GPI-linked proteins, acetylcholinesterase and LFA-3.

20. Ans. b. Autoimmune hemolytic anemia
Ref: Hoffman's 6/e p616-7

The diagnosis of AIHA is established by the presence following pentad: normocytic or macrocytic anemia, reticulocytosis, low haptoglobin, elevated lactate dehydrogenase (LDH), and elevated unconjugated bilirubin. Additional findings are increased urobilinogen and spherocytes. Automatic flow cytometric methods are more precise, reliable, and convenient for detecting reticulocytosis. Reticulocytosis is often (up to 25%) not present at the onset of AIHA, mostly because of the delayed initial bone marrow response of erythrocytosis. Haptoglobin may be falsely normal or increased, particularly in patients with malignant or immune disease, because haptoglobin is an acute phase reactant. Haptoglobin may be falsely low in case of haplotype H_0H_0 and in patients with severe liver disease. Both increased bilirubin and LDH have limited sensitivity and specificity.

21. Ans. d. Gallstones *Ref: Hoffman's 6/e p596-7*

In chronic hemolysis, there can be development of gallstones. All other features are not seen in hemolysis. If a patient is suspected of pigment stones and hemolysis is suspected and is planned for cholecystectomy, it should always be done with splenectomy; otherwise the stone will be formed in bile duct which can lead to cholangitis which is a potentially life-threatening complication.

22. Ans. a. Rhesus incompatibility
Ref: Hoffman's 6/e p583, 630-635, 1728

Rh incompatibility causes acute extravascular hemolysis manifested by fever, indirect hyperbilirubinemia, and post-transfusion increment lower than what is expected. Acute intravascular hemolysis causes fever, chills, dyspnea, hypotension, tachycardia, flushing, vomiting, back pain, hemoglobinuria, and hemoglobinemia. Delayed intravascular hemolysis is caused by Kidd system incompatibility. Delayed extravascular hemolysis is caused by Duffy system incompatibility. Other causes of intravascular hemolysis are PNH, hemoparasites, mechanical trauma, cardiopulmonary bypass, venoms, bites, stings, toxins, copper poisoning, and G6PD deficiency.

23. Ans. a. Jaundice *Ref: Hoffman's 6/e p1728*

Jaundice is a feature of extravascular hemolysis and all others are features of intravascular hemolysis.

24. Ans. c. Splenectomy is the treatment
Ref: Hoffman's 6/e p596-7

Splenectomy is curative in almost all cases of HS. Only population-based Chinese data is available, and this shows slight female preponderance. HS is caused by a defect in red cell membrane protein.

25. Ans. d. Varying concentrations of saline
Ref: Dacie and Lewis 10/e p206-7

The principle of osmotic fragility is the lysis of red cells when mixed with varying concentrations of saline. Small volumes of blood are mixed with a large excess of buffered saline solutions of varying concentrations. The fraction of red cells lysed at each saline concentration is determined colorimetrically.

26. Ans. a. Hereditary spherocytosis (HS)
Ref: William's 7/e p590-594; Hoffman's 6/e p597

Most HS patients have either mild-to-moderate anemia or no anemia at all. Some patients of nondominant HS can have very severe anemia. MCV of HS cells is low normal or slightly low and the MCHC is usually increased (>35 g/dL). The finding of an MCHC >35.4 g/dL combined with RDW <14% is an excellent screening test for HS. Usually, there are associated features of hemolysis such as high LDH, elevated indirect bilirubin, and reticulocytosis. Partial splenectomy (PS) shows characteristic spherocytes. A subset of HS patients show pincer-like RBCs which are sensitive and specific for band-3 deficiency. Surface spiculations and acanthocytic spherocytes are characteristically seen in β spectrin deficiency. Frequent sphero-ovalocytes and stomatocytes have been reported in Japanese patients with protein 4.2 deficiency.

In HE, there is presence of cigar-shaped elliptocytes. These normocytic, normochromic elliptocytes may number from a few to 100% and the degree of hemolysis does not correlate with the number of elliptocytes present, but in case of HS the degree of hemolysis correlates with the percentage of spherocytes. Osmotic fragility is abnormal in severe HE and HPP.

In HPP, in addition to the blood film findings seen in HE, many HPP erythrocytes are bizarrely shaped, with fragmentation or budding. Microspherocytosis is common, and MCV usually is low (50–70 fL).

In AIHA, the osmotic fragility is normal and MCV is usually high.

Dehydrated hereditary stomatocytosis, also known as hereditary xerocytosis or dessicocytosis, is associated with red cell dehydration and decreased osmotic fragility. Laboratory features include increased MCHC (feature of red cell dehydration) and MCV is mildly increased. The effects of splenectomy have been variable so they should be carefully selected.

27. Ans. c. G6PD *Ref: Hoffman's 6/e p581-7*

Hereditary nonspherocytic anemia, when inherited as autosomal recessive trait, is associated with defects in membrane, or porphyrin synthesis, or in the breakdown of sugars. The symptoms are jaundice, Heinz bodies in RBCs, or moderate-to-severe anemia. The most common cause is G6PD deficiency; other causes are pyruvate kinase deficiency, hexokinase deficiency, and aldolase A deficiency. This entity usually excludes hemoglobinopathies.

28. **Ans. d. All of the above**

Ref: Paula HB Bolton-Maggs. Guidelines for the diagnosis and management of hereditary spherocytosis – 2011 update. BJH, 2011

There is a shift in the osmotic fragility curve to right indicating the presence of spherocytes. When positive, it merely confirms the presence of spherocytes, regardless of the etiology (hereditary or acquired/autoimmune). It can be positive in hereditary spherocytosis (HS), hereditary elliptocytosis, hereditary stomatocytosis and autoimmune hemolytic anemia. Furthermore, a normal osmotic fragility test does not exclude HS, since 10% to 20% of HS cases are negative for the test. Cell dehydration of spherocytes in an HS patient is one of the causes of normal osmotic fragility test. Given the typical clinical presentation and the similar family history, the most probable diagnosis is HS.

The osmotic fragility test is useful for diagnosis of hereditary spherocytic hemolytic anemia. Spherocytes are osmotically fragile cells that rupture more easily in a hypotonic solution than do normal RBCs. Because these cells have a low surface area:volume ratio, they lyse at a higher solution osmolarity than do normal RBCs with discoid morphology. After incubation in a hypotonic solution, a further increase in hemolysis is typically seen in hereditary spherocytosis. Cells that have a larger surface area:volume ratio, such as target cells or hypochromic cells, are more resistant to lysing in a hypotonic solution. The osmotic fragility of freshly taken red cells reflects their ability to take up a certain amount of water before lysing. Characteristically, osmotic fragility curves from patients with HS who have not been splenectomized show a 'tail' of very fragile cells.

According to BCSH guidelines, for a newly diagnosed patient with a family history of HS, typical clinical features and laboratory investigations (spherocytes, raised mean corpuscular hemoglobin concentration [MCHC], increase in reticulocytes), additional tests are not required. In children undergoing splenectomy, the gallbladder should be removed concomitantly if there are symptomatic gallstones. When splenectomy is indicated, ideally it should be done after the age of 6 years. Splenectomy is very effective in reducing hemolysis and anemia, leading to a significant prolongation of the red cell life span.

29. **Ans. d. Hepatitis A**

Infections associated with cold agglutinin disease include M pneumoniae, EBV, HIV, rubella virus, influenza virus, varicella zoster virus and also secondary to autoimmune disorders like systemic sclerosis and rheumatoid arthritis.

30. **Ans. c. Hereditary xerocytosis (Somatocytosis)**

Ref: Hoffman, p645

Several patients with somatocytosis (both hydrocytosis and xerocytosis) have developed hypercoagulopathy after splenectomy leading to catastrophic thrombotic episodes or chronic pulmonary hypertension.

CHAPTER 11

Disorders of Red Cell Enzymes

1. Hemolysis in glucose-6-phosphate dehydrogenase (G6PD) is caused by all of the following, *except*:
   a. Primaquine
   b. Chloroquine
   c. Pyrimethamine
   d. Quinine

2. The most common cause of hereditary nonspherocytic hemolytic anemia is:
   a. Pyrimidine 5' nucleotidase deficiency
   b. Pyruvate kinase deficiency (PKD)
   c. Triose-phosphate isomerase deficiency
   d. Phosphofructokinase

3. All of the followings are associated with increased red cell adenosine deaminase (ADA) levels, *except*:
   a. Diamond-Blackfan anemia (DBA)
   b. Severe combined immunodeficiency
   c. Acquired immunodeficiency syndrome (AIDS)
   d. Hereditary nonspherocytic hemolytic anemia

4. All of the following red cell enzyme deficiencies are inherited as autosomal recessive, *except*:
   a. G6PD deficiency
   b. PKD
   c. Triose-phosphate isomerase deficiency
   d. Glucose phosphate isomerase deficiency

5. Which of the following is normal form of G6PD?
   a. G6PD B
   b. G6PD A$^-$
   c. G6PD A$^+$
   d. G6PD mediterranean

6. Which of the following is true about G6PD?
   a. Drug-induced hemolysis begins after 7 days
   b. Heinz bodies are seen in red blood cells (RBCs)
   c. In the A-form of G6PD, hemolytic anemia is self-limited
   d. Common (polymorphic) forms have no clinical manifestations

7. All of the followings are true about red cell enzyme defects, *except*:
   a. Basophilic stippling in red cell is characteristic of pyrimidine's nucleotidase deficiency
   b. Jaundice of glucose phosphate isomerase deficiency responds to phenobarbital
   c. Patients with glucose phosphate isomerase deficiency respond better to splenectomy
   d. Phosphoglycerate kinase deficiency is autosomal recessive

8. Which one of the following is a feature of chronic extravascular hemolysis?
   a. Raised serum conjugated bilirubin
   b. Low reticulocyte count
   c. Hypocellular bone marrow
   d. Gallstones

9. Which of the following is not a cause of intravascular hemolysis?
   a. Rh incompatibility
   b. ABO incompatibility
   c. G6PD deficiency
   d. Red cell fragmentation syndrome

10. A 10-year-old child presented with severe hemolytic anemia after febrile illness. There was marked reticulocytosis and lactate dehydrogenase (LDH) of 10,000 IU/mL. His total bilirubin was 0.3 mg/dL with direct fraction of 0.2 mg/dL. The most likely diagnosis is:
    a. Heme oxygenase deficiency
    b. Ferrochelatase deficiency
    c. Biliverdin reductase deficiency
    d. Aminolevulinic acid (ALA) dehydratase deficiency

11. Which of the following is not a feature of intravascular hemolysis?
    a. Jaundice
    b. Hemosiderin in urine
    c. Absent haptoglobin
    d. Hemoglobin in urine

12. Which of the following is not true about G6PD deficiency?
    a. Commonly presents as chronic hemolytic anemia
    b. Leads to intravascular hemolysis after certain infections
    c. Protects against malaria
    d. Carrier females have approximately 50% G6PD levels
    e. It is a cause of neonatal jaundice

13. Extravascular hemolysis is best characterized by all, *except*:
    a. Increased LDH
    b. Splenomegaly
    c. Jaundice
    d. Increased plasma hemoglobin

14. **In G6PD deficiency, the morphological feature of red cell is:**
    a. Heinz body
    b. Cabot ring
    c. Crescent body
    d. Howell-Jolly body
    c. Spherocytes
    d. Bite cells
    e. Pencils cells

15. **A 15-year-old boy presented with weakness and shortness of breath. Blood test showed macrocytes with reticulocytosis. Genetic analysis showed G6PD deficiency. What is the most common cell type seen in PS of this patient?**
    a. Schistocytes
    b. Target cells

16. **Which of the following is false about pyrimidine 5' nucleotidase -1 deficiency?**
    a. Autosomal recessive inheritance
    b. Acquired deficiency is found in acute lead toxicity
    c. Marked basophilic stippling is seen on peripheral blood film
    d. It does not require magnesium for its activity

ANSWERS WITH EXPLANATIONS

1. Ans. c. Pyrimethamine   *Ref: Harrison 18/e p879*

	Definite risk	Possible risk	Doubtful risk
Anti-malarials	Primaquine dapsone/ chlorproguanil	Chloroquine	Quinine
Sulfonamides	Sulfamethoxazole	Sulfasalazine sulfadimidine	Sulfisoxazole sulfadiazine
Antibiotics	Clotrimazole, nalidixic acid, nitrofurantoin, niridazole	Ciprofloxacin norfloxacin	Chloramphenicol, p-aminosalicylic acid
Analgesics	Acetanilide, phenazopyridine	Acetylsalicylic acid high dose (>3 g/day)	Acetaminophen phenacetin aspirin (<3 g/d)
Others	Naphthalene methylene blue	Vitamin K analogs Ascorbic acid >1 g Rasburicase	Dexoxibicin Probenecid

2. Ans. b. Pyruvate kinase deficiency (PKD)
Ref: William's 8/e p648

The most common enzyme abnormalities are G6PD and PK. The most common form of G6PD is the polymorphic form in which the hemolysis occurs only under stress. Chronic hemolysis in the absence of stress occurs rarely in the functionally severe forms of G6PD deficiency. Triose phosphate isomerate (TPI) deficiency also causes hereditary nonspherocytic hemolytic anemia but is less common that G6PD or PKD and is also associated with severe neuromuscular disorder.

3. Ans. b. Severe combined immunodeficiency (SCID)
Ref: William's 8/e p653

Severe combined immunodeficiency is associated with deficiency of adenosine deaminase. Hereditary increase in activity of red cell adenosine deaminase results in depletion of adenosine triphosphate (ATP) and causes nonspherocytic hemolytic anemia. For unknown reasons, red cell adenosine deaminase levels are high in AIDS and DBA.

4. Ans. a. G6PD deficiency

Most red cell enzyme deficiencies are inherited as autosomal recessive and present as hereditary nonspherocytic hemolytic anemia. G6PD and phosphoglycerate kinase deficiencies are X-linked.

5. Ans. a. G6PD B   *Ref: William's 8/e p656-8*

G6PD B is the normal variant of G6PD which represent the most common type of enzyme encountered in all population groups. Among persons of African descent, a mutant enzyme with normal activity is very prevalent known as G-6PD A$^+$ which migrates electrophoretically more rapidly than the normal B enzyme. G6PD A$^-$ is the principal deficient variant found in people of African origin. Among Caucasians G6PD deficiency is most common in Mediterranean countries and the most common enzyme variant is G6PD Mediterranean.

There are usually no clinical manifestations (hemolysis occurs only with stress) in individuals who inherit the common (polymorphic) form of G6PD deficiency, such as G6PD B and G6PD Mediterranean.

6. Ans. a. Drug-induced hemolysis typically begins after 7 days   *Ref: Williams 8/e p662-3*

Drug-induced hemolysis in G6PD typically begins 1-3 days after drug administration. In severe cases abdominal and back pain may occur. The urine may turn dark and black. Heinz bodies are seen in RBCs. Hemolytic anemia is self-limited in the A-type of G6PD deficiency because the young red cells produced in response to hemolysis have nearly normal G6PD levels and are relatively resistant to hemolysis. Hemolysis is not self-limited in the more severe Mediterranean type of deficiency.

7. Ans. d. Phosphoglycerate kinase deficiency is autosomal recessive   *Ref: William's 8/e p658-9*

Phosphoglycerate kinase deficiency is inherited as X-linked disorder. Basophilic stippling in RBCs is characteristically seen in pyrimidine 5 nucleotidase deficiency.

Jaundice of glucose phosphate isomerase deficiency responds more favorably to splenectomy.

Splenectomy should be considered in following setting—(1) severity of the disease, (2) family history of response to splenectomy, (3) underlying defect (GPI deficiency).

A single dose of Sn-mesoporphyrin, potent inhibitor of heme oxygenase activity and thus of bilirubin production, has been advocated to eliminate the need for phototherapy.

8. Ans. d. Gallstones

9. Ans. a. Rh incompatibility

Ref: William's 8/e p451, 452, 2265

Intravascular destruction occurs if the red cell membrane is breached in the circulation which occurs in ABO incompatibility, paroxysmal nocturnal hemoglobinuria (PNH), prosthetic valve hemolysis, and microangiopathic hemolytic anemia. It also occurs in anti-Jka and anti-Jkb antibodies. ABO, anti-Jka and anti-Jkb antibodies are strongly expressed on RBCs and these antibodies bind complement efficiently. Intravascular hemolysis is also caused by G6PD and other enzyme abnormalities.

Extravascular hemolysis occurs when the red cells become damaged or senescent which result in decreased deformability and/or altered surface properties. Deformability is decreased in hereditary spherocytosis, hereditary elliptocytosis, autoimmune hemolytic anemia (due to decreased surface to volume ratio) and in sickle cell disease and hemoglobin C disease (the internal viscosity of the cell is increased). Altered surface properties of RBC membrane can be altered by binding of antibodies, complements and by chemical alteration (particularly oxidative damage to membrane components as occurs in sickled cells and thalassemic cells). Extravascular hemolysis occurs with IgG1 and IgG3 antibodies that react at body temperature and is seen in Rh, Kidd, kell, Duffy or Ss antigens.

10. Ans. a. Heme oxygenase deficiency *Ref: Internet*

In extravascular hemolysis RBCs are degraded within the macrophages so hemoglobin is not released free into the plasma and therefore, hemoglobinemia or hemoglobinuria are not seen in extravascular hemolysis. Hemoglobin breaks down to heme and globin in macrophages. In lysosomes globin is broken into amino acids. Oxidation of porphyrin ring of heme by microsomal heme oxygenase produces biliverdin and CO, and releases Fe^{3+} which may get incorporated in transferrin or stored in ferritin. With time ferritin in excess may be oxidized and degraded to hemosiderin. Biliverdin is reduced by biliverdin reductase to unconjugated bilirubin (water insoluble). It is released into plasma where it can bind to albumin or hemopexin. From them it is taken by hepatocytes for conjugation.

The above-mentioned case is having defect in bilirubin synthesis and is classically seen in heme oxygenase-1 deficiency. Heme oxygenase has two isoenzymes: (1) heme oxygenase-1 (inducible), and (2) heme oxygenase-2 (constitutive). First case of human heme oxygenase-1 deficiency was described in 1999 and is characterized by hemolysis (endothelial damage) and disseminated intravascular coagulation (DIC). It may also be associated with congenital asplenia and nephritis.

Recent studies have shown that bilirubin has cytoprotectant effects by having antioxidant properties.

11. Ans. a. Jaundice *Ref: Hoffbrand 7/e*

	Intravascular	Extravascular
Peripheral smear	Schistocytes (may be)	Spherocytes (may be)
Haptoglobin	Decreased/absent	Mild decrease
Hemosiderinuria	++	–
Hemoglobinuria	++	–
DCT	Usually negative	++++
LDH	High	High
Jaundice	Absent	Present
Iron stones	Decreased	Normal/increased
Splenomegaly	Usually absent	Present

(LDH: lactate dehydrogenase).

Hemolytic anemia is defined as increased destruction of red cells in the peripheral blood without evidence of ineffective erythropoiesis. After haptoglobin is saturated, excess hemoglobin is filtered in kidneys and reabsorbed in proximal tubules where iron is converted to ferritin or hemosiderin. Hemoglobinuria indicates severe intravascular hemolysis overwhelming the absorbing capacity of renal tubular cells.

12. Ans. a. Commonly presents as chronic hemolytic anemia *Ref: Hoffman 6/e p583-4*

The common (polymorphic) form present as hemolysis under stress (mainly drugs, fever, and infection) only. It protects against malaria.

13. Ans. d. Increased plasma hemoglobin

The diagnosis of hemolysis is established by reticulocytosis, increased unconjugated bilirubin and LDH, decreased haptoglobin, and peripheral blood smear findings. Premature destruction of erythrocytes occurs intravascularly or extravascularly. Extravascular hemolysis occurs when RBCs are phagocytized by macrophages in the spleen, liver and bone marrow.

14. Ans. a. Heinz body *Ref: William's 7/e p488, 618*

In severe cases of megaloblastic anemia basophilic stippling and nuclear remnants such as Cabot rings and Howell-Jolly bodies are seen. Heinz bodies are often found in RBCs of G6PD deficient patients. Sometimes bite cells are also seen. Crescent cells are ghost red cells where in all the hemoglobin content is absent, and this is usually seen in cases of severe parasitic infection, e.g., falciparum.

15. Ans. d. Bite cells *Ref: William's 7/e p378-9*

In G6PD deficiency bite cells are seen, which are characteristics and can also be seen in other hereditary nonspherocytic anemias.

16. Ans. d. It does not require magnesium for its activity
Ref: Hoffmann, p621

Pyrimidine 5' nucleotidase-1 deficiency is inherited in an Autosomal recessive inheritance. Acquired deficiency is found in acute lead toxicity because of lead outcompeting the essential cofactor magnesium. The ribosomal aggregates are visible as the characteristic coarse basophilic stippling seen on PBF.

CHAPTER 12

Sickle Cell Anemia

1. A patient with sickle cell anemia should avoid the following:
   a. Swimming
   b. Dehydration
   c. Pneumococcal immunization
   d. Early antibiotics for respiratory infection

2. Which of the following may constitute high risk during surgery?
   a. β-thalassemia minor
   b. Hemoglobin (Hb) S homozygous
   c. Hb D Punjab
   d. Hb E trait

3. A patient of sickle cell disease (SCD) presented with priapism. Which of the following is contraindicated?
   a. Hydralazine   b. Atenolol
   c. Shunt surgery   d. Etilefrine

4. In an SCD patient to cause vaso-occlusive crisis, HbS level should be:
   a. 20%   b. 40%
   c. 60%   d. 30%

5. The least severe form of SCD is:
   a. HbSS
   b. HbSβ^0
   c. HbSβ$^+$
   d. SCD with hereditary persistence of fetal hemoglobin (S/HPFH)

6. The least common cause of death in an adult with SCD is:
   a. Pulmonary hypertension
   b. Sudden death of unknown etiology
   c. Renal failure
   d. Infection
   e. Myocardial infarction

7. Which is least implicated in the pathophysiology of SCD?
   a. Neutrophils
   b. Nitric oxide (NO)
   c. Platelets and coagulation factors
   d. Free hemoglobin

8. Events which precipitate veno-occlusive crises are:
   a. Dehydration
   b. Infection
   c. Extreme temperature
   d. Emotional stress
   e. All of the above

9. Not true regarding acute chest syndrome (ACS) is:
   a. Pulmonary infiltrates are seen
   b. Risk of mortality increases
   c. Hydroxyurea is indicated
   d. Pulmonary hypertension is an important cause

10. True regarding central nervous system involvement in SCD is:
    a. Microvasculature is commonly involved
    b. Chronic transfusion does not help much
    c. Cognitive impairment is not seen
    d. Transcranial Doppler (TCD) is helpful
    e. Nearly all patients have clinical manifestations

11. True regarding sickle cell trait are all, *except*:
    a. Is associated with normal growth and life expectancy
    b. The ratio of HbA to HbS is 50:50
    c. Impaired urine-concentrating ability and hematuria can occur
    d. Splenic infarction is possible at very high altitudes

12. True regarding the sickling test is:
    a. Can distinguish sickle cell trait from sickle cell anemia
    b. Can be used for primary diagnosis of HbSS
    c. Can quantify HbS
    d. All of the above
    e. None of the above

13. Hydroxycarbamide (hydroxyurea) therapy in SCD results in reduction of all, *except*:
    a. Acute chest syndrome
    b. Acute painful crises
    c. Leg ulcers
    d. Transfusion requirements
    e. All of the above

14. HbC disease is characterized by the presence of:
    a. Sickle cells   b. Target cells
    c. Burr cells   d. Spur cells

SECTION 2 | Benign Hematology

15. A young boy is worried about his general health in view of a positive family history of SCD and hypertension. On evaluation, his general and systemic examinations were normal. Which of the following tests would be done to investigate for SCD?
   a. Ham's test
   b. Sodium metabisulfite test
   c. Schilling test
   d. Osmotic fragility test
   e. Coomb's test

16. Crizanlizumab and voxelotor are Food and Drug Administration (FDA)—approved drugs that are used for which of the diseases?
   a. Thrombotic thrombocytopenic purpura
   b. Thalassemia major
   c. Sickle cell disease
   d. Hemophilia A

17. Mechanism of action of crizanlizumab is:
   a. P-selectin inhibitor
   b. HbF inducer
   c. Vascular endothelial growth factor (VEGF) inhibitor
   d. Selectively increases NO in lungs preventing ACS

18. Mechanism of action of voxelotor in SCD is:
   a. Decreases deoxyhemoglobin polymerization
   b. Decreases the total leucocyte count
   c. HbF induction
   d. Decreases inflammatory mediators

19. The following are complications of sickle cell trait, *except*:
   a. Increased risk of urinary tract infection (UTI)
   b. Increased risk of pneumonia
   c. Splenic infarction at high altitude
   d. Exercise-related sudden death

20. A 10-year-old girl is a case of sickle cell disease and having recurrent painful crisis, so she was started on hydroxyurea. After 6 months, all of the findings can be seen in her, *except*:
   a. Rise in hemoglobin
   b. Fall in WBC count
   c. Increased reticulocyte count
   d. Increase in HbF concentration
   e. MCV of 108 fL

ANSWERS WITH EXPLANATIONS

1. Ans. b. Dehydration Ref: William's 7/e p673-4

Factors that influence the severity of SCD are:
- *Intravascular:*
  - Concentration of HbS in RBCs (no symptoms if HbS <50%)
  - Coexistent α-thalassemia
  - Presence of HbC and HbD
  - Polymorphism in endothelial nitric oxide synthase (eNOS) (e.g., T786C polymorphism)
  - High 2, 3-bisphosphoglycerate (BPG) level.
- *Extravascular:*
  - Deoxygenation (e.g., high altitude, asthma)
  - Vascular stasis
  - Low temperature
  - Acidosis
  - Dehydration [due to increased mean corpuscular Hb concentration (MCHC) and vascular stasis]
  - Infection.

2. Ans. b. Hemoglobin (Hb) S homozygous
Ref: William's 8/e p728-30

HbD Punjab and HbD Los Angeles have the same biochemical structure (glutamic acid is replaced by lysine at 121 position in β chain). Heterozygous state is essentially asymptomatic. Homozygous HbD is very rare. SCD is relatively less associated with by HbS-D Punjab/Los Angeles.

Mutation in β chain by virtue of which glutamic acid is replaced by lysine at the 26th position in β chain causes HbE. In the HbE carrier state, 30–45% of the Hb is HbE, and such carriers are asymptomatic but show microcytosis. Homozygous E disease is associated with marked microcytosis and hypochromia, but the anemia is usually mild. It clinically resembles β-thalassemia minor. HbE with HbD heterozygous state is variable in severity.

3. Ans. b. Atenolol Ref: William's 7/e p682

Management of priapism in SCD patients are:
- Surgical intervention (shunt surgery) (particularly done after puberty)
- Hydration and exchange transfusion
- Adrenergic agents (e.g., Etilefrine)
- Sildenafil.

4. Ans. c. 60% Ref: William's 7/e p673

The red cells of sickle cell carrier, who is virtually asymptomatic, always contain <50% HbS. The remainder is largely normal adult Hb.

5. Ans. d. SCD with hereditary persistence of fetal hemoglobin (S/HPFH) Ref: Hoffman's 7/e

Sickle cell disease results from any combination of the sickle cell gene with any other abnormal β-globin gene. There are many types of SCD but most common types include SCD (HbSS), sickle beta-thalassemias (HbS/β), and SCD with S/HPFH. HbSS is the most common form of SCD. Patients with HbS/β⁰ in general, have the most severe forms of SCD including lower Hb levels and more frequent vaso-occlusive and hemolytic complications. The second most common form of SCD is sickle-C (Hb SC) disease. Patients with this type of SCD generally have a more benign clinical course than do patients with HbSS or sickle/β⁰-thalassemia. Likewise, patients with sickle/β⁺-thalassemia and S/HPFH also generally have a more benign clinical course and patients with S/HPFH may actually have Hb levels that are or approximately normal.

6. Ans. e. Myocardial infarction   *Ref: Hoffman's 7/e*

The most common causes of death in adults from SCD reported are pulmonary hypertension, sudden death of unknown etiology, renal failure, and infection. The most common causes of death in childhood from SCD are infection, ACS, and stroke.

7. Ans. c. Platelets and coagulation factor
Ref: William's 8/e p711-5

The pathophysiologic processes that lead to SCD-related complications result from a combination of hemolysis and vaso-occlusion. Hemolysis occurs as a result of repeated episodes of Hb polymerization/depolymerization as sickle red blood cells pick up and release oxygen in the circulation. Red blood cell membranes become abnormal from this process and red blood cells have a shortened lifespan. Hemolysis can occur both chronically and during acute painful vaso-occlusive crises and also results in the release of substantial quantities of free Hb into the vasculature. The consumption of significant quantities of NO by this resultant free ferrous Hb, in turn, leads to abnormal regulation in vascular homeostasis. Moreover, neutrophils play a key role in the tissue damage which occurs as both neutrophil numbers are increased and evidence suggests that they are abnormally activated and adherent. Likewise, as suggested by recent data, sickle red cells induce adhesion of lymphocytes and monocytes to the endothelium such that these may contribute to the pathogenesis of vascular occlusion. Platelet activation also occurs in SCD but is least implicated among the given options.

8. Ans. e. All of the above   *Ref: William's 8/e p713*

Dehydration, infection, extreme temperature, low pH, hypoxia, high intracellular Hb concentration, 2,3-BPG levels, and emotional stress are the common triggers for vaso-occlusive crises. However, often no identifiable cause is found and pain often occurs without warning. Painful events are unpredictable and often severe resulting in repeated hospitalizations, missed days of school or work, and very poor health-related quality of life as well as an increased mortality rate.

9. Ans. d. Pulmonary hypertension is an important cause   *Ref: William's 8/e p718*

The ACS refers to a new pulmonary infiltrate accompanied by fever and/or symptoms or signs of respiratory disease in a patient with SCD. It is a relatively common cause of frequent hospitalizations and death and a common indication for transfusion and treatment with hydroxyurea. The etiology of ACS is multifactorial. Although many episodes of ACS develop without an obvious cause, studies indicate that infection, fat emboli, and pulmonary infarction are all commonly associated with its development. Treatment usually involves antimicrobials to cover both common causes of pneumonia such as *Streptococcus pneumoniae* and *Chlamydia pneumoniae* and atypical pathogens such as mycoplasma. Chronic pulmonary problems seen in SCD are restrictive and obstructive lung disease, hypoxemia, and pulmonary hypertension. Pulmonary hypertension is more frequent among patients with high rates of chronic hemolysis, reflected by marked elevation in plasma lactate dehydrogenase (LDH). Pulmonary hypertension is not the cause of ACS, but frequent ACS can lead to pulmonary hypertension.

10. Ans. d. Transcranial Doppler (TCD) is helpful
Ref: William's 8/e p719

Central nervous system disease is common in SCD and usually manifests as stroke and/or vasculopathy in those with the disease. Overt stroke usually involves large cerebral vessels that affect large regions of the brain and occurs in up to 10% of children with the disease. Silent stroke which occurs in at least 22% of those with SCD is defined as an infarct on imaging studies with a normal neurological examination. Elevated TCD velocities detected in large intracerebral vessels are associated with an increased risk of an overt stroke and it is the best predictor. For patients who received chronic red blood cell transfusions to decrease the concentration of HbS, the risk was significantly decreased and this therapy has now been accepted as standard of care for patients with elevated TCD velocities. Children suffer cognitive impairment that impacts their academic achievement.

11. Ans. b. The ratio of HbA to HbS is 50:50
Ref: Hoffman's 7/e

Sickle cell trait (HbAS) is a benign condition that has no hematological manifestations and is associated with normal growth and life expectancy. The ratio of HbA to HbS is 60:40. Impaired urine concentrating ability and hematuria can occur, and an increased incidence of UTI is observed in pregnant women with sickle cell trait. Splenic infarction is possible at very high altitudes and varies in severity from mild discomfort to occasional splenic rupture.

Condition	Hemoglobin (g/dL)	MCV (fL)	HbS	HbA	Symptoms
Sickle cell trait	Normal	80–100	40%	60%	Very rare
Sickle cell anemia	6–9	80–100	100%	0	Veno-occlusive and pain crises
Sickle beta 0 thal (β⁰)	6–9	60–80	100%	0	Veno-occlusive crises
Sickle beta + thal (β⁺)	9–13	70–80	60%	40%	Rare
HbSC	9–13	80–100	50%	0	HbC 50%, Rare crises

(MCV: mean corpuscular volume; thal: thalassemia).

12. Ans. e. None of the above   *Ref: William's 8/e p715*

Sickling of red cells can be induced by sealing a drop of blood under a coverslip to exclude oxygen or by adding 2% sodium metabisulfite. This test cannot be used for primary diagnosis since it is unable to distinguish sickle cell trait from sickle cell anemia. Identification and quantification of HbS and other hemoglobins can be done using high performance liquid chromatography (HPLC).

13. Ans. c. Leg ulcers   *Ref: William's 8/e p722, 725*

Hydroxycarbamide is a very important drug in the management of patients with SCD who have severe clinical manifestations. Hydroxycarbamide inhibits ribonucleotide reductase, leading to S-phase arrest of replicating cells and is used in SCD because of its ability to stimulate production of HbF. The myelo-suppressive effect of hydroxycarbamide induces stress erythropoiesis as a result of which HbF increases. Patients on hydroxycarbamide experience 50% reduction in the incidence of acute painful episodes and ACS. Transfusion needs, frequency of hospital admissions, and risk of death are also decreased. Leg ulcers are not improved by hydroxycarbamide; rather it has been implicated in the causation of leg ulcers. It is started at a dose of 20 mg/kg/day and increased by 5 mg/kg every 2–3 months until the absolute neutrophil count is close to 2,500/μL.

14. Ans. b. Target cells   *Ref: Hoffman's 6/e p609-11*

Target cells or codocytes are bell-shaped cells which are characteristically seen in liver disease, thalassemia syndromes (HbC, HbD, HbE disease), and lecithin-cholesterol acyltransferase deficiency (LCAT deficiency).

15. Ans. b. Sodium metabisulfite test
    Ref: Dacie and Lewis 10/e p292, 323; Hoffman's 6/e p662

Sodium metabisulfite is the oxidizing agent used most commonly for inducing sickling in red cells. Ham's test is diagnosis of paroxysmal nocturnal hemoglobinuria (PNH). Similarly, Schilling test is for megaloblastic anemia, pancreatic insufficiency, and osmotic fragility for hereditary spherocytosis and Coomb's test is for autoimmune hemolytic anemia (AIHA).

16. Ans. c. Sickle cell disease

Crizanlizumab is an anti-P-selectin antibody. P-selectin is a protein found on the surface of endothelial cells and in platelets. P-selectin normally works to control the flow of white blood cells through blood vessels and how they adhere to blood vessel walls during periods of inflammation and tissue repair, such as after injury. In SCD, P-selectin contributes to the adhesion of sickle red blood cells to blood vessels, preventing blood flow through smaller vessels. This causes inflammation and vaso-occlusive pain crises. By blocking P-selectin, crizanlizumab prevents this adhesion molecule from starting the process that leads to blood vessel occlusion, inflammation, and pain and helps to maintain normal blood flow.

Voxelotor is an inhibitor of deoxygenated sickle Hb polymerization, which is the central abnormality in SCD. This drug makes sickle cells less likely to bind together and form the sickle shape, which can cause low Hb levels due to red blood cell destruction.

17. Ans. a. P-selectin inhibitor

See explanation to Q. No. 16.

18. Ans. a. Decreases deoxyhemoglobin polymerization

See explanation to Q. No. 16.

19. Ans. b. Increased risk of pneumonia
    Ref: Hoffman's 6/e p542-7

There are a few clinical complications of sickle cell trait such as splenic infarction at high altitude, hyposthenuria, hematuria, recurrent UTI, increased risk of thrombosis and in armed forces recruits' age-dependent risk of exercise-related sudden death.

20. Ans. c. Increase in reticulocyte count
    Ref: Qureshi, A., et al. Guidelines for the use of hydroxycarbamide in children and adults with sickle cell disease: A British Society for Haematology Guideline. Br J Haematol. 2018;181(4):460-475.

Hydroxyurea is an antimetabolite which works by inhibiting enzyme ribonucleotide reductase. The therapeutic effect of hydroxycarbamide is mainly via an increase in the proportion of fetal hemoglobin (HbF) and a reduction of intercellular adhesions.

Besides the increase in HbF, it also:
- Increases the MCV and hemoglobin concentration
- Reduces the absolute reticulocyte, white blood cell, and platelet counts.

Patients started on hydroxycarbamide should have their full blood count checked: 2 weeks after starting treatment, at every dose increment, and at least every 8–12 weeks afterwards.

Chapter 13: Methemoglobinemia

1. Which of the following is not true about methemoglobinemia?
a. Cyanosis due to abnormal hemoglobin (Hb) is inherited as autosomal recessive trait
b. Cyanosis due to nicotinamide adenine nucleotide phosphate (NADH) diaphorase deficiency is inherited as autosomal recessive trait
c. Most accurate method of diagnosing methemoglobinemia is by spectrophotometric analysis
d. Hereditary methemoglobinemia due to NADH-diaphorase deficiency is readily treated by ascorbic acid

2. When the circulating hemoglobin in blood is present with iron in an oxidized form (Fe^{3+}) instead of Fe^{2+} state, it is called:
a. Carboxymethemoglobinemia
b. Methemoglobinemia
c. Congenital dyserythropoietic anemia
d. Carboxyhemoglobinemia

3. Acquired causes of a methemoglobinemia are:
a. Aniline dye
b. Sulfonamide
c. Chloroquine
d. Dapsone
e. All of the above

4. Clinical manifestations of methemoglobinemia include:
a. Cyanosis
b. Hemolysis
c. Normal PaO_2 in arterial blood gas analysis
d. All of the above

5. A 31-year-old man is brought to the emergency department after he had collapsed following a dental extraction in which prilocaine hydrochloride 3% was used as local anesthesia. On examination the patient had cyanosis despite a good respiratory effort, a clear airway, and bilateral clear breath sounds. His level of consciousness keeps on deteriorating. Oxygen saturation was 60% with the patient breathing room air. He was intubated and assisted ventilation started, but this did not improve his cyanosis or level of consciousness. There was no family or personal history of such incidence. This patient should be treated with:
a. Exchange transfusion
b. Hyperbaric oxygen
c. Methylene blue
d. Dialysis

6. Methemoglobinemia is a condition in which:
a. Iron in the Hb molecule is oxidized to a ferric state
b. Iron in the Hb molecule is reduced to a ferrous state
c. Hb is methylated
d. Hb is carboxylated

ANSWERS WITH EXPLANATIONS

1. Ans. a. Cyanosis due to abnormal hemoglobin (Hb) is inherited as autosomal recessive trait
Ref: William's 8/e p743-7

Methemoglobinemia is due to abnormal Hb and NADH-diaphorase deficiency, which are autosomal dominant and autosomal recessive, respectively. It can be misinterpreted when automated instruments designed to estimate levels of reduced Hb, oxygenated Hb, Met Hb, and carboxy Hb are used. Direct spectrophotometric analysis is required to diagnose methemoglobinemia or sulfhemoglobinemia. For hereditary methemoglobinemia due to NADH-diaphorase deficiency, treatment is ascorbic acid, 300–600 mg/day. Acute toxic methemoglobinemia is treated with methylene blue. NADPH rapidly reduces methylene blue to leukomethylene blue which nonenzymatically reduces Met-Hb to Hb. Dose is 1–2 mg/kg over 5 minutes for rapid action. Cimetidine is a selective inhibitor of M-hydroxylation, so it is used in methemoglobinemia produced by dapsone. Unlike methemoglobinemia, sulfhemoglobin cannot be converted to Hb.

2. Ans. b. Methemoglobinemia
Ref: William's 8/e p744-5

Methemoglobinemia can occur due to abnormal Hb (called HbM) or due to deficiency of NADH-diaphorase.

In most HbM, tyrosine is substituted for either proximal or distal histidine and this tyrosine can form iron-phenolate complex that resists reduction to a divalent iron state by the NADH-diaphorase enzyme.

3. Ans. e. All of the above *Ref: William's 8/e p744*

Acquired methemoglobinemia can be caused due to multiple drugs and toxins including aniline dyes, benzene, chloroquine, dapsone, local anesthetic agents, Reglan, primaquine, phenazopyridine, sulfonamides, acetanilid, alloxan, benzocaine, bivalent copper, bismuth subnitrate, bupivacaine hydrochloride, chlorates, chloroquine, chromates, clofazimine, dimethyl sulfoxide, dinitrophenol, exhaust fumes, ferricyanide, flutamide, hydroxylamine, lidocaine hydrochloride, metoclopramide, methylene blue, naphthalene, nitrates, nitric oxide, nitrites, nitrofuran, nitroglycerin, sodium nitroprusside, phenacetin, phenazopyridine hydrochloride, phenytoin, prilocaine, rifampin, silver nitrate, sodium valproate, smoke inhalation, and sulfasalazine trinitrotoluene. HbM is used to designate several variants of abnormal Hb associated with genetic methemoglobinemia. In most of the HbM, tyrosine has been substituted for either the proximal or the distal histidine. This results in reduced capacity of the enzymatic machinery of the erythrocyte to efficiently reduce the iron to the divalent form and thus predisposes to methemoglobinemia. These Hb variants are associated with cyanosis, which is present from early life.

4. Ans. d. All of the above *Ref: William's 8/e p745*

Methemoglobinemia may be acute or chronic. The physiologic level of met-Hb in the blood is 0–2%. Met-Hb concentrations of 10–20% are tolerated well, but levels above this are often associated with symptoms. Levels above 70% may cause death. Symptoms also depend on the rapidity of its formation. Many patients with lifelong methemoglobinemia are asymptomatic, but patients exposed to drugs and toxins who abruptly develop the same levels of methemoglobinemia may be severely symptomatic. Dyspnea, nausea, and tachycardia occur at met-Hb levels of 30% or more. Lethargy, stupor, and deteriorating consciousness occur as met-Hb levels approach 55%. Higher levels may cause cardiac arrhythmias and circulatory failure. Drug-induced methemoglobinemia may be followed by hemolytic anemia, especially with exposure to dapsone, sulfasalazine, or phenacetin. Heinz bodies (precipitated Hb or globin subunits due to denaturation of Hb in erythrocytes) and fragmented red blood cells characterize this type of anemia. Acute intravascular hemolysis may occasionally lead to renal failure. Blood containing high concentrations of met-Hb appears chocolate brown. Subjects with methemoglobinemia may have normal partial pressures of oxygen, despite life-threatening methemoglobinemia. The oxygen saturation values, measured by a pulse oximeter, are falsely elevated.

5. Ans. c. Methylene blue *Ref: William's 8/e p747*

The possible diagnosis of methemoglobinemia should be suspected because the patient is cyanosed, the cyanosis is unresponsive to ventilation, there is no prior history of respiratory problems, and the patient had been exposed to a topical anesthetic that is known to cause methemoglobinemia. Cyanosis, low Hb oxygen saturation on pulse oximetry (typically 85–89% representing the absorbance spectrum of met-Hb), normal PaO$_2$ on arterial blood gas (ABG), and appearance of "chocolate blood" are suggestive of methemoglobinemia. Co-oximetry of ABG will quantify the percent of methemoglobinemia in a fresh arterial sample. For methemoglobinemia due to drug exposure, the traditional first-line therapy consists of an infusion of methylene blue (1%; 1–2 mg/kg IV over 5 minutes), whose action depends on the availability of reduced NADPH within the red blood cells. After an acute exposure to an oxidizing agent, treatment should be considered when the met-Hb is 30% in an asymptomatic patient and 20% in a symptomatic patient. Patients with anemia or cardiorespiratory problems should be treated at lower levels of met-Hb. Dextrose should be given because the major source of NADH in the red blood cells is the catabolism of sugar through glycolysis. Dextrose is also necessary to form NADPH through the hexose monophosphate shunt, which is necessary for methylene blue to be effective. Exchange transfusion is reserved for patients in whom methylene blue therapy is ineffective.

6. Ans. a. Iron in the Hb molecule is oxidized to a ferric state *Ref: Hoffman's 6/e p941-5*

Methemoglobinemia results from oxidation of the iron moieties in Hb from the ferrous to the ferric state. Normal oxygenation of the Hb causes a partial transfer of an electron from the iron to bound oxygen. Iron in this state resembles ferric iron and oxygen resembles superoxide (O_2^-). Deoxygenation returns the electron to the iron, with release of oxygen.

CHAPTER 14: Immune Hemolytic Anemia

1. Which of the following is not true about hemolytic anemia?
   a. The degree of spherocytosis does not correlate with the severity of hemolysis
   b. Alloimmune hemolytic anemia is characterized by positive indirect Coombs test (ICT)
   c. In autoimmune hemolytic anemia (AIHA), the most common target is rhesus (Rh) antigen
   d. Therapy should not be stopped until the direct Coombs test (DCT) becomes negative

2. All of the following are associated with cold-type autoantibody, *except*:
   a. Mycoplasma pneumonia
   b. Donath-Landsteiner hemolytic anemia
   c. Infectious mononucleosis
   d. Hodgkin lymphoma

3. In chronic lymphocytic leukemia (CLL), the AIHA is due to:
   a. Warm antibody
   b. Cold antibody
   c. Mixed cold and warm antibody
   d. Occurs only with treatment with purine analog

4. Which of the following is not true about AIHA associated with α-methyldopa?
   a. Positive DCT is found in 8–36% of patients
   b. Lag period of 3–6 months is present between the start of therapy and the development of positive DCT
   c. Less than 1% of patients develop hemolytic anemia
   d. Hemolytic anemia is due to hapten mechanism

5. In CLL patients, the risk factors for the development of AIHA after purine analog treatment are all, *except*:
   a. Previous exposure prior to purine analogs
   b. Positive direct antiglobulin test (DAT) prior to therapy
   c. Hypogammaglobulinemia
   d. High β-2 microglobulin

6. Which of the following is true about cold agglutinin disease?
   a. Usually the antibodies are of immunoglobulin M (IgM) type
   b. Occurs in infectious mononucleosis
   c. In vitro agglutination is maximum at 0–5°C
   d. Infectious mononucleosis has cold agglutinin with anti-D specificity

7. Which of the following is not true about AIHA?
   a. May be due to drugs
   b. Associated with pernicious anemia (PA)
   c. May complicate B-cell CLL
   d. May be associated with IgM antibodies in serum

8. What is detected by ICT?
   a. Antibodies in serum
   b. Antibodies on red blood cell (RBC) surface
   c. Antigens on RBC surface
   d. Antibodies in plasma
   e. Associated with positive DCT

9. Which of the following is not true about DCT-negative AIHA?
   a. Polyspecific antihuman globulin (AHG) may not be able to detect this type of AIHA if the type of antibody is IgA or IgM
   b. Low-affinity IgG autoantibodies
   c. Low titer IgG autoantibodies
   d. Gel card is not able to detect rare IgA-only AIHA

10. Direct Coombs' test may be positive in:
    a. Immediate post-transfusion
    b. Thalassemia major
    c. Hereditary spherocytosis
    d. Paroxysmal nocturnal hemoglobinuria (PNH)

11. Polyspecific antisera in DCT is:
    a. Anti-IgG and IgA
    b. Anti-IgG and C3
    c. Anti-IgG, IgM, and IgA
    d. Anti-IgM and C3

12. In a patient, ICT is positive but DCT is negative. What is the most likely explanation for this?
    a. Autoimmune antibody present
    b. Alloimmune antibody present
    c. Autoimmune antibody associated with CLL
    d. Autoimmune antibody associated with infectious mononucleosis

13. All of the following drugs can cause immune-mediated hemolysis, *except*:
    a. Penicillin
    b. Quinine
    c. Methyldopa
    d. Chloramphenicol

14. Anti-D is useful in all, *except*:
    a. Abortion before 12 weeks of pregnancy
    b. Delivery of an Rh-positive baby within 3 days

c. Threatened abortion with a live fetus of 12 weeks gestation
d. After chorionic villous sampling

15. Hemoglobinuria is not seen in:
a. Paroxysmal nocturnal hemoglobinuria
b. Glucose-6-phosphate dehydrogenase (G6PD) deficiency
c. Autoimmune hemolytic anemia
d. Malaria

16. The antibody type present in chronic cold agglutinin hemolytic disease is:
a. IgG
b. IgM
c. IgA
d. Mixed

17. The antibody type responsible for paroxysmal cold hemoglobinuria (PCH) is:
a. IgG
b. IgM
c. IgA
d. Mixed

18. A 35-year-old lady, who is a known case of systemic lupus erythematosus (SLE), presented to ER with shortness of breath. On evaluation, she was found to be having Hb 4.5, mean corpuscular volume (MCV) 145 fL, mean corpuscular hemoglobin concentration (MCHC) 36 g/dL, reticulocyte count of 7%, lactate dehydrogenase (LDH) 400 IU/L. What should be the next test to diagnose her cause of anemia?
a. Direct Coombs' test
b. Incubated osmotic fragility test
c. Test for antiphospholipid antibodies workup
d. Serum vitamin B_{12} and folate levels

19. An 18-years-old female presented with weakness, easy fatigability and jaundice for 4 weeks. Her Hb was 6.2 g/dL and had indirect hyperbilirubinemia. Her direct Coombs' test (DCT) using polyspecific IgG was done as shown below.

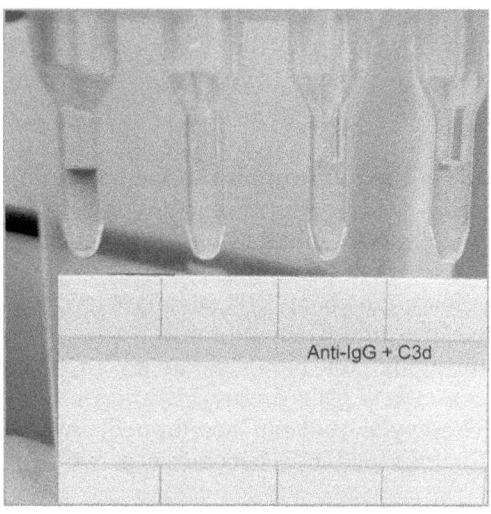

Courtesy: Dr Rasika Setia, MD

Which of the following statement is true about the test?
a. The DAT is performed using heparin-anticoagulated blood
b. It is the conventional test tube method
c. It is only for anti-IgG and not for anti-complement
d. Non-agglutinated RBC are trapped
e. None of the above

ANSWERS WITH EXPLANATIONS

1. Ans. a. The degree of spherocytosis does not correlate with the severity of hemolysis
Ref: William's 8/e p782, 787-90

Spherocytosis is a very important diagnostic feature of AIHA and the degree of spherocytosis correlates well with the severity of hemolysis. ICT +ve and DCT –ve are usually seen in alloimmunization due to prior sensitization with blood transfusion or pregnancy, and in drug-induced hemolytic anemia or low titer antibodies. Nearly half of all AIHA patients have autoantibodies specific for epitopes on Rh proteins. The other antigens are band-3 anion transporter or glycophorin A. Steroid therapy should be continued till DCT becomes negative.

2. Ans. d. Hodgkin lymphoma   *Ref: William's 8/e p778*

3. Ans. a. Warm antibody   *Ref: William's 8/e p778*

Autoimmune cytopenia complicating CLL is usually caused by polyclonal T-cell-dependent mechanisms that result from the loss of self-tolerance. The pathogenic antibodies responsible for about 90% of cases of AIHA and immune thrombocytopenic purpura (ITP) are produced by nonmalignant B cells and are polyclonal high-affinity IgG directed against RBC or platelet antigens. These antibodies can ligate antigens on RBC and platelets and the opsonized cells are then destroyed via an antibody-dependent cellular cytotoxicity (ADCC) mechanism mediated predominantly by fixed macrophages in the spleen and liver. Although CLL cells can produce monoclonal autoantibodies that are detectable in the serum, these are rare and responsible for <10% of cases of autoimmune cytopenia. These monoclonal autoantibodies are usually IgM directed against the I antigen and cause AIHA by both complement-dependent cytotoxicity and ADCC.

4. Ans. d. Hemolytic anemia is due to hapten mechanism
Ref: William's 8/e p783, 784

α-methyldopa induces the formation of autoantibodies reactive with autologous (or homologous) RBCs in the absence of instigating drug. Diclofenac, procainamide, fludarabine, pentostatin, 2-CDA, L-dopa, mefenamic acid, teniposide, and cephalosporins are other important drugs in this category. Positive DCT (with anti-IgG reagents) in patients taking α-methyldopa varies from 8 to 36%. A lag period of 3–6 months exists between the start of therapy and development of positive DCT, but only <1% patients develop hemolytic anemia. Development of hemolytic anemia does not depend on drug dose. They typically have strong +ve DCT and ICT. Frequently, the autoantibodies are reactive with determinants of the Rh complex.

	Hapten/drug adsorption	Ternary complex formation	Autoantibody binding	Nonimmunologic protein adsorption
Prototype drug	Penicillin	Quinidine	α-Methyldopa	Cephalothin
Role of drug	Binds to red cell membrane	Forms ternary complex with Ab and red cell membrane-component	Induces Ab-formation to native red cell Ag	Possibly alters red cell membrane
Drug affinity to cell	Strong	Weak		Strong
Ab to drug	Present	Present	Absent	Absent
Ab class	IgG	IgM or IgG	IgG	None
Proteins detected by DCT	IgG, rarely complement	Complement	IgG, rarely complement	Multiple plasma proteins
Dose of drug associated with positive DCT	High	Low	High	High
Presence of drug required for ICT	Yes (coating red cells)	Yes (added to test medium)	No	Yes (added to test medium)
Mechanism of red cell destruction	Splenic sequestration of IgG coated RBC	Direct lysis by complement plus splenic-hepatic clearance of C3b–coated RBCs	Splenic sequestration	None

(DCT: direct Coombs' test; ICT: indirect Coombs test).

5. Ans. d. High β-2 microglobulin
Ref: William's 8/e p784

High β-2 microglobulin is a poor prognostic marker in CLL but is not a risk factor for the development of AIHA. Other options are known risk factors.

6. Ans. d. Infectious mononucleosis has cold agglutinin with anti-D specificity
Ref: William's 8/e p779, 782, 789

Cold agglutinin disease is less common than warm type, accounting for 10–20% of all cases of AIHA. It is more common in women. Secondary cold agglutinin disease occurs most commonly in adolescents and young adults as a self-limiting process mostly associated with mycoplasma infection or infectious mononucleosis. Idiopathic (primary) chronic cold agglutinin disease has its peak incidence at the age of 50 years with presence of monoclonal IgM protein. In vitro agglutination is maximum at 25°C, but complement fixations by these antibodies are optimal at 20–25°C. Cold agglutinins with anti-I specificity are seen in infectious mononucleosis and in some cases of lymphomas.

7. Ans. b. Associated with pernicious anemia (PA)
Ref: William's 8/e p548

Pernicious anemia is a disease of insidious onset that generally begins in middle age or later (usually after 40 years). It is an autoimmune disease. Although antiparietal cell antibodies are found in 90% of PA patients, they are not thought to be responsible for pathogenesis. Antibodies to intrinsic factors (type I or blocking type) or the intrinsic factor–Cbl complex (type II or binding type) are highly specific to PA patients. Type I antibodies are found in 70% of the patients. Type II antibodies are found in 50% of cases. The rest of all the statements about AIHA are true.

8. Ans. a. Antibodies in serum
Ref: Dacie and Lewis 10/e p241

Warm antibodies present freely in the patient's serum are best detected by means of ICT or by use of enzyme-treated (e.g., trypsinized or papainized) red cells.

9. Ans. d. Gel card is not able to detect rare IgA-only AIHA
Ref: Dacie and Lewis 10/e p248-249

Polyspecific AHG contains antibodies against IgG and C3d complement, so it will not be able to detect IgA or IgM autoantibody type AIHA. The incidence of IgA-only warm AIHA is 0.2–2.7%. 2–6% of patients with clinical and hematological features of AIHA have DCT negative on repeated analysis. Low-affinity IgG autoantibodies dissociate from RBC during the washing phase in tube technique, resulting in negative DCT.

Low-titer IgG autoantibodies (threshold is 300–4000 molecules per RBC) may also be missed in the tube technique, which can be overcome by a more sensitive technique such as column agglutination method, ELISA (enzyme-linked immunosorbent assay), or flow cytometry.

The Diamed DAT gel card, which contains a set of monospecific AHG reagents (i.e., anti-IgG, -IgA, -IgM, -C3c, -C3d, and inert control), can also be used. There is no washing phase in this, so it detects low-affinity IgG, IgA, and IgM. A gel card can also pick up the rare IgA-only AIHA.

10. Ans. a. Immediate post-transfusion
Ref: Dacie and Lewis 10/e p239, 247

Direct Coombs' test may be positive in autoimmune diseases, recent blood transfusions, recent infections, and exposure to toxins or drugs.

11. **Ans. b. Anti-IgG and C3** *Ref: William's 8/e p786*

Broad-spectrum or polyspecific Coombs reagent contains antibodies directed against human IgG and complement component, principally C3.

12. **Ans. b. Alloimmune antibody present**
Ref: William's 8/e p782, 787-90

ICT +ve and DCT –ve are usually seen in alloimmunization due to prior blood transfusion, pregnancy, or in drug-induced AIHA.

13. **Ans. d. Chloramphenicol** *Ref: William's 8/e p9, 780*

14. **Ans. c. Threatened abortion with a live fetus of 12 weeks gestation** *Ref: William's 8/e p811*

Postpartum anti-RhD immunoglobulins to all nonsensitized Rh –ve women who deliver an Rh +ve baby decrease the incidence of Rh isoimmunization from 12-2%.

It can further be reduced to 0.1% if prophylaxis is given at 28 weeks gestation.

The standard dose is 300 μg Rh Ig which affords protection against a fetomaternal transfusion of 15 mL of Rh +ve red cell and 30 mL of whole blood.

The recommended dose should be administered as soon as possible, within 72 hours of delivery. Some protection can still be obtained up to 13 days and possibly up to 28 days after delivery.

Rh Ig is indicated following pregnancy termination, miscarriage, amniocentesis, chorionic villous sampling, or other manipulations during surgery.

Rh Ig is ineffective once alloimmunization to Rh D has occurred.

A smaller dose is adequate (50 μg) if pregnancy is terminated at <12 weeks of gestation.

No definite evidence-based recommendation is available regarding administration of Rh Ig to women with threatened abortion and a live fetus or embryo at or before 12 weeks of gestation.

If therapeutic or spontaneous abortion occurs after the first trimester, the standard 300 μg dose is recommended.

15. **Ans. c. Autoimmune hemolytic anemia**

Hemoglobinuria is a feature of intravascular hemolysis and in AIHA hemolysis in extravascular.

16. **Ans. b. IgM** *Ref: William's 8/e p780-2*

Cold agglutinins directly agglutinate saline-suspended human RBCs at low temperatures, maximally at 0-5°C. Cold agglutinins are characteristically IgM; others are rare.

17. **Ans. a. IgG** *Ref: William's 7/e p780-2*

In PCH, the DCT is positive during and briefly following an acute attack because of the coating of surviving RBCs with complement, mainly C3d fragments. The Donath-Landsteiner antibody is responsible for complement deposition on the cells which is a nonagglutinating IgG that binds RBC only in cold. The Donath-Landsteiner antibody has specificity for the P blood group antigen (also present on lymphocytes and fibroblasts).

18. **Ans. a. Direct Coombs' test**
Ref: Hoffman 5/e p296; Dacie and Lewis 10/e p239

This lady is definitely having hemolytic anemia as evident by low Hb, high LDH, and reticulocytosis. If the MCV is very high (145 fL) and MCHC is also high (36 g/dL), then it means that there is presence of spherocytosis or autoagglutination. This patient most likely is having AIHA so Coombs test should be performed. Usually, if MCV is very high (>125 fL), then AIHA should be suspected. In cases of megaloblastic anemia, the MCV is usually in the range of 110-125 fL, and MCV is usually <110 fL in cases of other causes of macrocytic anemias. The MCV can be mildly elevated as well, where there is no autoagglutination, and this is because the reticulocytes are bigger than normal RBCs.

19. **Ans. e. None of the above**
Ref: Zantek ND. The direct antiglobulin test: A critical step in the evaluation of hemolysis. Am J Hematol. 2012

The direct antiglobulin test (DAT or DCT) is a laboratory test that detects immunoglobulin and/or complement on the surface of red blood cells. The utility of the DAT is to sort hemolysis into an immune or nonimmune etiology. The DAT is performed with polyspecific antiglobulin reagent containing antibodies to IgG and the C3d component of complement. Several methods for performing the DAT exist, including the conventional test tube (CTT) method and the more sensitive gel microcolumn. In the gel microcolumn method, RBCs are filtered through a gelatinous matrix mixed with antihuman globulin reagents. The gel traps the agglutinated RBCs and non-agglutinated RBCs pass through the column. DAT can help classify causes of hemolysis, Including autoimmune hemolytic anemia, transfusion-related hemolysis, hemolytic disease of the fetus/newborn, drug-induced hemolytic anemia, passenger lymphocyte syndrome, and DAT-negative hemolytic anemia. The principle of the DAT is that antihuman globulin (AHG) agglutinates, or clumps, antibody-coated cells. Testing typically starts with polyspecific AHG containing both anti-IgG and anti-complement with positive reactions repeated with monospecific AHG to individually detect IgG and complement. The DAT is performed using ethylene-diamine-tetra-aceticacid-(EDTA) anticoagulated blood, which inhibits complement binding to RBC in vitro and ensures the detection of only in vivo bound complement. The direct antiglobulin test is also referred as the direct Coombs' test since it is based on the test developed by Coombs.

CHAPTER 15
Primary Immunodeficiency Diseases

1. A 12-year-old female child weighing 20 kg is having recurrent respiratory infections since 5 years of age. Her complete blood count was normal. Her quantitative serum immunoglobulins (g/L) and lymphocyte ($\times 10^9$/L) subset analysis showed following results:
- IgG: 3.15 (7.2–19.0)
- IgA: 0.11 (0.8–5.0)
- IgM: 0.66 (0.5–2.0)

Total lymphocyte count: 1.6 (1.5–3.5)
- CD3: 1.31 (0.9–2.8)
- CD4: 0.89 (0.6–1.2)
- CD8: 0.41 (0.4–1.0)
- CD19: 0.1 (0.2–0.4)

Which is most appropriate diagnosis?
 a. Hyper IgM syndrome
 b. Common variable immunodeficiency
 c. Bruton agammaglobulinemia
 d. Severe combined immunodeficiency

2. A male child was born at term by Cesarean section and weighed 3 kg. He is the sixth child of non-consanguineous parents. At the age of 4 weeks, he developed an abscess in groin area which healed spontaneously. He had a total white-cell count of 45×10^9/L, of which 90% were neutrophils. He had recurrent hospital admissions for large staphylococcal abscesses, requiring surgical incision and systemic antibiotics. His three elder brothers had died of infections at ages ranging from 7 months to 3 years, but his parents and two sisters were healthy. On examination his height and weight were below the third centile. He had bilateral axillary and inguinal lymphadenopathy with marked hepatosplenomegaly. The laboratory investigations showed following results:

Quantitative serum immunoglobulins (g/L):
- IgG: 17.8 (5.5–10.0)
- IgA: 4.8 (0.3–0.8)
- IgM: 2.0 (0.4–1.8)

Nitroblue tetrazolium (NBT test)
- Stimulated: 10% (normal >90%)

Which is most appropriate diagnosis?
 a. Hyper IgM syndrome
 b. Common variable immunodeficiency
 c. Leukocyte adhesion defect
 d. Chronic granulomatous disease

3. Which gene is most likely affected in X-linked chronic granulomatous disease?
 a. CYBA
 b. CYBB
 c. NCF1
 d. NCF2

4. A male child was born after an uneventful pregnancy and weighed 3.1 kg. At 4 months, he developed otitis media and an upper respiratory tract infection. At the age of 5 months, he was admitted to hospital with *Haemophilus influenzae* pneumonia. The infections responded promptly to the appropriate antibiotics. He is the fourth child of unrelated parents. His three sisters showed no predisposition to infection. He has been immunized as per schedule. Examination at the age of 18 months showed a pale, thin child whose height and weight were below the third centile. There were no other abnormal features.

His quantitative serum immunoglobulins (g/L):
- IgG: 0.17 (5.5–10.0)
- IgA: 0.1 (0.3–0.8)

Blood lymphocyte subpopulations ($\times 10^9$/L)
Total lymphocyte count: 3.5 (2.5–5.0)
T lymphocytes (CD3): 3.02 (1.5–3.0)
B lymphocytes (CD19): <0.1 (0.3–11.0)

Which is the most appropriate diagnosis?
 a. Bruton's agammaglobulinemia
 b. Common variable immunodeficiency
 c. Leukocyte adhesion defect
 d. Chronic granulomatous disease

5. A 6-month-old child is having recurrent infections. His X-ray chest showed characteristic abnormality in the superior mediastinum. His absolute lymphocyte count is 0.9×10^9/L. Which immune defect is most likely in this child?
 a. Humoral immunodeficiency
 b. DiGeorge syndrome
 c. Neutrophil function defect
 d. Complement pathway defect
 e. Bruton's agammaglobulinemia

SECTION 2 | Benign Hematology

6. Which gene is most likely affected in DiGeorge syndrome?
   a. 22q11
   b. 11q23
   c. P53
   d. 7q21

7. One of the following is not considered as warning signs of primary immunodeficiency in children:
   a. 8 or more new ear infections in 1 year
   b. 2 or more serious sinus infections in 1 year
   c. 2 episodes of pneumonias in 5 years
   d. Persistent thrush in the mouth in 2-year-old child

8. A 1-year-old male infant, born of consanguinity, is having history of ecchymotic spots over body and recurrent episodes of bleeding from gums. He is also having history of recurrent otitis media and impetigo, and on examination he is having generalized dermatitis. The gene most likely affected in this child is:
   a. *BTK* gene
   b. *WAS* gene
   c. *LYST* gene
   d. *CYBB* gene

9. True about leukocyte adhesion deficiency (LAD) are all, *except*:
   a. LAD type I is the result of mutations in a gene CD18
   b. LAD type I may be treated by bone marrow transplantation
   c. LAD type II can be treated by eating large amount of fucose sugar
   d. LAD type III is caused by mutation of *BTK* gene

10. Which one is not phagocytic disorder?
   a. Chronic granulomatous disease
   b. Leukocyte adhesion defect
   c. Chediak-Higashi syndrome
   d. Hyper IgE syndrome (Job syndrome)
   e. Wiskott-Aldrich syndrome

11. A 4-year-old girl was brought with multiple suppurative lymphadenopathy of two months duration. She developed BCG adenitis at 6 months of age which was treated with anti-tuberculous medications. She is the first born child to non-consanguineous parents. Investigations revealed—highly elevated ESR and positive CRP. Ultrasonogram revealed multiple retroperitoneal lymph nodes with pressure effect on the left kidney causing moderate hydronephrosis. Cervical node biopsy was consistent with tuberculosis but the cultures of the lymph node material were negative for AFB and fungus. Anti-tuberculous treatment as per the 5 drug regimen started to treat multidrug resistant TB. HIV screening was negative. T and B cell numbers were normal. Immunoglobulin levels were normal. NBT test for chronic granulomatous disease was negative. 8 months later she had progressively increasing swelling over the left lumbar region of 15 days duration and needed drainage of a psoas abscess. Histopathology of the abscess wall revealed granulomatous inflammation consistent with histoplasmosis. She responded to antifungals.

What is the most probable diagnosis?
   a. Chronic granulomatous disease
   b. Common variable immune deficiency
   c. Severe combined immunodeficiency
   d. IL-12 deficiency

ANSWERS WITH EXPLANATIONS

1. Ans. b. Common variable immunodeficiency
   Ref: Salzer U. Common variable immunodeficiency: an update. Arth Res Ther. 2012;14:223.

Common variable immunodeficiency (CVID) represents the most common primary immunodeficiency. The most common symptoms are severe, recurrent and sometimes chronic bacterial infections mainly of the respiratory and gastrointestinal tracts. The diagnosis of CVID can be made if the following criteria are fulfilled: (1) a male or female patient who exhibits a marked decrease of IgG and of at least one of the IgM or IgA isotypes, (2) onset of immunodeficiency at greater than 2 years of age, (3) absence of isohemagglutinins and/or poor response to vaccines, and (4) other defined causes of hypogammaglobulinemia have been excluded. An inexpensive, quantitative determination of serum immunoglobulins is the first and most important step in the diagnosis of CVID. The next stage of diagnosis is flow cytometric analysis of lymphocyte subpopulations, including total T, B and natural killer cells. The total number of peripheral B cells is slightly reduced in about 40–50% of CVID patients. In some patients elevated numbers of B cells are reported. T cell abnormalities can also be seen in some patients. The immunoglobulin replacement therapy is the mainstay of therapy; 90% of CVID patients are on either intravenous (IVIg) or subcutaneous (SCIg) immunoglobulin treatment. The child mentioned here has recurrent infections and decreased IgG, IgA and B cells (CD19 positive cells).

2. Ans. d. Chronic granulomatous disease
   Ref: Arnold DE. A review of chronic granulomatous disease. Adv Ther. 2017;34:2543-57.

Chronic granulomatous disease (CGD), an inherited disorder of phagocytic cells, results from defective NADPH oxidase leading to an inability of phagocytes to produce bactericidal superoxide anions (O^{2-}). This consequently impairs the production of hydrogen peroxide (H_2O_2), hypochlorous acid (HOCl), and hydroxyl radicals (OH•), products that play a critical role in killing certain pathogenic bacterial and fungal agents. These deficits lead to recurrent, life-threatening bacterial and fungal infections as well as the formation of granulomas in tissue. In addition, most patients with CGD have dysregulated T helper (Th)-17 lymphocyte-controlled inflammation. Children with CGD are often healthy at birth, but develop severe infections in infancy or early childhood. The most common form of CGD is genetically inherited in an X-linked manner, affecting boys. There are also autosomal recessive forms of CGD that affect both sexes. The nitroblue tetrazolium (NBT) and dihydrorhodamine (DHR) tests, as well as genetic testing, are indicated in the workup of chronic granulomatous disease.

3. Ans. b. CYBB

Ref: Leiding JW. Chronic granulomatous disease. Gene Rev. 2016.

Chronic granulomatous disease is diagnosed by tests that measure neutrophil superoxide production via the nicotinamide adenine dinucleotide phosphate (NADPH) oxidase complex: the DHR test has largely replaced the NBT test, the oldest and most recognized diagnostic test for CGD. CGD is caused by pathogenic variants in one of five genes that encode the subunits of phagocyte NADPH oxidase: biallelic pathogenic variants in CYBA, NCF1, NCF2, and NCF4 cause autosomal recessive CGD (AR-CGD); mutation of CYBB causes X-linked CGD.

4. Ans. a. Bruton's agammaglobulinemia

Ref: Conley ME. X-linked agammaglobulinemia. Clin Rev Aller Immunol. 2000;19:183-204.

Bruton's X-linked agammaglobulinemia (XLA) is a disease of the immune system in which there is defective development of the B lymphocytes due to which the production of gamma globulins is markedly reduced. This results in immunodeficiency and high vulnerability to contract fatal infections. XLA is known to be caused by mutation in the *BTK* (B-lymphocyte tyrosine kinase) gene. *BTK* gene mutation results in markedly reduced levels of B lymphocytes and immunoglobulins, and these are the confirmatory laboratory findings for the diagnosis of XLA. Children with XLA are usually healthy for the first 1 or 2 months of life because they are protected by antibodies acquired before birth from their mother. After this, the maternal antibodies are cleared from the body, and the affected child begins to develop recurrent infections. Colonel Ogden Bruton identified the first XLA patient in 1952.

5. Ans. b. DiGeorge syndrome

At age of 6 months the X-ray shows absent thymus which is the characteristic feature of DiGeorge Syndrome. Absolute lymphocyte count is also very low. DiGeorge syndrome is a primary immunodeficiency disease caused by abnormal migration and development of certain cells and tissues during fetal development. As part of the developmental defect, the thymus gland may be affected and T-lymphocyte production may be impaired, resulting in low T-lymphocyte numbers and frequent infections. The 22q11 deletion syndrome, also known as DiGeorge or velocardiofacial syndrome, is one of the most common microdeletion syndromes in humans.

6. Ans. a. 22q11

Approximately 90% of patients with DGS have a small deletion in chromosome number 22 at position 22q11.2. Thus, another name for this syndrome is the 22q11.2 deletion syndrome.

7. Ans. c. 2 episodes of pneumonias in 5 years

The child should be evaluated when there is the presence of ≥2 of the following 10 warning signs (Jeffrey Modell Foundation's warning signs):
- ≥8 ear infections in 1 year
- ≥2 severe sinus infections in 1 year
- ≥2 months treatment of antibiotics with little effect
- ≥2 pneumonias per year
- Insufficient weight gain or growth delay
- Recurrent deep skin or organ abscesses (e.g. liver, lungs)
- Persistent thrush in mouth or fungal infection on skin
- Need for intravenous antibiotics to clear infections
- ≥2 deep seated infections (e.g. septicemia, meningitis)
- Family history of a primary immunodeficiency.

8. Ans. b. *WAS* gene

As per history this child is having recurrent infections, bleeding, and eczema. Most probable diagnosis is Wiskott-Aldrich syndrome (WAS) which is a rare X-linked recessive disease characterized by eczema, bleeding due to thrombocytopenia (low platelet count) and recurrent infections due to immune deficiency. Gene affected is *WAS* gene. *BTK* gene is affected in X-linked agammaglobulinemia, LYST gene in Chédiak-Higashi syndrome and *CYBB* gene in CGD.

9. Ans. d. LAD type III is caused by mutation of *BTK* gene

Leukocyte adhesion deficiency type I (LAD1) is the result of mutations in a gene CD18. Patients with the severe phenotype have <1% of normal expression of CD18 on neutrophils. LAD1 is by far the most common cause of leukocyte adhesion deficiency and it is usually corrected by bone marrow transplantation. However, milder forms of LAD1 can sometimes be managed with antibiotics alone. Leukocyte adhesion deficiency type II (LAD2) is due to mutations in an enzyme that attaches fucose (a type of sugar) to proteins. These patients can be treated by eating large amounts of fucose. Leukocyte adhesion deficiency type III (LAD3) is caused by mutations in a gene called FERMT3.

10. Ans. e. Wiskott-Aldrich syndrome

Ref: McCusker C. Primary immunodeficiency. Allergy Asthma Clin Immunol. 2011;7:S11.

Following defects are found in various phagocytic disorders:

- *Phagocytosis defect:* Leukocyte adhesion defect
- *Chemotaxis defect:* Hyper IgE syndrome
- *Degranulation defect:* Chediak-Higashi syndrome
- *Respiratory burst pathway defect:* Chronic granulomatous disease
- *Combined immunodeficiency:* Wiskott-Aldrich syndrome.

11. Ans. d. IL-12 deficiency

Ref: Picard C. Inherited interleukin-12 deficiency: IL12B genotype and clinical phenotype of 13 patients from six kindreds. Am J Hum Genet. 2002;70(2):336-48

Interleukin-12 (IL12) is a cytokine that is secreted by activated phagocytes and dendritic cells and that induces interferon-γ production by natural-killer and T lymphocytes. IL12 deficiency is principally associated with infectious diseases caused by Mycobacteria. Children inoculated with live BCG vaccine develop clinical infection. Laboratory studies, including a comprehensive evaluation of immunological parameters, are normal, with the exception that the patients exhibit an impressive and consistent deficiency in the production of the cytokine IL-12. Recurrent infections with mycobacterium, salmonella and histoplasma are common. Gamma interferon therapy helps reduce infective episodes.

CHAPTER 16

Thalassemia Syndromes

1. Thalassemia major is characterized by all of the following, *except*:
   a. Splenomegaly
   b. Microcytic hypochromic anemia
   c. Presence of target cells in peripheral blood smear
   d. Increased osmotic fragility

2. Hemoglobin E is seen most often in:
   a. South-East Asia
   b. Central Africa
   c. Eastern Africa
   d. South America

3. Thalassemia control has been most successful in:
   a. USA
   b. Cyprus
   c. Iraq
   d. Thailand

4. Major cause of death in thalassemia major is due to:
   a. Endocrinopathies
   b. Cardiomyopathies
   c. Liver failure
   d. Infection

5. A 6-month-old untransfused child presented with lethargy, failure to thrive and looking pale. Complete blood count (CBC) is showing Hb of 5.6 g/dL, mean corpuscular volume (MCV)—58 fl and peripheral blood picture showing micro-cytic hypochromic red cells, target cells and anisopoikilocytosis. Hb high-pressure liquid chromatography (HPLC) is showing Hb F of 100%. The most likely diagnosis is:
   a. Delta-beta thalassemia
   b. Hb Bart's
   c. β-Thalassemia major
   d. Hereditary persistence of fetal Hb (HPFH)

6. Hb H inclusion seen in α-thalassemia is composed of:
   a. γ-4 tetramers
   b. β-4 tetramers
   c. δ-4 tetramers
   d. ε-4 tetramers

7. The most common infection in hemochromatosis is:
   a. *Vibrio vulnificus*
   b. *Staphylococcus aureus*
   c. *Yersinia enterocolitica*
   d. Salmonella
   e. *Listeria monocytogenes*

8. The most common cause of beta thalassemia is:
   a. Point mutation
   b. Insertion
   c. Deletion
   d. All are equally distributed

9. The most common cause of alpha thalassemia is:
   a. Point mutation
   b. Insertion
   c. Deletion
   d. All are equally distributed

10. True in beta thalassemia are all, *except*:
    a. Reduced beta chain production
    b. Increased delta chain production
    c. Increased alpha chain production
    d. Increased gamma chain production
    e. All of the above

11. The coinheritance of alpha thalassemia with beta thalassemia:
    a. Increases the severity of symptoms
    b. Decreases the severity of symptoms
    c. Does not effect
    d. Variable effects

12. True regarding blood transfusion in thalassemia are all, *except*:
    a. Pretransfusion hemoglobin level should be 9–10 g/dL
    b. Whole blood should be preferred
    c. Leukocyte depleted blood should be preferred
    d. All of the above

13. True regarding iron overload in thalassemia major patients are all, *except*:
    a. Each unit of transfused blood contains about 200–250 mg iron
    b. Serum hepcidin levels are high
    c. Nontransferrin bound iron is toxic
    d. All of the above are true

14. Side effects of desferrioxamine is:
    a. Retinal toxicity
    b. Growth impairment
    c. *Yersinia enterocolitica* infection
    d. All of the above

15. Drug more effective in reducing cardiac iron overload is:
    a. Desferrioxamine
    b. Deferiprone
    c. Deferasirox
    d. All are equally effective

16. Marked clinical variability in hemoglobin E-beta thalassemia is due to:
   a. Type of beta-thalassemia mutation
   b. Coinheritance of alpha-thalassemia
   c. Serum erythropoietin (EPO) in response to anemia
   d. Associated XMNL polymorphism
   e. All of the above

17. True about alpha thalassemia trait is:
   a. Diagnosed by Hb-HPLC
   b. HbA2 level is low
   c. Asymptomatic splenomegaly is common
   d. None of the above

18. The anemia that is microcytic and hypochromic but not iron deficient is:
   a. Thalassemia
   b. Hereditary spherocytosis
   c. Sickle cell anemia
   d. Hereditary xerocytosis

19. A 21-year-old female is being evaluated for anemia. On examination she had spleen 3 cm below costal margin and liver 2 cm below costal margin. Peripheral blood film showed marked aniso-poikilocytosis with microcytic hypochromic cells, target cells, tear drop cells and 13 nRBCs/100 WBCs. Her CBC and hemoglobin-HPLC are given below.

Complete blood count:

Parameter		Results	Reference range
Hb	(g/dL)	9.8	12–16
RBC	(mill/µL)	5.27	4.20–5.40
PCV	(%)	32.9	37–47
MCV	(fl)	62.4	82–97
MCH	(pg)	18.6	27–33
MCHC	(g/dL)	29.8	32–36
TLC	(per µL)	10,120	4,000–10,000
Platelets	(per µL)	1,60,000	1,50,000–4,50,000
RDW	(%)	26.1	11.5–14.5

HPLC (BioRad "Variant" System—Thalassemia Short Program):

Fraction	Retention time (minutes)	%	Normal range (%)
F	1.17	90.8	0.1–1.5
Hb A	2.44	6.4	
Hb A2	3.62	3.6	1.5–3.5

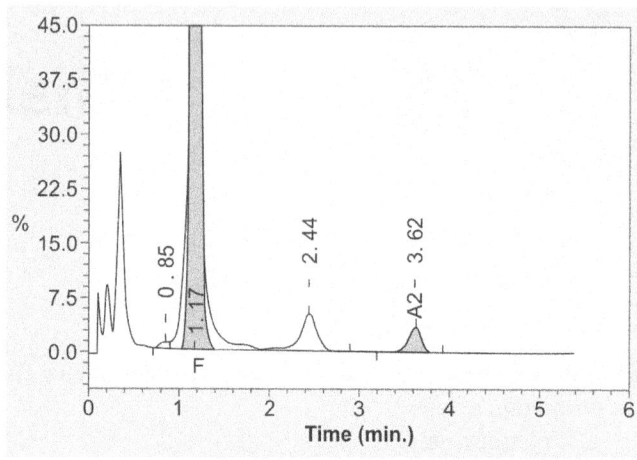

Courtesy: Dr Tina Dadu, MD

What is the probable diagnosis?
   a. Beta-thalassemia intermedia
   b. Homozygous delta-beta thalassemia
   c. Compound heterozygous delta-beta thalassemia and HPFH
   d. Compound heterozygous beta thalassemia with HPFH
   e. All of the above

20. The perinatal screening of a 24-year-old with 5 weeks' gestation revealed the below mentioned CBC and Hb HPLC results. What advice will you give to the patient?

Complete blood count:

Parameter		Results	Reference range
Hb	(g/dL)	12.7	12–16
RBC	(mill/µL)	4.73	4.20–5.40
PCV	(%)	37.7	37–47
MCV	(fl)	79.7	82–97
MCH	(pg)	26.8	27–33
MCHC	(g/dL)	33.6	32–36
TLC	(per µL)	6,520	4,000–10,000
Platelets	(per µL)	2,75,000	1,50,000–4,50,000
RDW	(%)	14.0	11.5–14.5

HPLC (BioRad "Variant" System-beta Thalassemia Short Program):

Fraction	Retention time (minutes)	%	Normal range (%)
F	1.09	5.3	Adult: < 1
P2	1.32	4.0	
P3	1.71	5.1	
Hb A	2.38	83.7	
Hb A2	3.29	2.7	1.9–3.5

a. The female has hereditary persistence of fetal hemoglobin (HPFH) and should undergo termination of pregnancy
b. The patient has thalassemia minor and should undergo chorionic villous sampling for fetal evaluation
c. It is normal and she should be re-assured
d. Patient should be evaluated for rare hematological malignancies

21. An 18-year-old boy presented with generalized weakness and breathlessness on exertion. On physical examination there is mild pallor, mild icterus and spleen tip is palpable. CBC shows Hb of 8.5 g/dL, Hct of 24.1%, MCV of 65 fL, WBC count 10000/cumm and platelet count 2,50,000/cumm. His serum ferritin is 3740 ng/mL. A bone marrow was done which showed M:E ratio of 1:4, and there is 4+ stainable iron. Which of the following is the most likely diagnosis?
a. Beta thalassemia
b. Sickle cell disease
c. Hereditary spherocytosis
d. Anemia of chronic disease
e. Iron deficiency anemia

22. E-beta thalassemia is characterized by all of the following, *except*:
a. Caused by G to A substitution at codon 26 of beta globin gene
b. It behaves like mild beta thalassemia
c. Mahidol score helps in assessing severity
d. It is a structurally abnormal Hb but synthesized at normal rate

23. Which of the following is true about modifiers in beta thalassemia?
a. Coinheritance of alpha thalassemia decreases severity
b. Deletion and nondeletion HPFH muatation having high HbF reduces thalassemia severity
c. Excess of alpha globin genes may increase severity of thalassemia
d. All of the above

ANSWERS WITH EXPLANATIONS

1. Ans. d. Increased osmotic fragility
Ref: Dacie and Lewis 10/e p210

Osmotic fragility is decreased in thalassemia because of unusually flattened RBCs (leptocytes) which are present in thalassemia. The osmotic fragility is decreased since these cells are resistant to osmotic lysis. The remaining three features are characteristically seen in thalassemia if they are not adequately transfused.

2. Ans. a. South-East Asia *Ref: William's 8/e p729-30*

HbE is common in South-East Asia. The highest prevalence of carriers is in some parts of Thailand, in Cambodia and in Laos.

3. Ans. b. Cyprus *Ref: William's 8/e p702*

4. Ans. b. Cardiomyopathy *Ref: William's 8/e p693*

In thalassemia major, death usually occurs in the second or third decade as a result of cardiac siderosis. Cardiac siderosis may cause acute cardiac death with arrhythmia or intractable cardiac failure.

5. Ans. c. β-thalassemia major
Ref: William's 8/e p694, 695, 698

- The child is having β-thalassemia major
- HPFH does not present with severe anemia
- δ-β thalassemia presents with thalassemia intermedia syndrome with presentation in later childhood and not at 6 months of age
- α-thalassemia presents with Hb Bart's hydrops fetalis syndrome and manifests intranatally, but HbH disease can present with severe anemia and behaves such as thalassemia major, but most patients have a much milder course.

6. Ans. b. β-4 tetramers *Ref: William's 7/e p634*

In fetal life, reduced rate of α-chain synthesis results in an excess of γ-4 chains, which form γ-4 tetramers or Hb Bart's. A deficiency of α-chains in adult life, results in an excess of β-chains, which form β-4 tetramers or Hb H.

7. Ans. c. *Yersinia enterocolitica* *Ref: William's 8/e p691*

Yersinia enterocolitica, is normally a nonvirulent pathogen that can produce its own siderophore and hence can thrive in iron excess. *Vibrio vulnificus* and *Listeria* are the other pathogens which are particularly common in iron overload states.

8. Ans. a. Point mutation *Ref: Hoffman 6/e p506*

The vast majority of beta thalassemia mutations are point mutations (i.e. single-base substitutions) and small insertions or deletions of one to two bases. These may involve any step in globin chain production: transcription, translation or post-translational modification of the globin gene product. The beta gene is completely inactivated by approximately half of these mutations with no beta globin production resulting in beta-0 thalassemia. Mutations that allow the production of some beta globin cause beta + or beta ++ thalassemia depending on whether there is a marked or mild reduction in the output of beta chains. The five common mutations—IVS 1-5 G → C, IVS 1-1

G → T, Codon 41/42 (- TCTT), Codon 8/9 and the 619 bp deletion account for over 90% of the mutations in beta-thalassemia patients. The most common beta-thalassemia allele in the Indian population is IVS-I-5 (G → C).

9. Ans. c. Deletion *Ref: Hoffman 6/e p530*

Alpha thalassemia occurs because of mutation leading to reduced production of one or more of the four alpha globin chains. Generally, the alpha globin chains are structurally normal but are produced in reduced quantities. Most alpha thalassemia mutations result in gene deletion; with nondeletional point mutations being less common. As a result of deletions there is a loss of alpha globin chains. The larger the deletions the more is the loss of alpha globin genes (from 1 to 4 alpha chains), the more severe the thalassemia. Molecular analysis of DNA using polymerase chain reaction (PCR) has now replaced hemoglobin H inclusion test. The PCR test can also identify nondeletional point mutations leading to alpha plus thalassemia.

10. Ans. c. Increased alpha chain production *Ref: William's 6/e p696-8*

The molecular defects in beta thalassemia result in absent or reduced beta chain production while alpha chain synthesis is unaffected. The imbalance in globin chain production leads to an excess of alpha chains. The free alpha globin chains are highly unstable and precipitate in red cell precursors, forming intracellular inclusions that interfere with red cell maturation. Those red cells which mature and enter the circulation contain alpha chain inclusions that interfere with their passage through the microcirculation, particularly in the spleen. Cells which make relatively more gamma chains in the bone marrow of beta thalassemics are partly protected against the deleterious effect of alpha chain precipitation. The F cells which produce the gamma chains come under selection in the marrow and peripheral blood and thus individuals with beta thalassemia have variable increases in Hb F due to selective survival of these F cells. The disorder is characterized by a relative or absolute increase in HbA2 (alpha-2–delta-2) production since delta chain synthesis is unaffected.

11. Ans. b. Decreases the severity of symptoms *Ref: William's 6/e p693-4*

Coinheritance of alpha thalassemia reduces chain imbalance and disease severity in individuals who have inherited two copies of beta thalassemia alleles, the increased output of alpha globin through coinheritance of extra alpha globin genes in beta thalassemia heterozygotes increases chain imbalance, converting a typically asymptomatic state to that of thalassemia intermedia.

12. Ans. b. Whole blood should be preferred *Ref: William's 6/e p700-01*

The aim of regular transfusions is to correct anemia and suppress the abnormal erythroid hyperplasia, aiming for a pretransfusion Hb of 9-10 g/dL. This can usually be achieved by regular red cell transfusions every 2-4 weeks, with a post-transfusion Hb target of 13-15 g/dL. Ideally transfusions are with packed red cells Leukodepleted blood reduces the risk of transfusion reactions and cytomegalovirus infection, and should be used where available.

13. Ans. b. Serum hepcidin levels are high *Ref: William's 6/e p700-01*

Each unit of transfused blood contains about 200-250 mg iron (about 1 mg per mL), compared with the 1 mg iron normally absorbed each day. Inspite of the increased iron, serum hepcidin remains inappropriately low, which further contributes to iron loading through increased intestinal iron absorption. Iron is initially stored in macrophages within the liver, and is transferred around the body bound to transferrin. As transferrin becomes saturated, labile, more toxic forms of iron appear in cells and plasma, referred to as nontransferrin bound iron (NTBI). This NTBI is responsible for most of the iron toxicity, including iron loading into cardiac and endocrine tissues. Once in cells, the iron causes oxidative tissue damage, mostly through the generation of free radicals.

14. Ans. d. All of the above *Ref: William's 6/e p701*

Ocular and retinal toxicity, growth impairment, and cartilaginous dysplasia are some of the important side-effects of desferrioxamine. *Yersinia enterocolitica* infection is increased in iron overload, particularly if desferrioxamine is also used [3 O toxicities with desferrioxamine–ocular, osteoporosis, and ototoxicity, 3 A toxicities with deferiprone-agranulocytosis, arthropathy and aspartate aminotransferase/alanine aminotransferase (AST/ALT) elevation].

15. Ans. b. Deferiprone *Ref: William's 6/e p701*

Heart failure mainly related to iron-induced toxicity remains the leading cause of morbidity and mortality in thalassemia major patients. The oral chelating agent deferiprone has been proved to be more effective than subcutaneous desferrioxamine for removing heart iron, measured by T2*MRI, and in improving survival. desferrioxamine and deferasirox appear to be more effective in removing or preventing iron deposition in the liver.

16. Ans. e. All of the above *Ref: William's 6/e p711, Internet*

Hemoglobin E/beta-thalassemia results from coinheritance of a beta-thalassemia allele from one parent and the structural variant Hb E from the other.

Hb E results from a G→A substitution in codon 26 of the β *globin* gene, which produces a structurally abnormal Hb. The disorder is characterized by marked clinical variability, ranging from a mild and asymptomatic anemia to a life-threatening disorder requiring transfusions from infancy. Genetic factors influencing the severity of this disorder include the type of beta-thalassemia mutation, the coinheritance of alpha-thalassemia, and polymorphisms (XMNL) associated with increased production of fetal Hb. Other factors, including a variable increase in serum EPO in response to anemia, previous or ongoing infection with malaria, previous splenectomy and other environmental influences, may be involved. A modified "natural history" study of Hb E/beta-thalassemia in children highlighted the instability of phenotype over the first 10 years of life, during which there was a variable, and changing, pattern of anemia and erythroid expansion. In many patients, the phenotype became more stable later in development, and it was frequently possible to stop blood transfusion in a proportion of older patients with no apparent subsequent effects on activities of daily living, or quality of life. Coinheritance of alpha thalassemia appears to be a major genetic factor modifying clinical phenotype, including the finding that a considerable number of patients who coinherit alpha-thalassemia may be diagnosed later in life. The XMNL polymorphism appears to be an important modifying factor in Hb F synthesis. Chronic hyperbilirubinemia, gallstone formation, and gall bladder disease may significantly worsen the phenotype of patients with Hb E/beta-thalassemia, the inherited variability in the function of the gene for UDP-glucuronosyltransferase-1 (UGT1*1, the enzyme responsible for hepatic glucuronidation of bilirubin) may underlie the chronic hyperbilirubinemia. Changes in EPO responsiveness to severe anemia may also have important implications in Hb E/β-thalassemia. Hb E/beta-thalassemia patients have been divided into five groups—Group 1 included those patients who had undergone only minimal transfusion and had normal growth and sexual maturity; Group 1 children had adequate growth and all patients rated quality of life as exceeding 5 on the 10-point scale. Group 2 comprised patients similar to those in group 1, except for transfusion history: these patients had a longer history of transfusions. Group 3 included patients who had undergone splenectomy with a beneficial response and during the 2 years following splenectomy an improvement in quality of life and increase in height velocity were observed. Group 4 included those patients who, while maintained off transfusions, were struggling as evidenced by poor growth, delayed sexual maturation, and marginal self-reported quality of life (less than 5 on the 10-point scale). Group 5 comprised those patients who were unable to function off transfusions, because of problems similar to those observed in group 4 patients.

17. Ans. d. None of the above   *Ref: Hoffman's 6/e p530-2*

Alpha thalassemia trait is characterized by very mild hypochromic anemia with red cell indices similar to those of beta thalassemia trait; the mean corpuscular hemoglobin (MCH) is less than 25 pg, MCV less than 80 fl and the HbA2 level is normal. Occasional HbH bodies may be present in the red cell on supravital staining. There are no diagnostic tests with which to identify this condition with certainty except DNA analysis. Except for mild anemia no clinical findings are usually present. Hemoglobin electrophoresis is usually normal and not helpful in the differential diagnosis.

18. Ans. a. Thalassemia   *Ref: Hoffman's 6/e p423, 438*

The differential diagnoses for microcytic anemia are—thalassemia, iron deficiency anemia (IDA), sideroblastic anemia, and anemia of chronic disease. In sickle cell anemia, the MCV is usually normal. In both hereditary spherocytosis and xerocytosis the MCV is normal with increased mean corpuscular hemoglobin concentration (MCHC).

19. Ans. e. All of the above

There is a major peak within F window (retention time 1.17 minutes) of 90.8% with markedly reduced Hemoglobin A. In view of CBC findings and above HPLC features, beta-thalassemia syndrome is a likely possibility. Possibilities include: (1) beta-thalassemia intermedia; (2) Homozygous delta-beta thalassemia; (3) Compound heterozygous delta-beta thalassemia and HPFH; (4) Compound heterozygous beta thalassemia with HPFH; (5) Compound heterozygous beta thalassemia with delta-beta thalassemia. Definite diagnosis can be achieved with DNA analysis or amino acid sequencing. Family studies should also be done.

20. Ans. c. It is normal and she should be re-assured

Hemoglobin F is elevated (5.3%). Mild elevation of Hb F (1.0–5.0 %) may be seen (1) sporadically in the general population; (2) some heterozygotes/homozygotes for Hb variant; (3) some hematological disorders; (4) pregnancy; (5) stress hematopoiesis. HbF levels might become slightly increased during pregnancy. This can be due to physiological erythropoietic processes in the mother, eventually associated with the described polymorphisms causing a moderate increase in HbF or HbF cells. A more pronounced increase could, however, be due to a serious fetal-maternal transfusion. Fetal cells from maternal origin can then be distinguished from the fetal cells coming from the fetus by the presence of carbonic anhydrase. HbF may remain elevated after birth due to pathological conditions such as beta-thalassemia major or in potentially pathological beta-thalassemia minor, delta beta-thalassemia, or in non-pathological conditions such as hereditary persistence of fetal hemoglobin (HPFH).

HbF may also become slightly or substantially elevated sometime in life as a consequence of erythropoietic stress, in a number of bone marrow malignancies and in pregnancy.

So, if a an otherwise healthy pregnant lady is found to have raised HbF then:
a. If the level of Hb F is under 5%. The results can be reported as normal.
b. If the level of Hb F is between 5 and 10% and the rest of the woman's hemoglobinopathy screening results are normal. The results can again be reported as normal.
c. A level of Hb F over 10%. This is more unusual and requires follow-up even if everything else is normal. In this case the husband should also be screened for hemoglobinopathy. If the father is not available for testing, the mother can be offered DNA testing to help establish if she has a mutation that might put the child at increased risk. In some women, DNA testing may find that the increased level of Hb F is not caused by a delta beta thalassaemia but by a benign HPFH mutation that does not present any significant health risks to her or her baby.

21. Ans. a. Beta thalassemia *Ref: Hoffman's 6/e p 438, 509*

This child is most likely having beta thalassemia as seen by RBC microcytosis, hypochromia, ineffective erythropoiesis, and excessive iron absorption leading to iron overload. He is most likely having thalassemia intermedia, seeing the age of presentation. Anemia of chronic disease may also have same picture but jaundice and splenomegaly is unusual. There is chronic anemia, because the major hemoglobin A1 is produced insufficiently. The nature of the mutation, typically affecting RNA transcript production, determines the severity of the disease. Hereditary spherocytosis and sickle cell disease will have typical picture on peripheral smear.

22. Ans. d. It is a structurally abnormal Hb but synthesized at normal rate

Hemoglobin E is caused by a G-to-A substitution in codon number 26 of the β-globin gene, which produces a structurally abnormal hemoglobin and an abnormally spliced nonfunctional mRNA. Hemoglobin E is synthesized at a reduced rate and behaves like a mild β+-thalassemia.

23. Ans. d. All of the above
Ref: Danjou F. Genetic modifiers of β-thalassemia and clinical severity as assessed by age at first transfusion. Haematologica, 2012;97:989–93

The extent of globin chain imbalance is the main determinant of clinical severity in β-thalassemia. Therefore, the presence of factors able to reduce the globin chain imbalance results in a milder form of thalassemia. One of the most common and consistent mechanisms is homozygosity or compound heterozygosity for two β+-thalassemia mild and silent mutations. Examples of these alleles are the silent –101 C→T and the mild IVS-1-6 T→C mutation in the Mediterranean population, the –28 A→G in Southeast Asian population and the –29 A→G in Africans. Other factors able to ameliorate the phenotype are the coinheritance of α-thalassemia or of genetic determinants that increase gamma-chain production. Deletion and nondeletion HPFH mutations, associated with a high HbF level in carriers, when in genetic compounds with severe β-thalassemia alleles, result in mild thalassemia intermedia. A mild phenotype may also be determined by co-inheritance of genetic determinants associated with gamma chain production, mapping outside the β-globin cluster. Recently, several studies using genome-wide association studies (G-WAS) have identified two quantitative trait loci (Bcl11A on chromosome 2p16 and HBS1L-MYB intergenic region on chromosome 6q23) that account for 20–30% of the common variation in HbF levels in healthy adults and are associated with the mild thalassemia intermedia phenotype and with a delayed need of transfusions in patients with homozygous β-zero thalassemia. Furthermore, Bcl11A seems to be involved in the regulation of the hemoglobin switching process. In some instances, heterozygous β-thalassemia may lead to the thalassemia intermedia phenotype instead of the asymptomatic carrier state.

Most of these patients have excess functional α-globin genes (α-gene triplication or quadruplication) which increases the imbalance in the ratio of α/non-α globin chain synthesis. Moreover, rare mutations that result in the synthesis of extremely unstable β-globin variants which precipitate in erythroid precursors causing ineffective erythropoiesis may be associated with thalassemia intermedia in the heterozygotes (dominant thalassemia).

CHAPTER 17

Eosinophilic Disorders

1. A patient presented with intermittent hemoptysis for 2 years with peripheral blood showing eosinophil count of 3,000/mm³. X-ray chest is showing multiple nodules and cavitations with bronchoalveolar lavage (BAL) fluid showing eggs. Likely diagnosis:
   a. Chronic eosinophilic leukemia
   b. Löffler's syndrome
   c. Paragonimiasis
   d. Toxoplasmosis

2. Which of the following is not a cause of eosinophilia?
   a. Eczema
   b. Steroid therapy
   c. Hookworm
   d. Hodgkin lymphoma

3. Which of the following will not respond to imatinib?
   a. FIP1L1/PDGFR α-positive chronic eosinophilic leukemia
   b. Chronic myeloid leukemia (CML)
   c. Gastrointestinal stromal tumor
   d. Kit mutation (D816V) positive mast cell neoplasm

4. Which cytokine is not involved in the development and maturation of eosinophils?
   a. Interleukin 3 (IL3)
   b. IL5
   c. IL6
   d. Granulocyte-macrophage colony-stimulating factor (GM-CSF)

5. Severe eosinophilia is defined as absolute eosinophil count more than:
   a. 500/µL
   b. 1,000/µL
   c. 3,000/µL
   d. 5,000/µL

6. Diagnosis of hypereosinophilic syndrome (HES) includes:
   a. A sustained absolute eosinophil count (AEC) >1,500/µL is present, which persists for longer than 4 weeks
   b. No identifiable etiology for eosinophilia is present
   c. Patients must have signs and symptoms of organ involvement
   d. All of the above

7. Treatment of FIP1L1-PDGFRA positive HES patients is:
   a. Vincristine
   b. Imatinib
   c. Prednisolone
   d. Hydroxyurea

8. True about hypereosinophilic syndrome is:
   a. More common in females
   b. More common in black population
   c. More common in elderly
   d. All of the above
   e. None of the above

9. All of the following can lead to eosinophilia, *except*:
   a. Strongyloidosis
   b. Visceral leishmaniasis
   c. Churg-Strauss syndrome
   d. Drug hypersensitivity
   e. Visceral larva migrans (toxocariasis)

10. Which of the following is not a criterion for idiopathic HES?
   a. Eosinophil count ≥1,500/mm³
   b. Absence of reactive causes
   c. Presence of tissue damage
   d. Other clonal myeloid neoplasms have been ruled out
   e. Presence of PDGFR mutation

ANSWERS WITH EXPLANATIONS

1. Ans. c. Paragonimiasis
Ref: Barruentos MA. NEJM. 2012;366

Features are of lung fluke infection, *Paragonimus westermani*. Eggs are not found in Löffler's syndrome (Immunologic phenomenon), toxoplasma. Chronic eosinophilic leukemia does not have infective pathology.

2. Ans. b. Steroid therapy *Ref: Williams 8/e p905*

Eosinophilia is defined as AEC is >500/mm³. Mild is 500–1,500/mm³, moderate is 1,500–5,000/mm³ and severe is >5,000/mm³. Causes of eosinophilia can be primary or secondary. Secondary is usually due to allergy, worm infestation or hematological malignancies (T cell lymphomas or Hodgkin lymphoma).

3. Ans. d. Kit mutation (D816V) positive mast cell neoplasm
Ref: Hoffman 6/e p1109

Mast cell neoplasm with kit mutation (D816V) is predictive of nonresponse, otherwise imatinib has very good response.

4. Ans. c. IL6
Ref: William's 8/e p899

Three cytokines: IL3, IL5, and GM-CSF are involved in eosinophil development and maturation. These three hemopoietic growth signaling polypeptides are encoded by genes linked on chromosome 5, produced by T-helper cells. IL5 is considered to be the most important eosinophilopoietin. It is in particular IL5 which mobilizes eosinophils from the bone marrow to the blood.

5. Ans. d. 5,000/μL
Ref: William's 8/e p904

Blood eosinophil count above the upper reference limit (in adults more than 500/μL) is the hallmark of eosinophilia. Eosinophilia is considered as mild if blood AEC is 500–1,500/μL, moderate if the count is between 1,500 and 5,000/μL and severe, if the count is more than 5,000/μL. The most common cause of eosinophilia in the western world is allergy and in the developing countries invasive parasite infections.

6. Ans. d. All of the above
Ref: William's 8/e p907

The idiopathic HES is defined (Chusid's criteria) as—(1) persistent eosinophilia of more than 1,500 μL for longer than 6 months, or death before 6 months associated with signs and symptoms of hyper eosinophilic disease; (2) a lack of evidence for parasites, allergies, or other known causes of eosinophilia; and (3) presumptive signs and symptoms of organ involvement. Despite aggressive therapy, some patients with HES developed severe, often fatal complications, including endomyocardial fibrosis and neurologic involvement. Hypereosinophilic syndrome induces organ damage due to the eosinophilic infiltration of the tissues accompanied by the mediator release from the eosinophil granules. Hence, organ damage is not truly reflected by the level of eosinophilia. Patients presenting with potentially life-threatening complications, including cardiac or neurologic involvement, and marked eosinophilia should be treated empirically with high-dose corticosteroids (e.g. intravenous methylprednisolone at a dose of 1 mg/kg per day) to prevent progression of end-organ damage. The mainstay of treatment for symptomatic idiopathic HES, whether constant or episodic, remains glucocorticoids, though imatinib, hydroxyurea, and vincristine have also been used.

7. Ans. b. Imatinib
Ref: William's 8/e p909

The best described clonal aberration is the interstitial deletion on chromosome 4q12, resulting in fusion of the 5′ portion of the *FIP1L1* gene to the 3′ portion of the *PDGFRA* gene. This fusion gene encodes for the FIP1L1-PDGFR alpha protein, the constitutively activated tyrosine kinase activity that induces eosinophilia. Patients with HES with the PDGFRA mutation have a very high incidence of cardiac involvement and carry a bad prognosis without therapy. Fortunately, imatinib therapy in such cases of HES gives results which are very encouraging. The FIP1L1-PDGFRA fusion is 50-fold more sensitive to imatinib than BCR/ABL, and molecular remission can be maintained in most patients with FIP1L1-PDGFRA positive disease with low doses of imatinib (as little as 100 mg/week in some series). Nevertheless, data from CML suggest that initiation of therapy with higher doses (e.g. 400 mg/day) leads to longer remission. Thus, it seems prudent to initiate therapy with imatinib 400 mg/day and to taper the dose only after a complete and stable clinical, hematologic, and molecular remission has been achieved. Because of cardiac side-effects, it is recommended that patients with known cardiac manifestations or an elevated serum troponin should receive high-dose corticosteroids during the first 2 weeks of imatinib therapy.

8. Ans. e. None of the above
Ref: William's 8/e p907-09

There is a male predominance in HES, with a male-to-female ratio of 9:1. HES is most commonly diagnosed in patients aged 20–50 years, with a peak incidence in the fourth decade. It is rare in children. The incidence of HES seems to decrease in the elderly population. No racial predilection is reported for HES.

9. Ans. b. Visceral leishmaniasis
Ref: Barruentos MA. NEJM. 2012 p366

The recognized causes of reactive eosinophilia are:
- Filarial worms
- Tapeworms
- Strongyloidosis
- Toxocariasis (visceral larva migrans)
- Schistosomiasis
- Trichinella spiralis
- Intestinal nematodes
- Hydatid disease
- Hookworm
- Fascioliasis
- Tropical pulmonary eosinophilia (usually results from hypersensitivity to microfilariae).

10. Ans. e. Presence of PDGFR mutation
Ref: WHO Classification, Revised 4/e p56

Idiopathic HES can be diagnosed only in fully investigated patients and only when:
- Eosinophil count ≥1,500/mm³ persisting for ≥6 months
- Reactive eosinophilia have been ruled out after thorough investigations
- Other clonal myeloid neoplasms have been ruled out, e.g., acute myeloid leukemia (AML), MPN, MDS, MDS/MPN overlap syndromes, and systemic mastocytosis
- A cytokine-producing immunophenotypically aberrant T-cell population has been excluded
- Tissue damage as a result of hypereosinophilia.

If criteria 1–4 are met but there is no tissue damage, the appropriate diagnosis is idiopathic hypereosinophilia.

CHAPTER 18

Neutrophilic Disorders

1. An 1-year-old child presented with history of recurrent pneumonia, otitis media, and sinusitis. He was found to have neutropenia with normal hemoglobin and platelet count. He also had family history of similar illness in mother. Peripheral smear showed neutrophils with pyknotic nuclei abnormal thin filaments connecting lobes and cytoplasmic lobulation. Most likely diagnosis is:
   a. Kostmann syndrome
   b. Myelokathexis
   c. Cyclical neutropenia
   d. Shwachman–Diamond syndrome

2. Which of the following granulocyte stage is not capable of division (mitosis)?
   a. Myelocyte
   b. Promyelocyte
   c. Metamyelocytes
   d. Myeloblast

3. Specific/secondary granules appear at which stage of granulocyte development?
   a. Myeloblast
   b. Metamyelocyte
   c. Myelocyte
   d. Promyelocyte

4. Hypersegmented neutrophils are seen in all of the following, *except*:
   a. Vitamin B_{12} and folate deficiency
   b. Patient on hydroxyurea
   c. Glucocorticoid therapy
   d. Chronic myeloid leukemia (CML)

5. Which of the following is not found in primary granules?
   a. Myeloperoxidase (MPO)
   b. Elastase
   c. Proteinase-3
   d. Lactoferrin

6. Which of the following is found in all the types of granules in granulocytic stages (viz., primary, secondary, and tertiary)?
   a. Defensin
   b. Myeloperoxidase
   c. Lysozyme
   d. Lactoferrin

7. Which of the following organisms do not cause infection in chronic granulomatous disease (CGD) patients?
   a. *Pneumococci*
   b. *Staphylococci*
   c. *Escherichia coli*
   d. *Klebsiella*

8. Treatment of chronic idiopathic neutropenia of adults is:
   a. Steroids
   b. Granulocyte-colony stimulating factor (G-CSF)
   c. Cyclosporine
   d. Folic acid

9. Risk of invasive aspergillosis is maximum, if:
   a. Neutropenia duration <7 days
   b. Neutropenia duration 7–10 days
   c. Neutropenia duration >10 days
   d. None of the above

10. Cytoplasm of mature neutrophil contains:
    a. Primary granules
    b. Secondary granules
    c. Both
    d. None of the above

11. Myeloperoxidase is:
    a. Located in primary and secondary granules of neutrophils
    b. A lipophilic dye
    c. Not inhibited by heparin
    d. Not seen in eosinophilic granule

12. Primary (azurophilic) granules start appearing at which stage of granulocyte development?
    a. Promyelocyte
    b. Myeloblast
    c. Metamyelocyte
    d. Myelocyte

13. G-CSF increases the neutrophil by all of these mechanisms, *except*:
    a. Induction of neutrophil differentiation
    b. Suppression of apoptosis of myeloid cells
    c. Increased neutrophil proliferation
    d. Reduction in self-renewal capacity of hematopoietic stem cells

14. Neutrophil alkaline phosphatase activity is found in:
    a. Neutrophil
    b. Eosinophil
    c. Myeloblast
    d. Monocyte

15. Which is not true about neutropenia?
    a. Found in aplastic anemia
    b. May be associated with rheumatoid arthritis (RA)
    c. Associated with mouth ulcers
    d. Can be caused by ibuprofen

16. Which of the following is not true of neutrophilia?
 a. Trauma
 b. Myocardial infarction
 c. Steroid therapy
 d. Asthma

17. The abnormality of failure of neutrophil to form more than two segments is:
 a. Pelger-Huet anomaly
 b. May-Hegglin anomaly
 c. Alder-Reilly anomaly
 d. Chediak-Higashi anomaly

18. Hypersegmented, macrocytic neutrophils are seen in:
 a. Pelger-Huet anomaly
 b. Pernicious anemia
 c. Acute myelogenous leukemia (AML)
 d. Acute lymphoblastic leukemia

19. May-Hegglin like inclusions containing rough endoplasmic reticulum are:
 a. Döhle bodies
 b. Auer rods
 c. Barr body
 d. Y tag

ANSWERS WITH EXPLANATIONS

1. Ans. b. Myelokathexis *Ref: Williams 8/e p941*

The peripheral smear findings are typical of myelokathexis. Myelokathexis (from the Greek, meaning 'retained in the bone marrow') is a congenital disorder associated with severe chronic neutropenia. Bone marrow (BM) shows maturation arrest with absent band forms and neutrophils. Caused by mutation in *CXCR 4* gene and inherited as autosomal-dominant pattern.

Kostmann syndrome is also an autosomal dominant disease with BM showing maturation arrest but the characteristic peripheral smear findings on neutrophils will be absent.

Cyclical neutropenia is characterized by the presence of typical cyclical pattern of neutropenia every 21 days. This also manifests as autosomal dominant inheritance pattern. Neutropenic period usually lasts 3-6 days with fever, malaise, oral ulcerations, and cervical lymphadenopathy.

2. Ans. c. Metamyelocytes *Ref: Williams 8/e p891*

Myeloblasts, promyelocytes, and myelocytes are capable of replication and constitute the mitotic compartment of marrow neutrophils. Metamyelocytes, bands and mature neutrophils, none of which replicate, constitute the maturation storage compartment.

3. Ans. c. Myelocyte *Ref: Williams 8/e p891*

During the myelocyte stage, normal specific granules appear.

4. Ans. d. Chronic myeloid leukemia
 Ref: Williams 8/e p895

Hypersegmentation of neutrophils is a characteristic of vitamin B_{12} and folate, but can also be seen after hydroxyurea and glucocorticoid therapy and iron-deficiency anemia in children.

5. Ans. d. Lactoferrin *Ref: Williams 8/e p883-4*

Primary or azurophilic granules contain MPO, lysosomal enzymes, elastase, proteinase-3 and α1-antitrypsin, defensins, azurophill-derived bactericidal factors, and bactericidal permeability increasing protein. Lactoferrin is present in secondary or specific granules. Peroxidase, lysozyme, B_{12}-binding proteins, and other proteins are the other contents of secondary granules.

6. Ans. c. Lysozyme *Ref: Williams 8/e p884*

Lysozyme is present in all three types of granules viz. primary, secondary, and tertiary.

7. Ans. a. *Pneumococci* *Ref: Williams 8/e p976*

Chronic granulomatous disease is the most commonly encountered immunodeficiency involving the phagocyte, and is characterized by repeated infections with bacterial and fungal pathogens, as well as the formation of granulomas in tissue. The disease is the result of a disorder of the NADPH oxidase system, culminating in an inability of the phagocyte to generate superoxide, leading to the defective killing of pathogenic organisms. This can lead to infections with *Staphylococcus aureus*, *Psedomonas* species, *Nocardia* species, and fungi (such as *Aspergillus* species and *Candida albicans*).

8. Ans. b. Granulocyte-colony stimulating factor (G-CSF) *Ref: Williams 8/e p942*

Chronic idiopathic neutropenia predominantly affects young adult women aged 18–35 years (female to male ratio: 8:1). The condition is acquired. Erythrocytes, reticulocytes, and platelets are normal. Marrow shows normal cellularity to selective hypoplasia of neutrophil series. It is the result of accelerated apoptosis of neutrophils and their precursors mediated via the Fas-ligand or interferon-γ.

9. Ans. c. Neutropenia duration >10 days
 Ref: IDSA Guidelines

Risk of invasive aspergillosis or any other fungal infection is unusual if the expected duration of neutropenia is <7 days. The risk of infection increases with the duration of neutropenia, so the best option here is c with neutropenia duration >10 days.

10. Ans. c. Both *Ref: Williams 8/e p884*

Mature neutrophils contain primary, secondary, tertiary granules, and secretory vesicles.

11. Ans. c. Not inhibited by heparin
Ref: Williams 8/e p884; Dacie and Lewis 10/e p318-20

Secondary (specific) granules by definition do not contain peroxidase, and thus specific granules are also called peroxidase negative granules. MPO in eosinophilic granules is cyanide resistant. 3,3′-diaminobenzidine is the preferred chromogen used in MPO staining. MPO is not inhibited by heparin, oxalate, or ethylenediaminetetraacetic acid. Films should be made within 12 hours of sample collection.

12. Ans. a. Promyelocyte
Ref: Williams 8/e p875; Hoffman 6/e p281

In the promyelocyte stage, the azurophilic or primary granules, which are large peroxidase positive granules that stain metachromatically (reddish-purple) with a polychromatic stain such as Wright stain, are formed.

13. Ans. d. Reduction in self-renewal capacity of hematopoietic stem cells
Ref: Hoffman 6/e p282-3

The major role of G-CSF is thought to be induction of neutrophil proliferation and differentiation. G-CSF delays neutrophil apoptosis by inhibition of calpains upstream of caspase-3.

14. Ans. a. Neutrophil
Ref: Dacie and Lewis 10/e p320-2

Alkaline phosphatase activity is predominantly found in mature neutrophils with some activity in metamyelocytes. Other leukocytes are generally negative. Cytochemically demonstrable activity may be seen in some lymphoid malignancies. BM macrophages are positive.

The reaction is graded from 0 to 4 depending on the intensity of staining, so the overall possible score ranges from 0 to 400 per 100 cells. Normal range varies from laboratory to laboratory. In normal individuals, it is rare to find any neutrophil with a score of 3, and a score of 4 should not be present.

15. Ans. d. Can be caused by ibuprofen
Ref: Williams 8/e p943, 945

Neutropenia is associated with RA only in 3% cases. Felty syndrome comprises leukopenia, deforming RA, and splenomegaly. Indomethacin, phenylbutazone, phenytoin, carbamazepine, and antithyroid drugs are the common drugs associated with neutropenia.

16. Ans. d. Asthma
Ref: Williams 8/e p943, 947

The causes of neutrophilia can be divided into acute and chronic.

Acute	Chronic
Physical stimuli: Cold, heat, exercise, pain, labor, seizure	Infections
Emotional stress: Panic, rage, stress	*Inflammation*: Colitis, dermatitis, nephritis, RA, rheumatic fever
Infections: Acute bacterial, mycotic, rickettsial, spirochetal	*Tumors*: Gastric, bronchogenic, breast, renal, uterine, squamous cell carcinoma
Inflammation: Burns, electric shock, trauma, infarction, vasculitis	*Drugs*: Lithium
Drugs: G-CSF, epinephrine, steroids, smoking tobacco	*Hematologic*: Asplenia, myeloproliferative disorders, chronic hemolysis

17. Ans. a. Pelger-Huet anomaly
Ref: Dacie and Lewis 10/e p106-07

The Pelger-Huet anomaly is a benign inherited condition in which neutrophil nuclei fail to segment properly. The majority of neutrophils have only two discrete equal sized lobes connected by a thin chromatin bridge. A similar acquired anomaly, known as pseudo-Pelger cells or the acquired Pelger-Huet anomaly, is seen in myelodysplastic syndromes, AML with dysplasia, or the chronic granulocytic leukemia.

18. Ans. b. Pernicious anemia
Ref: Hoffman's 6/e p175-6

Hypersegmented and big neutrophils are characteristically seen in megaloblastic anemia and is an early sign. Red blood cells have increased mean corpuscular volume and PS show macrocytosis with macro-ovalocytosis.

19. Ans. a. Döhle bodies
Ref: Dacie and Lewis 10/e p105

In May-Hegglin anomaly, Döhle bodies like inclusions are seen in all leukocytes except lymphocytes. Döhle bodies are small, round or oval, blue-gray structures found at the periphery of neutrophil. They consist of ribosomes and endoplasmic reticulum.

CHAPTER 19

Hemophilia and Other Coagulation Factor Defects

1. Which factor has the shortest half-life?
   a. VII
   b. VIII
   c. V
   d. XIII

2. Joint hematoma (hemarthrosis) can be seen in all, *except*:
   a. Hemophilia A
   b. Hemophilia B
   c. Bernard-Soulier syndrome (BSS)
   d. Type III von Willebrand disease (VWD)

3. Recurrent abortions are seen in:
   a. Factor IX deficiency
   b. Factor XIII deficiency
   c. von Willebrand disease
   d. Factor VIII deficiency

4. All of the following can be done in a patient of severe hemophilia A with inhibitor presenting with major bleeding, *except*:
   a. Recombinant factor VII
   b. Porcine factor VIII concentrate
   c. Immune tolerance therapy
   d. Intermediate purity plasma-derived factor VIII

5. Treatment of factor VIII deficiency can be done with all of the following, *except*:
   a. Cryoprecipitate
   b. Fresh blood
   c. Factor VIII concentrate
   d. Fresh frozen plasma (FFP)

6. A 15-year-old girl presented with menorrhagia since menarche and also has history of gum bleeding, purpura, and prolonged bleeding from cut injury. His brother is also having similar complaints from cut injury. On evaluation, his factor VIII level is 15% and vW:Ag level is 60 IU/mL. What is the diagnosis of this patient?
   a. Type 2B VWD
   b. Type 2N VWD
   c. Type 3 VWD
   d. Type 1 VWD

7. The chances of the daughter of a severe hemophilia A to be a carrier are:
   a. 75%
   b. 25%
   c. 50%
   d. 100%

8. A 65-year-old woman planned for cataract surgery. She is having history of prolonged bleeding after dental extraction for which she was given 2 units of blood. Her one sibling died of postoperative hemorrhage during childhood. There is history of prolonged bleeding in a number of relatives, both males and females. During preanesthetic workup, her prothrombin time (PT) is normal, activated partial thromboplastin time (APTT) is markedly prolonged, and bleeding time is normal. The most likely diagnosis is deficiency of:
   a. Factor VII
   b. Factor VIII
   c. Factor XI
   d. Factor XII

9. A 15-year-old girl develops massive bleeding from a wound site 4 weeks after a large cyst has been removed from her right thigh. Local measures to control bleeding were unsuccessful. There is no family history of increased bleeding. Her PT, APTT, thrombin time (TT), platelet count, and bleeding time are normal. Which of the following tests is to be ordered further?
   a. Factor IX assay
   b. Factor XII assay
   c. Urea clot lysis test
   d. Mixing studies

10. In a patient of type III VWD, the treatment of choice is:
    a. Intermediate purity plasma-derived factor VIII
    b. Fresh frozen plasma
    c. Highly purified plasma-derived factor VIII
    d. DDAVP

11. Which of the following is not true about stabilization of platelet plug by fibrin?
    a. Plasminogen and tissue plasminogen activator (tPA) stabilize the clot
    b. Platelets provide membrane phospholipids to accelerate coagulation cascade
    c. Thrombin generated at injury site converts fibrinogen to insoluble fibrin
    d. After vascular injury, formation of extrinsic X-ase complex initiates coagulation

12. Which of the following drugs cause thrombocytopenia?
    a. Heparin
    b. Amphotericin B
    c. Imipenem
    d. Paracetamol
    e. All of the above

13. Which of the following is not indicated for the treatment of idiopathic thrombocytopenic purpura (ITP)?
    a. Rituximab
    b. Eltrombopag
    c. Cyclosporine
    d. Vincristine
    e. Cytosine

14. Hereditary hemorrhagic telangiectasia is associated with:
    a. Gastrointestinal (GI) bleeding
    b. Thrombocytopenia
    c. Renal failure
    d. Intracranial bleed

15. Which of the following statements is not true regarding treatment of hemophilia A?
    a. Plasma-derived factors should be heat and solvent-detergent treated
    b. Cryoprecipitate is the treatment of choice
    c. DDAVP infusion can raise the factor VIII level by—two to four times
    d. Factor VIII concentrate is given twice-daily dose

16. Which of the following statements is not correct about VWD?
    a. It is the most common inherited bleeding disorder and has autosomal dominant inheritance
    b. Cryoprecipitate is the treatment of choice in most cases
    c. VWD has an associated low factor VIII level
    d. It may be of a quantitative or a qualitative defect

17. Which of the following is true about vitamin K deficiency?
    a. Vitamin K is abundant in meat products
    b. Breastfed babies are at a less risk of hemorrhagic disease of newborn
    c. Hemorrhagic disease of newborn has a peak incidence from 2nd to 4th day of life
    d. There is prolongation of PT and with normal APTT
    e. Vitamin K is required for glycosylation of II, VII, IX, X, and proteins C and S

18. Which of the following is not true regarding thromboelastography (TEG)?
    a. It can be used as the only test for primary hemostatic disorder
    b. It is used for global assessment for hemostasis
    c. r-time presents the time of latency from the start of test to initial fibrin formation
    d. α-angle measures the speed of fibrin build-up and cross-linking

19. A 17-year-old girl underwent tonsillectomy at the age of 3 years and had no bleeding. Now she is planned for elective major surgery and during preanesthetic workup, she was found to be having prolonged APTT with normal PT. There is no family history of any bleeding diathesis. The diagnosis is:
    a. Factor XII deficiency
    b. Mild hemophilia A
    c. Hemophilia B Leiden
    d. Liver disease

20. A 36-year-old female presented with prolonged APTT with normal PT and platelet count. There is no history of any bleeding. She had a major surgery done 3 years ago without any bleeding complication. What next test should be done in this patient?
    a. Factor VIII assay
    b. Ristocetin cofactor assay
    c. Dilute Russell's viper venom time (dRVVT)
    d. Factor X assay

21. Which of the following tests may help in differentiating hemophilia A from VWD?
    a. Prothrombin time
    b. APTT
    c. Bleeding time
    d. Factor VIII levels

22. Bleeding in disseminated intravascular coagulation (DIC) is due to:
    a. Raised thrombin time
    b. Low fibrinogen levels
    c. Raised fibrin degradation product (FDP) levels in blood
    d. Prolonged prothrombin time

23. All of the following hematological malignancies are associated with DIC, *except*:
    a. Acute promyelocytic leukemia
    b. Acute myeloid leukemia (AML) with t(9;11)
    c. Acute lymphocytic leukemia (ALL) with t(9;22)
    d. Aggressive natural killer (NK) cell leukemia

24. A neonate is born with a large cephalohematoma after full-term normal vaginal delivery. His screening coagulogram is showing normal PT and platelet count with prolonged APTT. There is no family history of any bleeding. The preferred next course of action would be:
    a. Desmopressin
    b. Collect sample for specific factor assay and give FFP
    c. Recombinant factor VIII as hemophilia A is most likely
    d. Give vitamin K

25. An elderly gentleman is diagnosed with amyloid light-chain (AL) amyloidosis. His screening coagulogram shows prothrombin time 20 seconds (normal 12 seconds), APTT 48 seconds (normal 35 seconds), and thrombin time 18 seconds (normal 19 seconds). What is the most likely explanation for this coagulation abnormality?
    a. Factor X deficiency
    b. Prothrombin deficiency
    c. Combined factor V and VII deficiency
    d. Factor V deficiency

26. Heparin inhibits the blood from clotting by inactivating:
    a. Thrombin
    b. Platelet
    c. Fibrinogen
    d. Ionized calcium

27. A 12-year-old boy presented with bleeding into the gums while brushing and occasional epistaxis. On examination, he was also found to have some skin bruises. On evaluation, he was found to be having normal platelet count and PT. The bleeding time and APTT are prolonged. The most likely diagnosis is:
    a. Liver disease
    b. von Willebrand disease
    c. Glanzmann thrombasthenia
    d. Bernard-Soulier disease

28. Mechanism of action of luspatercept is as follows:
    a. JAK 2 inhibition
    b. HbF induction
    c. Activin receptor trap ligand
    d. Immunomodulation

29. Emicizumab is used for the treatment of:
    a. Newly diagnosed hemophilia B
    b. Hemophilia A with inhibitors
    c. ITP
    d. Factor XIII deficiency

30. Mechanism of action of emicizumab is:
    a. Factor X activation
    b. Monoclonal antibody which brings factors IX and V together
    c. Monoclonal antibody which brings factors IX and X together
    d. Factor XI upregulation

31. Fitusiran is a drug used for hemophilia which is a:
    a. Small interfering RNA (siRNA)
    b. mRNA
    c. Monoclonal antibody
    d. Nanobody

32. Hemophilia C is due to deficiency of:
    a. Factor IX
    b. Factor VIII
    c. Factor X
    d. Factor XI

33. Concizumab is:
    a. Anti-tissue factor pathway inhibitor (anti-TFPI)
    b. Anti-AT
    c. Anti-factor V
    d. Anti-allophycocyanin (anti-APC)

34. Frequency of hemophilia is about:
    a. 1 in 1,000 births
    b. 1 in 10,000 births
    c. 1 in 50,000 births
    d. 1 in 100,000 births

35. Spontaneous mutations resulting in hemophilia are seen in what percentage of patients?
    a. 5%
    b. 10%
    c. 20%
    d. 30%

36. The triad of groin pain, hip flexure, and cutaneous sensory loss over the femoral nerve distribution is seen in:
    a. Sickle cell anemia
    b. Myelofibrosis
    c. Hemophilia
    d. Lymphoma
    e. Avascular necrosis of hip

37. Which of the following statements is false?
    a. Levels of factor VIII increase significantly in pregnancy
    b. Immediate female relatives (mother, sisters, and daughters) of a person with hemophilia should have their clotting factor level checked, especially prior to any invasive intervention or if any symptoms occur
    c. Menorrhagia and bleeding after medical interventions are the most common manifestations among carriers with significantly low factor levels
    d. All of the above

38. True about FVIII assay is:
    a. It can be a one-stage assay
    b. It can be a two-stage assay
    c. It can be a chromogenic FVIII assay
    d. It is a modified APTT-based assay
    e. All of the above

39. The dose of factors VIII and IX needed to raise the plasma levels of respective factors is calculated by: Dose to be infused (IU) = Weight (kg) × Desired rise (IU/dL) × K,
    where K for FVIII and FIX, respectively, is:
    a. 0.5 and 1
    b. 1 and 0.5
    c. 1 and 2
    d. 2 and 1

40. True about desmopressin is:
    a. It acts on hepatocytes
    b. Effective in mild deficiency of both FVIII and FIX
    c. Given at a dose of 0.3 µg/kg body weight either by slow intravenous infusion over 20 minutes or by subcutaneous injection
    d. All of the above

41. True about development of FVIII inhibitors is:
    a. Most common in patients with mild-to-moderate hemophilia A
    b. Most likely to develop in the elderly
    c. Dependent on the underlying FVIII mutation
    d. All of the above

42. Desmopressin raises FVIII levels by:
    a. 1–2 times
    b. 3–6 times
    c. 6–10 times
    d. 10–15 times

43. Which of the following is true about hemophilia A?
    a. Prophylaxis was conceived from the observation that moderate hemophilia patients with clotting factor level >1 IU/dL seldom experience spontaneous bleeding and have much better preservation of joint function

b. Prophylaxis prevents bleeding and joint destruction and should be the goal of therapy to preserve normal musculoskeletal function
c. Prophylactic replacement of clotting factor has been shown to be useful even when factor levels are not maintained above 1 IU/dL at all times
d. All of the above

44. Secondary prophylaxis in hemophilia is:
a. Regular continuous treatment initiated in the absence of documented osteochondral joint disease, determined by physical examination and/or imaging studies, and started before the second clinically evident large joint bleed and age 3 years
b. Regular continuous treatment started after two or more bleeds into large joints and before the onset of joint disease documented by physical examination and imaging studies
c. Regular continuous treatment started after the onset of joint disease documented by physical examination and plain radiographs of the affected joints
d. Treatment given to prevent bleeding for periods not exceeding 45 weeks in a year

45. The dose of factors used in Malmö protocol is:
a. 10–25 IU/kg per dose   b. 25–40 IU/kg per dose
c. 40–60 IU/kg per dose   d. 60–80 IU/kg per dose

46. All of the following are the obligate carriers of hemophilia, *except*:
a. Daughters of a person with hemophilia
b. Mother of one son with hemophilia and who have at least one other family member with hemophilia
c. Sisters of two or more brothers with hemophilia
d. Mothers of two or more sons with hemophilia

47. True about the Nijmegen assay is:
a. Factor VIII assay   b. Factor IX assay
c. FVIII inhibitor assay
d. Less specific than Bethesda assay

48. True about FVIII treatment is:
a. Each unit of FVIII/kg infused intravenously raises the plasma FVIII level approximately by 2 IU/dL
b. The half-life of FVIII is approximately 8–12 hours
c. The patient's factor level should be measured 15 minutes after the infusion to verify the calculated dose
d. All of the above

49. True about emicizumab are all, *except*:
a. Is a monoclonal antibody against FVIII inhibitor
b. Has long half-life
c. Can be given subcutaneously
d. All of the above

ANSWERS WITH EXPLANATIONS

1. Ans. a. VII   *Ref: William's 8/e p1816 (Table)*

Factor VII has the shortest half-life of approximately 3–6 hours.

2. Ans. c. Bernard-Soulier syndrome (BSS)
Ref: William's 8/e p1885

Bernard-Soulier syndrome is an inherited platelet disorder, which is transmitted in an autosomal recessive manner. This syndrome is characterized by variable thrombocytopenia and large defective platelets. BSS often presents early with bleeding symptoms, such as epistaxis, ecchymosis, menometrorrhagia, and gingival or GI bleeding. Diagnosis can be confirmed by platelet aggregation studies and flow cytometry. Joint bleedings are usually not a feature of BSS.

3. Ans. b. Factor XIII deficiency
Ref: William's 8/e p2044

Bleeding from the umbilical cord stump during the first few days of life is common and intracranial hemorrhage is more commonly seen than in other bleeding disorders. Ecchymosis, muscle hematomas, hemarthrosis, delayed wound healing, and recurrent abortions are also common in factor XIII deficiency.

4. Ans. d. Intermediate purity plasma-derived factor VIII   *Ref: William's 8/e p2022, Table-124.6*

The various treatment options available in a patient of hemophilia A with inhibitor are:
- Recombinant factor VII
- FEIBA (factor eight inhibitor bypass activity)
- Prothrombin complex concentrates
- Porcine factor VIII concentrates
- Immune tolerance therapy.

5. Ans. b. Fresh blood   *Ref: William's 8/e p2018*

Cryoprecipitate contains approximately 80 units of factor VIII per 10 mL and is used for the treatment of bleeding in hemophilia A. Fresh whole blood is not recommended for any condition nowadays. In order to control the bleeding, both recombinant and plasma-derived factor VIII can be used. Recombinant factors are preferred but have high cost.
Fresh frozen plasma can be used, but it has the disadvantage of large volume and at a time the plasma level can only be raised by 20%.

6. Ans. b. Type 2N VWD   *Ref: Hoffman 5/e p1995*

A normal level of von Willebrand factor (VWF), a decreased level of factor VIII, and evidence against X-linked inheritance suggest a diagnosis of VWD type 2N, although assays of factor VIII-VWF binding (VWF:F VIII B) may be necessary to exclude hemophilia A. In VWD type 2N, the ratio FVIII:C/VWF:Ag generally is <0.5. This ratio in the present patient is 0.25 (15/60).

7. Ans. d. 100%

Male persons have only 1 X chromosome and in hemophiliacs, this single X chromosome carries the hemophilic gene. All females inherit one X from the father, so the chances of the daughter of a hemophilic being carrier are 100%.

8. Ans. c. Factor XI   *Ref: William's 8/e p2041-2, 1887*

Most bleeding in homozygotes and compound heterozygotes are injury related. Excessive bleeding can occur at the time of injury or begin several hours and days after trauma. Some may not even bleed after trauma. These patients have normal PT and platelet count with prolonged APTT.

9. Ans. c. Urea clot lysis test

Ref: William's 8/e p2044, 1887

This patient is having characteristic history of delayed bleeding from trauma after 4 weeks with normal PT, APTT, TT, and platelet count, which is typically seen in factor XIII deficiency. Because of increased fibrin breakdown, levels of FDP may be increased which can lead to minimally prolonged TT and this could be the clue to diagnosis.

10. Ans. a. Intermediate purity plasma-derived factor VIII   *Ref: William's 8/e p2081*

Heat-inactivated solvent-detergent-treated plasma-derived factor VIII is the treatment of choice in type 3 VWD and in the patients unresponsive to DDAVP. Humate P and Alphanate are both commercially acceptable VWF-containing plasma concentrates.

Fresh frozen plasma is not a better option because larger volumes are required for a desirable effect.

Highly purified and recombinant factor VIII concentrates do not contain VWF, so they are not advised. DDAVP usually does not work in type 3 VWD.

11. Ans. a. Plasminogen and tissue plasminogen activator (tPA) stabilize the clot

Ref: William's 8/e p2220-2222, 1835-8

Tissue plasminogen activator and urokinase plasminogen activator (UPA) are activators of plasminogen and convert it to plasmin which degrades fibrin polymer to FDPs.

$$\text{Plasminogen} \xrightarrow[\text{(PAI-1)}]{\text{tPA or UPA}} \text{Plasmin}$$

$$\text{Fibrin} \xrightarrow[\text{(PAI-2)}]{(\alpha 2\text{-antiplasmin})} \text{FDPs}$$

Platelets provide phospholipids which accelerate the coagulation cascade. The phosphatidyl serine present on the inner membrane moves to the outer membrane by the flip-flop mechanism once platelets are activated. Extrinsic X-ase complex (TF/VIIa) in the presence of IXa Ca^{2+} which is formed at the site of injury converts X to Xa and converts prothrombin to thrombin (I to Ia) which further clears fibrinogen to fibrin. Intrinsic X-ase is IXa/VIIIa.

12. Ans. e. All of the above   *Ref: William's 8/e p1914*

Drugs causing thrombocytopenia are gold, quinidine, quinine, heparin, amphotericin B, linezolid, and paracetamol though many other drugs have also been implicated.

13. Ans. e. Cytosine   *Ref: William's 8/e p1906-08*

The various second-line treatment options in chronic ITP are:
- Rituximab
- Splenectomy
- Cyclosporine
- Vinca alkaloids
- Danazol, dapsone, interferon-α
- Azathioprine
- Cyclophosphamide.

14. Ans. a. Gastrointestinal (GI) bleeding

Ref: William's 8/e p1874

Hereditary hemorrhagic telangiectasia, also known as Osler-Weber-Rendu syndrome, is an autosomal dominant disorder with a frequency of 1:10,000–50,000. It is manifested by widespread dermal, mucosal, and visceral telangiectasias. Telangiectasias are predominantly seen under tongue and on the face, lips, perioral lesion, nasal mucosa, fingertips, toes, and trunk.

Recurrent epistaxis is universally present and symptoms worsen with age. Beginning at puberty, cutaneous changes usually progress throughout life. Bleeding can occur in any organ with GI tract, oral, and urogenital system (more common). In the GI tract, the stomach and duodenum are more common than colon. Improvement in lesions has been reported in cases with antivascular endothelial growth factor and aspirin.

15. Ans. b. Cryoprecipitate is the treatment of choice

Ref: William's 8/e p2018-21

Factor VIII concentrates are usually sterilized by heating in solution, by superheating to 80°C after lyophilization, and by exposure to organic solvent-detergents that inactivate lipid-enveloped viruses including HIV and hepatitis B and C, but do not inactivate hepatitis A and parvovirus.

There is a risk of transmission of infection because of which cryoprecipitate is not the treatment of choice.

A dose of DDAVP (0.3 μg/kg), given IV or subcutaneous, can increase factor VIII levels by 2-4-folds in mild or moderate hemophilia A. Severe hemophilia A does not respond to DDAVP treatment. A concentrated intranasal spray of DDAVP can also be used (150 μg in each nostril for adults and 150 μg in one nostril for children weighing <50 kg).

Because of the half-life of 8–12 hours of factor VIII, it is given in twice-daily doses.

16. Ans. b. Cryoprecipitate is the treatment of choice in most cases

Ref: William's 8/e p2069, 2074, 2081

von Willebrand disease is the most common inherited bleeding disorder in humans and the most common type is type I which has an autosomal dominant type of inheritance. VWD also has an associated factor VIII defect. Types I and III are quantitative defects while type II is a qualitative defect. Cryoprecipitate and fresh frozen plasma contain functional von Willebrand factor (vWF) but should be avoided if at all possible because of the potential transmission of viral disease.

17. Ans. c. Hemorrhagic disease of newborn has a peak incidence from 2nd to 4th day of life

Ref: Hoffman 6/e p2125

Vitamin K is a necessary cofactor for γ-glutamyl carboxylase, which is required for γ-carboxylation of factors II, VII, IX, X, and proteins C, S, and Z. Neonates are at risk of vitamin K deficiency and the risk factors are maternal malabsorption, maternal drugs impairing vitamin K metabolism, exclusive breast feeding, and neonatal malabsorption.

Hemorrhagic disease of newborn occurs from day 2 to 7 of life. GI bleeding is the most common presentation. Bleeding occurring within 2 days of life is usually associated with maternal drugs (phenytoin, barbiturates, antibiotics, etc.). They have prolongation of both PT and APTT. These prolonged PT/APTT may also be because of decreased synthetic capacity of the liver of newborn. Vitamin K deficiency is indicated by elevation of abnormal (des γ-carboxy) prothrombin (PIVKA-II) antigen level as this form of prothrombin appears only when post-translation modification is impaired but not when protein synthesis is impaired. The source of vitamin K is plant products or it is produced normally by bacterial flora of gut.

18. Ans. a. It can be used as the only test for primary hemostatic disorder

Ref: EJP. 2012;171(1):1-10.

Thromboelastography provides an effective and convenient means of monitoring whole blood coagulation and evaluates the elastic properties of whole blood and provides a global assessment of hemostatic function. Vascular abnormalities, VWD, thrombocytopenia, and platelet dysfunction are the primary hemostatic disorders, which can cause mucocutaneous bleeding. Thus, TEG cannot be the only test to diagnose primary hemostatic disorder. There are several other tests, e.g., complete blood count, mean platelet volume, VWF:Ag, RiCoF or factor VIII activity, platelet aggregometry, and flow cytometry, which are useful.

In TEG trace, r time and K time are lag time from the start of test to fibrin formation and the time taken to achieve a certain level of clot strength, respectively. α angle is the speed at which fibrin build-up and cross-linking take place (clot strengthening), i.e., the rate of clot strengthening.

19. Ans. a. Factor XII deficiency

Ref: William's 8/e p1887, 2024-5

Options b and c are wrong as the patient is a girl, and it is very rare to have X-linked disease in a female patient. Since there are no signs or symptoms of liver disease, option d is also wrong and moreover liver disease patients will also have prolonged PT. Isolated prolonged APTT without bleeding occurs in deficiency of factor XII, high-molecular-weight kininogen (HMWK) or prekallikrein (PK), presence of lupus anticoagulant, or heparin. Hemophilia B Leiden phenotype is characterized by low levels of factor IX antigen and activity at birth and childhood but the level gradually rises to 60% following puberty, apparently in response to endogenous androgen synthesis. Several different mutations in the 5′ promoter region of factor IX gene disrupt binding of transcription factors, but this is overcome by androgen secretion following puberty.

20. Ans. c. Dilute Russell's viper venom time (dRVVT)

Ref: William's 8/e p1887

As the patient is a lady who is having prolonged APTT with normal PT, the possibility of factor VIII deficiency is unlikely because of female sex. Since the patient did not have any bleeding symptoms and she also had a major surgery done 3 years ago without any bleeding complication, ristocetin cofactor assay for the diagnosis of VWD is also unlikely. Factor X deficient patients will have both prolonged PT and APTT. The most likely diagnosis is lupus anticoagulant because this is a female patient with isolated prolonged APTT and no history of bleeding. Thus, the next approach will be to do dRVVT test.

21. Ans. c. Bleeding time   *Ref: William's 8/e p1887, 2078*

Bleeding time will be prolonged in VWD and is normal in hemophilia A. PT is normal in both VWD and hemophilia A, so it cannot differentiate. Similarly, APTT will be prolonged in both the conditions and factor VII level will also be low in both the conditions.

22. Ans. b. Low fibrinogen levels   *Ref: William's 8/e p2105*

Widespread generation of thrombin induces deposition of thrombin which leads to consumption of platelets, fibrinogen, factors V and VIII, proteins C and S, and components of the fibrinolytic system. Thus, raised PT and TT are indirect measures of low clotting factors. FDPs that exhibit anticoagulant and antiplatelet aggregation effects can promote bleeding. Thus, the best answer is low fibrinogen levels.

23. Ans. c. Acute lymphoblastic leukemia (ALL) with t(9;22)   *Ref: Haematologica. 2002;87(12):1343-5.*

Acute promyelocytic leukemia is well known to cause DIC. AML with t(9;11) may present with DIC. DIC, hemophagocytic syndrome, and multiorgan failure may complicate aggressive NK cell leukemia.

24. Ans. b. Collect sample for specific factor assay and give FFP

The possibility of a deficiency of hemophilia A, B, or other factors is also there since there is no family history of bleeding and the sex of the child is not mentioned. As the patient has major bleeding, the best thing to do is to collect a sample for specific factor assay and give FFP till the results are awaited.

25. Ans. a. Factor X deficiency *Ref: William's 8/e p1687*

Many clotting abnormalities have been described in AL amyloidosis. Factor X may bind to amyloid fibrils, leading to its rapid clearance from the blood, with subsequent prolongation of the PT and APTT.

26. Ans. a. Thrombin *Ref: Hoffman's 6/e p2106*

Heparin acts as an anticoagulant by activating antithrombin (AT III) and accelerating the rate at which it inhibits clotting enzymes, particularly thrombin and factor Xa.

27. Ans. b. von Willebrand disease
Ref: Hoffman's 6/e p1864

This patient is most likely having VWD as both the bleeding time and the APTT are prolonged. In cases of both Glanzmann thrombasthenia and BSS, the APTT will be normal. In case of liver disease, the platelet count is usually low and PT will be prolonged, but the APTT will be usually normal.

28. Ans. c. Activin receptor trap ligand

Luspatercept is an activin receptor trap ligand that is used in adults with beta thalassemia who require regular blood transfusion. The BELIEVE trial found that when this drug was administered subcutaneously once every 3 weeks, it showed 33% reduction from baseline in transfusion requirement with at least 2 units from week 13 to week 24. The most common side effects were headache, bone pains, arthralgia, fatigue, cough, and abdominal pain. The recommended starting dose is 1 mg/kg once every 3 weeks.

Activin receptor traps belong to the transforming growth factor beta (TGF-β) superfamily ligands. Luspatercept is an erythroid maturating agent that neutralizes select TGF-βa superfamily ligands to inhibit aberrant SMAD 2/3 signaling and enhance late-stage erythropoiesis. It has also been tried in low-risk myelodysplastic syndrome.

29. Ans. b. Hemophilia A with inhibitors

Emicizumab is a recombinant humanized bispecific antibody for the treatment of hemophilia A with or without inhibitors. It substitutes for the cofactor function of activated factor VIIIa by bridging activated factor IX and factor X. It is indicated for routine prophylaxis to prevent or reduce the frequency of bleeding episodes in adults and children of all ages.

30. Ans. c. Monoclonal antibody which brings factors IX and X together

See explanation to Q. No. 29.

31. Ans. a. Small interfering RNA (siRNA)

Fitusiran is a siRNA targeting antithrombin in liver. It interferes with AT translation and blocks AT synthesis. Because AT is a regulatory natural anticoagulant targeting thrombin, fitusiran blocks AT synthesis and interferes with thrombin breakdown, thereby promoting hemostasis.

32. Ans. d. Factor XI *Ref: Hoffman's 6/e p1973*

Hemophilia C is a rare genetic disorder caused by missing or defective blot clotting protein called factor XI.

33. Ans. a. Anti-tissue factor pathway inhibitor (anti-TFPI)

Tissue factor (TF) activates the initial phase of coagulation after tissue damage via the extrinsic coagulation pathway. The major inhibitor of TF-initiated coagulation is endogenous TFPI. A novel strategy to promote hemostasis is to inhibit TFPI by the novel monoclonal antibody, anti-TFPI, and a single-chain polypeptide that inhibits TF-VIIa-initiated coagulation. TFPI is a kunitz-type protease inhibitor consisting of three kunitz domains which bind protein S. It results in increased thrombin generation in hemophilia.

34. Ans. b. 1 in 10,000 births
Ref: Srivastava A. Guidelines for the Management of Hemophilia, 2nd edition. WFH 2012.

Hemophilia has an estimated frequency of approximately 1 in 10,000 births.

35. Ans. d. 30%

Both *F8* and *F9* genes are prone to new mutations, and as many as one-third of all cases are the result of spontaneous mutation where there is no prior family history. A family history of bleeding is obtained in about two-thirds of all patients.

36. Ans. c. Hemophilia *Ref: Hoffbrand 7/e p716*

In hemophilia, muscle bleeding can be seen in any anatomical site, but it most often presents in the large load-bearing groups of the thigh, calf, posterior abdominal wall, and buttocks. Local pressure effects often cause entrapment neuropathy, particularly of the femoral nerve with iliopsoas bleeding. This causes a common symptom triad of groin pain, hip flexure, and cutaneous sensory loss over the femoral nerve distribution.

37. **Ans. d. All of the above**

Ref: Srivastava A. Guidelines for the Management of Hemophilia, 2nd edition. WFH 2012.

FVIII levels usually rise into the normal range during the second and third trimesters and should therefore be measured in carriers during the third trimester of pregnancy to take decisions for factor coverage during delivery. In carriers with significantly low factor levels (<50 IU/dL), clotting factor replacement is necessary for surgical or invasive procedures including delivery. Desmopressin is particularly useful in the treatment or prevention of bleeding in carriers of hemophilia A.

38. **Ans. e. All of the above**   *Ref: Hoffbrand 7/e p716*

In most laboratories, the FVIII assay is a modified APTT which is often referred to as a "one-stage assay" because the activation of FVIII and coagulation are performed in a single step. However, it is also possible to do a "two-stage assay" in which the FVIII is activated in a first step and its activity is measured in a second separate step. Chromogenic FVIII assays also use a two-stage procedure. The two assays normally give similar results. In severe cases, both assays should be done and compared.

39. **Ans. a. 0.5 and 1**

On average, FVIII infusion produces a plasma increment of 2 IU/dL per unit infused per kilogram body weight and FIX a rise of 1 IU/dL. Therefore, K is 0.5 for FVIII concentrate and 1 for FIX concentrate.

40. **Ans. c. Given at a dose of 0.3 μg/kg body weight either by slow intravenous infusion over 20 minutes or by subcutaneous injection**

Desmopressin (1-deamino-8-D-arginine vasopressin) can be used to treat mild hemophilia A and provides a nonplasma alternative to concentrates. It has no effect on FIX deficiency. It acts via the V_2 receptors on endothelial cells to stimulate exocytosis of Weibel-Palade bodies, which contain VWF and also FVIII.

41. **Ans. c. Dependent on the underlying FVIII mutation**
Ref: Hoffbrand 7/e p721

Antibodies to FVIII (inhibitors) are most common in patients with severe hemophilia A and are most likely to develop during childhood within the first 20 exposures to FVIII, after which they are infrequent. Inhibitors in moderate and mild hemophilia are far less common. In severe hemophilia A, inhibitors are detected in around 25–30% of patients at some stage in their treatment. The likelihood of an individual developing an inhibitor is strongly dependent on the underlying FVIII mutation. Inhibitors in hemophilia B are much less common than in hemophilia A. Only about 2–3% of patients with severe hemophilia B develop inhibitors.

42. **Ans. b. 3–6 times**

Administration of desmopressin (DDAVP) can raise FVIII level adequately (3–6 times baseline levels) to control bleeding in patients with mild, and possibly moderate, hemophilia A. Testing for DDAVP response in individual patients is appropriate.

43. **Ans. d. All of the above**

Ref: Srivastava A. Guidelines for the Management of Hemophilia, 2nd edition. WFH 2012.

Prophylaxis was conceived from the observation that moderate hemophilia patients with clotting factor level >1 IU/dL seldom experience spontaneous bleeding and have much better preservation of joint function. Prophylaxis prevents bleeding and joint destruction and should be the goal of therapy to preserve normal musculoskeletal function. Prophylactic replacement of clotting factor has been shown to be useful even when factor levels are not maintained >1 IU/dL at all times.

44. **Ans. b. Regular continuous treatment started after two or more bleeds into large joints and before the onset of joint disease documented by physical examination and imaging studies**

Ref: Srivastava A. Guidelines for the Management of Hemophilia, 2nd edition. WFH 2012.

Option a is primary prophylaxis, option b is secondary prophylaxis, option c is tertiary prophylaxis, and option d is intermittent prophylaxis. Prophylaxis does not reverse established joint damage; however, it decreases the frequency of bleeding and may slow progression of joint disease and improve quality of life.

45. **Ans. b. 25–40 IU/kg per dose**

The Malmö protocol is a prophylaxis protocol for hemophilia patients. Accordingly, 25–40 IU/kg per dose of factor is administered three times a week for those with hemophilia A and twice a week for those with hemophilia B.

46. **Ans. c. Sisters of two or more brothers with hemophilia**

An obligate carrier is an individual who may be clinically unaffected but must carry a gene based on analysis of the family history. It usually applies to disorders inherited in an autosomal recessive and X-linked recessive manner. Most carriers are asymptomatic.

47. **Ans. c. FVIII inhibitor assay**

The Nijmegen modification is used for FVIII inhibitor assay and it offers improved specificity and sensitivity over the original Bethesda assay.

48. **Ans. d. All of the above**

The short half-life requires prophylaxis treatment to be given every other day to maintain a trough level >1% to achieve adequate hemostasis.

49. **Ans. a. Is a monoclonal antibody against FVIII inhibitor**

Ref: Balkaransingh P. Novel therapies and current clinical progress in hemophilia A. Ther Adv Hematol. 2018;9(2):49-61.

Emicizumab is a bispecific monoclonal antibody which mimics the function of the activated FVIII (FVIIIa) molecule by binding to FIXa with one variable region and to FX with the other. It is given subcutaneously and has a half-life of 4–5 weeks. The long half-life as well as the mode of administration offers possible solutions to address the unmet needs regarding treatment burden previously described. While emicizumab mimics the function of FVIII, it does not resemble FVIII structurally or immunologically and thus is not affected by inhibitors.

CHAPTER 20

Inherited Bone Marrow Failure Syndromes and Aplastic Anemia

1. Which of the following does not cause pancytopenia?
  a. Iron deficiency
  b. Folate deficiency
  c. Aplastic anemia
  d. Acute myeloid leukemia (AML)
  e. Cyclophosphamide

2. Which of the following is not associated with red cell aplasia?
  a. High reticulocyte count
  b. Parvovirus infection
  c. Thymoma
  d. Chronic lymphocytic leukemia (CLL)

3. A male child presented with neutropenia, exocrine pancreatic insufficiency, and short stature. Serum biochemistry showed deranged liver function tests. The disease manifests as autosomal recessive trait and has a propensity to transform to myelodysplastic syndrome (MDS) or AML. Which of the following best suits the diagnosis?
  a. Fanconi anemia
  b. Shwachman-Diamond syndrome
  c. Diamond-Blackfan syndrome (DBA)
  d. Cystic fibrosis

4. Which of these is false regarding congenital dyserythropoietic anemia (CDA)?
  a. WBC and platelet count are normal
  b. Show ineffective erythropoiesis and erythroblast multinuclearity
  c. Often triggered by parvovirus infection
  d. Anemia is usually first noted in infancy or childhood

5. Which is true regarding Fanconi anemia?
  a. It is due to mutation in *ATM* gene
  b. Physical development is always normal
  c. It has sex-linked inheritance
  d. Diagnostic test is clastogenic stress cytogenetic test

6. What is the sequence of response to androgen therapy in Fanconi anemia?
  a. WBC → Hb → platelet
  b. Platelet → WBC → Hb
  c. Hb → WBC → platelet
  d. Hb → platelet → WBC

7. Which of the following inheritance pattern can be seen in dyskeratosis congenita?
  a. Autosomal dominant   b. X-linked recessive
  c. Autosomal recessive   d. All of the above

8. A 40-year-old male patient presented with pancytopenia and is diagnosed to have severe aplastic anemia. The best treatment for him would be:
  a. Antithymocyte globulin (ATG) + cyclosporine
  b. Cyclosporine alone
  c. Allogenic hematopoietic stem cell transplantation (HSCT)
  d. Stanozolol + cyclosporine

9. Bone marrow biopsy is superior to aspirate in diagnosing all of the following, *except*:
  a. Aplastic anemia
  b. Granuloma involving bone marrow
  c. Myelofibrosis
  d. Iron stores

10. A child of 5 years of age presented with severe anemia, reticulocytopenia, febrile illness associated with typical cutaneous emptions, arthralgia, and arthritis. Bone marrow test showed giant pronormoblast. The most likely etiological agent in this condition is:
  a. Hepatitis B virus infection
  b. Cytomegalovirus (CMV) infection
  c. Parvovirus B_{19} infection
  d. Inherited marrow failure syndrome

11. Which of the following is not the etiological agent for aplastic anemia?
  a. Hepatitis B virus
  b. Hepatitis C virus (HCV)
  c. Non-A non-B virus
  d. Hepatitis A virus

12. For very severe aplastic anemia, the absolute neutrophil count should be:
  a. $<200/mm^3$ b. $<500/mm^3$
  c. $<100/mm^3$ d. $<1,000/mm^3$

13. Clastogenic agents are all of the following, *except*:
  a. Mitomycin C   b. Diepoxybutane
  c. Radiation   d. Cyclosporine

14. Chronic cyclosporine toxicity includes all, *except*:
   a. Hypertension
   b. Seizure
   c. Myocardial infarction
   d. *Pneumocystis carinii* infection

15. Predictors of response to glucocorticoids in inherited pure red cell aplasia (DBA) are all, *except*:
   a. Older age at presentation
   b. Positive family history
   c. Normal platelet count
   d. Younger age at presentation

16. All are adverse effects of erythropoietin therapy, *except*:
   a. Hypertension
   b. Seizure
   c. Pure red cell aplasia (PRCA)
   d. Osteopenia

17. Which is not a feature of paroxysmal nocturnal hemoglobinuria (PNH)?
   a. Occurs due to *PIG-A* gene mutation
   b. Cells are deficient in glycosylphosphatidylinositol (GPI)-linked proteins
   c. Never associated with MDS
   d. Patients can present with thrombosis

18. All of the following have a low leukocyte alkaline phosphatase (LAP) score, *except*:
   a. Paroxysmal nocturnal hemoglobinuria
   b. Chronic myeloid leukemia (CML)—chronic phase
   c. Hereditary hypophosphatasia
   d. Polycythemia vera

19. Paroxysmal nocturnal hemoglobinuria is associated with all of the following, *except*:
   a. Aplastic anemia
   b. Increased LAP score
   c. Venous thrombosis
   d. Iron deficiency

20. All of the following statements about Fanconi anemia are true, *except*:
   a. Autosomal dominant inheritance
   b. Hypocellular bone marrow
   c. Congenital anomalies
   d. Normocytic/macrocytic red cells

21. The following is not a feature of Fanconi anemia:
   a. Short stature
   b. Hypopigmented spots and café-au-lait spots
   c. Abnormality of thumb
   d. Hypogonadism
   e. Macrocephaly

22. The most common solid malignancy in Fanconi anemia is:
   a. Lung cancer
   b. Squamous cell carcinoma of head and neck
   c. Genitourinary malignancy
   d. Skin cancers

23. The peak age of presentation in Fanconi anemia is:
   a. <1 year
   b. 1–5 years
   c. 5–15 years
   d. 15–20 years

24. The triad of dyskeratosis congenita includes all, *except*:
   a. Aplastic anemia
   b. Hyperpigmented rash
   c. Nail dystrophy
   d. Mucosal leukoplakia

25. Dyskeratosis congenita is inherited as:
   a. X-linked trait
   b. Autosomal dominant trait
   c. Autosomal recessive trait
   d. All of the above

26. True about Shwachman-Diamond syndrome are:
   a. Conversion mutations which recombine portions of the pseudogene and *SBDS* gene resulting in dysfunctional *SBDS* gene
   b. Autosomal recessive disorder
   c. It is a ribosomal disorder
   d. All of the above

27. Which statement is correct?
   a. TAR (thrombocytopenia with absent radius) syndrome has normal thumb
   b. In Fanconi anemia, when radii are absent, thumb is preserved
   c. Barth syndrome is related to platelet
   d. Shwachman-Diamond syndrome is characterized by endocrine pancreatic insufficiency

28. Which of the following may not be seen in pure red cell aplasia?
   a. Reticulocytopenia
   b. Splenomegaly
   c. Reduction in erythroid series cells in bone marrow aspirate
   d. Lymphoid aggregates in bone marrow biopsy

29. All of the statements are true regarding PNH, *except*:
   a. It is an acquired clonal stem cell disorder
   b. Jaundice is the common presenting feature
   c. Complement is activated via alternate or classical pathway
   d. All PNH cells are sensitive to complement-mediated lysis

30. The sensitivity of Ham test can be improved by addition of:
   a. Magnesium
   b. Calcium
   c. Potassium
   d. Low ionic-strength saline (LISS)

31. The genetic defect in PNH is:
   a. Somatic mutation
   b. Translocation
   c. Deletion
   d. Telomere shortening

CHAPTER 20 | Inherited Bone Marrow Failure Syndromes and Aplastic Anemia

32. A 20-year-old girl presented high-grade fever for 1 week and on evaluation she was looking unwell. Blood tests reveal neutropenia with normal Hb and platelet count. The bone marrow did not show any abnormality. There is no organomegaly and lymphadenopathy. The most likely diagnosis in this case is:
 a. Acute myeloid leukemia
 b. Acute lymphoblastic leukemia (ALL)
 c. Bacterial infection
 d. Thrombotic thrombocytopenic purpura (TTP)
 e. Aplastic anemia

33. A 35-year-old male presents with recurrent fever, weakness, and breathlessness for 1 month. He was found to have petechial rashes on legs and large splenomegaly. Blood tests showed pancytopenia. Which of the following tests would help in differentiating between aplastic anemia and hypersplenism?
 a. Direct Coombs test b. Reticulocyte count
 c. USG whole abdomen d. Osmotic fragility test

34. In the NIH study evaluating standard immunosuppression plus eltrombopag therapy for aplastic anemia, which of the following is false?
 a. In the cohort which used eltrombopag from day 1 to 6 months was most beneficial
 b. 58% CR and 94% overall response rate was achieved in most effective therapy group
 c. Cyclosporine was continued for 6 months
 d. Dose of eltrombopag was 150 mg once daily in East or Southeast Asian patients

35. Regarding telomeropathies which of the following is incorrect?
 a. Telomerases are enzymes which reduce the length of telomeres by removing guanine rich repetitive sequences
 b. Telomerase activity is exhibited in gametes, stem cells and tumor cells
 c. Imetelstat is a telomerase inhibitor
 d. In DKC a telomeropathy the risk for pulmonary fibrosis and cryptogenic liver cirrhosis is not reduced even after HSCT

ANSWERS WITH EXPLANATIONS

1. Ans. a. Iron deficiency

2. Ans. a. High reticulocyte count
 Ref: William's 8/e p488

Classification of pure red cell aplasia:
- Fetal red cell aplasia (nonimmune hydrops fetalis):
  - Parvovirus B_{19} in utero.
- Inherited (DBA)
  - RPS 19 mutation (25% cases).
- Acquired:
  - Transient
  - Acute parvovirus infection
  - Transient erythroblastopenia of childhood.
- Chronic:
  - Idiopathic
  - Large granular lymphocytic leukemia
  - CLL
  - Thymoma
  - Collagen vascular disease
  - Post stem cell transplant
  - Drug induced
  - Pregnancy
  - Antierythropoietin antibodies.

3. Ans. b. Shwachman-Diamond syndrome
 Ref: Hoffman 6/e p316-8

Shwachman-Diamond syndrome is an autosomal recessive disorder caused by mutation in *SBDS* gene (found in 90% cases). For diagnosis, a patient must have two essential features: pancreatic insufficiency and one or more cytopenias. Delayed appearance of secondary ossification centers is common. It can be differentiated from Pearson (marrow-pancreas) syndrome by the presence of ringed sideroblasts with decreased erythroblasts and vacuolization of erythroid and myeloid precursors. Chances of malignant transformation are seen in 7–33%. Isochromosome 7q [i(7q)] is a fairly specific marker of MDS secondary to Shwachman-Diamond syndrome.

Fanconi anemia and DBA: They do not have pancreatic insufficiency.

In cystic fibrosis, cytopenias are not a feature.

4. Ans. c. Often triggered by parvovirus infection
 Ref: Hoffman 5/e p343-7

Congenital dyserythropoietic anemia is characterized by ineffective erythropoiesis, marrow erythroid multinuclearity, and secondary hemosiderosis irrespective of transfusional iron overload. Granulopoiesis and thrombopoiesis are normal. Type I and type II are autosomal recessive while type III is autosomal dominant.

Types of congenital dyserythropoietic anemia:
- *Type I:* It presents with macrocytosis, megaloblastic erythroid precursors (2–5% binucleate forms), and internuclear chromatin bridges. Ham test is negative. Gene for CDA I is present on chromosome 15q15 and is called CDAN1 which encodes Codanin 1 which may be involved in nuclear membrane integrity. About 80% require blood transfusion

during the neonatal period. Peripheral smear shows red cell anisopoikilocytosis and occasionally Cabot rings (unique to CDA I). Electron microscopy shows nuclear membrane pore space with cytoplasmic invagination into nucleus, spongy appearance of nuclear chromatin. Interferon (IFN) alpha 2a, alpha 2b, and Peg IFN alpha 2a should be given in mildly severe or moderately severe anemia in CDA I.

- *Type II:* It has normocytic, normoblastic erythroid maturation (10–35% binucleate forms) and positive Ham test. An abnormality in the glycosylation pathway may be the possible etiology. There may be alpha-mannosidase II deficiency, N-acetyl glucosamyl transferase II deficiency, or galactosyl transferase deficiency. All three deficiencies lead to abnormal oligosaccharides on band 3 on RBC membranes. The magnitude of anemia is usually severe, and karyorrhexis is common. Electron microscopy shows a double nuclear membrane appearance due to excess of endoplasmic reticulum parallel to nuclear membrane. CDA II cells are lysed by ABO-compatible acidified sera of a normal patient but not from the same patient (reverse is seen in PNH). There is expression of i and I antigens on the red cell membrane. Splenomegaly is present, and these patients respond to splenectomy.
- *Type III:* It is most common followed by type I and then type II CDA. Anemia is mild to moderate. Biomicroscopy shows giant erythroblasts with up to 12 nuclei. Electron microscopy shows nuclear clefts and blebs, autolytic areas in cytoplasm, and iron-laden mitochondria. Elevated thymidine kinase is found in all patients but is normal in siblings.
- *Type IV:* Morphologically type II but negative Ham test.

5. Ans. b. Physical development is always normal
Ref: Hoffman 5/e p310-311, 316

Fanconi anemia is inherited as an autosomal recessive pattern in 99% cases and rarely may have sex-linked inheritance in mutant *FANC B* gene cases. About 75% of patients are between 3 and 14 years of age. 70% have mutant *FANC A*, 10% *FANC C*, 10% *FANC G*, 5% *FANC E*, and rest others. The most common anomaly is skin hyperpigmentation (with or without café-au-lait spots) followed by short stature. Diepoxybutane testing is gold standard, but mitomycin C is still used. About 10–15% may have negative stress cytogenetics with diepoxybutane (DEB) or mitomycin C (MMC). Usually, they have high alpha-fetoprotein. The rate of malignant transformation is 16%. The most common solid tumor is squamous cell carcinoma of head and neck. Response with androgens is approximately 50%. First, hemoglobin rises, then WBC followed by platelet. Corticosteroids are added to androgens to prevent androgen-induced growth acceleration and to prevent thrombocytopenic bleeding.

6. Ans. c. Hb → WBC → platelet
Refer to explanation of Q. No. 5.

7. Ans. d. All of the above
Ref: Hoffman 5/e p321-2

The diagnostic triad of dyskeratosis congenita is reticulate skin pigmentation, mucosal leukoplakia, and nail dystrophy. Aplastic anemia occurs in up to 50% of cases and usually in the second decade. 73% are males with X-linked recessive inheritance, caused by mutation in *DKC 1* gene (protein-dyskerin). 16% are autosomal recessive linked to mutation in telomerase-associated protein NOP10. 11% are autosomal dominant with germline mutation in *TERC*, *TERT*, and *TINF2* genes. Malignant transformation occurs in 10–15% of cases. Granulocyte-colony stimulating factor (G-CSF) plus androgen is not recommended because of the risk of splenic peliosis and rupture.

8. Ans. c. Allogenic hematopoietic stem cell transplantation (HSCT)
Ref: William's 8/e p472

Transplantation could be considered a first-choice therapy for up to the age of 50 years for a patient with HLA allele-level matched sibling donor. For patients <20 years, even matched unrelated donors (MUD) transplant is a good option. Results of transplantation are 80–90% in a patient <20 years of age and the result is 50% in patients >40 years of age.

9. Ans. d. Iron stores

10. Ans. c. Parovirus B_{19} infection
Ref: William's 8/e p486-8

The child is most likely having PRCA secondary to parvovirus B_{19} infection. Usually, this infection causes PRCA [transient aplastic crisis (TAC)] in younger children who are chronically anemic due to hereditary spherocytosis, sickle cell disease, or other hemolytic anemias. It should be differentiated from transient erythroblastopenia of childhood (TEC).

Comparison between TAC and TEC.

Transient aplastic crisis	Transient erythroblastopenia of childhood
Occurs in the setting of previous hemolytic anemia	Occurs in a previously well child
Age of presentation is 1–3 years	Can occur in the first year through adolescence

(TAC: transient aplastic crisis; TEC: transient erythroblastopenia of childhood).

Comparison between inherited PRCA (DBA) and transient erythroblastopenia of childhood.

Inherited PRCA (DBA)	TEC
Presentation is always younger (esp. in 1st year of life)	Presents at older age
Physical abnormalities may be present	Physical abnormalities are absent
Does not resolve spontaneously	Resolves spontaneously
ADA levels are high	ADA levels are normal
Expression of i antigen and Hb F may be high	Red cells do not show stress pattern of fetal Hb or i antigens
Family history is positive	Family history is negative

(DBA: Diamond-Blackfan anemia; PRCS: pure red cell aplasia; TEC: transient erythroblastopenia of childhood).

Parvovirus is a small DNA virus and is tropic for the erythroid progenitor cell through P antigen or globoside. There can be two types of presentation:

1. *Fifth disease:* IgM Ab is present in blood, virus levels are low, or symptoms and signs of typical "slapped check" cutaneous eruptions and arthralgia or arthritis (which are secondary to immune complexes).
2. *Transient aplastic crisis:* High concentration of viruses is present in blood, and patients do not develop fifth disease.

Bone marrow typically shows giant pronormoblasts.

Aplastic anemia secondary to hepatitis B virus infection will have preceding jaundice and virus serology will be positive. CMV infection usually presents with mononucleosis syndrome in childhood associated with lymphocytosis and reactive lymphocytes in peripheral blood. It does not cause cytopenia.

11. Ans. b. Hepatitis C virus (HCV)

Ref: William's 8/e p422

Hepatitis C virus is not a frequent cause of aplastic anemia. Among these choices, HCV seems the most appropriate answer.

12. Ans. a. <200/mm³

Ref: Guidelines for diagnosis and management of aplastic anemia. BJH. 147, 43–70

Definition of aplastic anemia: Two of the following symptoms should be present:
1. Hb <10 g/dL
2. Platelet count <50,000/mm³
3. Neutrophil count <1500/mm³.

Severity grading is as follows:
- *Severe aplastic anemia:* BM cellularity <25% or 25–50% with <30% residual hematopoietic cells with two of these three findings—neutrophil count <500, platelet count <20,000/mm³ and reticulocyte count <20,000/mm³.
- *Very severe aplastic anemia:* As per severe but neutrophil <200/mm³.
- *Nonsevere aplastic anemia:* Not fulfilling the criteria for severe or very severe aplastic anemia.

13. Ans. d. Cyclosporine *Ref: Hoffman 6/e p312*

The top three options are all clastogenic agents which cause DNA breaks. Cyclosporine is a calcineurin inhibitor and has immunosuppressive action which is used for the treatment of acquired aplastic anemia. Homozygous FA cells are hypersensitive to many oncogenic and mutagenic inducers such as ionizing radiations, SV40 viral transformation, and alkylating and chemical agents, including cyclophosphamide, nitrogen mustard and platinum compounds but DEB, and mitomycin C have supplanted them for diagnostic testing.

14. Ans. c. Myocardial infarction *Ref: William's 8/e p473*

The side effects of cyclosporine are renal impairment, moderate hypertension, gum hypertrophy, convulsions, hypercholesterolemia, tingling, numbness, hyperkalemia, hepatotoxicity, and increased risk of bacterial and fungal infection.

15. Ans. d. Younger age at presentation

Ref: William's 8/e p438

16. Ans. d. Osteopenia *Ref: William's 8/e p500-1*

Adverse effects of erythropoietin are hypertension, seizures, thrombosis of arteriovenous fistula, hyperkalemia, and PRCA secondary to anti-erythropoietin (EPO) antibodies.

17. Ans. c. Never associated with MDS

Paroxysmal nocturnal hemoglobinuria is an acquired clonal stem cell disorder caused by mutation in X-linked *PIG-A* gene. The cells are deficient in GPI-anchor proteins, e.g., alkaline phosphatase, CD55, CD59, acetylcholinesterase CD16, CD58, and CD14. The risk of thrombosis increased with the number of PNH cells.

18. Ans. d. Polycythemia vera

Causes of low and high leukocyte alkaline phosphatase (LAP) score are:

Low LAP	High LAP
PNH	Leukemoid reaction
Hereditary hypophosphatasia	CML in AP/myeloid BT
CML in CP	Aplastic anemia
	Hodgkin lymphoma
	Polycythemia vera

(AP: accelerated phase; CML: chronic myeloid leukemia; CP: chronic phase; PNH: paroxysmal nocturnal hemoglobinuria).

19. Ans. b. Increased LAP score

Leukocyte alkaline phosphatase score is decreased in PNH, and usually they have associated iron deficiency because of hemoglobinuria. In PNH, thrombosis usually occurs at unusual sites, e.g., Budd–Chiari syndrome, cortical venous thrombosis, splenic/mesenteric vein thrombosis. In fact, in any patient presenting as thrombosis at these sites, PNH should always be looked for.

20. Ans. a. Autosomal dominant inheritance

See explanation of Q. No. 5.

21. Ans. e. Macrocephaly *Ref: Hoffman 6/e p311*

Morphological features of Fanconi anemia are:
- Skin hyperpigmentation (most common) (55%)
- Short stature (51%)
- Hypogonadism (35%)
- *Upper limb abnormalities* (43%): Hypoplastic, supernumerary, bifid or absent thumb
- Hypoplastic or absent radii are always associated with hypoplastic and absent thumb in contrast to TAR in which thumbs are always present.
- Head/face, neck, spine abnormality
- Microcephaly, small eyes, epicanthal folds, abnormal size, shape, and positioning of ears
- Renal abnormalities (21%)
- Ectopic, pelvic, or horseshoe kidney
- Gastrointestinal and cardiopulmonary malformation (11%)
- Hips, legs, feet, toes abnormality (10%).

22. Ans. b. Squamous cell carcinoma of head and neck

Fanconi anemia (FA) predisposes to hematologic disorders and myeloid neoplasia in childhood and to solid cancers, mainly oral carcinomas, in early adulthood. The most common types of solid tumors that occur in patients with FA include head and neck squamous cell carcinomas. The estimated cumulative probability of development of a solid tumor in FA patients is 76% by the age of 45 years. A severe subset, due to mutations in FANCD1/BRCA2, has a cumulative incidence of cancer (hematological and solid) of 97% by age 7 years.

23. Ans. c. 5–15 years

Hematologic abnormalities occur in virtually all patients with FA at a median age of 7 years (maximum chances are within 5–15 years, however, range is from birth to 50 years).

24. Ans. a. Aplastic anemia

Refer to explanation of Q. No. 7.

25. Ans. d. All of the above

Refer to explanation of Q. No. 7.

26. Ans. d. All of the above

Shwachman-Diamond syndrome (SDS) is an autosomal recessive ribosomopathy caused mainly by compound heterozygous mutations in SBDS. Most SBDS mutations occur within a approximately 240-bp region of exon 2 and result from gene conversion due to recombination with a pseudogene, SBDSP.

27. Ans. a. TAR (thrombocytopenia with absent radius) syndrome has normal thumb

In Barth syndrome, the most common hematologic abnormality is neutropenia. Anemia and thrombocytopenia are not seen. Shwachman-Diamond syndrome is characterized by exocrine (not endocrine) pancreatic insufficiency.

28. Ans. b. Splenomegaly *Ref: William's 8/e p488-9*

Pure red cell aplasia is characterized by anemia with reticulocytopenia and very few erythroid precursors in bone marrow. Lymphoid aggregates may be seen in bone marrow biopsy in case of lymphoma and CLL-associated PRCA.

29. Ans. d. All PNH cells are sensitive to complement-mediated lysis *Ref: Dacie and Lewis 10/e p260-1*

Paroxysmal nocturnal hemoglobinuria is an acquired clonal stem cell disorder resulting from somatic mutation in the stem cell. It classically presents as nocturnal hemoglobinuria, jaundice, and hemosiderinuria. Complements are activated in vivo via both the alternate and the classical pathways. In vitro, classical pathway-mediated lysis is seen in acidified serum (Ham), inulin, and cobra-venom test. Alternate pathway-mediated lysis is seen in cold-antibody test. Sucrose lysis test activates both alternate and classical pathways.

Only a proportion of PNH cells are hypersensitive to lysis by complement. Three types of PNH populations can be found in the same patient:
1. Very sensitive (type III) cells
2. Medium sensitive (type II)
3. Normal sensitive (type I).

In vivo, the proportion of type III cells parallels the severity of hemolysis. Type III cells have complete deficiency of CD59, so CD59 is largely responsible for complement-mediated hemolysis.

30. Ans. a. Magnesium *Ref: Dacie and Lewis 10/e p494-5*

In the standard Ham test, when 4 mmol (final concentration) of $MgCl_2$ is added, the sensitivity of test is markedly improved.

Agglutination or lysis (owing to complement action) is a visible indication (end-point) of antigen–antibody reaction and it occurs in two stages:
1. *First stage:* Antibody binds to red cell antigen (sensitization) and is reversible. It is influenced by temperature (different for cold and warm antibody), pH, and ionic strength (LISS increases the rate of antibody binding).

2. *Second stage:* Involves agglutination (or lysis) of the sensitized cells through antibody-dependent cellular cytotoxicity (ADCC), immune complex mediated, or complement mediated. Red cells are mainly lysed through complement-mediated mechanisms.

31. Ans. a. Somatic mutation

Refer to explanation of Q. No. 29.

32. Ans. c. Bacterial infection   *Ref: Harrison 18/e p2228*

This girl presented with high fever so she must be having sepsis, and in severe sepsis there can be both leukocytosis and leukopenia. Bone marrow test has already been done which is essentially normal, so the possibility of AML, ALL, or aplastic anemia is ruled out. TTP is not possible at all as the hemoglobin and platelets are normal.

33. Ans. b. Reticulocyte count   *Ref: Hoffman's 5/e p1899*

In hypersplenism, the reticulocyte count is normal or slightly elevated, but in aplastic anemia it is low which is the characteristic. However, to confirm the differentiation between these two, bone marrow aspirate and biopsy should be done.

34. Ans. d. Dose of eltrombopag was 150 mg once daily in East or Southeast Asian patients
Ref: N Engl J Med. 2017;20:376

Ninety two consecutive patients in a prospective phase 1–2 study of immunosuppressive therapy plus eltrombopag were evaluated. The three consecutively enrolled cohorts differed with regard to the timing of initiation and the duration of the eltrombopag regimen (cohort 1 received eltrombopag from day 14 to 6 months, cohort 2 from day 14 to 3 months, and cohort 3 from day 1 to 6 months). The rate of complete response at 6 months was 33% in cohort 1, 26% in cohort 2, and 58% in cohort 3. The overall response rates at 6 months were 80%, 87%, and 94%, respectively. The complete and overall response rates in the combined cohorts were higher than in our historical cohort, in which the rate of complete response was 10% and the overall response rate was 66%. Eltrombopag was administered at a dose of 150 mg daily in patients who were 12 years of age or older, at a dose of 75 mg daily in patients who were 6 to 11 years of age, and at a dose of 2.5 mg per kg of body weight per day in patients who were 2 to 5 years of age. East or Southeast Asian participants were administered 50% of the eltrombopag dose because of higher eltrombopag exposure due to differences in pharmacokinetics observed in this ethnic group.

35. Ans. a. Telomerases are enzymes which reduce the length of telomeres by removing guanine rich repetitive sequences   *Ref: Hoffman 7/e, p366*

Telomerase is the enzyme responsible for maintenance of the length of telomeres by addition of guanine-rich repetitive sequences. Telomerase activity is exhibited in gametes and stem and tumor cells. Critically short telomeres cause senescence, following crisis and cell death. Imetelestat is a telomerase inhibitor. DKC a telomeropathy, also known as Zinsser-Engman-Cole syndrome, was first described in 1906. It is a rare, progressive bone marrow failure syndrome characterized by the triad of reticulated skin hyperpigmentation, nail dystrophy, and oral leukoplakia in first decade, bone marrow failure in second decade, pulmonary fibrosis and cryptogenic liver cirrhosis in fourth decade. The risk for pulmonary fibrosis and cryptogenic liver cirrhosis is not reduced even after HSCT.

CHAPTER 21: Mast Cell/Basophilic Disorders

1. Increased basophils can be seen in all of the following, *except*:
 a. Chronic myeloid leukemia (CML)
 b. Acute myeloid leukemia (AML) with t(6;9)
 c. AML with t(3;6)
 d. AML with 12p abnormalities
 e. AML with t(8;21)

2. Urticaria pigmentosa is associated with which cell disorder?
 a. Basophil   b. Neutrophil
 c. Mast cell   d. Macrophages

3. True about mast cells is:
 a. KIT (CD117) positive
 b. Contains tryptase/chymase
 c. Mediate IgE-dependent hypersensitivity
 d. Produce TNF-α
 e. All of the above

4. Mast cell cytoplasmic granules are stained by all, *except*:
 a. Hematoxylin-eosin   b. Giemsa stain
 c. Toluidine blue   d. Chloroacetate esterase

5. Following all are true about cutaneous mastocytosis, *except*:
 a. Common in elderly population
 b. Symptomatic treatment
 c. Benign
 d. All of the above

6. Mast cells found in tissues resemble:
 a. Basophil   b. Eosinophil
 c. Monocyte   d. Neutrophil

7. White cell with lysosomes containing phosphatases, esterases, lysozymes, and arylsulfatase is:
 a. Basophil
 b. Eosinophil
 c. Monocyte
 d. Neutrophil

8. White cell with granule containing heparin, 5-hydroxytriptamine, and histamine is:
 a. Basophil
 b. Eosinophil
 c. Monocyte
 d. Neutrophil

ANSWERS WITH EXPLANATIONS

1. Ans. e. AML with t(8; 21)   *Ref: William's 8/e p885*

All the above conditions are associated with basophilia except t(8;21). AML with inv(16) or t(16;16) may be associated with large basophilic granules but these granules represent abnormal eosinophilic granules.

2. Ans. c. Mast cell   *Ref: William's 8/e p923*

WHO classification of systemic mastocytosis
- Cutaneous mastocytosis:
  - Urticaria pigmentosa
  - Diffuse cutaneous mastocytosis
  - Solitary mastocytoma of skin
- Indolent systemic mastocytosis
- Systemic mastocytosis (SM) with associated clonal, hematologic, nonmast cell lineage disease (SM-AHNMD)
- Aggressive systemic mastocytosis:
  - Mast cell leukemia
  - Mast cell sarcoma
  - Extracutaneous mastocytoma.

3. Ans. e. All of the above

Mast cells are tissue-based inflammatory cells of hematopoietic origin that respond to signals of innate and adaptive immunity with immediate and delayed release of inflammatory mediators. They are located primarily in association with blood vessels and at epithelial surfaces. Mast cells are central to the pathogenesis of diseases of immediate hypersensitivity, but are also implicated in host responses to pathogens, autoimmune diseases, fibrosis, and wound healing. Human mast cells are divided into two major subtypes based on the presence of tryptase (MCT cells) or tryptase and mast cell-specific chymase (MCTC cells), each predominating in different locations. Tryptase staining identifies all mast cells and is the primary method for identifying tissue mast cells. Mast cells are KIT (CD117)+ (receptor for stem cell factor) and FcεR1+; they express other cell surface receptors depending on their location and stage of differentiation and activation. Mast cells increase in number several-fold in association with IgE-dependent immediate hypersensitivity reactions, including rhinitis, urticaria, and asthma; connective tissue disorders, such as rheumatoid arthritis; infectious diseases, such as parasites; neoplastic diseases, such as lymphoma and leukemia; and osteoporosis, chronic liver disease, and chronic renal disease. The most striking increase in mast cells occurs in parasitic diseases and in mastocytosis (associated with gain-of-function mutations in KIT). TNF-α is a major cytokine stored and released by mast cells. Mast cells also release histamine which is involved in the inflammatory response.

4. Ans. a. Hematoxylin-eosin

Ref: Dacie and Lewis 10/e p329

Mast cells originate from pluripotential hemopoietic bone marrow stem cell. They are spindle-shaped cells that normally present in small numbers in the vicinity of dermal capillaries. Mast cell contains numerous cytoplasmic granules that do not stain with routine stains like hematoxylin-eosin. Instead, these granules stain metachromatically with methylene blue (Giemsa stain) and toluidine blue. Histochemical stains using chloroacetate esterase reaction are also used to identify mast cell granules.

5. Ans. a. Common in elderly population

Ref: William's 8/e p925-7

The most frequent site of organ involvement in patients with any form of mastocytosis is the skin. Cutaneous mastocytosis tends to appear early in life; 50% of cases present before the age of 2 years and another 15% before the age of 15. Adult onset mastocytosis occurs and represents a segment of the mastocytosis spectrum, which differs in many aspects from childhood onset mastocytosis. Mastocytosis can be diagnosed without difficulty when it presents with the typical rash and the classical Darier's sign. Adult patients are more prone to develop systemic mastocytosis (25%) than children. The target organs include bone marrow, skeleton, gastrointestinal tract, liver, spleen, and lymph node. In regard to prognosis adults' disease tends to persist in contrast to mastocytosis in children, which tends to regress spontaneously. There is no definite cure for mastocytosis, and treatment is aimed to alleviate symptoms and reduce cutaneous lesions by antihistamines and steroids.

6. Ans. a. Basophils

Ref: Hoffman's 6/e p1095

Normal mast cells originate from a $CD34^+$ cell population in the bone marrow. Mast cells are released into the circulation in a primitive state and undergo terminal maturation and differentiation after migrating into tissues, where they ultimately reside. Mast cells share several features with basophils, namely presence of cytoplasmic basophilic granules, expression of high affinity IgE receptors and release of histamine upon stimulation. But these two cells are different.

7. Ans. c. Monocyte

Ref: William's 7/e p964

As the monocyte matures into the macrophage, the cell enlarges in size, and the lysosomal content and the amount of hydrolytic enzymes (e.g., phosphatases, esterases, beta-glucuronidase, lysozyme, arylsulfatase) increase.

8. Ans. a. Basophil

Ref: Dacie and Lewis 10/e p107

Basophils contain distinctive, large, variably sized, dark blue or purple granules of the cytoplasm often obscure the nucleus. They are rich in histamine, serotonin, and heparin substance.

CHAPTER 22

Monocyte/Macrophage Disorders

1. **Which one of the following is not a tissue macrophage?**
   a. Kupffer cell
   b. Microglia
   c. Gaucher cell
   d. Mast cell

2. **In which of the following, blasts have oil red O positive vacuoles?**
   a. ALL-L1
   b. ALL-L2
   c. ALL-L3
   d. NK cell leukemia

3. **All are derived from monocytes, *except*:**
   a. Kupffer cells
   b. Langerhan cells
   c. Osteoblasts
   d. Dendritic cells (DCs)
   e. Microglia

4. **True regarding phagocytic killing by macrophages are all, *except*:**
   a. Nicotinamide adenine dinucleotide phosphate (NADPH) required
   b. Respiratory burst
   c. Mitochondrial mediated
   d. Free hydroxyl radical generated
   e. All of the above are true

5. **The following are associated with neutropenia, *except*:**
   a. Hyper-IgM syndrome
   b. Reticular dysgenesis
   c. Dyskeratosis congenita
   d. Leukocyte adhesion deficiency (LAD)

6. **True about pure white cell aplasia is:**
   a. Not associated with thymoma
   b. Erythroid and megakaryocytic precursors are not affected
   c. Ibuprofen can cause it
   d. All of the above

7. **Which of the following becomes tissue macrophage after a short stay in blood?**
   a. Neutrophil
   b. Monocyte
   c. Lymphocyte
   d. Plasma cell

8. **Reticuloendothelial cell is composed of:**
   a. Kupffer cells of liver
   b. Reticulum cells of spleen
   c. Reticulum cells of liver
   d. All of the above

ANSWERS WITH EXPLANATIONS

1. **Ans. d. Mast cell** *Ref: William's 8/e p990*

2. **Ans. c. ALL-L3**
   Ref: Clinical Laboratory Medicine by Kenneth D McClatchey 2/e p900

   Oil red O stains lipid material is an excellent marker for ALL-L3 or Burkitt leukemia/lymphoma. The oil red O stain distinctly stains the vacuoles that are seen in this subtype of leukemia/lymphoma.

3. **Ans. c. Osteoblasts** *Ref: William's 8/e p990-2*

   Tissue macrophages have a broad role in the maintenance of tissue homeostasis, through the clearance of senescent cells and the remodeling and repair of tissues after inflammation. They are generally considered to be derived from circulating monocytes and show a high degree of heterogeneity. The heterogeneity reflects the specialization of function that is adopted by macrophages in different anatomical locations, including the following: the ability of osteoclasts to remodel bone, the high expression of pattern recognition receptors and scavenger receptors by alveolar macrophages, which are involved in clearing microorganisms, viruses, and environmental particles in the lungs; and the positioning of thymic macrophages and tingible body macrophages in the germinal center for clearance of apoptotic lymphocytes that are generated during the development of an acquired immune response. The gut is one of the richest sources of macrophages in the body, and isolation of macrophages from the lamina propria has highlighted a unique macrophage phenotype that is characterized by high phagocytic and bactericidal activity but weak production of proinflammatory cytokines. This phenotype can be induced in peripheral blood-derived macrophages by intestinal stromal-cell products, indicating that the tissue microenvironment can markedly influence the phenotype of tissue-resident macrophages. Langerhan cells are present in epidermis. Kupffer cells are an important component of the mononuclear-phagocyte system that is present in the liver. The mononuclear phagocyte system has historically been categorized into monocytes, DCs, and macrophages on the basis of functional and phenotypical characteristics. Dendritic cells are antigen-presenting cells which play a critical role in the regulation of the adaptive immune response. DCs are capable of capturing antigens, processing them, and presenting them on the cell surface along with appropriate costimulation molecules.

4. Ans. c. Mitochondrial mediated
Ref: William's 8/e p999-1005

Activation of phagocytes is associated with a rapid and dramatic increase in oxygen consumption described as the respiratory burst. This process is nonmitochondrial and is mediated by the activation of a latent enzyme system referred as NADPH oxidase, which transfers a single electron to molecular oxygen to form the superoxide anion. The superoxide anion then dismutates to hydrogen peroxide (H_2O_2), a process occurring either spontaneously or through the catalytic function of superoxide dismutase. H_2O_2 then reacts with superoxide anion, forming the highly reactive hydroxyl radical (OH•), which is highly microbicidal.

5. Ans. d. Leukocyte adhesion deficiency.
Ref: William's 8/e p966-7

Leukocyte adhesion deficiency is a congenital disorder that presents with persistent leukocytosis, delayed separation of the umbilical cord, recurrent infections, impaired wound healing, and defects of neutrophil activation. The condition is caused by defects in adhesion of neutrophils to blood vessel walls. As a result, phagocytes do not migrate from the bloodstream to sites of infection. Because of the defect in neutrophil migration, abscesses and other sites of infection are devoid of pus despite the striking neutrophilia. Reticular dysgenesis is associated with neutropenia, lymphoid hypoplasia, and thymic hypoplasia with normal erythropoiesis and megakaryopoiesis. Dyskeratosis congenital is a rare disease characterized by abnormal skin pigmentation, nail dystrophy, and mucosal leukoplakia. More than 80% of the affected individuals develop bone marrow failure, which is the major cause of death. The disorder is caused by defective telomere maintenance in stem cells. Neutropenia has been seen with immunological abnormalities such as hyper-IgM syndrome and X-linked agammaglobulinemia. Hyper-IgM syndrome is an X-linked disorder characterized by lymphoid hyperplasia, low concentrations of IgG and IgA but high concentration of IgM, and severe neutropenia. A genetic defect in the T-cell CD40 ligand has been implicated as the cause of the disease.

6. Ans. d. All of the above

Pure white cell aplasia is a rare condition associated with recurrent pyogenic infections and with thymoma in 70% of the affected patients. There is almost complete absence of myeloid precursors without any abnormality of erythroid or megakaryocytic precursors in the marrow. The disorder has been associated with therapy with ibuprofen, certain natural remedies, and chlorpropamide. If associated with thymoma, surgical removal of the thymus gland can partially correct the neutropenia. Other treatment options include corticosteroids, cyclosporine, cyclophosphamide, and intravenous immunoglobulin.

7. Ans. b. Monocyte
Ref: Hoffman's 6/e p289

Survival of monocyte in blood is short, approximately 8–72 hours. Monocytes then enter into the tissues, where they develop into macrophages that may survive for 2–3 months. Tissue-fixed macrophages are found in lung (alveolar macrophages), the liver (Kupffer cells), the spleen, and the central nervous system (glial cells).

8. Ans. d. All of the above
Ref: William's 7/e p482

Vascular endothelium, reticular cells, and dendritic cells of lymphoid germinal centers comprised the previously described term reticuloendothelial system. Monocytes and macrophages comprise the functional system formerly known as reticuloendothelial system.

Chapter 23: Paroxysmal Nocturnal Hemoglobinuria

1. The paroxysmal nocturnal hemoglobinuria (PNH) affects:
   a. White blood cells
   b. Red blood cells
   c. Platelets
   d. All of the above

2. The causes of thrombosis in PNH are all, *except*:
   a. Nitrous oxide depletion
   b. Complement-mediated platelet activation
   c. Exposure of the procoagulant interior of the red cell membranes
   d. Leukocytosis

3. Not a feature of PNH is:
   a. Chronic kidney disease
   b. Pulmonary hypertension
   c. Stroke
   d. Dactylitis

4. Following are the indications for the evaluation for PNH, *except*:
   a. Iron-deficiency anemia
   b. Coombs' negative hemolytic anemia
   c. Coombs' positive hemolytic anemia
   d. All of the above

5. True about detection of PNH clone in aplastic anemia is:
   a. It signifies good response to the treatment
   b. It signifies poor response to the treatment
   c. It has no significance
   d. It has significance in aplastic anemia but not in myelodysplastic anemia

6. Ham's test for PNH is based on:
   a. Acid hemolysis
   b. Sucrose hemolysis
   c. Incubated osmotic fragility
   d. Flow cytometry (FCM)

7. Ravulizumab is approved for use in:
   a. Paroxysmal nocturnal hemoglobinuria
   b. Hemolytic uremic syndrome
   c. Mantle cell lymphoma
   d. Thalassemia

8. All are treatment options for PNH, *except*:
   a. Splenectomy
   b. Steroids
   c. Autologous stem cell transplant
   d. Anticoagulants

9. Alternative targets for inhibition of complement pathway in PNH are all, *except*:
   a. C3
   b. Factor D
   c. Factor B
   d. Factor H

10. The cause of resistance to eculizumab is:
   a. Polymorphism of C5
   b. Bone marrow failure
   c. Extravascular hemolysis
   d. All of the above

11. The indications of stem cell transplant (SCT) in PNH are:
   a. Nonavailability of eculizumab
   b. Heterozygous c.2654G → A mutations in C5
   c. PNH with aplastic anemia
   d. All of the above

12. Cause of thrombosis in PNH is:
   a. Scavenging of nitric oxide (NO)
   b. Complement activation
   c. Defective fibrinolysis
   d. Absence of DC55 and CD59 on platelets leads to prothrombotic microparticles
   e. All of the above

ANSWERS WITH EXPLANATIONS

1. Ans. d. All of the above

The pathogenesis of PNH has revealed that the disease arises from chronic and uncontrolled complement activation, causing dysfunction in all three blood cell lines: (1) red blood cells; (2) white blood cells (both granulocytes and monocytes); and (3) platelets.

2. Ans. d. Leukocytosis

Ref: Moyo VM. Natural history of paroxysmal nocturnal haemoglobinuria using modern diagnostic assays. Br J Haematol. 2004;126(1):133-8.

The combination of nitrous oxide depletion, complement-mediated platelet activation, and exposure of the procoagulant interior of the red cell membranes makes PNH an extremely hypercoagulable state. In fact, thrombosis is the leading cause of death among patients with PNH, and accounts for 40–67% of the mortality from the disease. A history of even one thrombotic event is associated with a 5-fold to 10-fold higher risk of death for PNH patients. Leukocytosis is a risk factor for thrombosis in sickle cell disease.

3. Ans. d. Dactylitis

Chronic kidney disease has been reported to occur in a majority of PNH patients. Pulmonary hypertension occurs in nearly half of PNH patients and often manifests as dyspnea, which can be moderate to severe. Stroke is a common cause of morbidity and mortality in PNH, and it is almost exclusively a result of cerebral venous thrombosis. Dactylitis is the manifestation of sickle cell disease in children.

4. Ans. c. Coombs' positive hemolytic anemia

Paroxysmal nocturnal hemoglobinuria screening is not necessary for patients with antibody-mediated Coombs positive hemolytic anemia. Routine PNH testing should be performed; however, in patients with Coombs-negative hemolytic anemia and in patients who have no other obvious cause for hemolysis, particularly when it is associated with abdominal pain or dyspnea. Iron-deficiency in patients with PNH is most often due to urinary losses of iron secondary to chronic intravascular hemolysis.

5. Ans. a. It signifies good response to the treatment
Ref: Sugimori C. Origin and fate of blood cells deficient in glycosylphosphatidylinositol-anchored protein among patients with bone marrow failure. Br J Haematol. 2009;147(1):102-12.

The presence of a PNH clone is a marker for response to immunosuppressive therapy among patients with bone marrow failure syndromes, and it has been shown that both aplastic anemia and myelodysplastic syndrome patients with detectable PNH clones of any size have an improved response to such treatment as compared with those who do not have such clones.

6. Ans. a. Acid hemolysis
Ref: Krauss JS. Laboratory diagnosis of paroxysmal nocturnal hemoglobinuria. Ann Clin Lab Sci. 2003;33:401-6.

The Ham's test is based on the fact that complement will attach to RBCs at somewhat acid pH and that PNH RBCs are sensitive to complement fixation. Whole defibrinated blood collected in heparin is utilized. Cells from the patient and controls are tested for hemolysis with—(1) unmodified serum, (2) acidified serum (pH 6.8), (3) heat-inactivated serum (55°C for 3 min), and (4) heated serum with guinea pig complement. So, the Ham's test involves placing RBCs in mild acidic medium and a positive result (increased RBC fragility) indicates PNH. Flow cytometry has recently replaced Ham's test as the definitive test for PNH. Usually, CD55 and CD59 are both measured by FCM; depressed levels of both of these glycoproteins are consistent with PNH. The sucrose lysis test is based on the fact that low ionic strength isotonic sucrose causes serum globulin aggregates to fix complement on the RBC surface. Consequently, a scant amount of serum added to this solution will lyse PNH RBCs preferentially to normal RBCs.

7. Ans. a. Paroxysmal nocturnal hemoglobinuria
Ref: Lee JW. Ravulizumab (ALXN1210) vs eculizumab in adult patients with PNH naive to complement inhibitors: the 301 study. Blood. 2019;133:530-9.

Ravulizumab exhibits a reduced target-dependent drug disposition and a longer half-life as compared to its parental molecule eculizumab, becoming an attractive long-acting anti-C5 mAb to be used in the clinic. It has been generated through specific amino acid modifications of eculizumab aiming to improve its pharmacokinetic profile. It is a new complement component C5 inhibitor administered every 8 weeks and is noninferior to eculizumab administered every 2 weeks in PNH. Patients with PNH may be safely and effectively switched from eculizumab (900 mg administered every 2 weeks) to ravulizumab administered every 8 weeks while maintaining the high level of efficacy, safety, and quality-of-life previously achieved with eculizumab.

8. Ans. c. Autologous stem cell transplant
Ref: Brodsky RA. How I treat paroxysmal nocturnal hemoglobinuria. Blood. 2009;113(26):6522-7.

Main treatment of PNH includes blood product support and steroids during acute phase of hemolysis. Rarely splenectomy may be considered although with marginal benefits, since the hemolysis is mainly intravascular. PNH patients are at risk for increased thrombosis, so anticoagulants are needed for many patients who develop clinical thrombosis. Allogeneic SCT is the only curative treatment for patients with PNH; however, autologous transplant is of no use.

9. Ans. d. Factor H

At the moment, there are three strategies of proximal complement inhibition: (1) anti-C3 agents; (2) anti-factor D agents; and (3) anti-factor B agents. These agents are available either subcutaneously or orally and have been investigated in monotherapy or in association with eculizumab in PNH patients. Complement factor H is a soluble complement regulator essential for controlling the alternative pathway in blood and on cell surfaces.

10. Ans. d. All of the above
Ref: Risitano MA. Anti-complement treatment for paroxysmal nocturnal hemoglobinuria. Front Immunol. 2019:10;1157.

Intrinsic resistance to eculizumab has been reported, albeit rare, and it is associated with inherited polymorphism of C5 which prevents eculizumab binding. Bone marrow function can also contribute to the impaired effect of eculizumab, since immune-mediated bone marrow failure is a key element of the pathophysiology of PNH. Impaired bone marrow function may become clinically meaningful even without overt aplastic anemia, given the lack of a compensatory increase in erythropoiesis with continuous hemolysis. Third is the occurrence of C3-mediated extravascular hemolysis. Residual anemia, presumably due to C3-mediated extravascular hemolysis of surviving PNH erythrocytes, has emerged as a common clinical manifestation during eculizumab treatment, eventually limiting the hematological benefit of this treatment. Moreover, some residual intravascular hemolysis is detectable in most PNH patients on eculizumab. In fact, 25–35% of patients continue to require red cell transfusions despite treatment with eculizumab. The most common reason for continued transfusions is extravascular hemolysis. An increase in the percentage of PNH red cells after eculizumab therapy correlates with response but also with extravascular hemolysis. About 50% of PNH patients (Coombs negative at diagnosis) become Coombs positive (IgG neg and C3 pos) after treatment with eculizumab.

11. Ans. d. All of the above

Ref: Brodsky RA. Paroxysmal nocturnal hemoglobinuria. Blood. 2014;124:2804-11.

Stem cell transplant should not be offered as initial therapy for patients with classical PNH given the risks of transplant-related morbidity and mortality. Exceptions are PNH patients in countries where eculizumab is not available. SCT is also a reasonable option for patients who do not respond to eculizumab therapy due to heterozygous 2654G→A mutations in C5 or the rare patient where eculizumab does not entirely block intravascular hemolysis due to persistent inflammation. Patients meeting criteria for severe aplastic anemia with PNH clones continue to be good candidates for SCT if they are young and have a suitable donor. Allogeneic stem cell transplantation is probably not a suitable treatment option for life-threatening thromboembolism in PNH.

12. Ans. e. All of the above

Ref: Brodsky RA. Paroxysmal nocturnal hemoglobinuria. Blood. 2014;124:2804-11.

There are multiple causes of thrombosis in PNH. The absence of CD55 and CD59 on PNH platelets leads to prothrombotic microparticles. High levels of free hemoglobin lead to scavenging of NO, which has been implicated in contributing to platelet activation and aggregation. Complement activation also contributes to the prothrombotic tendency of PNH patients. Specifically, C5a may result in proinflammatory and prothrombotic processes by generating inflammatory cytokines such as interleukin-6, interleukin-8, and tumor necrosis factor-α. Complement inhibition is the most effective strategy to stop thrombosis in PNH. Defective fibrinolysis resulting from deficiency or absence of GPI-linked proteins, such as urokinase-type plasminogen antivator receptor or heparan sulfate, has been speculated to contribute to the thrombophilic state in PNH. Anticoagulation and eculizumab are indication for acute thrombotic events.

CHAPTER 24

von Willebrand Disease

1. Defects in von Willebrand factor (VWF) can cause bleeding by:
   a. Impairing platelet adhesion
   b. Reducing the concentration of factor VIII (FVIII)
   c. Reduced binding to collagen
   d. All of the above

2. True about VWF are all, *except*:
   a. VWF levels are approximately 25% lower in blood group O individuals than in non-O
   b. A VWF activity <30 IU/dL is usually associated with bleeding symptoms
   c. The incidental finding of VWF activity <30 IU/dL should be taken to indicate von Willebrand disease (VWD) or acquired von Willebrand syndrome
   d. von willebrand disease can be excluded by a normal activated partial thromboplastin time (APTT)

3. The VWF-FVIII binding assay is useful for the diagnosis of:
   a. Type 2A VWD   b. Type 2B VWD
   c. Type 2M VWD   d. Type 2N VWD

4. True about type 1 VWD are all, *except*:
   a. Normal multimeric pattern
   b. Ratio of function to antigen (VWF:RCo/VWF:Ag) is < 0.6
   c. Mostly autosomal dominant inheritance
   d. Most common type of VWD
   e. All of the above

5. Platelet type pseudo-VWD should be differentiated from:
   a. Type 2A VWD   b. Type 2B VWD
   c. Type 2M VWD   d. Type 2N VWD

6. Which type of VWD should be distinguished from mild hemophilia A?
   a. Type 2A VWD   b. Type 2B VWD
   c. Type 2M VWD   d. Type 2N VWD

7. Ristocetin-induced platelet aggregation is increased in:
   a. Type 2A VWD   b. Type 2B VWD
   c. Type 2M VWD   d. Type 2N VWD

8. Desmopressin is contraindicated in:
   a. Type 2A VWD   b. Type 2B VWD
   c. Type 2M VWD   d. Type 2N VWD

9. Causes of acquired von Willebrand syndrome are all, *except*:
   a. IgG paraprotein
   b. Severe aortic stenosis
   c. Myeloproliferative disease
   d. Hypothyroidism
   e. Disseminated intravascular coagulation

10. Which of the following is not the first level test for VWD diagnosis?
   a. FVIII coagulant activity (FVIII:C)
   b. The VWF antigen level (VWF:Ag)
   c. Ristocetin cofactor activity (VWF:RCo)
   d. Ristocetin-induced platelet aggregation

11. True about type 3 VWD is:
   a. Complete deficiency of VWF in both plasma and platelets
   b. Inhibitor to VWF (anti-VWF alloantibodies) should be excluded in type 3 VWD patients
   c. VWF:Ag, VWF:RCo, and VWF:CB values are <1 IU/dL
   d. FVIII:C levels are very low (<10 IU/dL)
   e. All of the above

12. Ristocetin-induced platelet aggregation should be performed in all of the conditions, *except*:
   a. When VWF multimers are absent
   b. VWF:RCo/VWF:Ag ratio is reduced
   c. VWF:CB/VWF:Ag ratio is reduced
   d. Thrombocytopenia

13. True about VWD is:
   a. A function: antigen ratio of <0.6 should be used to identify patients with type 2 VWD
   b. Multimer analysis should be used to distinguish between types 2A and 2M
   c. VWF and FVIII levels increase with age
   d. All of the above

14. Which of the following is tissue factor pathway inhibitor (TFPI)?
   a. Emicizumab   b. FEIBA, Baxalta
   c. Concizumab   d. Fitusiran

15. Regarding acquired hemophilia, all are true, *except*:
a. Low FVIII level associated with the presence of a time-dependent inhibitor in the plasma
b. Only males are affected
c. Activated prothrombin complex concentrate (e.g., FEIBA) or recombinant activated factor VII (NovoSeven) can be used to control bleeding episodes
d. Immunosuppression with steroids is usually effective at reducing inhibitor production
e. None of the above

16. True about von Willebrand disease is:
a. VWF protect FVIII from early inactivation by the activated protein C
b. VWF is synthesized by liver
c. The gene coding for VWF is located at chromosome 11p
d. All of the above

17. True regarding vonicog alfa are all, *except*:
a. It is a recombinant VWF concentrate
b. It is a highly purified product
c. It contains all of the VWF multimers present in normal plasma and the ultra-large fraction
d. The ultra-large multimers are rapidly cleaved postinfusion by the enzymatic activity of patients' own plasma ADAMST13
e. High-risk of thrombosis has led to its discontinuation

18. Severe VWD is defined as:
a. VWF activity levels <1 IU/dL and/or FVIII levels <1 IU/dL
b. VWF activity levels <1 IU/dL and/or FVIII levels <5 IU/dL
c. VWF activity levels <5 IU/dL and/or FVIII levels <10 IU/dL
d. VWF activity levels <10 IU/dL and/or FVIII levels <20 IU/dL

19. For patients getting infusion of VWF/Factor VIII concentrate, the monitoring should include:
a. APTT monitoring
b. VWF:RCo monitoring
c. FVIII concentration monitoring
d. Both VWF:RCo and FVIII concentration monitoring

20. All of the following are VWF only concentrates, *except*:
a. Willfact
b. Vonvendi
c. Alphanate
d. None of the above

ANSWERS WITH EXPLANATIONS

1. Ans. d. All of the above

Defects in VWF can cause bleeding by impairing platelet adhesion or by reducing the concentration of FVIII. It also binds to collagen at sites of vascular injury and serves as a mediator for platelet adhesion.

2. Ans. d. von Willebrand disease can be excluded by a normal activated partial thromboplastin time (APTT)

Ref: Laffan MA. The diagnosis and management of von Willebrand disease. BCSH guidelines. BJH. 2014;167:453-65.

The plasma level of VWF in normal individuals varies over a sixfold range, from 0.40 to 2.40 IU/mL (40–240 IU/dL), and VWF levels are approximately 25% lower in blood group O individuals than in non-O. A VWF activity <0.30 IU/mL (<30 IU/dL) is usually associated with bleeding symptoms and is more likely to be associated with a mutation in VWF; however, these associations are less strong for VWF levels between 0.30 and 0.50 IU/mL (30–50 IU/dL). The incidental finding of VWF activity <0.30 IU/mL should be considered to indicate VWD or acquired von Willebrand syndrome. VWD cannot be excluded by a normal APTT.

3. Ans. d. Type 2N VWD

Ref: Stufano F. Diagnosis of von Willebrand disease. World Federation of Hemophilia; 2017

The VWF-FVIII binding assay (VWF:FVIIIB) evaluates the capacity of VWF to bind to FVIII. This assay is crucial to differentiate a diagnosis of VWD type 2N from mild hemophilia A since both conditions are associated with a moderate reduction in FVIII plasma levels, and normal levels of VWF:Ag. In the differential diagnosis, the results obtained from this assay can be: (1) a normal capacity of VWF to bind FVIII, resulting in a diagnosis of mild hemophilia A or, (2) a markedly reduced capacity of VWF to bind FVIII, resulting in a diagnosis of VWD type 2N.

4. Ans. b. Ratio of function to antigen (VWF:RCo/VWF:Ag) is <0.6
Ref: Hoffbrand 7/e p726

In contrast to hemophilia where there is only quantitative defect in factors, i.e., the only problem is varying severity of absence of FVIII or FIX, in case of VWD, there can be two types of defects in VWF. The first is quantitative deficiency of VWF causing either type 1 (mild-to-moderated deficiency) or type 3 VWD (severe deficiency), or type 2 VWD where defective VWF is produced, which loses its function to bind to platelets or FVIII **(Table 1)**. Type 1 VWD is defined as a quantitative deficiency of VWF, and the VWF present should be functionally normal with a normal multimeric pattern. The ratio of function to antigen (VWF:RCo/VWF:Ag) should be >0.6. Most common VWD is type 1 VWD.

Table 1: Classification of von Willebrand disease (VWD).

VWD type	Type of defect	Diagnosis	Inheritance
1	Partial quantitative decrease in VWF	VWF present is functionally normal with a normal multimeric pattern VWF:RCo/VWF:Ag >0.6	Autosomal dominant inheritance 75% of total VWD cases
2A	Selective deficiency of high-molecular-weight multimers	Multimer analysis helps in the diagnosis	Mostly autosomal dominant
2B	Defect in VWF such that there is increased affinity of VWF for platelet receptor GPIb, resulting in the clearance of high-molecular-weight multimers and platelets from the circulation due to formation of platelet aggregates	There is decreased VWF:RCo to VWF:Ag ratio and absence of high-molecular-weight multimers, but in contrast to 2A, ristocetin-induced platelet aggregation (RIPA) reveals increased sensitivity to low doses of ristocetin	Autosomal dominant RIPA is helpful in the diagnosis
2M	Defect in VWF such that it cannot bind platelet receptor GPIb despite the presence of normal VWF multimeric size	There is reduced ratio of VWF:RCo to VWF:Ag but a normal multimer pattern	Autosomal dominant
2N	Defect in VWF such that it cannot bind FVIII, but can bind platelets and collagen	Should be distinguished from mild hemophilia A, as FVIII level decreases because it requires VWF for stabilization. There is a disproportionate decrease in the FVIII level relative to the VWF level with a resultant reduction in the FVIII/VWF:Ag ratio	Autosomal recessive N refers to Normandy
3	Nearly complete deficiency of VWF	VWF < 30 IU/dL This condition is characterized by prolongation of the APTT, undetectable levels of VWF:Ag and VWF:RCo, and FVIII levels less than 10 IU/dL	Autosomal recessive

5. Ans. b. Type 2B VWD *Ref: Hoffbrand 7/e p726*

Type 2B VWD is characterized by increased affinity for platelet GPIb. It should be distinguished from platelet type pseudo-VWD, using either platelet agglutination tests or genetic testing. The increased affinity of this VWF variant for platelet GPIbα leads to spontaneous binding of VWF to platelets in vivo, resulting in the formation of aggregates with consequent loss of high-molecular-weight multimers, and occasionally thrombocytopenia **(Table 1)**.

6. Ans. d. Type 2N VWD *Ref: Hoffbrand 7/e p729*

Type 2N VWD is associated with markedly decreased binding of VWD with FVIII **(Table 1)**. FVIII and VWF circulate together as a complex in which VWF protects FVIII from degradation, so a deficiency in VWF or a reduction in its ability to bind FVIII will result in a low plasma level of FVIII. Therefore, deficiency of VWF can give rise to a dual hemostatic defect: reduced plasma levels of FVIII (due to its shorter half-life in the absence of VWF) and a defect in primary hemostasis because of the failure in assisting platelets to adhere to the cut edges of small blood vessels.

7. Ans. b. Type 2B VWD *Ref: Hoffbrand 7/e p729*

In type 2B, VWF binds prematurely with platelets in the circulation. This results in the loss of high-molecular-weight multimers and platelets from the circulation due to formation of platelet aggregates and to increased cleavage of platelet-bound VWF by ADAMTS13. The abnormality is detected in the laboratory by agglutination of platelets at a low concentration of ristocetin (0.5–0.7 mg/mL) that does not cause agglutination with normal VWF. Thus, RIPA should be routinely performed as part of the diagnostic work-up for type 2 VWD to detect type 2B VWD, which does not always show up in the other tests.

8. Ans. b. Type 2B VWD *Ref: Hoffbrand 7/e p730*

Desmopressin is generally contraindicated in type 2B VWD, as the released abnormal VWF will cause circulatory platelet aggregates to form, with a further fall in the platelet count.

9. Ans. e. Disseminated intravascular coagulation
Ref: Hoffbrand 7/e p731

A paraprotein can bind to VWF and accelerates its clearance, producing a type 2A or type 3 VWD. Severe aortic stenosis can cause sufficient shear stress on VWF to accelerate ADAMTS13 cleavage and cause an acquired von Willebrand syndrome that resolves immediately after valve replacement. A similar phenomenon occurs in myeloproliferative neoplasm when thrombocytosis is present and excess platelet binding promotes cleavage. In hypothyroidism, VWF synthesis is reduced.

10. Ans. d. Ristocetin-induced platelet aggregation
Ref: Stufano F. Diagnosis of von Willebrand disease. World Federation of Hemophilia; 2017.

First level tests measure the plasma level of FVIII coagulant activity (FVIII:C), the VWF antigen level (VWF:Ag), and platelet-dependent VWF function (VWF-platelet GPIbα-binding activity) usually measured as ristocetin cofactor activity (VWF:RCo). Second level tests are necessary for defining and classifying VWD variants. They are applied when low levels of VWF are detected and/or when a discrepancy between the concentration of VWF protein and its platelet-dependent functions is found (i.e., VWF:RCo/VWF:Ag <0.6). Only a few biochemical methods have been reported to distinguish VWD type 2B from the other VWD types (e.g., VWD type 2A or type 1). Among these methods, RIPA is the most widely used. Other second level tests are VWF:collagen binding assay, VWF:FVIII binding assay, and VWF multimer analysis.

11. Ans. e. All of the above
Ref: Stufano F. Diagnosis of von Willebrand disease. World Federation of Hemophilia; 2017.

von Willebrand disease type 3 is characterized by virtually complete deficiency of VWF in both plasma and platelets. VWD type 3 is inherited as a recessive trait. VWF:Ag, VWF:RCo, and VWF:CB values are <1 IU/dL, and FVIII:C levels are also very low (<10 IU/dL). It is very important to exclude the presence of an inhibitor to VWF (anti-VWF alloantibodies) in VWD type 3 patients. There are no reports of VWF alloantibody development in either VWD type 1 or type 2.

12. Ans. a. When VWF multimers are absent
Ref: Stufano F. Diagnosis of von Willebrand disease. World Federation of Hemophilia; 2017.

If it is not practical to perform RIPA on all cases, then it should always be performed when the VWF:RCo/VWF:Ag or VWF:CB/VWF:Ag ratio is reduced or if thrombocytopenia is present, bearing in mind that this may miss some mild forms of type 2B VWD.

13. Ans. d. All of the above
Ref: Stufano F. Diagnosis of von Willebrand disease. World Federation of Hemophilia; 2017.

Low-resolution VWF multimer analysis can detect the loss of HMWM, allowing patients with VWD type 1 to be distinguished from type 2, and to distinguish type 2A (loss of HMWM and intermediate molecular weight multimers) from type 2M (normal multimeric pattern). Both VWF and FVIII levels increase with age. In adults, VWF increases approximately 1–2% per year.

14. Ans. c. Concizumab
Ref: Non-factor replacement therapy for haemophilia, a current update. Blood Transfuse; 2018.

Emicizumab is a chimeric bispecific humanized antibody directed against factor IXa and factor Xa (FXa). FEIBA is FVIII inhibitor bypassing agent. Fitusiran is an antithrombin inhibitor.

Tissue factor pathway inhibitor is a potent inhibitor of the coagulation initiation phase, more specifically the activation of factor X to FXa by the TF/FVIIa complex. Concizumab has a high affinity for the KPI-2 domain of TFPI (the binding site of FXa), by preventing FXa binding to TFPI, concizumab also prevents TFPI inhibition of the TF-FVIIa complex, resulting in enhanced tenase and thrombin formation.

15. Ans. b. Only males are affected

Acquired hemophilia is a rare condition that is due to the production of autoantibodies, in adult life, which inactivate FVIII. Both the sexes are affected equally in acquired hemophilia. Typical clinical manifestations of the acquired form are extensive cutaneous purpura and internal hemorrhage; bleeding into the joints is not a prominent feature.

16. Ans. a. VWF protect FVIII from early inactivation by the activated protein C
Ref: Castaman G. Principles of care for the diagnosis and treatment of von Willebrand disease. Haematologica. 2013;98:667-74

VWD is caused by the deficiency or abnormality of VWF, which is required for platelet adhesion to subendothelium to occur and serves as carrier of FVIII, protecting it from early inactivation by the activated protein C. VWF is synthesized by endothelial cells and megakaryocytes. The gene coding for VWF is located at chromosome 12p13.

17. Ans. e. High-risk of thrombosis has led to its discontinuation
Ref: Mannucci PM. New therapies for von Willebrand disease. Blood Adv. 2019;3(21):3481-7

Vonicog alfa is a recombinant VWF concentrate and is a highly purified product. It contains all of the VWF multimers present in normal plasma and the ultra-large fraction. The ultra-large multimers are rapidly cleaved postinfusion by the enzymatic activity of patients' own plasma ADAMST13. These peculiarities have the potential advantage of supplying bleeding patients with the multimeric fraction most active in primary hemostasis. No thrombotic complication has been described in the early postinfusion period, at a time when these hyperactive multimers circulate for a short time period.

18. Ans. d. VWF activity levels < 10 IU/dL and/or FVIII levels < 20 IU/dL
Ref: Leebeek FG. How I manage severe von Willebrand disease. BJH. 2019;187(4):418-30

Unlike in hemophilia, in which the severity of disease is based on factor VIII (FVIII) or factor IX (FIX) levels, there is no uniformly accepted definition for mild, moderate or severe VWD. Federici classified patients with VWF: Ristocetin cofactor activity (VWF:RCo) levels <10 IU/dL and FVIII coagulant activity (FVIII:C) <20 IU/dL as severe; VWF:RCo 10-30 IU/dL and FVIII:C 20-40 IU/dL as moderate and VWF:RCo 30-50 IU/dL and FVIII:C 40-60 IU/dL as mild VWD. This includes type 3 VWD patients with a complete absence of VWF and most type 2B VWD patients, who generally also have a severe bleeding phenotype.

19. Ans. d. Both VWF:RCo and FVIII concentration monitoring

Ref: Leebeek FG. How I manage severe von Willebrand disease. BJH. 2019;187(4):418-30

During surgery or repeated VWF/FVIII concentrate infusions, it is recommend to measure both VWF:RCo and FVIII:C daily to ensure that the target levels of VWF and FVIII are reached. Despite the fact that it is still disputed whether normalization of VWF, FVIII or both are needed to achieve adequate hemostasis in VWD patients. An important physiological mechanism that should be considered in treatment with VWF/FVIII concentrates is that VWD patients have normal FVIII synthesis, but increased FVIII proteolysis because of reduced FVIII binding to VWF, resulting in low FVIII levels. In patients with severe VWD, FVIII levels may be less than 10 IU/dL, thereby worsening the bleeding phenotype and increasing the bleeding risk during interventions. Therefore, an increase of both VWF and FVIII by infusion of VWF/FVIII concentrates is needed. However, increase of VWF levels after administration of concentrates will also lead to an increment of endogenous FVIII, because of reduced FVIII proteolysis. This may lead to high FVIII levels after several days of treatment with VWF/FVIII concentrate. These high FVIII levels may be associated with an increased risk of thrombosis, especially after major surgery. Therefore, it is important to measure VWF and FVIII:C regularly to assess the risk for developing thrombosis and to adjust dosing. Pure VWF concentrates increase VWF levels immediately, whereas FVIII levels increase gradually over time. By binding of endogenous FVIII to the exogenous VWF, FVIII is stabilized and FVIII degradation prevented, thereby gradually increasing circulating FVIII levels. If pure VWF (without FVIII) is used in case of planned surgery, the first dose of pure VWF can be given the evening prior to surgery. However, additional FVIII should be co-administered if pure VWF concentrates are administered in emergency situations, such as severe bleeding or shortly before emergency surgery in patients with severe VWD, in order to increase FVIII levels immediately.

20. Ans. c. Alphanate *Ref: ASH 2019 Education Book, New herapies for VWD p592*

Willfact is a plasma derived VWF only concentrates which does not contain ultra large VWF multimers and deficient in HMWM's. Vonvendi is a recombinant VWF only concentrates which contain ultra large VWF multimers and HMWM's. On the other hand Alpanate, Wilate, Immunate, Hemate, Biostate contain both factor VIII and VWF.

SECTION 3: Malignant Hematology

25. Acute Lymphoblastic Leukemia
26. Acute Myeloid Leukemia
27. Acute Promyelocytic Leukemia
28. Chronic Lymphocytic Leukemia
29. Chronic Myeloid Leukemia
30. Hodgkin Lymphoma
31. Non-Hodgkin Lymphoma
32. Multiple Myeloma and Amyloidosis
33. Hairy Cell Leukemia
34. Myeloproliferative Neoplasms
35. Myelodysplastic Syndrome
36. Tumor Lysis Syndrome

CHAPTER 25

Acute Lymphoblastic Leukemia

1. **Diagnosis of acute lymphoblastic leukemia (ALL) in bone marrow requires:**
   a. 15% blasts
   b. 20% blasts
   c. 25% blasts
   d. 30% blasts

2. **A patient had blasts with immunophenotype CD13+, membrane CD19+, CD79a+, and cytoplasmic CD22+, CD10−, and CD20−. The most likely diagnosis is:**
   a. Early precursor B ALL
   b. Common ALL
   c. Late pre-B ALL
   d. Mixed phenotype acute leukemia

3. **True about the treatment outcomes in precursor B-cell ALL/lymphoblastic lymphoma (LBL) is:**
   a. In infants, many cases have translocations involving the mixed-lineage leukemia (MLL) gene at 11q23, which is associated with a poor prognosis
   b. Adult precursor B-ALL t(9;22) or/and t(v11q23) has/have poor prognosis
   c. Older children more often have t(12;21), which confers a better prognosis
   d. Myeloid antigen expression does not seem to be an independent prognostic factor in ALL
   e. All of the above

4. **In precursor T-cell LBL/ALL, the lymphoblasts on histochemistry show positivity most commonly for:**
   a. Periodic acid Schiff (PAS) staining
   b. Nonspecific esterase (NSE)
   c. Sudan black B (SBB)
   d. All of the above

5. **True regarding induction therapy for ALL is:**
   a. Rapid restoration of bone marrow function in order to prevent the emergence of resistant subclones
   b. Aims to reduce the total body leukemia cell population from approximately 10^{12} to below the cytologically detectable level of about 10^9 cells
   c. A substantial burden of leukemia cells persists undetected leading to relapse if no further therapy were administered
   d. Prophylactic treatment of sanctuary sites
   e. All of the above

6. **Anthracyclines are useful in ALL because:**
   a. Patients who receive daunorubicin demonstrate superior complete remission (CR) rates
   b. Median remission duration is prolonged
   c. Additive effect when used along with vincristine and prednisolone
   d. All of the above

7. **Asparaginase is one of the components of the following ALL regimens, *except*:**
   a. CALGB (Cancer and Leukemia Group B) ALL regimen
   b. BFM (Berlin, Frankfurt, Muenster) regimen
   c. GRAAL (Group for Research on Adult Acute Lymphoblastic Leukemia) 2003 regimen
   d. Hyper-CVAD (cyclophosphamide, vincristine, adriamycin, and dexamethasone) regimen

8. **Half-life of *Escherichia coli* asparaginase is:**
   a. 14 hours
   b. 24 hours
   c. 36 hours
   d. 6 days

9. **Structural abnormalities in childhood ALL associated with a poor outcome include the following, *except*:**
   a. t(9;22) BCR/ABL
   b. t(1;19) E2A/PBX1
   c. t(4;11) MLL/AF4
   d. t(1;14) TAL1/TCR
   e. All of the above

10. **Children with the following genetic diseases are at increased risk of ALL, *except*:**
    a. Down syndrome
    b. Neurofibromatosis type 1
    c. Bloom syndrome
    d. Ataxia telangiectasia
    e. Retinoblastoma

11. **The following are the risk factors for thrombosis during induction in childhood ALL, *except*:**
    a. Asparaginase
    b. Use of central venous catheters
    c. Prednisone
    d. Anthracycline
    e. Dexamethasone

12. **True about the use of asparaginase in ALL is:**
    a. Increases the risk of thrombosis
    b. Increase synthesis of procoagulants
    c. Pegylated (PEG)-asparaginase use does not reduce the risk of thrombosis
    d. All of the above

13. Cytarabine can be administered:
   a. Intravenously
   b. Subcutaneously
   c. Intrathecaly
   d. All of the above

14. Acute lymphoblastic leukemia accounts for what percentage of all childhood cancers?
   a. 25%
   b. 40%
   c. 55%
   d. 64%

15. True regarding renal involvement in ALL is:
   a. An enlarged kidney can be detected in 5% of patients
   b. It has no prognostic or therapeutic implications
   c. Ultrasound or CT scan should be done for assessment of renal involvement
   d. Radiotherapy is the treatment of choice
   e. All of the above are true

16. True regarding CNS involvement in ALL is:
   a. Leukemic blast in the cerebrospinal fluid (CSF) at diagnosis is seen in one-third of children with ALL
   b. Most patients have no neurological symptoms
   c. The presence of any leukemic cells in CSF predicts an increased risk of ALL relapse
   d. All of the above

17. The pre-B immunophenotype is defined by:
   a. Presence of surface immunoglobulins
   b. Presence of cytoplasmic immunoglobulins
   c. Presence of both surface immunoglobulins and cytoplasmic immunoglobulins
   d. Presence of surface CD 20

18. Good risk in pediatric ALL includes:
   a. Hyperdiploidy with 51–65 chromosomes
   b. Near-triploidy with 69–81 chromosomes
   c. Near-tetraploidy with 82–94 chromosomes
   d. All have equal prognosis

19. All are true regarding childhood ALL, *except*:
   a. Leukocyte count has prognostic significance in B-lineage but not T-lineage ALL
   b. About 20% of patients with low-risk B-lineage ALL may relapse
   c. Boys have a worse outcome than girls
   d. All are true

20. The methods for measuring minimal residual disease (MRD) in ALL are:
   a. Flow cytometric profiling of aberrant immunophenotypes
   b. Polymerase chain reaction (PCR) amplification of fusion transcripts and chromosomal breakpoints
   c. PCR amplification of antigen–receptor genes
   d. All of the above

21. What percentage of childhood ALL constitutes BCR-ABL positive ALL?
   a. 3%
   b. 10%
   c. 17%
   d. 23%

22. What percentage of ALL patients presents with central nervous system (CNS) involvement?
   a. 4%
   b. 11%
   c. 17%
   d. 25%

23. True regarding the use of granulocyte colony-stimulating factor (G-CSF) in ALL is:
   a. It can stimulate the leukemic growth
   b. Reduces the induction mortality
   c. Increases overall survival
   d. All of the above

24. Which drug in the induction regimen does not affect complete remission response?
   a. Prednisolone
   b. Vincristine
   c. Daunorubicin
   d. Asparaginase

25. The term "leukemia" was coined by:
   a. Aristotle
   b. Hippocrates
   c. Virchow
   d. Ehrlich

26. True regarding relapse in ALL are all, *except*:
   a. Most relapses occur during treatment or within the first 2 years after its completion
   b. The marrow remains the most common site of relapse in ALL
   c. Patients with CNS relapse do not require systemic treatment
   d. All of the above

27. True regarding the use of growth factors in ALL treatment are:
   a. Growth factors can stimulate leukemic cell growth
   b. Do not reduce the incidence and duration of febrile neutropenia
   c. Can be given simultaneously with chemotherapy
   d. Improve overall survival
   e. All of the above

28. Which of the following is not true regarding the blood culture samples taken during induction chemotherapy in case of febrile neutropenia?
   a. A sample of 20 mL blood from a peripheral vein and, when present, samples of 20 mL from each lumen of an indwelling vascular catheter should be taken
   b. Each sample is to be divided between an aerobic and an anaerobic bottle
   c. It identifies the cause of fever in 20–30% of cases
   d. The sample should be taken at the time of nadir of neutropenia
   e. All of the above

29. True regarding mature B-cell leukemia are all, *except*:
   a. Designated as L3 by French, American, and British (FAB) system
   b. Mature B-cell ALL is a disseminated form of Burkitt lymphoma
   c. Treatment is like precursor B-cell ALL
   d. Has good prognosis
   e. All of the above

30. True regarding BCR-ABL1–like ALL is:
   a. These cases lack BCR-ABL1 translocations
   b. They carry gene expression signature nearly identical to that of BCR-ABL1-positive ALL
   c. These patients are at very high-risk of treatment failure
   d. There is deletion of the Ikaros tumor suppressor gene
   e. All of the above

31. True regarding L-asparaginase is:
   a. L-asparaginase has a half-life of 4 hours
   b. Peripheral neuropathy is a common side effect
   c. It has minimal bone marrow toxicity
   d. All of the above

32. True regarding early T-cell precursors (ETP) ALL is:
   a. Gene expression profile of ETP ALL is similar to that of myeloid leukemia
   b. T-lineage cell surface markers CD1a and CD8 are present
   c. Associated with good prognosis
   d. All of the above

33. Blinatumomab is a monoclonal antibody against:
   a. CD3 and CD19
   b. CD3 and CD20
   c. CD4 and CD22
   d. CD4 and CD79

34. True about chimeric antigen receptor (CAR)-T cells is:
   a. They use allogeneic T cells
   b. Approved for upfront use in high-risk ALL
   c. Result in T-cell aplasia
   d. All of the above
   e. None of the above

35. The prevalence of BCR-ABL1–like ALL (Ph-like ALL) is:
   a. <2%
   b. 2–4%
   c. 10–15%
   d. 20–25%

36. Tisagenlecleucel is used for the treatment of:
   a. Precursor T-ALL
   b. B-ALL
   c. ETP-ALL
   d. Peripheral T-cell lymphoma

37. True about intrachromosomal amplification of chromosome 21 (iAMP21) are all, *except*:
   a. Defined as the presence of three or more RUNX1 signals on an abnormal chromosome 21
   b. Associated with good prognosis in children with ALL
   c. Fluorescence in situ hybridization (FISH) is the most common method used to identify it
   d. Not associated with T-cell ALL

38. True about ALL with t(4;11) (q21;q23) is:
   a. Common in infants
   b. Is associated with MLL gene translocation
   c. Associated with poor prognosis
   d. All of the above

39. A 33 years old male presented with fever and neck swelling for 2 months. CT scan of chest showed anterior mediastinal mass and LDH was 1600 U/l. The bone marrow aspirate shows 90% blasts. Next step should include:
   a. Biopsy of mediastinal mass
   b. Whole body PET CT scan
   c. Starting CHOP chemotherapy immediately
   d. Immunophenotyping
   e. Wait for biopsy report

40. Which of the following is not an anti-CD22 monoclonal antibody?
   a. Denintuzumab mafodotin
   b. Epratuzumab
   c. Inotuzumab ozogamicin
   d. Moxetumomab pasudotox

41. Which of the following is not considered high-risk ALL relapse?
   a. B-ALL early isolated marrow elapse
   b. Early/late B-ALL combined relapses
   c. T-ALL early marrow relapse
   d. T-ALL late marrow relapse

42. Which of these is the least preferred for CNS prophylaxis in children?
   a. CNS irradiation
   b. Intrathecal MTX
   c. Systemic high-dose therapy with MTX
   d. All are equally preferred

ANSWERS WITH EXPLANATIONS

1. Ans. b. 20% blasts *Ref: WHO 2017 Revised Edition*

The diagnosis of ALL requires ≥20% bone marrow lymphoblasts. The 2017 World Health Organization (WHO) classification lists ALL and LBL as the same entity, distinguished only by the primary location of the disease. The diagnosis of LBL is made when the disease is restricted to a mass lesion primarily involving nodal or extranodal sites with no or minimal involvement in blood or bone marrow, defined as more than 20% lymphoblasts in the marrow. A patient with LBL is treated as ALL. In many treatment protocols, a value of >25% marrow blasts is used to define leukemia.

2. Ans. a. Early precursor B ALL *Ref: Williams 7/e Table 91-4*

The antigens associated with various stages of differentiation in ALL are early precursor B (pro-B-ALL)—membrane CD19+, CD79a+, and cytoplasmic CD22+; common ALL—CD10+; and late pre-B ALL—CD20+, cytoplasmic μ heavy chain expression. In earlier studies, cases of B-cell precursor ALL were subdivided into those which were CD10-positive (so-called common ALL) and those which were CD10-negative (pre-pre-B, pro-B, or CD10-negative B-cell precursor) leukemias. Co-expression of myeloid antigens is seen in up to 30% of cases, most commonly CD13 (14%) and/or CD33 (16%). The presence of myeloid antigens in ALL does not have any effect on treatment but can be useful in immunologic monitoring of patients for minimal residual leukemia, as the presence of these aberrant markers in treated patients signifies residual disease.

3. Ans. e. All of the above *Ref: Williams 8/e Chap 91*

The outcome is less favorable in infants <1 year of age and in adults and more favorable in children. In infants, many cases have translocations involving the *MLL* gene at 11q23, which is associated with a poor prognosis. Adult precursor B-ALL, more often associated with the poor-prognosis, has t(9;22) or t(v11q23), and survival is much poorer than in childhood cases. Older children more often have hyperdiploidy and t(12;21), which confer a better prognosis. Myeloid antigen expression does not seem to be an independent prognostic factor in ALL. Age and leukocyte count are used for risk classification in nearly all pediatric clinical trials involving B-cell precursor ALL. Hyperdiploidy (>50 chromosomes) and *TEL-AML1* fusion, seen primarily in children aged 1-9 years, is associated with a favorable prognosis. *MLL* gene rearrangements, which occur in about 70% of infants <1 year and in 10% of adults, and Philadelphia chromosome, which is found in 3-5% of children but in 25-30% of adult patients, confer a poor outcome.

Another useful measure in risk assessment of ALL is the response to early treatment, as measured by the rate of clearance of leukemic cells (MRD) from the blood or marrow with the use of flow cytometric detection of aberrant immunophenotype or analysis by PCR of receptor gene rearrangements.

4. Ans. a. Periodic acid Schiff (PAS) staining *Ref: Williams 8/e*

Examination of bone marrow aspirate and biopsy is preferred for diagnosis of ALL because about 10% of patients do not demonstrate circulating blasts in the peripheral blood at the time of diagnosis and because bone marrow cells are better than blood cells for cytogenetic studies. The cytochemical stains needed to distinguish between the ALL and acute myeloid leukemia (AML) are the SBB stain and the stains for myeloperoxidase (MPO) and the NSE, including -naphthyl butyrate and -naphthyl acetate esterase. Stains for these esterases generally do not react with leukemic lymphoblasts. The granules seen in some of the lymphoblasts are usually amphophilic (which stain fuchsia), which can be readily distinguishable from the primary myeloid granules (which stain deep purple). Staining with PAS is positive in more than 70% of lymphoblasts.

5. Ans. e. All of the above *Ref: Williams 8/e; Hoffbrand 7/e*

Induction chemotherapy is given with the goals of rapid restoration of bone marrow function, using multiple chemotherapy drugs at acceptable toxicities, in order to prevent the emergence of resistant subclones. Use of adequate initial and prophylactic treatment of sanctuary sites such as the CNS is important, since CNS relapse is associated with a poor prognosis. Induction therapy aims to reduce the total body leukemia cell population from approximately 10^{12} to below the cytologically detectable level of about 10^9 cells. A substantial burden of leukemia cells persists undetected (e.g. MRD), leading to relapse if no further therapy were administered. The ALL induction regimen includes glucocorticoids (prednisolone or dexamethasone), vincristine, and L-asparaginase and anthracycline. Induction therapy is intensified based on the concept that more rapid and complete reduction of the leukemic cell burden also prevents the development of drug resistance. Because of its increased penetration into the CNS and because of its longer half-life, dexamethasone, when used in induction and continuation therapy, provides better control of systemic and CNS disease than does prednisone in children with ALL. However, it is more toxic.

6. Ans. d. All of the above
Ref: Cancer and leukemia group B studies in acute lymphoblastic leukemia.

The importance of an anthracycline in the treatment of adults with ALL was demonstrated by the randomized trial (CALGB 7612) that incorporated the anthracycline daunorubicin during the first 3 days of induction therapy into a chemotherapy program that included vincristine, prednisone, and L-asparaginase; patients who received daunorubicin demonstrated superior CR rates (83 vs. 47%) and median remission duration (18 vs. 5 months) when compared with those who did not receive daunorubicin. The results indicate that anthracyclines may offer the best survival chance when used at full dosage during induction and early consolidation treatment.

7. Ans. d. Hyper-CVAD (cyclophosphamide, vincristine, adriamycin, and dexamethasone) regimen
Ref: Kantarjian. Cancer. 101:2788, 2004

Asparaginase is a key component to the ALL regimens for children leading to superior CR and disease-free survival rates. It is a component of the CALGB ALL regimen, the BFM regimen, and the GRAAL 2003 regimen but not hyper-CVAD. The median overall survival of patients who demonstrated plasma asparagine depletion was significantly longer when compared with patients who still had measurable plasma asparagine (31 vs. 13 months, respectively). Hyper-CVAD developed by MD Anderson Cancer Center is used in adult ALL as it does not contain asparaginase which some adults cannot tolerate. Hyper-CVAD is one of the most frequently used adult ALL regimens in routine practice. With the hyper-CVAD regimen, the CR rate in adult ALL is 90% with a 5–10-year survival rate of 40–50%. In Ph+ ALL, the hyper-CVAD + imatinib regimen has shown encouraging data with 3-year survival rates of 60%. In Burkitt ALL, hyper-CVAD + rituximab has produced event-free survival rates of 80–90%. This continues to be the current frontline regimen.

8. Ans. b. 24 hours
Ref: Williams 8/e

Native *E. coli* asparaginase—half-life approximately 1 day. *Erwinia* asparaginase—half-life approximately 14 hours. PEG *E. coli* asparaginase—half-life approximately 6 days. Three forms of L-asparaginase, each having different pharmacokinetic profiles, are available: one derived from *Erwinia chrysanthemi*, another prepared from *E. coli*, and a third made of a polyethylene glycol form of the *E. coli* product (pegaspargase). The dosages of these three preparations are based on their half-lives. PEG *E. coli* asparaginase, which has the longest half-life, is usually administered at 2500 IU/m^2 every other week for two doses in cases of ALL. The *Erwinia* preparation, which has the shortest half-life, is administered at 20,000 IU/m^2 three times per week for 6–12 doses. The doses of *E. coli* L-asparaginase range from 5,000 to 10,000 IU/m^2, administered two to three times per week for 6–12 doses. Intramuscular administration causes less frequent and less severe hypersensitivity reaction than intravenous injection of L-asparaginase. L-asparaginase does not affect CR rate but improves leukemia-free survival (LFS).

9. Ans. e. All of the above
Ref: Williams 8/e

All of these cytogenetic abnormalities are associated with poor outcome. Approximately 75–80% of adult and childhood ALL cases can be readily classified into prognostically or therapeutically relevant subgroups based on the chromosome number, specific chromosomal rearrangements, and molecular genetic changes. t(12;21) ETV6/RUNX1 is associated with good outcome. More aggressive treatment regimens are recommended for children with any of these cytogenetic or molecular findings. Patients with t(1;19) respond well to treatment strategies, whereas the addition of tyrosine kinase inhibitor therapy should be considered in patients with t(9;22). Patients with the t(4;11) MLL rearrangement have a significantly poorer treatment outcome than those without this abnormality. Hence, they are treated with more intensive chemotherapy and/or hematopoietic cell transplantation.

10. Ans. e. Retinoblastoma
Ref: Williams 8/e; Hoffman 5/e p1019

Children with Down syndrome have a 20–30 times greater risk of developing leukemia; acute megakaryocytic (AML-M7) leukemia predominates in patients <3 years and ALL is predominant in older children. Autosomal recessive genetic diseases associated with increased chromosomal fragility and a predisposition to ALL include ataxia-telangiectasia, Nijmegen breakage syndrome, and Bloom syndrome. Patients with ataxia-telangiectasia have a 60–70 times greater risk of leukemia and about 250 times greater risk of T-cell lymphoma. In almost all other cases of ALL, lymphoblasts have acquired genetic changes, 75% of which have prognostic and therapeutic significance.

11. Ans. e. Dexamethasone
Ref: Blood 2006, Caruso et al and British Journal of Haematology, 2007, Jeanette H. Payne

Most of the thrombotic events occur during the induction phase of ALL therapy. In a study by Caruso et al., lower doses of asparaginase for long periods were associated with the highest incidence of thrombosis, as were anthracyclines and prednisone (instead of dexamethasone). The presence of central lines and of thrombophilic genetic abnormalities also appeared to be frequently associated with thrombosis. The cytotoxicity of asparaginase is mediated by depletion of the essential amino acid asparagine. In comparison with normal cells, lymphoblasts lack the enzyme asparagine synthetase, which makes them particularly susceptible. Asparaginase also reduces circulating levels of several hemostatic proteins including plasminogen, fibrinogen, and antithrombin by a combination of reduced hepatic production and increased clearance. Prednisolone leads to elevation of factor VIII, von Willebrand factor (vWF), prothrombin, and antithrombin levels. Although there are no randomized studies comparing the hemostatic effects and thrombosis risk associated with different glucocorticosteroids, a historical comparison of two BFM studies indicated that the risk during induction was much lower with dexamethasone than with prednisolone.

12. Ans. d. All of the above

Asparaginase depletes plasma asparagine, thereby inhibiting protein synthesis in leukemic cells and synthesis of many other plasma proteins, which results in deficiencies of albumin, thyroxine-binding globulin, and various coagulation proteins, including prothrombin, factors V, VII, VIII, IX, X, XI, fibrinogen, antithrombin, protein C, protein S, and plasminogen. These deficiencies result in prolongation of the prothrombin time, activated partial thromboplastin time (aPTT), thrombin time, and hypofibrinogenemia, with levels often <100 mg/dL. These coagulation abnormalities resolve within 1-2 weeks after cessation of the drug. PEG-asparaginase and L-asparaginase appear to have equivalent risk of severe thrombosis.

13. Ans. d. All of the above

Cytarabine can be given intravenously, subcutaneously, and intrathecaly. Cytarabine is converted intracellularly to the active metabolite cytarabine triphosphate. It inhibits DNA polymerase by competing with deoxycytidine triphosphate resulting in inhibition of DNA synthesis and is incorporated into DNA chain resulting in termination of chain elongation; cell cycle-specific for the S-phase of cell division. Cytarabine is indicated alone or in combination for induction of remission and/or maintenance in patients with AML, ALL, erythroleukemia, blast crises of chronic myeloid leukemia (CML), diffuse histiocytic lymphomas [non-Hodgkin's lymphomas (NHL) of high malignancy], meningeal leukemia, and meningeal neoplasms. Cytarabine has been given intrathecally at doses of 10-30 mg/m^2 three times a week until CSF findings return to normal.

14. Ans. a. 25% *Ref: Hoffbrands 6/e p448*

ALL is the most common childhood malignancy diagnosed in patients <15 years, accounting for 23% of all cancers and 76% of all leukemias in this age group.

15. Ans. b. It has no prognostic or therapeutic implications

An enlarged kidney can be detected in about 30-50% of patients but has no prognostic or therapeutic implications. Liver dysfunction due to leukemic infiltration occurs in 10-20% of patients, is usually mild, and has no important clinical or prognostic consequences. Abnormalities of the bone, such as metaphyseal banding, periosteal reactions, osteolysis, osteosclerosis, or osteopenia, can be revealed by radiography in half of the patients. As these changes do not affect treatment and outcome, routine diagnostic imaging studies (except for chest radiography to rule out mediastinal mass) are not necessary.

16. Ans. d. All of the above

Ref: CH Pui. ASH Education program. 2006

Leukemic blast cells can be detected at diagnosis in the CSF of about one-third of children with ALL. Most of these patients have no neurological symptoms. CNS leukemia is defined by the presence of at least 5 leukocytes per microliter of CSF and the detection of leukemic blast cells, or by the presence of cranial nerve palsy. The presence of any leukemic cells in CSF (even from iatrogenic introduction due to a traumatic lumbar puncture) predicts an increased risk of ALL relapse. The following presenting features are associated with an increased risk of CNS relapse in pediatric patients: (1) T-cell immunophenotype, (2) hyperleukocytosis, (3) high-risk genetic abnormalities such as the Philadelphia chromosome and t(4;11), and (4) the presence of leukemic cells in CSF (even from iatrogenic introduction due to a traumatic lumbar puncture). Patients with T-cell ALL and a baseline leukocyte count of more than 100×10^9/L have the highest risk of CNS relapse. Early intensive systemic and intrathecal chemotherapy could reduce the CNS relapse to a negligible level, permitting the omission of cranial irradiation in most of the patients.

17. Ans. b. Presence of cytoplasmic immunoglobulins

Ref: Williams 8/e

The pre-B immunophenotype is defined by the presence of cytoplasmic immunoglobulin μ heavy chains with no absence of surface immunoglobulins and is found in approximately 20-25% of cases. Pre-B ALL expresses CD19, CD22, and CD79 and, usually, CD10 and terminal deoxynucleotidyl transferase (TdT) but only two-thirds express CD34. In many cases of pre-B ALL, surface CD20 is absent or is weakly expressed. Early pre-B ALL cells lack expression of surface and cytoplasmic immunoglobulins.

18. Ans. a. Hyperdiploidy with 51-65 chromosomes

Williams 8/e; Hoffman 5/e

ALL with hyperdiploidy with the chromosome number of 51-65 represents a group of subset of B-lineage ALL with an excellent overall prognosis. ALL lymphoblasts with this karyotype have a marked propensity to accumulate greater quantities of methotrexate and its active polyglutamate metabolites leading to extensive apoptosis of leukemic blasts and thus favorable prognosis. These features help to explain the relatively low leukemic burden at presentation and the favorable prognosis of this ALL with hyperdiploidy with the chromosome number of 51–65. Among chromosomes that are over-represented, only the trisomies of chromosomes 4, 10, and 17 are associated with a favorable prognosis. In contrast to the overall favorable prognosis of cases with 51–65 chromosomes, cytogenetics showing near-triploidy (69–81 chromosomes) have a response to therapy similar to that of nonhyperdiploid ALL; cases with near-tetraploidy (82–94 chromosomes) have a high frequency of T-cell immunophenotype. Hypodiploidy (<45 chromosomes) occurs in less than 2% of ALL cases and is associated with a poor outcome. So not all hyperdiploidy are associated with a favorable prognosis.

19. Ans. d. All are true   *Ref: Hoffman 6/e; Williams 8/e*

Different systems have been used to classify childhood ALL risk. In one of the more common systems, children with ALL are divided into standard-risk, high-risk, or very high-risk groups, with more intensive treatment given for higher risk patients. Children at low-risk have a better outlook than those at very high-risk. Presenting clinical and biological features are commonly used to define subtypes of ALL with different risk of relapse. Presenting age and leukocyte count have prognostic significance in B-lineage but not T-lineage ALL. As many as 20% of patients with B-lineage ALL who are considered at lower risk of relapse by these criteria (e.g., age 1–9 years with leukocyte count < 50,000/μL) may relapse. Moreover, cases with a very high-risk of relapse cannot be reliably distinguished by these criteria. Boys have a worse outcome than girls. Children between the ages of 1 and 9 years with B-cell ALL tend to have better cure rates. Children <1 year and children ≥10 years are considered high-risk patients. The prognosis in T-cell ALL is not affected much by age. Children with pre-B or early pre-B-cell ALL generally do better than those with mature B-cell (Burkitt) leukemia. The prognosis for T-cell ALL seems to be about the same as that for B-cell ALL as long as treatment is intense.

20. Ans. d. All of the above   *Ref: ASH Education 2018 book*

A slow response to the initial induction therapy (e.g., poor prednisolone response or MRD positivity at the end of induction therapy) is associated with a poor treatment outcome and poor overall survival. Response to therapy, as assessed by morphological examination of bone marrow and peripheral blood smears, has limited sensitivity and accuracy. Advances in the methods for detecting MRD, which are at least 100 times more sensitive than conventional morphological techniques, have introduced a new way to monitor response to treatment and guide further therapy in high-risk groups. The most reliable methods for measuring MRD include flow cytometric profiling of aberrant immunophenotypes, PCR amplification of fusion transcripts and chromosomal breakpoints, and PCR amplification of antigen–receptor genes.

The prognostic importance of MRD in childhood ALL has been well established by the results of numerous studies. Patients who had MRD of 0.01% or more in bone marrow during or at the end of remission induction therapy had a significantly higher risk of relapse, while those with MRD of 1% or more at the end of remission induction therapy and those with MRD of 0.1% or more during continuation therapy had an extremely high relapse risk. Treatment is now stratified based on the MRD levels.

21. Ans. a. 3%

Ref: Fielding AK. How I treat Ph+ ALL. Blood, 2010

Polymerase chain reaction analyses have revealed that BCR–ABL-positive ALL occurs in 20–30% of adult patients compared with 3% of children. One-third of adult ALL patients with a Ph chromosome show M-BCR rearrangements (resulting in a 210-kDa protein), similar to patients with CML, whereas two-thirds have m-BCR rearrangements (resulting in a 190-kDa protein). The molecular aberration BCR–ABL is more frequently detected than the chromosome abnormality t(9;22) because of occasional difficulties in obtaining adequate material for cytogenetic analysis. In Ph+ ALL, there are many additional epigenetic changes, copy number abnormalities, and mutations downstream of *BCR-ABL* that contribute to the very aggressive clinical course of Ph+ ALL compared to CML. In the case of molecular diagnosis of *BCR-ABL*, screening for both potential transcripts, p190 and p210, should be undertaken.

22. Ans. a. 4%

Although 7% of ALL patients at presentation can have CNS involvement (demonstrated by leukemic blast cells in the CSF), only 4% initially have CNS symptoms such as headache, vomiting, lethargy, nuchal rigidity, and cranial or peripheral nerve dysfunction.

23. Ans. b. Reduces the induction mortality

The use of hemopoietic growth factors such as G-CSF is an effective supportive therapy during the treatment of ALL. There is no indication that these CSFs stimulate leukemic cell growth in a significant manner. Most clinical trials have demonstrated that the prophylactic administration of G-CSF significantly accelerates neutrophil recovery, and several prospective randomized studies have also shown that this is associated with a substantially reduced incidence and duration of febrile neutropenia and of severe infections and reduced induction mortality. However, a benefit in terms of long-term outcome due to increased dose intensity achieved by using G-CSF has not yet been demonstrated in any trial. G-CSF may even be given in parallel with chemotherapy without aggravating the myelotoxicity of these specific regimens.

24. Ans. d. Asparaginase   *Ref: Hoffbrands 7/e*

Standard induction therapy for ALL includes the four commonly used drugs—prednisone, vincristine, anthracyclines (mostly daunorubicin), and also asparaginase. Prednisolone used as a prophase is an important component of ALL induction therapy and day 8 prednisolone response is used for risk stratification of patients. Anthracycline dose intensity and schedule also play an important role in the induction therapy of ALL. Asparaginase does not affect CR rate but improves LFS. If asparaginase is not used during induction therapy, then it is often included in the consolidation treatment, particularly in adult ALL patients, who cannot tolerate asparaginase, because of increased toxicity.

25. Ans. c. Virchow *Ref: Williams 8/e*

In 1847, Virchow coined the term "leukemia." He differentiated it into two types—splenic and lymphatic—that could be distinguished from each other based on splenomegaly and enlarged lymph nodes and on the morphologic similarities of the leukemic cells to those normally found in these organs. In 1891, Ehrlich's introduction of staining methods allowed further distinction of leukemia into the subtypes.

26. Ans. c. Patients with CNS relapse do not require systemic treatment *Ref: Williams 8/e*

Relapse in ALL is defined as the reappearance of lymphoblasts at any site in the body. When the relapse occurs in marrow or blood, it is called medullary relapse and when it occurs outside the bone marrow, it is called extramedullary relapse. Most relapses occur during the treatment period or within the first 2 years after its completion. The bone marrow remains the most common site of relapse in ALL. Leukemic relapse occurring at extramedullary sites includes the CNS, testis, eye, ear, ovary, uterus, bone, muscle, tonsil, kidney, and paranasal sinus. In patients who develop hematologic relapse while on therapy or shortly thereafter, allogeneic hematopoietic stem cell transplantation is the treatment of choice. Although extramedullary relapse, e.g., in CNS or testis, occurs frequently in isolation, most if not all occurrences are associated with MRD in the marrow and will ultimately have frank relapse. Hence, patients with extramedullary relapse require intensive systemic treatment to prevent subsequent hematologic relapse.

27. Ans. c. Can be given simultaneously with chemotherapy *Ref: Hoffbrand 7/e*

Growth factors do not stimulate leukemic cell growth in a clinically significant manner. Most clinical trials have shown that the prophylactic administration of G-CSF significantly improves neutrophil recovery, and this is associated with a substantially reduced incidence and duration of febrile neutropenia and of severe infections and reduced induction mortality. G-CSF may even be given in parallel with chemotherapy without aggravating the myelotoxicity of these regimens, and this scheduling is an important determinant of clinical efficacy. A benefit in terms of long-term outcome due to increased dose intensity achieved by using G-CSF has not yet been demonstrated in any trial. The overall survival is not affected by the use of growth factors.

28. Ans. d. Sample should be taken at the time of nadir of neutropenia *Ref: Hoffbrand 7/e*

The sample should be taken at the time of fever and not at the peak of neutropenia. The specificity of blood cultures is increased if samples are taken from at least two separate sites, preferably including all lumina of a central venous catheter. Ideally, blood should be drawn from a peripheral vein and from the central venous catheter to confirm the significance of flora on skin commensals such as the gram-positive coagulase-negative *staphylococci*. Other isolates including gram-negative bacilli and viridans streptococci seldom, if ever, colonize the lumen of a central venous catheter because they normally originate from the oral cavity and gut in the setting of mucositis. Mucositis is a major risk factor for gram-negative septicemia. The total amount of blood sampled at any one time constitutes a single blood culture. In adults, the ideally recommended blood sample is at least 20 mL, and preferably 30 mL (to increase sensitivity and specificity), of blood taken from each sampling site and is divided between an aerobic and an anaerobic bottle to detect the majority of common pathogens. Culture and histological examination of skin punch–biopsy specimens are very helpful in diagnosing disseminated infections due to *Candida* spp., *Trichosporon* spp., and *Fusarium* spp. There is no point in undertaking surveillance cultures unless the results are used to guide therapeutic or prophylactic choice. Obtaining nasal swabs to detect *Staphylococcus aureus* is useful as there is a strong association between carriage and subsequent bacteremia. As per American Society of Clinical Oncology (ASCO) guidelines, high-risk regimens are those which have risk of infection leading to febrile neutropenia greater than 20% for any chemotherapy regimen, intermediate risk at 10–20%, and low-risk at less than 10%.

29. Ans. c. Treatment is like precursor B-cell ALL *Ref: Hoffman 7/e Chap 64*

Mature B-cell ALL was earlier termed Burkitt leukemia. It is a disseminated form of Burkitt lymphoma. It is designated as L3 in the FAB system. Mature B-cell ALL does not respond well to chemotherapy traditionally used for childhood ALL. However, good outcomes have been obtained with treatments designed for Burkitt lymphoma.

30. Ans. e. All of the above
Ref: Boer JM. BCR-ABL1-like acute lymphoblastic leukaemia: from bench to bedside. Eur J Cancer. 2017

Analysis of the gene expression signatures of patients with ALL has led to the identification of a new subtype of precursor B-cell ALL, termed BCR-ABL1-like or Ph chromosome-like (Ph-like) ALL. These cases were identified because they lack BCR-ABL1 translocations yet are characterized by a gene expression signature nearly identical to that of BCR-ABL1-positive ALL. These patients are at very high-risk of treatment failure. One common genetic feature common to both BCR-ABL and BCR-ABL-like ALL is the deletion of the Ikaros tumor suppressor.

31. Ans. c. It has minimal bone marrow toxicity
Ref: Egler RA. L-asparaginase in the treatment of patients with acute lymphoblastic leukemia. J Pharmacol Pharmacother. 2016

Asparaginase is an enzyme used in the treatment of ALL. It has minimal bone marrow toxicity. Its major side effects are anaphylaxis, pancreatitis, diabetes, coagulation abnormalities, and thrombosis, especially intracranial. Depletion of L-asparagine from plasma by L-asparaginase results in inhibition of RNA and DNA synthesis with the subsequent blastic cell apoptosis. Current treatment protocols include *E. coli* asparaginase or PEG asparaginase for first-line treatment of ALL. The parenteral administration of asparaginase results in rapid and complete deamination of the amino acid asparagine leading to depletion of asparagine, especially in the plasma and, in part, the cerebrospinal fluid. Native *E. coli* asparaginase has half-life of approximately 1 day, *Erwinia* asparaginase has half-life of approximately 14 hours, and PEG *E. coli* asparaginase has half-life of approximately 6 days. Peripheral neuropathy is common with vincristine.

32. Ans. a. Gene expression profile of ETP ALL is similar to that of myeloid leukemia
Ref: Coustan-Smith E, Mullighan CG, Onciu M, Behm FG, Raimondi SC, Pei D, et al. Early T-cell precursor leukemia: a subtype of very high-risk acute lymphoblastic leukemia. Lancet Oncol. 2009;10(2):147-56.

Early T-cell precursor leukemias are characterized by the presence of a gene expression profile of both hematopoietic stem cells and myeloid progenitors. ETP ALL is characterized by lack of expression of the T-lineage cell surface markers CD1a and CD8, weak or absent expression of CD5, and aberrant expression of one or more myeloid (CD13, CD33, CD117, CD11b) or hematopoietic stem cell markers (CD34, HLA-DR). ETP ALL is associated with a dismal outcome because of its poor response to chemotherapy and high rate of resistance or early relapse. The regimens used to treat AML, such as those incorporating high-dose cytarabine, and/or targeted therapies that inhibit cytokine receptor and Janus kinase (JAK) signaling may be beneficial in ETP ALL.

33. Ans. a. CD3 and CD19
Ref: Kantarjian H, Stein A, Gokbuget N, Fielding AK, Schuh AC, Ribdera JM, et al. Blinatumomab versus chemotherapy for advanced acute lymphoblastic leukemia. N Engl J Med. 2017;376(9):836-47.

Blinatumomab is a bispecific monoclonal antibody that enables CD3-positive T cells to recognize and eliminate CD19-positive ALL blasts. When blinatumomab concurrently binds CD3 and CD19, the T cells are activated and directed to CD19-expressing target B cells, resulting in a cytotoxic T-cell response. Treatment with blinatumomab results in significantly longer overall survival than chemotherapy among adult patients with relapsed or refractory B-cell precursor ALL.

34. Ans. e. None of the above
Ref: Mchayleh W, Bedi P, Sehgal R, Solh M. Chimeric antigen receptor T-cells: the future is now. J Clin Med. 2019;8(2):pii:E207.

Chimeric antigen receptor T cells are genetically engineered autologous T cells that express antigen receptors that result in recognition and killing of targeted malignant cells. The chimeric receptor CTL-019 binds CD19 on malignant B cells and leads to tyrosine kinase-mediated activation of the T cell which kills CD19-positive B cells. This leads to death of both malignant and native B cells leading to B-cell aplasia.

35. Ans. c. 10–15%
Ref: Hunger SP, Mullighan CG. Redefining ALL classification: toward detecting high-risk ALL and implementing precision medicine. Blood. 2015;125(26):3977-87.

Subtypes of B-ALL	Prevalence
Ph+ ALL	2–4%
Ph-like ALL	10–15%
Hyperdiploidy	20–30%
t(12;21)	15–25%
Hypodiploidy	2–3%

(ALL: acute lymphoblastic leukemia).

36. Ans. b. B-ALL
Tisagenlecleucel is a CAR-T cell therapy for both B-ALL and aggressive B-cell lymphomas. It is used for tumors that express the CD19 antigen. This CAR-T therapy targets the CD19 antigen on the B cells involved in the pathogenesis of B-ALL and the aggressive B-cell NHLs. Adoptive transfer of T cells engineered to express a CD19-targeted CAR is the most advanced CAR-modified T-cell technology. Normal lineage B cells are also eliminated after CD19 CAR-T infusion. This can cause long-lasting hypogammaglobulinemia, which requires monthly intravenous immunoglobulin replacement to prevent serious infections until the B-cell aplasia resolves.

37. Ans. b. Associated with good prognosis in children with ALL
Ref: Harrison CJ. An international study of intrachromosomal amplification of chromosome 21 (iAMP21): cytogenetic characterization and outcome. Leukemia. 2014;18:1015-21.

Amplification of RUNX1 occurs on a rearranged chromosome 21. FISH is the most common method used to identify iAMP21, which is defined as the presence of five or more total copies of RUNX1, with three or more extra RUNX1 signals on a single abnormal chromosome 21. The children are older, with a median age of 9–11 years, and generally have low white cell counts. iAMP21 is associated with poor outcome in children with ALL treated in contemporary standard-risk. Children with ALL often undergo blast FISH testing at diagnosis for the presence of the ETV6-RUNX1 fusion, which led to identification of intrachromosomal amplification of a region of chromosome 21 that included multiple copies of RUNX1 as a recurrent genetic lesion. First described in 2003, iAMP21 occurs in 1–3% of children. The Children's Oncology Group (COG) treats all patients with iAMP21, regardless of the risk group or MRD response, with a high-risk postinduction therapy.

38. Ans. d. All of the above

Ref: WHO revised edition, 2017.

The WHO classification of hematological myeloid neoplasms and acute leukemias identifies one subtype of B-ALL [termed as B lymphoblastic leukemia/lymphoma with t(v;11q23); *MLL* rearranged], which involves all translocations of *MLL* with one of the possible gene partners.

11q23 translocations [t(11q23)] are recurring cytogenetic abnormalities in both AML and ALL, involving the same gene, *ALL1* (or *MLL*). The prognosis of ALL with an 11q23 abnormality is particularly dismal in infants. Allogeneic transplantation with hemopoietic stem cells from an HLA-matched related donor does not seem to improve the clinical outcome in patients with t(4;11)-positive leukemia.

39. Ans. d. Immunophenotyping

The bone marrow aspirate exhibits 90% blasts. Since the diagnosis is evident by bone marrow examination, mediastinal mass biopsy is not required. Similarly there is no role of PET-CT scan in leukemia diagnosis. Immunophenotyping should be done for typing the leukemia and patient should be treated for leukemia. CHOP is not used to treat leukemia. Immunophenotyping by flow cytometry of bone marrow or peripheral blood samples can be used to help distinguish AML from ALL and further classify the subtype of AML/ALL.

40. Ans. a. Denintuzumab mafodotin

Epratuzumab is an unconjugated monoclonal antibody targeting CD22. Inotuzumab ozogamicin is a monoclonal antibody against CD22 that is conjugated to calicheamicin. Moxetumomab pasudotox is the third anti-CD22 monoclonal antibody, fused to Pseudomonas aeruginosa exotoxin A. Denintuzumab mafodotin is an anti-CD19 conjugated monoclonal antibody, where the antibody is linked to the microtubule-disrupting agent monomethyl auristatin F.

41. Ans. b. Early/late B-ALL combined relapses

Ref: Hunger SP. How I treat relapsed acute lymphoblastic leukemia in the pediatric population. Blood 2020

BFM and UK definitions of ALL relapse are—very early (<18 months from diagnosis), early (18 months from diagnosis but <6 months after completion of treatment), and late (≥6 months after completion of treatment). Early/late B-ALL combined (marrow plus CNS) relapses are considered as intermediate risk relapses. All T cell relapses (regardless of timing) are considered as high risk relapses.

42. Ans. a. CNS irradiation

Ref: Pui CH. Treating childhood acute lymphoblastic leukemia without cranial irradiation. N Engl J Med 2009; 360:2730-41

CNS prophylaxis can be achieved by CNS irradiation, intrathecal MTX in mono- or triple therapy (MTX, Cyt and steroids), and systemic high-dose therapy with MTX and/or cytarabine. CNS involvement at diagnosis requires both a standard chemotherapy model and intrathecal chemotherapy until spinal fluid cytology shows blast clearance. With effective risk-adjusted chemotherapy, prophylactic cranial irradiation can be safely omitted from the treatment of childhood ALL. In a growing proportion of patients, prophylactic cranial irradiation, once a standard treatment, is being replaced by intrathecal and systemic chemotherapy to reduce radiation-associated late complications such as second cancers, cognitive deficits, and endocrinopathy.

CHAPTER 26

Acute Myeloid Leukemia

1. 20% blasts are not required for the diagnosis of acute myeloid leukemia (AML) if following cytogenetic abnormalities are present, *except*:
   a. t(8;21)
   b. t(16;16)
   c. del 7
   d. All of the above

2. AML with t(8;21)(q22;q22) has all, *except*:
   a. Favorable prognosis
   b. Blasts with long thin Auer rods
   c. Highly sensitive to cytarabine
   d. Patients with RUNX1-RUNX1T1 detected by reverse transcription-polymerase chain reaction (RT-PCR) postinduction have poor prognosis

3. Megakaryoblastic leukemia is associated with:
   a. t(3;3)(q21;q26.2)
   b. t(1;22)(p13;q13)
   c. t(9;11)(p22;q23)
   d. t(6;9)(p23;q34)

4. Poor prognosis in acute myeloid leukemia is seen with the following molecular defects:
   a. AML with mutated NPM1
   b. AML with mutated CEBPA
   c. AML with mutations in FLT3
   d. None of the above

5. Acute myeloid leukemia is said to have evolved from myelodysplastic syndrome (MDS) if dysplasia is present in:
   a. More than 50% of cells
   b. More than 25% of cells
   c. More than 30% of cells
   d. More than 20% of cells

6. Acute myeloid leukemia-M0 may be positive for:
   a. CD117
   b. CD64
   c. Myeloperoxidase (MPO)
   d. Sudan black B (SBB)

7. Acute myeloid leukemia with maturation is negative for:
   a. MPO
   b. CD117
   c. CD64
   d. CD65
   e. None of the above

8. True regarding central nervous involvement in acute myeloid leukemia in children is:
   a. Prophylactic CNS directed chemotherapy or radiotherapy prolongs survival
   b. Blasts in the CSF at diagnosis in children with AML adversely affect prognosis
   c. Transplant in first remission is indicated
   d. None of the above
   e. All of the above

9. True regarding postremission therapy in acute myeloid leukemia is:
   a. Required in only intermediate- and high-risk patients
   b. Standard dose and high dose cytarabine are equally effective
   c. Maintenance therapy is not effective
   d. All of the above

10. Treatment of a child with acute myeloid leukemia with monosomy 7 should be:
    a. High dose cytarabine chemotherapy and transplant in second remission
    b. Autologous transplant in first remission
    c. Allogeneic transplant in first remission
    d. Any of the above

11. Treatment for myeloid sarcoma is:
    a. Radiotherapy
    b. Surgical excision
    c. Chemotherapy
    d. All of the above

12. Remission induction chemotherapy is aimed to reduce the burden of leukemic cells in the body from 10^{12} to:
    a. 10^3
    b. 10^6
    c. 10^9
    d. Zero

13. Consolidation chemotherapy is aimed to reduce the burden of leukemic cells in the body to:
    a. 10^3
    b. 10^6
    c. 10^9
    d. Zero

14. Most preferred agent to be used along with high dose cytarabine in consolidation for AML is:
    a. Etoposide
    b. Cyclophosphamide
    c. Mitoxantrone
    d. Daunorubicin
    e. None of the above

15. Allogeneic transplant in high risk AML is preferred in:
    a. First complete remission (CR)
    b. After completing 3 cycles of high dose cytarabine consolidation
    c. In second CR
    d. Any of the above

16. Remission induction therapy for high risk AML should be:
   a. High dose cytarabine
   b. 3 + 7 + 3 induction including etoposide
   c. High dose cytarabine plus mitoxantrone
   d. 3 + 7 induction

17. The high risk marker in acute promyelocytic leukemia (APL) is:
   a. Promyelocyte count
   b. Blast count
   c. Total leukocyte count
   d. Platelet count

18. True regarding therapy-related AML is:
   a. Alkylating agents or radiation therapy typically present after a latency period of approximately 5–7 years
   b. Topoisomerase II inhibitors have a considerably shorter latency period of 1–3 years
   c. Patients with t-AML have poor prognosis than patients with de novo AML
   d. All of the above

19. True regarding treatment of acute promyelocytic leukemia (APL) are, *except*:
   a. Best results are obtained by all-transretinoic acid (ATRA) induction plus two cycles of consolidation chemotherapy followed by ATRA maintenance
   b. Therapy-related APL has prognosis similar to primary APL
   c. Primary resistance is very uncommon
   d. Induction failure is defined as promyelocytic leukemia-retinoic acid receptor alpha (PML-RARa) positive after induction therapy

20. The following variants have been identified as ATRA-sensitive, *except*:
   a. NuMA/RARa and t (11;17)
   b. NPM1/RARa and t (5;17)
   c. FIP1L1/RARa
   d. STAT5b/RARa

21. True regarding retinoid acid syndrome is:
   a. Seen in 25% of APL patients
   b. Occurs 2–21 days after initiation of treatment
   c. More frequently in patients with a high white blood cell count at diagnosis
   d. All of the above

22. Lower dose of ATRA is used in children because of:
   a. Increased risk of ATRA syndrome in children
   b. Increased risk of headache and papilledema
   c. Prolongation of QT interval
   d. All of the above

23. The four factors that predict prognosis in a relapsed acute myeloid leukemia are all, *except*:
   a. Age at relapse
   b. Bone marrow transplant prior to relapse
   c. Cytogenetics at baseline
   d. Duration of remission
   e. Medullary or extramedullary relapse

24. Which one of the following is false about acute myeloid leukemia?
   a. It is most common in elderly
   b. It can be caused by chemotherapy
   c. More than 20% blast cells in the bone marrow are required for all cases of AML
   d. Disseminated intravascular coagulation can be a presenting feature

25. Which one of the following is not true about acute myeloid leukemia?
   a. AML M4 and M5 can have extramedullary sarcomas
   b. AML has a cure rate of >60% in some subtypes
   c. Allogeneic stem cell transplantation is needed in all patients less than 50 years old with an HLA matched donor
   d. Auer rods are seen in some but not all subtypes of AML

26. Which one of these is least valuable in the diagnosis of acute myeloid leukemia?
   a. Microscopic analysis of the bone marrow aspirate
   b. Immunophenotypic analysis of a bone marrow sample
   c. Cytogenetic analysis of peripheral blood
   d. Detection of clonal rearrangement of the immunoglobulin heavy chain gene

27. The word "leukemia" means:
   a. French word for "blood infection"
   b. Greek word for "white blood"
   c. Latin word for "white cell"
   d. Sanskrit word for "blood weakness"

28. Most common type of inherited leukemia is:
   a. Acute lymphoblastic leukemia (ALL)
   b. Acute myeloid leukemia
   c. Chronic lymphocytic leukemia
   d. Chronic myeloid leukemia (CML)

29. Which of the following cytogenetic abnormality is associated with spontaneous remission of leukemia?
   a. Monosomy 5
   b. Trisomy 18
   c. Trisomy 21
   d. Monosomy 7

30. The following diseases have been classified as Philadelphia negative chronic myeloproliferative neoplasms:
   a. CML and chronic myelomonocytic leukemia (CMML)
   b. Myelofibrosis and AML

c. Chronic lymphocytic leukemia (CLL) and lymphoma
d. Polycythemia rubra vera and essential thrombocythemia

31. JAK 2 mutation induces hemopoietic proliferation which is due to:
   a. Cytokine mediation
   b. Hypersensitivity of progenitor cells to erythropoietin and thrombopoietin
   c. Reactive marrow hyperplasia
   d. Stimulation of viral oncogene

32. Myeloperoxidase stains granules of all, *except*:
   a. Neutrophils
   b. Eosinophils
   c. Basophils
   d. Monocytes
   e. Auer rods

33. Periodic acid-Schiff stains:
   a. Neutrophils
   b. Lymphocytes
   c. Platelets
   d. Monocytes
   e. All of the above

34. Antibodies identifying antigens expressed mainly in hemopoietic precursors are all, *except*:
   a. CD34
   b. CD45
   c. HLA-DR
   d. Anti-terminal deoxynucleotidyl transferase (Anti-TdT)

35. True regarding Down syndrome is:
   a. Incidence of acute leukemia is 10–20 times that of individuals without trisomy 21
   b. Increased risk of acute megakaryoblastic leukemia (AMKL)
   c. Transient abnormal myelopoiesis is a spontaneously remitting leukemia-equivalent unique to Down syndrome patients
   d. All of the above

36. Core binding factor AML includes:
   a. AML with t(8;21)
   b. AML with t(15;17)
   c. AML with (12;21)
   d. All of the above

37. The best induction regimen for acute myeloid leukemia is daunorubicin with:
   a. Cytarabine 100–200 mg/m² for 7 days
   b. Cytarabine 400 mg/m² for 7 days
   c. Cytarabine 3,000 mg/m² for 3 days
   d. Depends upon cytogenetic risk factors

38. True regarding acute myeloid leukemia induction are all, *except*:
   a. If patients fail to achieve a substantial reduction in marrow blasts in the first course or fail to enter CR with a second course, they should be considered refractory
   b. The distribution of cytogenetic subtypes is related to age
   c. Remission rates are lower, if patients have antecedent hematological disorder
   d. Addition of etoposide increases remission rates
   e. All of the above

39. The response to induction chemotherapy in acute myeloid leukemia depends on all, *except*:
   a. Age
   b. Cytogenetics
   c. Lactate dehydrogenase
   d. WBC count at presentation
   e. All of the above

40. Which of the following is not associated with high risk acute myeloid leukemia?
   a. t(9;11)(p21.3;q23.3); MLLT3-KMT2A
   b. t(6;9)(p23;q34.1); DEK-NUP214
   c. t(v;11q23.3); KMT2A rearranged
   d. t(9;22)(q34.1;q11.2); BCR-ABL1

41. True regarding midostaurin is:
   a. It is a FLT3 inhibitor
   b. It also inhibits kinases other than FLT3
   c. It is superior regardless of internal tandem duplication (ITD) allelic ratio or whether the FLT3 mutation is an ITD or a tyrosine kinase domain (TKD)
   d. Midostaurin can be combined to standard chemotherapy
   e. All of the above

42. True regarding gemtuzumab ozogamicin is:
   a. It is an antibody against CD13
   b. Effective in AML other than APL
   c. Highly effective as a single agent
   d. Increases the risk of veno-occlusive disease
   e. All of the above

43. True regarding CPX 351 is:
   a. It is a combination of cytarabine and daunorubicin
   b. Used for therapy-related AML
   c. Used for AML with MDS-related changes
   d. Has side-effect profile similar to 3 + 7 chemotherapy
   e. All of the above

44. True about RAM immunophenotype-acute myeloid leukemia are all, *except*:
   a. High intensity CD56 expression
   b. Dim-to-negative expression of CD45 and CD38
   c. Negative for HLA-DR expression
   d. Good prognosis
   e. All of the above

45. The preferred treatment for a 72-year-old male with AML with 30% myeloblasts and normal molecular studies, who is not fit for 3 + 7 induction, is:
   a. Low-dose cytarabine
   b. Lenalidomide
   c. Decitabine
   d. Azacitidine plus venetoclax

46. A 56-year-old male with acute myeloid leukemia was treated with induction chemotherapy. On day 9 of induction chemotherapy he developed febrile neutropenia and received empirical antibiotics and voriconazole was added on day 11 as fever continued and HRCT chest showed fungal pneumonia. He subsequently became afebrile and blood count improved on day 21. His chest X-ray done on day 25 is shown below. The next step of treatment will be:

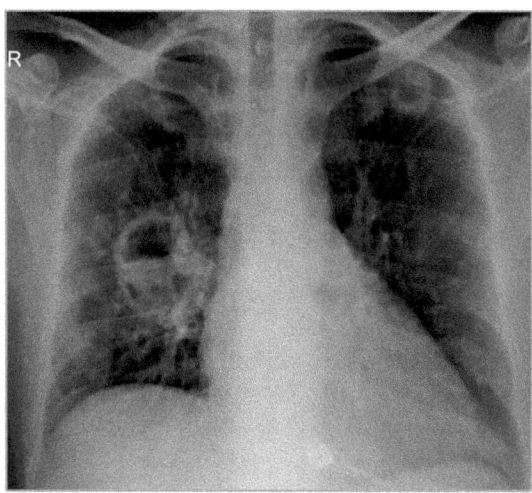

   a. Increase the dose of voriconazole
   b. Stop voriconazole and add another antifungal
   c. Continue voriconazole prophylaxis
   d. Add antibiotics to voriconazole

47. A 62-year-old male with acute myeloid leukemia developed fever and cough on day 13 of induction chemotherapy with daunorubicin and cytarabine. His high resolution computed tomography of chest showed right upper zone consolidation and CT guided fine needle aspiration cytology (FNAC) from the lesion is shown below.

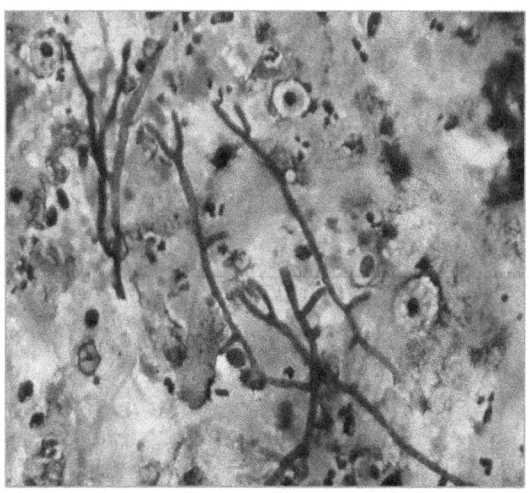

   The picture depicts:
   a. Aspergillus
   b. Mucorales
   c. Histoplasmosis
   d. Cryprosporidium

48. A 35-year-old lady was diagnosed as acute myeloid leukemia and was started on 3+7 induction chemotherapy. She was also on allopurinol, ondansetron and antifungal prophylaxis with fluconazole. There was no history of allergy to any drugs. On day six patient developed rash over both ears and face. What is the least probable cause of the rash?
   a. Leukemia cutis
   b. Cytarabine
   c. Allopurinol
   d. Fluconazole

49. True regarding colony-stimulating factor 1 receptor (CSF1R) are all, *except:*
   a. CSF1 receptor (CSF1R) is responsible for proliferation and differentiation of myeloid-lineage cells
   b. CSF1R is expressed on myeloid leukemic blasts
   c. Inhibition of CSF1R can be used to treat AML
   d. All of the above

50. Triplet therapy for AML includes:
   a. Decitabine, venetoclax and FLT3 inhibitor
   b. Cytarabine, decitabine and FLT3 inhibitor
   c. Venetoclax, glasdegib and FLT3 inhibitor
   d. Venetoclax, daunomycin and fludarabine

51. Mechanisms of resistance to FLT3 inhibitors is:
   a. Increased signaling through FGF2 and CXCL12/CXCR4
   b. Increased signaling through RAS–RAF–MEK–ERK pathways
   c. Increased signaling through PI3K–AKT–mTOR pathways
   d. Increased signaling through JAK–STAT5–PIM1 pathways
   e. All of the above

52. Ferrara criteria is used for:
   a. Assessing fitness for allogeneic stem cell transplant
   b. Assessing fitness for intensive chemotherapy in AML
   c. Assessing suitability for match unrelated donor (MUD) stem cell transplant
   d. Assessing fitness for surgical intervention in leukemia patients

ANSWERS WITH EXPLANATIONS

1. Ans. c. del 7

Ref: WHO classification of tumors of hematopoietic and lymphoid tissues, 2017 Revised Edition

Acute myeloid leukemia with certain genetic abnormalities such as those with t(8;21), inv(16), or t(16;16) and myeloid sarcoma are considered diagnostic of AML without regard to the blast count. Deletion 7 with less than 20% blasts is MDS not AML.

2. Ans. d. Patients with RUNX1-RUNX1T1 detected by reverse transcription-polymerase chain reaction (RT-PCR) postinduction have poor prognosis.

Acute myeloid leukemia with t(8;21)(q22;q22), RUNX1-RUNX1T1 (previously AML1-ETO) may not have 20% blasts, but can be identified if the cytogenetic abnormality is present. It typically has associated morphologic features that can suggest its diagnosis. These include blasts with long thin Auer rods, and maturation of the blasts to abnormal mature granulocytic elements with salmon colored cytoplasm with blue rims, and cytoplasmic globules, or Chediak-Higashi-like granules. This leukemia frequently has myeloid markers, but can also express CD19 and CD56. The leukemia is associated with a more favorable prognosis. The presence of c-KIT mutations is an adverse prognostic feature in patients with t(8;21). Patients can have transcripts of the RUNX1-RUNX1T1 detected by RT-PCR even in patients who have been in remission for many years. It has a limited clinical applicability since a persistent positivity has been observed in long survivors even after allogeneic stem cell transplantation.

3. Ans. b. t(1;22)(p13;q13)

AML-M7 (megakaryoblastic) with t(1;22)(p13;q13), RBM15-MKL1 is a rare AML, typically occurring in infants and is associated with poor prognosis. The t(1;22)(p13;q13), characteristic of AMKL, is restricted to infants. It has been reported as the sole chromosomal aberration in about 60% of AMKL cases below 6 months of age and above the age of 6 months, the t(1;22) is often associated with complex secondary chromosomal aberration including hyperdiploidy. In both cases, the prognosis appears to be poor.

4. Ans. c. AML with mutations in FLT3

Ref: WHO classification of tumors of hematopoietic and lymphoid tissues, 2017 Revised Edition

Leukemias with mutations of NPM1 are considered as a provisional entity. In almost all cases, the mutation is seen in AML with normal cytogenetics. The presence of the NPM1 mutation confers a better prognosis, but only if it is seen alone. When seen in conjunction with mutations in FLT3, it is associated with a poor prognosis. Mutations in CEBPA are seen in about 6-15% of AML, commonly in cases with a normal karyotype. Cases with this mutation are associated with a good prognosis. AML with mutations in FLT3 are seen in 30-40% of patients with AML and normal cytogenetics. Patients with this mutation often present with high WBC counts and poor prognosis.

5. Ans. a. More than 50% of cells

Ref: WHO classification of tumors of hematopoietic and lymphoid tissues, 2017 Revised Edition

Acute myeloid leukemia with morphologically identified multilineage dysplasia is defined as dysplasia present in ≥50% of cells in two or more hematopoietic lineages. AML that demonstrates these cytogenetic abnormalities, monosomy 5 or del(5q), monosomy 7 or del(7q), and isochromosome 17p, are also considered MDS-related AML. This secondary AML has poor prognosis.

6. Ans. a. CD117

Ref: WHO classification of tumors of hematopoietic and lymphoid tissues, 2017 Revised Edition

Acute myeloid leukemia M0 is AML with minimal differentiation. There are no cytoplasmic granules or Auer rods and they cannot be differentiated from ALL [i.e. French American British (FAB) L2 blasts] based upon morphology alone. The blasts are negative for the MPO or SBB reactions, but are considered myeloid due to the presence of myeloid associated markers. Most cases express antigens of early hematopoiesis (e.g. CD34, CD38, and HLA-DR) and the myeloid antigens CD13, CD117, and CD33. They lack antigens of more mature myeloid differentiation such as CD14, CD15, CD11b, and CD64.

7. Ans. c. CD64

CD34, CD38, and HLA-DR are markers of early hematopoiesis. CD13, CD33, CD65, and CD15 are myeloid-associated antigens. CD11c, CD14, and CD64 are monocytic markers. AML with maturation has myeloid markers but not monocytic markers, unlike myelomonocytic or monocytic leukemia.

8. Ans. d. None of the above

Ref: Williams 8/e; Hoffman 7/e

There is no evidence that CNS-directed therapy with either intrathecal chemotherapy alone or in combination with cranial irradiation prolongs disease-free survival in children with AML. Most pediatric AML studies, however, still include intrathecal chemotherapy because isolated CNS relapse occurred in approximately 10-20% of children with AML who did not receive any CNS-directed therapy. In contrast to ALL, the

9. Ans. c. Maintenance therapy is not effective

Ref: Williams 8/e; Hoffman 7/e

Without further treatment after standard induction chemotherapy, more than 90% of patients relapse within 1 year. Cytarabine is the single most active agent in AML, because laboratory and clinical studies have indicated that a log increase in its dose can overcome the mechanisms of resistance. Approximately 40% of patients with AML who are refractory to standard doses of cytarabine achieve a CR with high-dose cytarabine. The optimal number of consolidation chemotherapy cycles has not been determined, but is usually 3–4 cycles. Maintenance chemotherapy with oral thioguanine and standard doses of cytarabine given after consolidation chemotherapy have not been shown to further increase the proportion of patients in long-term remission. Patients who receive maintenance have a poor salvage rate if relapsed because of clinical drug resistance and so maintenance therapy is not recommended in AML.

10. Ans. c. Allogeneic transplant in first remission

Ref: Creutzig U. Diagnosis and management of acute myeloid leukemia in children and adolescents: recommendations from an international expert panel. Blood. 2012; Hoffman 7/e

The choice of chemotherapy versus hematopoietic stem cell transplantation (HSCT) in first remission depends on prognostic factors and the availability of a suitable donor. Matched-related or, if a sibling donor is unavailable, matched-unrelated or haploidentical HSCT is recommended for patients with high-risk features, including monosomy 7, FLT3 internal tandem duplication mutation, and patients with refractory disease after two courses of induction. Allogeneic HSCT in first remission should also be considered for non-Down syndrome patients with FAB M7 morphology because of poor outcomes with this subtype. Favorable-risk patients [i.e. Down syndrome M7, inv(16), t(15;17), t(8;21)] should be treated with chemotherapy alone. For these patients without high-risk features, matched-related or matched-unrelated HSCT should be reserved for relapsed disease. Auto-HSCT is not recommended for children with AML in first CR.

11. Ans. c. Chemotherapy

Ref: Bakst RL. How I treat extramedullary acute myeloid leukemia. Blood. 2011

Myeloid sarcoma may present simultaneously with or precede bone marrow disease. Sites of isolated myeloid sarcoma include bone, periosteum, soft tissues, and lymph nodes, and less commonly the intestine, mediastinum, epidural region, uterus, and ovary. The definitive diagnosis rests on identifying the tumor cells as myeloid with the use of MPO or lysozyme staining, flow cytometry, or immunophenotyping from tissue sections. The approach to treatment of patients with myeloid sarcoma without evidence of AML on bone marrow biopsy is similar to that for patients with overt AML.

12. Ans. c. 10^9

Ref: Williams 8/e; Hoffman 7/e

The aim of remission induction chemotherapy is the rapid restoration of normal bone marrow function and attainment of CR. Induction therapy aims to reduce the total body leukemia cell population from approximately 10^{12} to below the cytologically detectable level of about 10^9 cells, i.e., three log reduction. However, still a substantial burden of leukemia cells persists undetected (i.e., minimal residual disease), leading to relapse within a few weeks or months if no further therapy were administered. Postinduction or "remission consolidation" therapy usually comprises one or more courses of chemotherapy or hematopoietic cell transplantation (HCT). It is designed to eradicate residual leukemia, allowing the possibility of cure and to decrease the leukemic cell population further down, possibly zero.

13. Ans. d. Zero

Consolidation chemotherapy is designed to eradicate residual leukemia, allowing the possibility of cure.

14. Ans. e. None of the above

Ref: Rowe JM. How I treat acute myeloid leukemia. Blood. 2010. Williams 8/e

High dose cytarabine (HIDAC) has been the consolidation chemotherapy of choice in AML patients postinduction. Various studies attempted to improve on survival rates attained with HIDAC by substituting other agents with different mechanisms of action have not been successful. In a study, the use of three consolidation courses of HIDAC (3 g/m^2) was equally as effective as three courses of sequential multiagent chemotherapy (one course each of HIDAC with etoposide/cyclophosphamide/amsacrine/mitoxantrone). Cytarabine is one of the most effective agents available for the treatment of AML and is a key component of induction therapy. High dose cytarabine produces high intracellular drug concentrations, which saturate the deaminating metabolic enzyme pathway, leading to increased levels of the active agent ara-cytidine triphosphate. In this way, HIDAC can often effectively eliminate minimal residual disease that survived induction with cytarabine containing regimens. Consolidation chemotherapy with HIDAC produces superior survival rates than those seen with lower doses of cytarabine.

15. Ans. a. First complete remission (CR)

Ref: Rowe JM. How I treat acute myeloid leukemia. Blood. 2010; Williams 8/e

Allogeneic HCT should be performed after attainment of an initial CR. Postremission consolidation therapy with standard or high-dose cytarabine is not associated with improved outcome, compared with proceeding directly to allogeneic transplantation following successful induction therapy. Allogeneic HCT using a matched unrelated donor (MUD) is an option for younger adults who lack a sibling donor. Because myeloablative allogeneic HCT may lead to significant early morbidity and mortality in patients of higher age and those with comorbidities, nonmyeloablative HCT has been developed as an alternative strategy. Thus, older patients who are not candidates for myeloablative allogeneic HCT may be candidates for a nonmyeloablative HCT. This procedure relies less on the dose intensity of the pretransplant cytotoxic regimen and heavily upon the graft-versus-leukemia effect.

16. **Ans. d. 3 + 7 induction**   Ref: Hoffman 6/e; Williams 8/e

Gold standard for induction chemotherapy for AML remains treatment with an anthracycline and cytarabine irrespective of cytogenetics. Daunorubicin 60–90 mg/m2 for 3 days with cytarabine 100 mg/m^2 for 7 days (3 + 7) is a standard to which other regimens are compared. There is no definitive evidence that therapy with another anthracycline or anthracenedione is superior. Standard 3 + 7 regimen is effective for all cytogenetic or molecular subtypes. Increasing the dose of cytarabine from 100 to 200 mg/m^2 does not improve outcome. Continuous infusions of cytarabine are preferable to bolus administration. Intensifying induction by using higher doses of cytarabine or addition of etoposide does not affect the remission induction rate. High doses of cytarabine or addition of etoposide may prolong disease-free survival at the cost of toxicity, and overall survival is not affected.

17. **Ans. c. Total leukocyte count**

The most important factor predicting outcome in APL is the WBC count at initial presentation. The GIMEMA and PETHEMA cooperative groups used both WBC count and platelet count to identify patients at low risk (WBC ≤10,000/μL, platelet count >40,000/μL), intermediate risk (WBC ≤10,000/μL, platelet count <40,000/μL), or high-risk (WBC >10,000/μL, Sanz criteria) for relapse. Advanced age is another important unfavorable prognostic factor. In addition, the FLT-3 internal tandem duplication mutation occurs in approximately 35% of patients with APL and appears to confer an unfavorable prognosis in patients with APL.

18. **Ans d. All of the above**   Ref: Hoffman 7/e; Williams 8/e

Therapy related-AML after exposure to alkylating agents or radiation therapy typically presents after a latency period of approximately 5–7 years. Two-thirds of these patients are first recognized by evidence of myelodysplasia (usually trilineage dysplasia), marrow failure, and pancytopenia. The chromosomal abnormalities seen in these therapy-related AML (t-AML) often involve complex abnormalities and monosomies such as –5 or –7 that have been associated with unfavorable risk. Therapy related-AML that develops after the use of topoisomerase II inhibitors has a considerably shorter latency period of 1–3 years and most often presents with overt leukemia and rarely with MDS. The cytogenetic alterations typically apparent in these t-AML often involve 11q26 abnormalities, such as t(9;11), or 21q22 abnormalities, such as t(8;21) or t(3;21). Approximately 90% of cases of t-AML demonstrate clonal chromosomal abnormalities, most often complex in nature. Despite favorable cytogenetics, patients with t-AML do worse than patients with de novo AML in the same risk group.

19. **Ans. d. Induction failure is defined as PML-RARa positive after induction therapy**

Ref: Sanz MA. Management of acute promyelocytic leukemia: recommendations from an expert panel on behalf of the European LeukemiaNet. Blood. 2009.

The survival using various protocols in APL was—chemotherapy induction plus two cycles of consolidation chemotherapy followed by observation (16%); chemotherapy induction plus two cycles of consolidation chemotherapy plus ATRA maintenance (47%); ATRA induction plus two cycles of consolidation chemotherapy followed by observation (55%); and ATRA induction plus two cycles of consolidation chemotherapy followed by ATRA maintenance (74%). The duration of coagulopathy appears shortened when ATRA is added to induction chemotherapy (e.g. 3 days compared with 6 days with chemotherapy alone). Several trials have demonstrated better outcomes when chemotherapy is administered with ATRA during induction (simultaneous administration) rather than postponing chemotherapy until a CR is achieved with ATRA (sequential administration). Low-risk patients are now treated without chemotherapy, using only ATRA and arsenic. The goal of remission induction treatment in APL is the attainment of a morphological remission. Molecular remission is attained only after completion of consolidation therapy. Premature evaluation of response may be misleading and is discouraged. Blasts and promyelocytes may remain elevated in the marrow for many weeks and the RT-PCR signal of the fusion gene may remain detectable during a slow decline. Primary resistance is very uncommon. Approximately 90% of patients with newly diagnosed APL will achieve a CR with induction therapy. However, without additional cytotoxic therapy, virtually all of these patients will relapse. Consolidation therapy is directed at leukemia cells that survived induction therapy but are not detectable by conventional tests thereby converting patients with morphologic and cytogenetic CR into a more durable molecular remission and cure. A molecular CR takes time to achieve, and is usually attained only after completion of consolidation therapy. Patients who achieve molecular CR should proceed directly to maintenance therapy. Patients who have a positive RT-PCR test should have a second bone marrow aspirate and biopsy with RT-PCR testing repeated in 2-4 weeks. If this second test is negative, the patient may proceed to maintenance therapy. If the second RT-PCR is still positive, the patient should proceed to treatment for resistant disease.

20. Ans. d. STAT5b/RARa

STAT5b/RARa and interstitial chromosome 17 deletion, and PLZF/RARa and t(11;17) are resistant to ATRA.

21. Ans. d. All of the above

Ref: Hoffman 6/e; Williams 8/e; Tallman MS. How I treat APL. Blood. 2009

The differentiation syndrome ("retinoid acid syndrome") occurs in approximately 25% of APL patients within 2-21 days after initiation of treatment and is seen more frequently in patients with a high WBC count at diagnosis. It can occur in the absence of ATRA, and by arsenic trioxide also, and is characterized by fever, peripheral edema, pulmonary infiltrates, hypoxemia, respiratory distress, hypotension, renal and hepatic dysfunction, and serositis resulting in pleural and pericardial effusions. The symptoms of fever, hypotension, dyspnea, and pulmonary infiltrates can mimic sepsis. Early recognition and aggressive management with dexamethasone therapy (10 mg IV every 12 hours for 3 or more days) has been effective in most patients.

22. Ans. b. Increased risk of headache and papilledema

Idiopathic intracranial hypertension, commonly called pseudotumor cerebri, can complicate the treatment of APL with ATRA. Pseudotumor cerebri is more common in children and adolescents treated with ATRA and the incidence in this population decreases with the use of lower dose of ATRA (e.g. 25 mg/m^2/day). The diagnosis of pseudotumor cerebri is suspected in patients with headache, papilledema, and/or vision loss. Evaluation includes a physical examination including evaluation of the optic nerve, lumbar puncture, and cerebral imaging studies. The diagnosis is confirmed in patients with increased intracranial pressure, normal CSF, and negative cerebral imaging studies (e.g. computed tomography or magnetic resonance imaging scan). The pathogenesis of pseudotumor cerebri in patients with APL being treated with ATRA is thought to be similar to the mechanism in vitamin A overdose—overdosage of vitamin A is postulated to impair CSF absorption at the level of the arachnoid villi or granulations by altering the lipid constituents of choroid plexus and arachnoid villi. The treatment of pseudotumor cerebri includes suspension of ATRA until neurologic symptoms subside. For patients with pseudotumor cerebri whose neurologic complaints do not improve after withholding ATRA, use of acetazolamide, therapeutic high-volume lumbar punctures, dexamethasone, and analgesics may be useful. Patients may be rechallenged with ATRA once neurologic complaints improve, but symptoms recur in most cases.

23. Ans. e. Medullary or extramedullary relapse

Ref: Breems DA. Prognostic index for adult patients with acute myeloid leukemia in first relapse. JCO. 2005

European Prognostic Index (EPI) identified four risk factors in relapsed AML patients (ABCD—Age, BMT, Cytogenetics, and Duration of remission)—(1) Relapse-free interval from first CR (0, 3, and 5 points for >18, 7 to 18, and ≤6 months, respectively); (2) Cytogenetics at the time of diagnosis [0, 3, and 5 points for t(16;16) or Inv(16); t(8;21) with or without other abnormalities; and normal, intermediate, unfavorable, or unknown cytogenetics, respectively]; (3) Age at first relapse (0, 1, and 2 points for ≤35, 36 to 45, and >45 years, respectively); and (4) Autologous or allogeneic HCT before first relapse (0 and 2 points for no prior HCT or a prior HCT, respectively). Site of relapse is not a risk factor. Three risk groups were identified—favorable (1-6 points), intermediate (7-9 points), and high-risk (10-14 points), with 5-year overall survivals of 22-46%, 12-18%, and 4-6%, respectively, when the EPI was employed.

24. Ans. c. More than 20% blast cells in the bone marrow are required for all cases of AML

Ref: WHO 2017 Revised Edition

Acute myeloid leukemia is the most common acute leukemia in adults and accounts for approximately 80% of cases in this group. AML has been associated with environmental factors (e.g. exposure to chemicals, radiation, tobacco, or chemotherapy drugs), genetic abnormalities (e.g. trisomy 21, Fanconi's anemia, Bloom's syndrome), and other benign (e.g. paroxysmal nocturnal hemoglobinuria) and malignant (e.g. MDS and myeloproliferative disorders) hematologic diseases. In the current WHO classification system, blast forms must account for at least 20% of the total cellularity. Exceptions to this include AML with t(8;21), inv(16), and t(15;17). The diagnosis of therapy-related myeloid neoplasm (t-MN) is made when evaluation of the peripheral blood and bone marrow demonstrates morphologic, immunophenotypic, and cytogenetic changes consistent with the diagnosis of AML, MDS, or MDS/MPN in a patient with prior exposure to cytotoxic agents.

25. Ans. c. Allogeneic stem cell transplantation is needed in all patients less than 50 years old with an HLA matched donor

Acute myeloid leukemia M4 and M5 can have extramedullary sarcomas. Allogeneic transplant is needed only in high-risk patients. Auer rods, which are slender, fusiform cytoplasmic inclusions that stain red with Wright-Giemsa stain, are virtually pathognomonic of AML. Auer rods, needle-shaped intracytoplasmic azurophilic inclusion bodies are often, but not always seen in AML, particularly in M2 or M3 AML.

26. Ans. d. Detection of clonal rearrangement of the immunoglobulin heavy chain gene

Although well-established diagnostic criteria exist for mature B-cell neoplasms, a definitive diagnosis of a B-cell lymphoproliferative disorder cannot always be obtained using more conventional techniques such as flow cytometry immunophenotyping, conventional cytogenetics, fluorescence in situ hybridization, or immunohistochemistry. However, because B-cell malignancies contain identically rearranged immunoglobulin heavy chain genes, the PCR can be a fast, convenient, and dependable option to identify clonal B-cell processes.

27. Ans. b. Greek word for "white blood"

Leukemia is derived from Greek word, leukos meaning white and hemea meaning blood.

28. Ans. c. Chronic lymphocytic leukemia

A person's risk of developing CLL may be higher than average when there is a family history of this disease or other blood and bone marrow cancers. First-degree relatives of individuals with CLL have a 2- to 4-fold increased risk of developing CLL.

29. Ans. c. Trisomy 21

Ref: Gruber TA. The biology of pediatric acute megakaryoblastic leukemia. Blood. 2015;126(8):943-9.

Acute megakaryoblastic leukemia in infants and children may be associated with the presence of t(1;22), and Down syndrome (trisomy 21). AMKL in children with Down syndrome is characterized by a founding *GATA1* mutation that cooperates with trisomy 21, followed by the acquisition of additional somatic mutations. Down syndrome-AMKL is associated with transient abnormal myelopoiesis (TAM), a hematologic disorder of infancy. In this disorder, a clonal population of megakaryoblasts accumulates in the peripheral blood. These blasts are phenotypically indistinguishable from AMKL leukemic blasts, and in the majority of cases, remission is spontaneous within 3 months in the absence of treatment. In children, the disease is divided into two major subgroups: AMKL in patients with Down syndrome and AMKL in patients without Down syndrome. AMKL is the most frequent type of AML in children with Down syndrome, and the incidence in these patients is 500-fold higher than in the general population. AMKL with Down syndrome is both biologically and clinically distinct, with superior outcomes compared with non-Down syndrome-AMKL.

30. Ans. d. Polycythemia rubra vera and essential thrombocythemia. *Ref: WHO 2017 Revised Edition*

Myeloproliferative neoplasms (MPNs) are primarily separated by *BCR/ABL*-positive CML defined by the Philadelphia translocation t(9;22)(q34;q11)/*BCR-ABL* and in all other so-called *BCR/ABL*-negative MPN. According to the WHO, the latter are subdivided into polycythemia vera (PV), idiopathic myelofibrosis (IMF), essential thrombocythemia (ET), and unclassified MPN (MPN-U). The backbone in all cases of suspicious or proven MPN should be screening for the JAK2V617F, CAL-R, and MPL mutation status by PCR. The Philadelphia chromosome-negative chronic MPNs are PV, ET, and chronic IMF, and have overlapping clinical features but exhibit different natural histories and different therapeutic requirements.

31. Ans. b. Hypersensitivity of progenitor cells to erythropoietin and thrombopoietin

Myeloproliferative neoplasms are clonal disorders characterized by the autonomous proliferation of committed hematopoietic progenitors secondary to an aberrant activation of tyrosine kinase (TK) signaling pathways in combination with an exaggerated response to hematopoietic cytokines and growth factors. JAK2V617F occurs in the pseudokinase domain of the *JAK2* gene. The mutated pseudokinase domain is not able to negatively regulate the kinase domain of *JAK2*, resulting in an autonomous activation of the *JAK2* kinase domain with subsequently persistent phosphorylation of STAT and mitogen-activated protein kinase (MAPK) proteins and hyperstimulation of the cytokine signaling pathway. As a consequence, cells expressing the JAK2V617F mutation are hypersensitive to hematopoietic cytokine stimulation, resulting in an abnormal erythroid, myeloid, and thromboproliferation. Moreover, JAK2-deficient mice do not survive because of absence of erythropoiesis. Myeloid progenitors of these mice fail to respond to erythropoietin (EPO), granulocyte-macrophage colony stimulating factor (GM-CSF), and thrombopoietin stimulation. These experiments demonstrate that *JAK2* plays an essential role in the development of normal hematopoiesis.

32. Ans. c. Basophils

Myeloperoxidase stains primary and secondary granules of cells of neutrophil lineage, eosinophil granules (granules appear solid), granules of monocytes, and Auer rods. Granules of normal mature basophils do not stain by MPO. Detection of MPO (if present in ≥3% of blasts) indicates myeloid differentiation, but its absence does not exclude a myeloid lineage because early myeloblasts and monoblasts may lack MPO. SBB staining parallels MPO but is less specific. Nonspecific esterase (NSE) stains show diffuse cytoplasmic activity in monoblasts (usually >80% positive) and monocytes (usually >20% positive). In acute erythroid leukemia, a periodic acid-Schiff (PAS) stain may show large globules of PAS positivity.

33. Ans. e. All of the above

Periodic acid-Schiff stains cells of neutrophil lineage (granular, increasing with maturation), leukemic promyelocytes (diffuse cytoplasmic), eosinophil cytoplasm but not granules, basophil cytoplasm (blocks), monocytes (diffuse plus granules), megakaryocytes and platelets (diffuse plus granules), some T and B lymphocytes, and many leukemic blast cells (blocks, B more than T).

34. Ans. b. CD45

CD34 is expressed by B-lineage lymphoblasts, early T-cell precursors, myeloid progenitors, blast cells in most cases of AML, and undifferentiated acute leukemia. HLA-DR is a major histocompatibility complex, class II antigens; expressed on B lymphocytes and B-lymphocyte progenitors, activated T lymphocytes, blast cells of a small minority of cases of T lineage ALL, monocytes and their precursors, myeloid precursors, and blast cells of most cases of AML. Anti-TdT is expressed by blast cells of ALL (stronger in B-lineage than T-lineage blasts), more weakly expressed in blasts in 10–20% of AML. CD45 is a common leukocyte antigen. It is an antibody which identifies antigens expressed on all leukocytes. Use of CD45 permits gating on blast cells which express CD45 and have low sideways light scatter, however leukemic blast cells, particularly B-lineage lymphoblasts, may fail to express CD45 or may express it weakly; cells of neutrophil lineage show increased CD45 expression with maturation; monocytes and eosinophils show stronger expression than neutrophils.

35. Ans. d. All of the above

Ref: Williams 8/e; Hoffman 7/e, See Q. No. 29

Down syndrome has been recognized as one of the most important leukemia-predisposing syndromes and patients with Down syndrome and leukemia have unique clinical features and significant differences in treatment response and toxicity profiles compared to patients without Down syndrome. Down syndrome children with AML, and in particular, the acute megakaryocytic leukemia subtype have exceptionally high cure rates. On the other hand, the outcome of Down syndrome children with ALL has been historically considered worse than the outcome of ALL patients without Down syndrome. Down syndrome children with leukemia are more prone to suffer from significant toxicity to chemotherapy, particularly methotrexate. Acute leukemia is 10–20 times more common in Down syndrome than that of individuals without trisomy 21. Risk of AMKL is as high as about 600 times normal. Transient abnormal myelopoiesis is the clonal proliferation of myeloid blast cells which affects an estimated 5–10% of infants with Down syndrome. The majority of infants with transient abnormal myelopoiesis are asymptomatic and picked up incidentally on routine testing. Most cases of transient abnormal myelopoiesis resolve over the first few months of life, but 13–33% may go on to develop AML within the first 4 years of life. GATA-1 mutations, a transcription factor mutation integral to the normal development of erythroid, megakaryocytic, and basophilic cell lines, have been associated with transient abnormal myelopoiesis and AML in Down syndrome. Transient abnormal myelopoiesis is a unique disorder of Down syndrome infants that presents with clinical and morphologic findings indistinguishable from AML. The blasts have morphologic and immunologic features of megakaryocytic lineage.

36. Ans. a. AML with t(8;21)

Ref: WHO 2017 Revised Edition

Core binding factor (CBF) AML includes AML with t(8;21) and AML with inv(16)/t(16;16). These two AML cytogenetic groups are often grouped together based on involvement of related CBF machinery and relatively overall favorable prognosis. The CBF genes are RUNX1 and CBFB (16q22). AML with inv(16)/t(16;16) is defined by the translocation and/or molecular fusion of CBFB and MYH11 regardless of blast count. AML with t(15;17)(q22;q21)/PML-RARA is a distinct clinicopathologic entity defined by the presence of the PML-RARA fusion, regardless of blast count.

37. Ans. a. Cytarabine 100–200 mg/m^2 for 7 days

Ref: Williams 8/e; Hoffman 7/e

The backbone of treatment for 30 years has been the combination of daunorubicin and cytarabine. Usually daunorubicin is given for 3 days in a dose of 60–90 mg/m^2. Cytarabine is given for 7 days as a continuous infusion or by bolus doses of 100–200 mg/m^2 daily. Higher doses of cytarabine (3 g/m^2) in induction have been tested, with mixed results and no convincing evidence of overall benefit. Intermediate doses (400 mg/m^2 daily vs. 200 mg/m^2 daily) have been tested in younger patients without demonstrating a difference. The induction regimen does not depend upon cytogenetic risk factors. However, the type of consolidation therapy depends upon risk stratification-high dose cytarabine for low-risk and stem cell transplant for high-risk AML.

38. Ans. d. Addition of etoposide increases remission rates

If patients fail to achieve a substantial reduction in marrow blasts in the first course or fail to enter CR with a second course of induction chemotherapy, they should be considered refractory and treated with an alternative treatment schedule. Studies did not show any difference between etoposide or thioguanine when used as the third drug in combination with daunorubicin and cytarabine. A number of factors influence the chances of achieving remission. Age is a dominant and independent risk factor. The distribution of cytogenetic subtypes is related to age, with more responsive subtypes frequently seen in younger patients and less responsive subtypes aggregating in older patients. If patients have had an antecedent hematological disorder, e.g., myelodysplasia, then the remission rate will be about 20% lower than in age matched groups.

39. **Ans. b. Cytogenetics** *Ref: Hoffbrand 7/e*

A number of factors influence the prospects of achieving remission. Age is a dominant and independent risk factor and a continuous variable; 80% of patients under 60 years will achieve CR, but this prospect diminishes with age. A larger proportion of older patients will have a poorer risk score and therefore, the score has more predictive impact. The distribution of cytogenetic subtypes is related to age, with more responsive subtypes frequently seen in younger patients and less responsive subtypes aggregating in older patients. Tumor burden at diagnosis, as represented by white blood count, serum albumin or lactate dehydrogenase levels, will adversely impact on response to induction treatment. The type of consolidation is actually based on the risk stratification of the AML, the most common factor for that is cytogenetics.

40. **Ans. a. t(9;11)(p21.3;q23.3)); MLLT3-KMT2A is an intermediate-risk AML**

Ref: Estey EH. Acute myeloid leukemia: 2019 update on risk-stratification and management. Am J Hematol. 2018;93(10):1267-91.

41. **Ans. e. All of the above**

Ref: Estey EH. Acute myeloid leukemia: 2019 update on risk-stratification and management. Am J Hematol. 2018;93:1267-91.

About 25–30% of patients with AML had an activating mutation in the transmembrane tyrosine kinase FLT3. The more common ITD mutation is particularly ominous, leading to rapid relapse and short survival with standard chemotherapy. Midostaurin is a multikinase tyrosine kinase inhibitor acting against targets known to be expressed in hematologic malignancies, especially AML. Midostaurin combined with chemotherapy followed by single-agent maintenance therapy has shown statistically significant and clinically meaningful improvement in overall survival in patients with newly diagnosed FLT3-mutant AML. It is superior regardless of ITD allelic ratio or whether the FLT3 mutation is an ITD or a TKD. Midostaurin is an orally administered type III tyrosine kinase inhibitor which in addition to FLT3 inhibits c-kit, platelet-derived growth factor receptors, SRC, and vascular endothelial growth factor receptor.

42. **Ans. d. Increases the risk of veno-occlusive disease**

Ref: Wadleigh M, Richardson PG, Zahrieh D, Lee SJ, Cutler C, Ho V, et al. Prior gemtuzumab ozogamicin exposure significantly increases the risk of veno-occlusive disease in patients who undergo myeloablative allogeneic stem cell transplantation. Blood. 2003;102(5):1578-82.

The cell surface antigen CD33 is commonly expressed on the AML cell surface (including possibly in some cases AML "stem cells") as well as on normal myeloid cells but not on other normal cells, with the exception of sinusoidal cells in the liver. GO consists of an antibody to CD33 combined with the toxin calicheamicin. Used alone GO is highly effective against APL presumably because of the heavy expression of CD33 in APL. It is much less effective as a single agent in other AML with CR and CRi rates of only 13% each in relapsed disease. Prior gemtuzumab ozogamicin exposure significantly increases the risk of veno-occlusive disease in patients who undergo myeloablative allogeneic stem cell transplantation, as CD33 is present in sinusoidal cells.

43. **Ans. e. All of the above**

Ref: Feldman EJ, Lancet JE, Kolitz JE, Ritchie EK, Roboz GJ, List AF, et al. First-in-man study of CPX-351: a liposomal carrier containing cytarabine and daunorubicin in a fixed 5:1 molar ratio for the treatment of relapsed and refractory acute myeloid leukemia. J Clin Oncol. 2011;29(8):979-85.

CPX351 is a liposomal formulation of cytarabine and daunorubicin at a fixed 5:1 M ratio of cytarabine/daunorubicin. The liposomal encapsulation leads to prolonged exposure to the two drugs. It is Food and Drug Administration (FDA) approved for t-AML or AML with MDS-related changes. It has side-effect profile similar to 3 + 7 chemotherapy.

44. **Ans. d. Good prognosis**

Ref: Eidenschink Brodersen L, Alonzo TA, Menssen AJ, Gerbing RB, Pardo L, Voigt AP, et al. A recurrent immunophenotype at diagnosis independently identifies high-risk pediatric acute myeloid leukemia: a report from Children's Oncology Group. Leukemia. 2016;30(10):2077-80.

A newly described subtype of AML, with a distinct immunophenotype (referred to as RAM immunophenotype), was reported by Eidenschink Brodersen et al. It is characterized by high intensity CD56 expression, dim-to-negative expression of CD45 and CD38, and a lack of HLA-DR expression. Clinically, RAM cases showed a distinctly high induction failure rate and extremely poor outcome. The RAM phenotype has been named after the patient's initials (RAM).

45. **Ans. d. Azacitidine plus venetoclax**

Ref: NCCN AML guidelines version 2020.

B-cell lymphoma 2 (BCL-2) is an antiapoptotic protein involved in the survival and maintenance of AML, and it is overexpressed in the leukemia stem cell population. Venetoclax is an oral BCL-2 protein inhibitor recently approved by the United States FDA for use in combination with a hypomethylating agent (HMA) (azacitidine or decitabine) or low-dose cytarabine for front-line treatment of AML in older patients or those unfit for induction chemotherapy. Venetoclax plus HMA is increasingly being used in the treatment of AML, and is considered by many to now be the standard of care for this population.

46. **Ans. c. Continue voriconazole prophylaxis**

Ref: Abramson S. The air crescent sign. Radiology, 2001.

The chest X-ray is showing air-crescent sign suggestive of resolving fungal pneumonia. An air crescent sign describes the crescent of air that can be seen in invasive aspergillosis or other processes that cause pulmonary necrosis. It usually heralds recovery and is the result of increased granulocyte activity usually after two weeks of disease onset. In angioinvasive fungal infection, the nodules are composed of infected hemorrhagic and infarcted lung tissue. As the neutrophil count recovers and the patient mounts an immune response, peripheral reabsorption of necrotic tissue causes the retraction of the infarcted center and air fills the space in between. This creates an air crescent within the nodules and is a good prognostic finding because it marks the recovery phase of the infection. This sign is seen in ~50% of patients. So this patient has resolving fungal pneumonia and should be continued on voriconazole prophylaxis.

47. **Ans. a. Aspergillus**

Ref: Guarner J. Histopathologic diagnosis of fungal infections in the 21st century. Clin Microbiol Rev. 2011;24(2):247–80

Fine needle aspiration cytology from the lesion is showing hyphae branching at acute angle suggesting aspergillus. Aspergillus have nonpigmented (hyaline), septated hyphae with acute-angle branching. Mucorales have nonpigmented (hyaline), pauciseptate ribbon-like hyphae with right-angle branching. Histoplasma appears as small yeasts (2–4 μm) with narrow-based budding grouped in clusters inside macrophages. Cryptosporidium oocysts are 4–6 micron in diameter and exhibit partial acid-fast staining. The oldest specific preparation for microscopy is a concentrated (10–20%) potassium hydroxide (KOH) solution, which softens keratin and allows direct visualization of fungi and some morphology evaluation. Gram stains are less sensitive. Papanicolaou stains may be useful. Cytology slides may be stained with sliver or Gomori Methenamine Silver (GMS) stains. Immunofluorescence microscopy is the best method to detect Pneumocystis. Fluorescent brighteners (Calcofluor white, Blankophor or Tinopal UNPA-GX), which bind to chitin in the fungal cell wall, are a rapid means of scanning samples for fungal hyphae, and enhance morphology assessment.

48. **Ans. a. Leukemia cutis**

Ref: Wagner G. Leukemia cutis—epidemiology, clinical presentation, and differential diagnoses. JDDG, 2011;10:27-36.

Cytarabine, a pyrimidine analog, is used for treating various hematological malignancies such as acute leukemias and lymphomas. Side effects of cytarabine are dose dependent and include bone marrow suppression, fever, cerebellar toxicity, cardiomyopathy, hepato-renal insufficiency, necrotizing enterocolitis, pancreatitis, acute respiratory distress, corneal toxicity and dermatological side effects. Cytarabine can cause various skin reactions. Incidence of this cytarabine induced rash varies between 3–72% and is more commonly seen in patients receiving high doses of cytarabine. It has also been reported with low doses and in both adults and children. It may manifest as maculopapular or morbilliform rash or as hand-foot syndrome which presents as erythema of palms and soles, associated with pain, tingling and paresthesia. Allopurinol has been associated with severe cutaneous adverse reactions (SCAR), including drug reaction with eosinophilia and systemic symptoms (DRESS), toxic epidermal necrolysis, Stevens–Johnson syndrome and allopurinol hypersensitivity syndrome (AHS). These syndromes have similar clinical features, including fever, eosinophilia, hepatic and renal dysfunction and rash. Fixed drug eruption is an uncommon fluconazole-induced cutaneous reaction. Fixed drug eruption is a type of cutaneous drug reaction that occurs at the same sites upon re-exposure to specific medications. Leukemia cutis is a rare disorder that is distinguished by the infiltration of leukemic cells into the skin. Since leukemia cutis may be a sign of a systemic disorder that occurs before, after, or concurrently with the beginning of AML, treatments should focus on the eradication of systemic leukemia. Leukemia cutis is least likely among these options to present 6 days after starting chemotherapy.

49. **Ans. b. CSF1R is expressed on myeloid leukemic blasts**

Ref: Edwards DK. CSF1R inhibitors exhibit antitumor activity in acute myeloid leukemia by blocking paracrine signals from support cells. Blood. 2019;133(6):588–99

Colony-stimulating factor 1 (CSF1) receptor (CSF1R), a receptor tyrosine kinase responsible for survival, proliferation, and differentiation of myeloid-lineage cells. CSF1R is not expressed on the majority of leukemic blasts but instead on a subpopulation of supportive cells. CSF1R-expressing cells support the bulk leukemia population through the secretion of HGF and other cytokines. CSF1R is a novel therapeutic target of AML and provides a mechanism of paracrine cytokine/growth factor signaling in this disease and its inhibition is being used as treatment of AML.

50. **Ans. a. Decitabine, venetoclax and FLT3 inhibitor**

Ref: Daver N. New directions for emerging therapies in acute myeloid leukemia: the next chapter. Blood Cancer Journal. 2020.

As the treatment paradigm for multiple myeloma has expanded to include the combination of several agents in the induction and salvage setting to improve survival, so too there is interest in combination or sequential approaches for AML treatment. Triplet regimens of venetoclax, HMA, and FLT3 inhibitor is being studied in phase 1/2 trials. It is hoped that such triplets will enhance efficacy while maintaining an acceptable safety profile and, importantly, early mortality rates <5-10%.

51. **Ans. e. All of the above**

Ref: Daver N. New directions for emerging therapies in acute myeloid leukemia: the next chapter. Blood Cancer Journal. 2020.

Mechanisms of resistance to FLT3 inhibitors include: 1. Alterations of the leukemia microenvironment, including increased FGF2 and CXCL12/CXCR4 signaling, may protect *FLT3*-mutated progenitors. 2. Increased signaling through parallel prosurvival pathways, including RAS-RAF-MEK-ERK, PI3K-AKT-mTOR, and JAK-STAT5-PIM1 pathways. Agents targeting these pathways are in clinical trial development. 3. Resistant mutations are also commonly observed (30%–40%) in FLT3 inhibitor-resistant cases and may be treatment-emergent or due to expansion of a preexisting resistant subclone. These include *NRAS/KRAS* mutations, alternative *FLT3* mutations (e.g., D835, F691, and others), and *BCR–ABL* translocation. 4. Upregulation of antiapoptotic proteins, including BCL2 and MCL1, has been observed in cases of FLT3 inhibitor resistance, and a number of FLT3 inhibitors also inhibit MCL1, providing the rationale for combining FLT3 inhibitors with BCL2 inhibitors.

52. **Ans. b. Assessing fitness for intensive chemotherapy in AML**

Ref: Ferrara L. Consensus-based definition of unfitness to intensive and non-intensive chemotherapy in acute myeloid leukemia: a project of SIE, SIES and GITMO group on a new tool for therapy decision making. Leukemia. 2013;997–9.

In 2013, Ferrara and colleagues proposed a set of objective criteria for defining patients as "fit" or "unfit" for intensive chemotherapy for AML. The Ferrara criteria are widely used to identify patients with AML who would be most suitable for intensive chemotherapy. The predications from the Ferrara score were compared with those of the previously developed treatment-related mortality (TRM) score. The Ferrara score was more accurate compared with the TRM score at predicting day-28 and day-100 mortality. The criteria includes age >75 years, cardiac, renal, pulmonary and hepatic comorbidities, cognitive functions and ECOG performance status.

CHAPTER 27

Acute Promyelocytic Leukemia

1. **Risk of relapse in patients with acute promyelocytic leukemia (APL) is stratified by:**
   a. Prothrombin time and platelet count
   b. Leukocyte and platelet count
   c. Prothrombin time and fibrinogen
   d. Hemoglobin and platelet count

2. **Treatment of coagulopathies in acute promyelocytic leukemia includes all, *except*:**
   a. Immediate start of all-transretinoic-acid (ATRA) therapy
   b. Maintaining platelet count above 30,000/µL
   c. Maintaining fibrinogen concentration above 100 mg/dL
   d. Starting dexamethasone 10 mg twice daily

3. **True regarding induction treatment for acute promyelocytic leukemia is:**
   a. Induction with arsenic trioxide (ATO) is superior to induction with ATRA plus anthracycline
   b. Induction with ATRA plus anthracycline is superior to ATO
   c. Both ATRA and ATO are equally effective
   d. Not evaluated

4. **Risk factors for the development of differentiation syndrome are:**
   a. Age more than 60 years
   b. Female sex
   c. Morphological characteristics of blasts
   d. Concomitant use of chemotherapy
   e. None of the above

5. **True about differentiation syndrome is:**
   a. Can develop with either ATRA or ATO
   b. Incidence is up to 27% of cases of APL
   c. Begin at an interval of 7–14 days
   d. Include fever, weight gain, and pulmonary infiltrate, pericardial or pleural effusion
   e. All of the above

6. **A 7-year-old child with APL developed headache, vomiting, and blurring of vision after 15 days of starting treatment ATRA. The most effective intervention would be:**
   a. Give platelets for suspected intracranial bleed
   b. Give dexamethasone for ATRA syndrome
   c. Do lumbar puncture to rule out CNS leukemia
   d. Withhold ATRA and give acetazolamide

7. **Cytarabine is indicated in:**
   a. Low-risk APL
   b. Intermediate-risk APL
   c. High-risk APL
   d. None of the above

8. **Treatment for a relapsed APL patient in second molecular remission is:**
   a. ATRA maintenance
   b. ATO and ATRA maintenance
   c. Autologous transplant
   d. Allogenic transplant

9. **The method most effective in predicting relapse in APL is:**
   a. Flow cytometry
   b. Fluorescent in-situ hybridization (FISH)
   c. Real-time quantitative polymerase chain reaction (RQ-PCR) from peripheral blood
   d. RQ-PCR from bone marrow
   e. Any of the above

10. **Side-effects of ATO include:**
    a. QT prolongation
    b. Hypokalemia
    c. Hypomagnesemia
    d. All of the above

11. **Response to induction therapy in APL should be assessed at:**
    a. 7 days
    b. 14 days
    c. 28–30 days
    d. After 45 days

12. **Treatment of a pregnant female with APL in first trimester is:**
    a. ATRA
    b. ATO
    c. Daunorubicin
    d. Supportive care with platelets and fresh frozen plasma (FFP) transfusion
    e. None of the above

13. **True regarding therapy-related APL are all, *except*:**
    a. Breast carcinoma is the most frequent previous cancer
    b. Drugs most commonly implicated in therapy-related APL are epirubicin and mitoxantrone
    c. Latency period is less than 3 years

d. Occurs without a preceding myelodysplastic phase
e. Therapy-related APL has a very poor prognosis and requires aggressive chemotherapy

14. **True regarding ATRA + arsenic trioxide (ATO) in APL is, *except*:**
a. ATRA targets RARA and ATO targets PML
b. ATRA + ATO is superior to ATRA + chemotherapy for newly diagnosed low-risk APL
c. About 20% of patients have been reported to relapse after modern, risk-adapted ATRA and chemotherapy regimens
d. Treatment should be escalated in the presence of high-risk features like FLT3

15. **Which of the following APL variants is resistant to ATRA and ATO?**
a. NUMA/RARA
b. STAT5B/RARA
c. NPM/RARA
d. BCOR/RARA
e. FIP1L1/RARA

16. **The most common APL variant is:**
a. NUMA/RARA
b. STAT5B/RARA
c. NPM/RARA
d. ZBTB16/RARA
e. FIP1L1/RARA

17. **Managing increasing leukocytosis during induction in APL includes:**
a. Gemtuzumab ozogamicin in low- and intermediate-risk APL
b. Hydroxyurea in low- and intermediate-risk APL
c. Idarubicin in high-risk patients
d. All of the above

ANSWERS WITH EXPLANATIONS

1. **Ans. b. Leukocyte and platelet count**
Ref: Adès L. Treatment of newly diagnosed acute promyelocytic leukemia (APL): a comparison of French-Belgian-Swiss and PETHEMA results. Blood. 2008

The criteria used are called the Sanz criteria which include the leukocyte and platelet counts at the time of diagnosis. Patients are considered low-risk when, at diagnosis, the leukocyte count is less than 10,000/μL and the platelet count is more than 40,000/μL, intermediate-risk when the leukocyte count is less than 10,000/μL and the platelet count is less than 40,000/μL, and high-risk when the leukocyte count is more than 10,000/μL. Data suggests that the addition of cytarabine to ATRA and anthracyclines in high-risk patients may result in a trend toward lower incidence of relapse, and to better survival.

2. **Ans. d. Starting dexamethasone 10 mg twice daily**
Ref: Sanz MA. Management of acute promyelocytic leukemia: recommendations from an expert panel on behalf of the European LeukemiaNet. Blood. 2009

Intracerebral and pulmonary hemorrhages are relatively common life-threatening complications occurring in APL. The recommended treatment for bleeding disorders in patients with APL is the immediate start of ATRA therapy with support using blood products to keep the platelet count above 30,000/μL and the fibrinogen concentration above 100 mg/dL (using concentrated platelet, FFP, and cryoprecipitate transfusions). Dexamethasone is used in ATRA syndrome.

3. **Ans. c. Both ATRA and ATO are equally effective**
Ref: Lo Coco F. Retinoic acid and arsenic trioxide for acute promyelocytic leukemia. NEJM. 2013

There is no evidence of superiority of ATO compared to ATRA combined with an anthracycline in the induction treatment for APL. In the evaluation of ATRA (25–45 mg/m^2/day) associated with ATO (0.15–0.16 mg/kg/day) or ATO alone in patients with relapsed APL, no significant difference was found in the complete remission (CR) rate between combination therapy (89.8%) and single drug therapy (81.7%). Pilot studies of treatment with ATO with or without ATRA have shown high efficacy and reduced hematologic toxicity.

4. **Ans. e. None of the above**

Leukocytosis is a predictor for the development of differentiation syndrome when the WBC count is >20,000/μL. A body mass index above 30 kg/m^2 and creatinine above the normal value are also predictors for the development of differentiation syndrome. There is no evidence for age, gender, morphological and molecular subtypes, and concomitant systemic chemotherapy as risk factors for the development of the syndrome.

5. **Ans. e. All of the above**
Ref: Sanz MA. Management of acute promyelocytic leukemia: recommendations from an expert panel on behalf of the European LeukemiaNet. Blood. 2009

Differentiation syndrome is the main complication associated with therapy using agents that promote differentiation, such as ATRA and ATO, during induction therapy of APL. Because of the life-threatening nature of the full-blown syndrome, specific treatment with dexamethasone at a dose of 10 mg twice daily by intravenous injection should be started promptly at the very earliest symptom or sign. ATRA is well-tolerated, however, the incidence of differentiation syndrome has been described in up to 25–30% APL patients. In most reported cases, symptoms relating to differentiation syndrome began in a median of 9 days (range: 0–23 days) from the start of treatment. Differentiation syndrome includes the following according to the criteria of Frankel—three of the following signs in the absence of other causes: fever, weight gain, pulmonary infiltrate, pericardial or pleural effusion, hypotension, liver failure, and/or acute renal failure, with 37.9% of early deaths. On suspicion of symptoms related to differentiation syndrome, the early addition of high doses of dexamethasone reduces associated mortality from 30 to 5% or less. It is recommended to start dexamethasone using an intravenous dose of 10 mg twice daily until total regression of the symptoms. Most patients present a rapid improvement with the administration of the corticosteroid. But, there is no evidence supporting the prophylactic use of corticosteroids in patients with APL to prevent differentiation syndrome. ATRA should be stopped for 48–72 hours and reintroduced at a 50% dose with stepped increases until the full dose.

6. Ans. d. Withhold ATRA and give acetazolamide
Ref: Williams 8/e; Hoffbrand 7/e

The temporary suspension of ATRA is recommended when there is diagnostic suspicion of pseudotumor cerebri in patients with APL, particularly in children. ATRA can be reintroduced after improvement of the symptoms. Mannitol and acetazolamide together can be used with the suspension of ATRA to decrease the cerebrospinal fluid (CSF) pressure improving the headaches, diplopia, nausea, and vomiting. Pseudotumor cerebri is characterized by increased intracranial pressure with the presence of papilledema, normal or diminished ventricles, and with normal CSF. Bleeding at this time is unlikely as is primary CNS involvement by APL, though these rare possibilities can sometime happen. ATRA syndrome does not involve CNS. Although, some protocols include CNS prophylaxis, at least for patients with hyperleukocytosis, it should be noted that neither an increased incidence of CNS relapse nor a benefit of CNS prophylaxis has been established in children. To decrease the frequency of side effects associated with induction therapy including ATRA, particularly severe headache and pseudotumor cerebri, which are both frequently observed in children, most investigators have used a reduced dose of ATRA (e.g. 25 mg/m^2 instead of 45 mg/m^2) in the pediatric age group.

7. Ans. c. High-risk APL

ATRA in association with an anthracycline is the standard treatment for the induction phase of the treatment of APL. The role of cytarabine is controversial. The association of cytarabine to an anthracycline and ATRA in the consolidation therapy of patients diagnosed with APL is recommended for under 65-year-old high-risk patients based on the significant reduction in the relapse rate and the significant increases in event-free survival. There is no evidence to support this association for intermediate or low-risk patients.

8. Ans. c. Autologous transplant
Ref: Sanz MA. Management of acute promyelocytic leukemia: recommendations from an expert panel on behalf of the European LeukemiaNet. Blood. 2009

The European Group of Hematopoietic Stem Cell Transplantation recommends autologous stem cell transplantation (SCT) for cases of APL in second CR and SCT with a human leukocyte antigen (HLA)-identical related donor in the case of molecular persistent APL. Data suggests that autologous SCT is very effective in the treatment of APL for patients in second complete molecular remission. Allogeneic bone marrow transplant (BMT), though with a lower relapse rate, is associated with high transplant-related mortality and is preferred for those who do not achieve second remission or relapse after autologous transplant or had high-risk disease.

9. Ans. d. RQ-PCR from bone marrow

Molecular diagnosis of relapse in APL can be performed by FISH, RT-PCR, and RQ-PCR; RQ-PCR (quantitative real time polymerase chain reaction) is the most important to predict hematologic relapse and disease-free survival (DFS). In assessing the minimal residual disease (MRD) in APL with RQ-PCR, values less than 3 log after the end of consolidation treatment compared with values more than 3 log proved to be the most important predictor of relapse. PCR analysis of promyelocytic leukemia/retinoic acid receptor alpha (PML-RARA) is preferably carried out on RNA extracted from bone marrow samples. Recurrence of PCR positivity typically occurs first in the marrow, and occasionally *PML-RARA* transcripts do not become detectable in peripheral blood until time of hematologic relapse. Therefore, in some patients, the monitoring of peripheral blood alone (even if performed monthly) could reduce the opportunity for successful delivery of preemptive therapy to prevent disease progression.

10. Ans. d. All of the above *Ref: Williams 8/e; Hoffbrand 7/e*

Treatment with ATO is associated with several electrolyte abnormalities and QT prolongation that can lead to a torsade de pointes-type ventricular arrhythmia, which can be fatal. This requires careful monitoring to maintain the serum potassium above 4.0 mEq/L and serum magnesium above 1.8 mg/dL. In patients who reach an absolute QT interval value longer than 500 msec, ATO should be withheld, the electrolytes (potassium and magnesium) repleted, and other medications that may cause prolonged QT interval should be discontinued.

11. Ans. d. After 45 days
Ref: Sanz MA. Management of acute promyelocytic leukemia: recommendations from an expert panel on behalf of the European LeukemiaNet. Blood. 2009

Treatment with ATRA should be continued allowing sufficient time for terminal differentiation of blasts to occur. Molecular assessment by RT-PCR after induction has no clinical relevance, because PCR positivity at this early time point may simply reflect delayed maturation instead of resistance. Potentially misleading cytomorphologic features due to incomplete blast maturation are occasionally seen even after several weeks from treatment initiation (up to 40-50 days). CR is attained in virtually all patients with genetically proven PML-RARA APL. In contrast to the lack of clinical value of molecular assessment performed at the end of induction, RT-PCR of PML-RARA in bone marrow carried out on regeneration after the final course of chemotherapy is extremely relevant to determine the relapse risk in the individual patient.

12. Ans. c. Daunorubicin

Ref: Sanz MA. Management of acute promyelocytic leukemia: recommendations from an expert panel on behalf of the European LeukemiaNet. Blood. 2009

Both ATRA and ATO have teratogenic potential therefore therapeutic options for patients diagnosed during the first trimester are limited. ATRA (like retinoids) is considered highly teratogenic in first trimester. ATRA should be avoided during the first trimester. If elective abortion is unacceptable, administration of daunorubicin chemotherapy alone, without ATRA, is the only option during the first trimester. Among anthracyclines, it has been suggested that daunorubicin might be preferred because this agent is known to be effective in APL and there is more published experience of its use in pregnancy. If remission is achieved with chemotherapy and the pregnancy is progressing normally, treatment with ATRA could be administered during the second and third trimesters. ATO also has high potential for embryo toxicity and it cannot be recommended for use at any stage of pregnancy. Treatment with ATRA and anthracycline-based chemotherapy seem reasonably safe when applied to patients with APL presenting during the second or third trimester of pregnancy.

13. Ans. e. Therapy-related APL has a very poor prognosis and requires aggressive chemotherapy

Ref: Sanz MA. Management of acute promyelocytic leukemia: recommendations from an expert panel on behalf of the European LeukemiaNet. Blood. 2009

Breast carcinoma is the most common previous cancer, followed by lymphoma, with a large predominance of non-Hodgkin lymphoma compared with Hodgkin disease. The drugs most commonly implicated in therapy-related APL are epirubicin and mitoxantrone, but several cases have been reported to follow exposure to radiotherapy alone. The latency period between chemotherapy for previous cancer and development of therapy-related APL is less than 3 years and typically occurs without a preceding myelodysplastic syndrome. Hematologic and clinical findings do not differ from those observed in de novo APL. Patients with therapy-related APL have a relatively favorable prognosis. The treatment of therapy-related APL is same as that of de novo APL.

14. Ans. d. Treatment should be escalated in the presence of high-risk features like FLT3

Ref: Lo-Coco F, Cicconi L, Breccia M. Current standard treatment of adult acute promyelocytic leukemia. Br J Haematol. 2016;172(6):841-54.

ATRA and ATO have been shown to target RARA and PML, respectively, i.e., the two distinct moieties of the disease-specific oncoprotein PML/RARA. ATRA + ATO is superior to ATRA + chemotherapy for newly diagnosed low-risk APL resulting in 2-4 years event-free survival rates above 90% and very few relapses and considerably less hematological toxicity in patients receiving the chemotherapy-free approach. About 20% of patients have been reported to relapse after modern, risk-adapted ATRA and chemotherapy regimens. Standard induction therapy should not be modified based on the presence of leukemia cell characteristics that have variably been considered to predict a poorer prognosis (e.g. secondary chromosomal abnormalities, FLT3 mutations, CD56 expression, and BCR3 PML-RARA isoform).

15. Ans. b. STAT5B/RARA

Ref: Adams J, Nassiri M. Acute promyelocytic leukemia: review and discussion of variant translocations. Arch Pathol Lab Med. 2015;139(10):1308-13.

About 1-2% of APL cases are due to rare variant translocations, which typically involve *RARA*. No APL variants with PML involvement alone have been identified, thus, *RARA* is assumed to have a key role in the pathogenesis of APL. These variants have been found to involve the *RARA* gene on chromosome 17 but not the *PML* gene on chromosome 15, thus supporting the central role of *RARA* in the pathogenesis of APL. The variant translocations identified to date all involve RARA and include ZBTB16/RARA, NPM/RARA, NUMA/RARA, STAT5B/RARA, PRKAR1a/RARA, BCOR/RARA, and FIP1L1/RARA. Of these, ZBTB16/RARA and STAT5B/RARA are resistant to treatment with ATRA, ATO, and anthracyclines, and have poor prognosis. Apart from molecular variants, there are two morphologic variants of APL. These are hypergranular or "typical" APL [M3 by the French-American-British FAB classification] and hypogranular or "microgranular" APL (M3v by the FAB classification). Both forms have promyelocytes with abnormal bilobed nuclei. There is no link between molecular and morphologic variants.

16. Ans. d. ZBTB16/RARA

Ref: Adams J, Nassiri M. Acute promyelocytic leukemia. A review and discussion of variant translocations. Arch Pathol Lab Med. 2015;139(10):1308-13.

The most common APL variant is t(11;17)(q23;q21), which fuses ZBTB16 [formerly PLZF (promyelocytic leukemia zinc finger)] with RARA and results in the production of the ZBTB16-RARA fusion protein and the RARA-ZBTB16 reciprocal fusion protein. It is important to identify this variant translocation in APL because it alters patient treatment and prognosis. Diagnosis of t(11;17) APL can be difficult based on morphology alone because the blasts have a more regular nucleus compared with the bilobed nucleus typically found in APL.

17. Ans. d. All of the above

Ref: Osman AE. Treatment of Acute Promyelocytic Leukemia in Adults. J CO 2018

Gemtuzumab ozogamicin has been administered as a single dose of 6 or 9 mg/m^2 when WBC count rises to greater than 30,000/μL during induction in low- and intermediate-risk patients. Alternatively, hydroxyurea could be administered when WBC count rises to greater than 10,000/μL, starting with a dose of 500 mg every 6 hours. High-risk patients seem to benefit from substantial cytoreduction early during induction by using anthracyclines.

CHAPTER 28

Chronic Lymphocytic Leukemia

1. **What percentage of lymphocytes constitutes T cells in normal person?**
   a. 20%   b. 40%
   c. 70%   d. 90%

2. **Lymphocytes with villous projections are seen in:**
   a. Hairy cell leukemia
   b. Large granular lymphocytic (LGL) leukemia
   c. Mycosis fungoides
   d. Splenic marginal zone lymphoma

3. **Bone marrow involvement in chronic lymphocytic leukemia (CLL) is:**
   a. Stage 0   b. Stage I
   c. Stage III   d. Stage IV

4. **The diagnosis of CLL is confirmed by:**
   a. Peripheral smear
   b. Bone marrow aspirate and smear
   c. Immunophenotyping
   d. Cytogenetics

5. **The following are the markers of CLL, except:**
   a. CD19   b. CD23
   c. CD5   d. Strong CD20

6. **Most common presentation of CLL is in stage:**
   a. Stage 0 (lymphocytosis)
   b. Stages I to II (lymphadenopathy, organomegaly)
   c. Stages III to IV (anemia, thrombocytopenia)
   d. All stages have equal frequency of presentation

7. **The median survival from the time of diagnosis in stage III and IV CLL patients is:**
   a. 10 months
   b. 20 months
   c. 30 months
   d. 40 months

8. **True about CLL are all, except:**
   a. Short doubling time may favor more aggressive disease
   b. Diffuse pattern predicts a progressive course
   c. Beta-2 microglobulin levels correlate with disease stage and tumor burden
   d. CD38 is associated with an adverse prognosis
   e. Zeta-associated protein (ZAP-70) correlates with good survival

9. **True about mutated immunoglobulin heavy chain variable-region (IgVH) genes in CLL are all, except:**
   a. Develops from pregerminal center memory B-cells
   b. Lower expression of CD38 and ZAP-70
   c. Lower clinical stage
   d. Good response to therapy
   e. All of the above

10. **Autoimmune phenomena seen in CLL are all, except:**
    a. Coombs' positive autoimmune hemolytic anemia
    b. Idiopathic thrombocytopenic purpura
    c. Pure red cell aplasia
    d. Rheumatoid arthritis

11. **Cytogenetic abnormalities seen in CLL are all, except:**
    a. Trisomy 12   b. del6q
    c. del17p   d. del11p

12. **Indications for treatment in CLL are all, except:**
    a. Symptomatic anemia and/or thrombocytopenia
    b. Repeated episodes of infection
    c. Weight loss
    d. Autoimmune hemolytic anemia
    e. del17p

13. **Adverse prognostic features in CLL are, except:**
    a. ZAP-70   b. CD38
    c. Unmutated *IgVH* genes   d. del13q14

14. **Treatment of choice for patients with localized (stage I) small lymphocytic lymphoma is:**
    a. Observation
    b. Localized radiation therapy
    c. Chemotherapy
    d. Chemotherapy plus localized radiation therapy

15. **Patients with del (17p) or del (11q) are at high risk because of:**
    a. Not responding adequately to initial treatment
    b. Relapsing soon after achieving remission
    c. Requiring treatment early
    d. All of the above

16. **Regarding alemtuzumab therapy in CLL, true is:**
    a. Effective in CLL with del17p
    b. A survival benefit has not been demonstrated

c. Effective when maximum lymph nodes <5 cm in diameter
d. Can deplete bone marrow leukemic clone and achieve minimal residual disease (MRD) negativity
e. All of the above are true

17. Which of the following drugs are used in CLL?
a. Mitoxantrone   b. Pentostatin
c. Fludarabine   d. All of the above

18. Alemtuzumab is effective in CLL with chromosome 17p deletion because it:
a. Acts through IP3/mTOR pathway
b. Acts through heat shock proteins
c. Acts through p53 pathway of apoptosis
d. None of the above

19. Prolymphocytic leukemia (PLL) differs from CLL by:
a. PLL cells are large with prominent vesicular nucleolus
b. PLL cells do not express CD5
c. Prognosis is poor
d. All of the above

20. True regarding treatment of relapsed/refractory CLL are all, *except*:
a. Eligible patients should be considered for allogeneic transplant
b. Rituximab maintenance is preferred for patients who achieve second remission
c. Flavopiridol is effective
d. Radiotherapy is indicated

21. Complete remission (CR) in CLL is defined as:
a. Absence of constitutional symptoms
b. No lymph nodes >1.5 cm in diameter
c. No splenomegaly
d. Absolute neutrophil count >1,500/µL
e. All of the above

22. Regarding treatment with intravenous immunoglobulin (IVIG) in CLL patients true is:
a. There is a decrease in the incidence of major bacterial infections
b. Patients with repeated infections should be treated with prophylactic IVIG
c. The usual dose is 200–400 mg/kg by IV infusion
d. The serum IgG in treated patients should be kept above 500 mg/dL
e. All of the above

23. Cause of anemia in CLL is:
a. Gastrointestinal blood loss
b. Hypersplenism
c. Marrow suppression secondary to the use of alkylating agents
d. Red blood cell aplasia
e. All of the above

24. True regarding autoimmune hemolytic anemia (AIHA) in CLL is:
a. Treatment with fludarabine, cyclophosphamide, and rituximab eliminates the risk of developing AIHA
b. The incidence of AIHA may be lower following purine analog treatment
c. Patients with a history of fludarabine associated-AIHA have a low risk of recurrent AIHA if rechallenged with fludarabine
d. The reported incidence is about 10–15%
e. All of the above

25. When compared to chlorambucil, fludarabine resulted in the following, *except*:
a. Complete remission rates were higher with fludarabine
b. Overall remission rates (CR plus PR) were higher for fludarabine
c. Median duration of response for patients achieving CR or PR was longer with fludarabine
d. Overall survival (OS) was higher with fludarabine
e. All of the above

26. Which of the following patients with chronic lymphocytic leukemia (CLL) should not be treated with fludarabine/cyclophosphamide/rituximab (FCR) or bendamustine and rituximab (BR) regimens?
a. CLL with del11q23
b. CLL with del13q14
c. CLL with del17p13
d. CLL with unmutated *IgVH* genes

27. What is the significance of TP53 evaluation in chronic lymphocytic leukemia?
a. It is associated with poor prognosis
b. It does not respond to conventional treatment
c. It is associated with del17p13
d. All of the above

28. The side-effects of ibrutinib include all *except*:
a. Diarrhea
b. Bleeding
c. Thrombosis
d. Atrial fibrillation
e. All of the above

29. True regarding venetoclax is:
a. Single-agent venetoclax is approved for patients with relapsed/refractory CLL who have del17p by fluorescent in situ hybridization (FISH)
b. The combination of venetoclax and rituximab is approved for all patients with relapsed/refractory CLL regardless of the CLL FISH profile
c. The most common side-effect of venetoclax is neutropenia

d. Venetoclax plus rituximab may achieve MRD negative complete remission sooner than those treated with ibrutinib as a single agent
e. All of the above

30. Treatment of chronic lymphocytic leukemia progressing on ibrutinib is:
a. Idelalisib and rituximab
b. Venetoclax and rituximab
c. Chimeric antigen receptor (CAR)-T cell therapy
d. Reduced intensity conditioning (RIC)-allogeneic stem cell transplant
e. All of the above

31. Richter's transformation in chronic lymphocytic leukemia can result in:
a. Diffuse large B-cell lymphoma
b. Hodgkin lymphoma
c. Acute lymphoblastic leukemia
d. All of the above
e. Only a and b

32. Ibrutinib acts by inhibiting:
a. CYP3A4
b. BTK
c. JAK-STAT
d. BCL-2
e. BCL-6

33. True about venetoclax is:
a. BCL-6 inhibitor
b. Not effective in CLL with del17p
c. Antagonizes ibrutinib effect
d. None of the above
e. All of the above

34. A 67-year-old man with chronic lymphocytic leukemia stage 0 on FISH examination has been found to have del17p. What will be your advice to the patient?
a. Watchful waiting with 3 monthly follow-up
b. Start ibrutinib
c. Whole body PET-CT
d. Start prednisolone at 1 mg/kg/day

35. False about ibrutinib treatment in chronic lymphocytic leukemia is:
a. Ibrutinib does not cure CLL
b. Indefinite administration is required
c. up to 41-51% of CLL patients discontinue therapy
d. None of the above

36. True about treatment with ibrutinib is:
a. Ibrutinib should be started at a lower dose and titrated up
b. High lymphocyte count increases the risk of complications with ibrutinib
c. A previous diagnosis of atrial fibrillation or other cardiac arrhythmia is a contraindication to ibrutinib initiation
d. None of the above

37. True about ibrutinib induced bleeding is:
a. Ibrutinib prolongs prothrombin time
b. Major bleeding is seen in less than 1% of patients
c. Minor surgical procedures can be done without stopping the drug
d. Platelet transfusions are not indicated in the event of bleeding
e. None of the above

ANSWERS WITH EXPLANATIONS

1. Ans. c. 70%

Circulating blood lymphocytes include T-cells, B-cells, and natural killer (NK) cells. Their normal relative proportions in the blood are: T-cells (CD3+ cells)—60-80%, B-cells (CD20+ cells)—10-20%, and NK-cells (CD56+ cells)—5-10%. The normal relative proportions of T-cell subtypes in the blood are: helper/inducer T-cells (CD4+ cells)—60-70% and suppressor/cytotoxic T-cells (CD8+ cells)—30-40%.

2. Ans. d. Splenic marginal zone lymphoma

Ref: WHO 2017 Revised Edition

Lymphocytes with villous projections are seen in splenic marginal zone lymphoma. Normal appearing small lymphocytes, often with a large proportion of damaged lymphocytes ("smudge" cells), are seen in CLL. Lymphocytes with hairy projections are seen in hairy cell leukemia. Large granular lymphocytes are feature of LGL leukemia. Small lymphocytes with cleaved nuclei are seen in follicular lymphoma and mantle cell lymphoma and lymphocytes with "cerebriform" nuclei (Sezary cells) in mycosis fungoides.

3. Ans. a. Stage 0

Ref: Rai et al, Clinical staging of chronic lymphocytic leukemia. Blood. 1975

The Rai classification of CLL relies upon the fact that in CLL, there is a gradual and progressive increase in the body burden of atypical lymphocytes, starting in the blood and bone marrow (lymphocytosis), progressively involving lymph nodes (lymphadenopathy), spleen and liver (organomegaly), with eventual compromise of bone marrow function (anemia and thrombocytopenia). So, bone marrow involvement in CLL is an early manifestation.

Rai devised a method of clinical staging of CLL based on the concept that CLL is a disease of progressive accumulation of nonfunctioning lymphocytes: stage 0, bone marrow and blood lymphocytosis only; stage I, lymphocytosis with enlarged nodes; stage II, lymphocytosis with enlarged spleen or liver or both; stage III, lymphocytosis with anemia; and stage IV: lymphocytosis with thrombocytopenia. Analysis of 125 patients in the series reported by Rai et al. showed the following median survival times from diagnosis: stage 0, is greater than 150 months; stage I, 101 months; stage II, 71 months; stage III, 19 months; and stage IV, 19 months.

4. Ans. c. Immunophenotyping

Ref: Gribben JG. How I treat CLL upfront. Blood. 2010; Hoffbrand 7/e

Bone marrow aspirate and biopsy are not required for the diagnosis of CLL because the diagnosis can be made from the abnormal lymphocytes (monoclonal B cells more than 5,000/μL) present in the blood, by flow cytometric techniques. There can three types of infiltrative patterns of lymphocytes recognized in bone marrow biopsy: nodular, interstitial, and diffuse, these patterns have prognostic significance. Patients with diffuse infiltration of bone marrow tend to have advanced disease and a poorer prognosis. Flow cytometry is essential for diagnosis and shows CD5+ve, CD23+ve B monoclonal lymphocytes. Peripheral smear shows the leukemic cells that are typically small, mature appearing lymphocytes with a dense nucleus, partially aggregated chromatin, and without discernible nucleoli. Smudge cells may be seen but are not diagnostic of CLL. Cytogenetics helps in risk stratification and prognosis.

Bone marrow biopsy should be done if patient is considered for treatment. It is also done in the newly diagnosed patients when they present with cytopenias, since, this may be useful in evaluating whether cytopenias are immune mediated or caused by marrow replacement by CLL.

5. Ans. d. Strong CD20

Ref: Williams 8/e Chap 92; Hoffbrand 7/e Chap 29

There are three major characteristic immunophenotypic findings in CLL: (1) Expression of B-cell associated antigens including CD19, CD20, and CD23. Expression of CD20 is usually weak; (2) Expression of CD5, a T-cell associated antigen; and (3) Low levels of surface membrane immunoglobulin (i.e., SmIg weak). The immunoglobulin is most often IgM and only a single immunoglobulin light chain is expressed (i.e., either kappa or lambda but not both), confirming the clonal nature of these cells.

6. Ans. b. Stages I to II (lymphadenopathy, organomegaly)

Ref: Gribben JG. How I treat CLL upfront. Blood. 2010

The presentation of CLL according to stages is: Stage 0 (lymphocytosis)—25%; Stages I to II (lymphadenopathy, organomegaly)—50%; Stages III to IV (anemia, thrombocytopenia)—25%.

7. Ans. b. 20 months

Ref: Williams 8/e Chap 92

The median survival of patients with CLL from the time of diagnosis is: Stage 0—150 months, Stage I—101 months, Stage II—71 months, and Stages III and IV—19 months.

8. Ans. e. ZAP-70 correlates with good survival

Ref: Williams 8/e; Hoffbrand 7/e

Various prognostic markers are used for risk stratification in patients with CLL. The presence of a short doubling time favors more aggressive disease, and this is an indication for early treatment. A diffuse pattern in the marrow biopsy predicts a progressive course and a nondiffuse (interstitial and nodular) pattern predicts a more indolent course. Beta-2 microglobulin levels have been found to correlate with disease stage and tumor burden in patients with CLL, with increasing levels associated with a poorer prognosis. The presence of CD38 appears to be independently associated with an adverse prognosis. ZAP-70, a tyrosine kinase normally expressed by T cells, has been found in a subset of patients with CLL and appears to correlate with poor survival. Both CD38 and ZAP-70 are surrogate markers for unmutated IgVH status.

9. Ans. a. Develops from pregerminal center memory B-cells

Ref: Williams 8/e; Hoffbrand 7/e

The monoclonal B lymphocytes in CLL can be divided into two groups that differ in the extent to which their expressed *IgVH* genes have undergone somatic mutation, and this has significant clinical correlation. About 50% of all cases have monoclonal B lymphocytes that express nonmutated *IgVH* genes; the rest 50% express *IgVH* genes. CLL developing from postgerminal center memory B-cells has mutated *IgVH* genes. Mutated *IgVH* gene status correlates with the presence of more favorable chromosomal abnormalities, lowered expression of CD38 and ZAP-70, lower clinical stage, and good survival. CLL developing from pregerminal center B-cells has unmutated *VH* genes. It has less favorable chromosomal abnormalities, higher expression of CD38 and ZAP-70, higher clinical stage, greater tendency to disease progression, a poor response to treatment, and shorter survival.

10. Ans. d. Rheumatoid arthritis

Autoimmune phenomena seen in CLL are Coombs' positive autoimmune hemolytic anemia, idiopathic thrombocytopenic purpura, and pure red cell aplasia (PRCA). Rheumatoid arthritis is associated with LGL syndrome. Hypogammaglobulinemia is a common finding in CLL and autoimmune disorders occur in 20-25% of patients. AIHA occur in about 11% of patients with CLL, primarily in advanced disease, and ITP and PRCA in 2-3 and 6%, respectively, primarily occurring in early disease.

A positive Coombs' test direct antiglobulin test (DAT) is a predictor of the subsequent development of AIHA after treatment. Those who are DAT positive at entry achieve lower CR rates and have poor progression free survival (PFS) and OS, suggesting indirectly that DAT status may be a useful prognostic factor.

11. Ans. d. del11p *Ref: Hoffbrand 7/e*

The most common recurrent chromosomal abnormalities seen in CLL are del13q, del11q, trisomy 12, del17p, and del6q (not 11p deletion). 11q deletions are associated with extensive adenopathy, progressive disease, and shorter survival, particularly in patients under the age of 55. 17p deletion is one of the strongest predictor of poor survival. The most common abnormality is del13q. 14, which occurs in more than 50% of cases.

12. Ans. e. del17p

Ref: Williams 7/e Chap 92 (Table 92-4); Hoffbrand 7/e

Therapy in CLL is indicated for patients with the following features: (1) Disease-related complications—weakness, night sweats, weight loss, painful lymphadenopathy or fever, (2) Symptomatic anemia and/or thrombocytopenia (Rai stages III or IV; Binet stage C), (3) Autoimmune hemolytic anemia and/or thrombocytopenia that are poorly responsive to corticosteroid therapy, (4) Progressive disease, as demonstrated by increasing lymphocytosis with a lymphocyte doubling time less than 6 months, and/or rapidly enlarging lymph nodes, spleen, and liver and repeated episodes of infection.

Poor cytogenetic risk factors though indicate early time to treatment, poor response to therapy, and aggressive disease course are not indicators for treatment initiation per se. Hypogammaglobulinemia or increased WBC counts alone are not enough to initiate treatment. Similarly, younger age, the mere availability of a bone marrow donor, or poor prognosis biomarkers such as IgVH unmutated status or high ZAP-70 expression are not per se criteria to initiate treatment.

13. Ans. d. del13q14 *Ref: Hoffbrand 7/e*

Poor cytogenetic risk factors in CLL are del17p and del11q. Both CD38 and ZAP-70 are surrogate markers for unmutated IgVH status and indicate poor prognosis. The deletions of 13q14 confer a good prognosis (even better than no abnormality), but only provided they are found as the only change.

14. Ans. b. Localized radiation therapy

While observation is advocated for patients with early stage CLL, localized radiation (IFRT) therapy is the treatment of choice for patients with localized (stage I) SLL. This is principally based upon retrospective analyses that have demonstrated prolonged freedom from relapse with localized radiation therapy alone and extrapolation of data from other indolent non-Hodgkin lymphoma subtypes.

15. Ans. d. All of the above

Ref: Gribben JG. How I treat CLL upfront. Blood. 2010

Patients with CLL with del(17p) or del(11q) are at high risk because their disease does not respond adequately to initial treatment, relapses soon after achieving remission, and requires treatment early because of early progression. Poor-risk features for CLL are largely also predictive of poor response to the conventional therapy. There is not enough evidence to alter therapy based upon molecular features, but the one exclusion from this is the patients who present with 17p deletions (resulting in loss of TP53 tumor suppressor gene). These patients have poor response to chemotherapy and poor survival. These patients should ideally be treated in clinical trials which are examining agents that have efficacy in patients without functional p53 (del17p) or with alemtuzumab-based therapy.

16. Ans. e. All of the above are true

Alemtuzumab (Campath) is a humanized monoclonal antibody that targets the cell-surface marker CD52. It is highly expressed on the surface of both healthy B and T lymphocytes and CLL cells. The National Comprehensive Cancer Network (NCCN) Drug and Biologics Compendium (2010) includes indications for alemtuzumab in CLL/small lymphocytic lymphoma as a first-line therapy for stage II–IV disease. Alemtuzumab is also indicated for patients with CLL with del (17p)—resulting in loss of p53 tumor suppressor gene, who have nonbulky adenopathy and partial response following allogeneic stem cell transplant. In cases where FISH analysis reveals the presence of del(17p), standard treatments which rely on the p53 pathway for activity are less effective. Treatment with chlorambucil, fludarabine, and rituximab has shown poor response rates in patients with this cytogenetic abnormality. Alemtuzumab acts via a p53 independent mechanism, (bypassing p53 pathway), and therefore has beneficial results in patients with del(17p).

Though single agent alemtuzumab results in overall response and CR rates of approximately 83% and 24%, respectively, a survival benefit has not been demonstrated. It is effective when maximum lymph nodes <5 cm in diameter. It can deplete bone marrow leukemic clone and achieve MRD negativity. Concern about infectious complications has contributed to the limited use of alemtuzumab. Opportunistic infectious complications are significant with patients developing herpes simplex virus (HSV) reactivation, pneumonia, oral candidiasis, and cytomegalovirus (CMV) reactivation.

17. Ans. d. All of the above

All of these have been used in CLL—mitoxantrone, pentostatin, lenalidomide, ibrutinib, and fludarabine.

18. Ans. d. None of the above

Ref: Österborg A. Management guidelines for the use of alemtuzumab in chronic lymphocytic leukemia. Leukemia, 2009.

Alemtuzumab is effective in CLL with chromosome 17p deletion because it bypasses p53 pathway of apoptosis. Chemotherapeutic agents like cyclophosphamide and fludarabine act through p53 pathway and initiate apoptosis. In chr17p deletion, these agents cannot act through p53 pathway as there is loss of p53 in del17p, and thus cell apoptosis which is p53 dependent, cannot take place. Alemtuzumab does not require p53 to mediate cell apoptosis and is thus effective even in del17p. p53 is a tumor suppressor gene located on the short arm of chromosome 17; it is inactivated by deletion and/or point mutation in many human malignancies. The wild-type *p53* gene protein helps trigger apoptosis and acts as a check point regulator of cells entering into S phase.

19. Ans. d. All of the above *Ref: Williams 8/e*

The diagnosis of PLL is considered when at least 55% of the circulating leukemic lymphocytes have a prolymphocytic morphology. Prolymphocytes are both morphologically and immunophenotypically distinct from typical CLL cells. Compared with typical CLL cells, these are large cells with somewhat immature-appearing nuclear chromatin, a prominent vesicular nucleolus, and a moderate amount of cytoplasm. Prognosis is poor compared to CLL. More than 50% of patients are older than 70 years at diagnosis. More than three-fourths of patients have blood lymphocyte counts greater than 100,000/μL. In contrast to CLL B cells, PLL cells generally express very high levels of surface Ig, usually IgM. They also react strongly with the antibody FMC7. In addition, PLL cells express high levels of CD22 and often are negative for CD23. Treatments for patients with PLL are similar to those for patients with CLL.

20. Ans. b. Rituximab maintenance is preferred for patients who achieve second remission.

Ref: Hoffman 6/e; Williams 8/e

Nearly, all patients with CLL ultimately develop refractory disease. Chemotherapy is the main treatment modality used for refractory CLL, either alone or in combination with hematopoietic cell transplantation (HCT). RIC transplant is preferred since most of the patients are elderly and morbidity is increased with myeloablative regimens.

Alemtuzumab (Campath-1H), an antibody directed against CD52, can be used for the treatment of previously untreated or relapsed/refractory CLL. While responses may be seen in approximately one-third of patients with disease that is refractory to fludarabine, the majority of these responses are partial remissions. Alemtuzumab, alone or in combination with methylprednisolone, is the only FDA-approved agent that reportedly has activity in cells lacking p53 function, as seen in patients with CLL with17p deletion.

The major indication for radiation therapy in CLL is the presence of large, bulky lymphoid masses causing compression symptoms, especially if the CLL has been unresponsive to chemotherapy. CLL lymphocytes are extremely radiation sensitive; treatment usually results in a rapid shrinkage of lymphoid masses.

Rituximab, which is highly effective in follicular lymphoma, has not been found to be that effective in CLL as single agent both in initial management or in refractory cases, though with combination it is useful. Maintenance rituximab has been approved in follicular lymphoma not in CLL.

21. Ans. e. All of the above

Ref: Gribben JG. How I treat CLL upfront. Blood. 2010; Williams 8/e

The National Cancer Institute Working Group (NCI/WG) and the International Workshop Group on CLL (IWCLL) have developed joint formal criteria for evaluating the response to treatment in CLL. CR in CLL is defined as absence of constitutional symptoms attributable to CLL [i.e. ≥10% unintentional weight loss within the previous 6 months, fatigue that interferes with work or usual activities, fever greater than 100.5°F (>38°C) for ≥2 weeks, or night sweats for >1 month]. No lymph nodes >1.5 cm in diameter on physical examination. No hepatomegaly or splenomegaly by physical examination. Absolute neutrophil count >1,500/μL and platelet count >100,000/μL. Untransfused hemoglobin concentration >11 g/dL and no clonal lymphocytes in the peripheral blood by immunophenotyping.

22. Ans. e. All of the above

Ref: Gribben JG. How I treat CLL up front. Blood. 2010;115(2):187-97.

Infections are the major complications of CLL and account for up to 50% of all deaths from CLL. The immune deficiency of CLL is due to factors such as hypogammaglobulinemia, impaired T-cell function, and impaired opsonization. The incidence of significant hypogammaglobulinemia increases with time and with repeated treatments. Patients who receive high dose intravenous immune globulin have a decrease in the incidence of major bacterial infections, such as pneumonia or septicemia, and should be treated with prophylactic IVIG. The usual dose is 200–400 mg/kg by IV infusion, given at 3–4 week intervals. The trough serum IgG in treated patients should usually be above 500 mg/dL.

23. Ans. e. All of the above

The anemia of CLL is multifactorial and includes gastrointestinal blood loss secondary to the use of corticosteroids, hypersplenism, and marrow suppression secondary to the use of alkylating agents or replacement by atypical lymphocytes, hemolytic anemia (AIHA) or red blood cell aplasia.

24. Ans. d. The reported incidence is about 10–15%

The incidence of AIHA in CLL is about 10%, which increases with the use of fludarabine. Complete treatment with FCR does not eliminate the risk of development of AIHA. Patients with a history of fludarabine associated-AIHA have a very high risk of recurrent AIHA if rechallenged with fludarabine, though some have reported successful rechallenge with fludarabine.

25. Ans. d. Overall survival (OS) was higher with fludarabine
> *Ref: Rai KR. Fludarabine compared with chlorambucil as primary therapy for chronic lymphocytic leukemia. NEJM. 2000;343(24):1750-7.*

In CALGB 9011 trial, CR rates were higher in the fludarabine containing arms, being 20, 4, and 20% for patients receiving F, C, or F + C, respectively ($p <0.001$ for comparison of F vs. C and for F + C vs. C). Overall remission rates (CR plus PR) for the three groups were 63, 37, and 61%, respectively ($p <0.001$ for the comparison of F vs. C and for F+C vs. C). Median duration of response for patients achieving CR or PR was longer in the fludarabine treatment arm (25 months) than in the chlorambucil arm (14 months, $p <0.001$). Similarly, the median time to disease progression was longer in the group receiving fludarabine (20 vs. 14 months, $p <0.001$). At a median follow-up of 62 months, OS was similar in the three treatment arms, being 66, 56, and 55 months, respectively.

26. Ans. c. CLL with del 17p13

Patients with del17p13 have a short PFS and OS when treated with standard chemoimmunotherapy regimens such as FCR and BR, and are therefore not recommended for these patients. These patients should be treated with ibrutinib.

27. Ans. d. All of the above
> *Ref: Parikh SA. Chronic lymphocytic leukemia treatment algorithm 2018. Blood Can J. 2018;8(10):93.*

The TP53 status has been found to be one of the most important prognostic and predictive biomarkers in CLL. This should be ascertained using—(1) CLL FISH panel to look for evidence of del17p13 and (2) Sanger sequencing or next-generation sequencing panel to evaluate for TP53 mutations, with a cutoff of at least 10%. It is important to obtain both these tests, since ~3–5% patients will harbor a deleterious TP53 mutation on DNA sequencing in the absence of del17p13 on CLL FISH. These patients have equally poor outcomes. Patients with TP53 disruption have a short PFS and OS when treated with standard chemoimmunotherapy regimens such as FCR and BR, and are therefore not recommended for these patients. The improved response rates and excellent outcomes make ibrutinib the treatment of choice in this group of patients. All other mutations can be treated with FCR or BR.

28. Ans. c. Thrombosis

The most common nonhematologic toxicities (≥ grade 3) reported in the ibrutinib arm of RESONATE trial included pneumonia (10%), diarrhea (5%), fatigue (4%), and arthralgia (2%). Other toxicities reported were hypertension (~15%), atrial fibrillation (~10%), and major bleeding (~7%).

29. Ans. e. All of the above

Single-agent venetoclax is approved for patients with relapsed/refractory CLL who have del17p by FISH. The combination of venetoclax and rituximab was recently approved by the FDA for all patients with relapsed/refractory CLL (regardless of the CLL FISH profile). The most common side effects of venetoclax are neutropenia (occurring in ~ 50% patients), tumor lysis syndrome (for which a gradual ramp-up dosing schema should be followed), and serious infections. Venetoclax (particularly in combination with rituximab) may achieve MRD negative CR sooner than those treated with ibrutinib as a single-agent.

30. Ans. e. All of the above
> *Ref: Parikh SA. Chronic lymphocytic leukemia treatment algorithm 2018. Blood Can J. 2018;8:93*

Richter's transformation typically occurs in the first year of ibrutinib therapy whereas CLL progression occurs in the second year of ibrutinib therapy. Venetoclax is usually preferred over idelalisib and rituximab in patients who progress on or have intolerance to ibrutinib. However, given the low CR rate with single-agent venetoclax, it will be necessary to use combination strategies with either an anti-CD20 monoclonal antibody therapy or other novel agents. The combination of idelalisib and rituximab is approved for the treatment of relapsed CLL. However, idelalisib is associated with ≥ grade 3 toxicity including colitis, transaminitis, and pneumonitis, in addition to infectious complications such as reactivation of cytomegalovirus and Pneumocystis jirovecii pneumonia, making it less attractive if other options are available. CAR-T cell therapy has also shown remarkable efficacy in the management of CLL patients who have disease progression on ibrutinib. Cytokine release syndrome and neurotoxicity are the major side effects of CAR-T cell therapy. Consolidation with RIC allogeneic stem cell transplantation (SCT) has shown to improve outcomes in CLL.

31. Ans. e. Only a and b

Richter's transformation is the development of an aggressive B-cell neoplasm in CLL patients. The most common histology is diffuse large B-cell lymphoma (BCL) followed by Hodgkin lymphoma.

32. Ans. b. Bruton's tyrosine kinase (BTK)
> *Ref: Akinleye A. Ibrutinib and novel BTK inhibitors in clinical development. J Hematol Oncol. 2013;6:59.*

The B cell receptor (BCR) pathway regulates multiple cellular processes (such as proliferation, differentiation, and apoptosis) that are essential for the functioning and survival of both normal and malignant B cells. In B cell malignancies, such as CLL, aberrant BCR signaling plays a critical role in the pathogenesis of disease. Ibrutinib is an orally administered, highly potent, selective, and irreversible small-molecule inhibitor of BTK. It forms a covalent bond with a cysteine residue (CYS-481) at the active site of BTK, leading to inhibition of BTK enzymatic activity. Ibrutinib also abrogates the full activation of BTK by inhibiting its autophosphorylation at Tyr-223. This inhibition prevents downstream activation of the BCR pathway and subsequently blocks cell growth, proliferation, and survival of malignant B cells.

33. Ans. d. None of the above

Venetoclax is a small molecule targeted against the anti-apoptotic BCL-2 protein, the overexpression of which is one of the molecular hallmarks of CLL. The drug is suitable for oral long-term administration and allows to achieve the high rate of overall response including CR with manageable toxicity profile, in both treatment-naïve and relapsed/refractory CLL patients. It allows the eradication of MRD in a number of patients, which is postulated to have an impact on the patients' OS. Venetoclax displays the activity in patients with del17p/TP53 mutation and in patients failing on ibrutinib or other BCR pathway inhibitors. Combination of venetoclax with other targeted drugs, in particular with anti-CD20 monoclonal antibodies or BCR pathway inhibitors, seems to be very promising in CLL treatment. Combined venetoclax and ibrutinib has synergistic effects and is an effective oral regimen for high-risk and older patients with CLL.

34. Ans. a. Watchful waiting with 3 monthly follow-up

Ref: Hallek M. IW-CLL guidelines for diagnosis, indications for treatment, response assessment, and supportive management of CLL. Blood. 2018;131(25):2745-60.

The vast majority of CLL patients have early-stage asymptomatic disease at diagnosis and do not require treatment. Patients carrying deletion 17p and/or deletion 11q experience a more aggressive clinical course than patients with deletion 13q, trisomy 12, or no abnormality on FISH. FISH at diagnosis does not guide treatment and in asymptomatic CLL patients with any cytogenetic risk factors, treatment should not be started.

35. Ans. d. None of the above

Ref: Brown JR. How I treat CLL patients with ibrutinib. Blood. 2018;131:379-86.

Inhibition of BTK by ibrutinib blocks BCR signaling which removes growth and activation signals and induce apoptosis. Unfortunately, ibrutinib does not cure CLL, and its efficacy is dependent upon chronic BTK inhibition. At present, ibrutinib is thought to require indefinite administration to ensure continued clinical benefit. With publication of long-term follow-up of the initial studies, it has become apparent that up to 51% of CLL patients have discontinued ibrutinib therapy. Similarly, a retrospective study of ibrutinib-treated patients in a "real world" setting reported a 41% discontinuation rate.

36. Ans. d. None of the above

Ref: Brown JR. How I treat CLL patients with ibrutinib. Blood. 2018;131:379-86.

With some drugs used in CLL like lenalidomide, the best way to safely start the drug is to slowly titrate it upwards. But, this is not the case with ibrutinib because starting at a dose that is lower than the recommended (420 mg, 3 tablets) could be sub-therapeutic and predispose the CLL cells to becoming resistant to this over time. Patient with CLL should be started at 420 mg (3 tablets) given once daily. If side effects are observed, it is acceptable to decrease the dose by one tablet for a period of time. However, in most patients this is not necessary. Ibrutinib, and other drugs (idelalisib) which target B-cell receptor signaling, typically causes lymphocytosis early in therapy. Typically this occurs over the first 1-2 months, reaches a plateau, and then diminishes slowly over time. In general, the rise in the lymphocytes is greatest in patients who start with relatively low counts, whereas those with high counts (>200,000/mcl) generally have modest rises. Side effects from the white blood cell count rising early during treatment are quite rare. A previous diagnosis of AF or other cardiac arrhythmia a not a contraindication to ibrutinib initiation, though the patient should be under regular cardiology follow-up.

37. Ans. e. None of the above

Ref: Stephens D. How I manage ibrutinib intolerance and complications in patients with chronic lymphocytic leukemia. Blood. 2019;133(12):1298-1307.

Ibrutinib impairs platelet aggregation and adhesion. A review of patients treated with ibrutinib in clinical trials and clinical practice revealed a risk of minor bleeding in up to 66% of patients and a risk of major bleeding in up to 6% of patients. The concurrent use of ibrutinib and anticoagulants is not recommended secondary to increased risk of bleeding. Patients should be counseled about the risk of bleeding upon initiation of ibrutinib. This includes instructions to hold ibrutinib for 3 days before and after minor surgical procedures and 7 days before and after major surgical procedures. Management of bleeding typically involves holding ibrutinib and providing platelet transfusions, regardless of platelet count, to overcome the platelet function defect induced by ibrutinib.

29 Chronic Myeloid Leukemia

1. In chronic myeloid leukemia, t(9;22) results from translocation of:
   a. Long-arm of chromosome 9 to short-arm of chromosome 22
   b. Long-arm of chromosome 9 to long-arm of chromosome 22
   c. Short-arm of chromosome 9 to short-arm of chromosome 22
   d. Short-arm of chromosome 9 to long-arm of chromosome 22

2. IRIS trial compared:
   a. Hydroxyurea with imatinib
   b. Cytarabine with imatinib
   c. Interferon with imatinib
   d. Interferon and cytarabine with imatinib

3. Accelerated phase in chronic myeloid leukemia is defined by the following, except:
   a. 5–9% blasts in the peripheral blood or bone marrow
   b. Basophils ≥20%
   c. Platelets <100,000/μL, unrelated to therapy
   d. Platelets >1,000,000/μL, unresponsive to therapy
   e. All of the above

4. Treatment of choice for chronic myeloid leukemia blast crises is:
   a. Imatinib 800 mg once daily
   b. Dasatinib 70 mg twice daily
   c. Cytarabine plus interferon
   d. Allogeneic stem cell transplantation

5. Complete hematologic response in chronic myeloid leukemia include all, except:
   a. White blood cell count <10,000/μL
   b. No immature granulocytes
   c. No basophils on differential
   d. Platelet count <450,000/μL
   e. Spleen not palpable

6. Treatment failure in chronic myeloid leukemia is defined by the inability to reach the following threshold levels after the initiation of therapy, except:
   a. Complete hematologic response by 3 months
   b. Ph chromosome more than 35% at 6 months
   c. BCR-ABL more than 1% at 12 months
   d. Ph chromosome more than 0 at 12 months
   e. All of the above

7. A patient with CML-CP, who achieved complete molecular response with imatinib 400 mg daily was found to have BCR-ABL transcript of 0.098%, the next step would be:
   a. Increase the dose of imatinib to 600 mg daily
   b. Change to dasatinib 100 mg daily
   c. Counsel for allogeneic stem cell transplant
   d. None of the above

8. Treatment of patient with T315I mutation is:
   a. Imatinib 800 mg once daily
   b. Nilotinib 400 mg twice daily
   c. Dasatinib 70 mg twice daily
   d. Allogeneic stem cell transplantation
   e. None of the above

9. The treatment of patient with chronic myeloid leukemia with Y253H mutation:
   a. Imatinib
   b. Nilotinib
   c. Dasatinib
   d. None of the above

10. True about chronic myeloid leukemia are all, except:
    a. Basophilia is universal
    b. Eosinophilia is seen in about 90% of cases
    c. Fusion protein p190 is most common though p210 is also seen in some cases
    d. All of the above

11. A patient presented with weakness and heaviness left side of abdomen for 2 months. Examination revealed splenomegaly of 15 cm below left costal margin. Hemogram revealed hemoglobin 8.5 g/dL, total leukocyte count of 350,000/μL with left shift and blasts and basophils 4% each, LAP score was low but cytogenetic analysis revealed normal chromosome pattern. The patient:
    a. Does not have CML
    b. Has atypical CML
    c. Has MDS/MPN overlap syndrome
    d. Leukemoid reaction
    e. Needs further evaluation

12. Most common additional cytogenetic abnormality seen in chronic myeloid leukemia patient who proceeds to blast crises is:
   a. Trisomy 8
   b. Trisomy 19
   c. Duplication of the Ph chromosome
   d. Isochromosome 17q

13. Following is true for juvenile myelomonocytic leukemia:
   a. Fatal disorder of infancy
   b. Monocytic cells are hyper-responsive to granulocyte macrophage colony stimulating factor
   c. Mutations occur in genes including *PTPN11, NRAS*
   d. Progression to acute leukemia is rare
   e. All of the above

14. True about atypical chronic myeloid leukemia are all, *except*:
   a. Ph negative by cytogenetics
   b. RT-PCR for BCR-ABL negative
   c. Is a myelodysplastic/myeloproliferative neoplasm
   d. Prognosis is good

15. The Sokal score for chronic myeloid leukemia include all, *except*:
   a. Spleen size
   b. Blasts percent
   c. Basophil percent
   d. Age
   e. Platelet count

16. True regarding risk assessment for allogeneic stem cell transplantation in chronic myeloid leukemia is:
   a. Prognosis is affected by the phase of CML
   b. Related to time to HCT from diagnosis
   c. Depends on the age of the patients
   d. All of the above

17. True regarding chronic myeloid leukemia blast crises are following:
   a. The preferred initial treatment is the use of tyrosine kinase inhibitor followed by an allogeneic HCT
   b. Transplantation in blast crisis has poor results
   c. Imatinib treatment prior to transplantation has not been associated with an increase in transplant associated morbidity or mortality
   d. All of the above are true

18. Imatinib inhibits:
   a. Tyrosine kinase
   b. c-kit
   c. Platelet-derived growth factor receptor
   d. All of the above

19. Pregnant patient with chronic myeloid leukemia should be treated with:
   a. Imatinib
   b. Nilotinib
   c. Dasatinib
   d. Interferon

20. Criteria for chronic myeloid leukemia blast crises are all, *except*:
   a. Blasts ≥20% of peripheral smear
   b. Extramedullary blast proliferation
   c. Large foci or clusters of blasts in the bone marrow biopsy
   d. Additional cytogenetic abnormalities
   e. All of the above

21. Not correct for polycythemia vera:
   a. Splenomegaly may be presenting sign
   b. JAK-2 V617F is seen in >90% of patients
   c. Aquagenic pruritus is a distinguishing feature
   d. Erythropoietin levels are raised

22. Tear drop cells are seen in:
   a. Chronic myeloid leukemia
   b. Myelofibrosis
   c. Polycythemia
   d. Essential thrombocytosis

23. Nonmalignant cause of myelofibrosis are all, *except*:
   a. HIV infection
   b. Tuberculosis
   c. Hypoparathyroidism
   d. Essential thrombocytosis

24. Massive splenomegaly is not seen in:
   a. Myelofibrosis
   b. Polycythemia vera
   c. Essential thrombocytosis
   d. Chronic myeloid leukemia

25. All are causes of reactive thrombocytosis, *except*:
   a. Iron-deficiency anemia
   b. Surgery
   c. Essential thrombocytosis
   d. Hemorrhage
   e. All of the above

26. True about chronic neutrophilic leukemia is:
   a. Cytogenetic abnormalities are seen in about 90% cases
   b. WBC count should be more than 15,000/μL
   c. May be associated with multiple myeloma
   d. Granulocytes show significant dysplasia
   e. BCR-ABL may be positive

27. Hasford system is related with:
   a. Hodgkins disease
   b. Non-Hodgkin lymphoma
   c. Chronic myeloid leukemia
   d. Cutaneous lymphoma

28. Donor lymphocyte infusion is most commonly used for:
   a. Acute myeloid leukemia
   b. Acute lymphoblastic leukemia

c. Non-Hodgkin lymphoma
d. Chronic myeloid leukemia

29. Following are common side effects of imatinib, *except*:
a. Skin rashes
b. Leg edema
c. Diarrhea
d. Renal dysfunction

30. In chronic myeloid leukemia, BCR-ABL transcript seen commonly is:
a. p230
b. p190
c. p210
d. p240

31. In chronic myeloid leukemia, Philadelphia chromosome is present in:
a. Myeloid cell
b. B lymphocytes
c. T lymphocytes
d. All of the above

32. True regarding findings in chronic myeloid leukemia are all, *except*:
a. Leukocyte alkaline phosphatase is reduced
b. Serum potassium is raised
c. Vitamin B_{12} levels are raised
d. All of the above

33. Imatinib acts by:
a. Phosphorylation
b. Dephosphorylation
c. Demethylation
d. Methylation

34. All are the side effects of imatinib therapy, *except*:
a. Edema
b. Hair loss
c. Rashes
d. Bone pains

35. True regarding hydroxycarbamide in chronic myeloid leukemia are all, *except*:
a. Its pharmacological action is rapid and readily reversible
b. The leukocyte count starts to fall within days and the spleen reduces in size
c. Reduction in Ph-positive cells occurs after prolonged treatment
d. All of the above

36. BCR-ABL1 (IS) 0.1% refers to:
a. 0.1-log reduction
b. 1-log reduction
c. 2-log reduction
d. 3-log reduction

37. The mechanism of dasatinib-induced pleural effusion is:
a. Inflammatory
b. Cardiac
c. Fluid retention
d. Drug-induced pulmonary hypertension
e. All of the above

38. True regarding dasatinib-induced pleural effusion are all, *except*:
a. About 2–5% patients develop pleural effusion
b. Pleural effusions are usually exudative
c. Can develop years after treatment initiation, and can recur even at lower dosages
d. The role of diuretics and steroids in the management of dasatinib-related pleural effusions is unclear
e. All of the above

39. Which investigation in CML patient is usually not required at baseline?
a. Cytogenetics
b. FISH
c. Qualitative RT-PCR for BCR-ABL
d. Quantitative RT-PCR for BCR-ABL
e. All can be done

40. Treatment-free remission can be considered in all, *except*:
a. Optimal response to first-line therapy
b. Duration of TKI therapy >5 years
c. Complete cytogenetic response for >5 years
d. Duration of deep molecular response >2 years
e. Can be considered with any TKI

41. True regarding ponatinib is:
a. It is indicated in the presence of the T315I mutation
b. Can be used if there is resistance to other TKIs without the T315I mutation
c. Is useful in Ph +ve ALL
d. Can cause arterial occlusive disease
e. All of the above

42. True regarding CML blast crises is:
a. BCR-ABL is the driving force of progression
b. Clonal evolution indicates progression
c. Blast crises patients who achieve a second chronic phase have the best prognosis
d. Blast crises can be prevented by elimination or reduction of BCR-ABL
e. All of the above

43. The following features are true about chronic myeloid leukemia, *except*:
a. Philadelphia chromosome is shortened chromosome 22 containing BCR-ABL1 fusion gene
b. Rare cases with the p190 BCR-ABL1 isoform can mimic chronic myelomonocytic leukemia morphologically
c. Micro-megakaryocytes are frequently seen in the CML-CP cases
d. Presence of marrow fibrosis in TKI era doesn't substantially affect prognosis of the patient.

44. Deep molecular response means:
a. BCR-ABL1 levels ≤1%
b. BCR-ABL1 levels ≤0.1%
c. BCR-ABL1 levels ≤0.01%
d. Complete cytogenetic response

45. Gatekeeper residue of BCR-ABL is:
a. Threonine 315
b. Tyrosine 315
c. Isoleucine 315
d. Tryptophan 315

ANSWERS WITH EXPLANATIONS

1. Ans. b. Long-arm of chromosome 9 to long-arm of chromosome 22
Ref: Hoffbrand's 6/e p486

Chronic myeloid leukemia (CML) is associated with the Philadelphia chromosome t(9;22)(q34;q11) resulting in a *BCR-ABL* fusion gene. This genetic abnormality results in the formation of a unique gene product (*BCR-ABL*), which is a constitutively active tyrosine kinase. CML is associated with the fusion of two genes: *BCR* (on long-arm of chromosome 22) and *ABL1* (on long-arm of chromosome 9) resulting in the *BCR-ABL1* fusion gene. This abnormal fusion typically results from a reciprocal translocation between chromosomes 9 and 22, t(9;22)(q34;q11), that gives rise to an abnormal chromosome 22 called the Philadelphia (Ph) chromosome. The translocation involves long-arm of chromosome 9 to long-arm of chromosome 22.

2. Ans. d. Interferon and cytarabine with imatinib
Ref: SG O'Brien. N Engl J Med. 2003

International Randomized study of Interferon and STI571 (IRIS) trial compared interferon and cytarabine, which was the standard chemotherapeutic regime for CML at that time with imatinib. The IRIS trial was a phase III randomized, open-label, multicenter, crossover trial of imatinib (400 mg/day by mouth) versus interferon (5 million units/m² per day) plus cytarabine (20 mg/m² per day for 10 days/month) in 1,106 patients with newly diagnosed chronic phase CML. Patients receiving imatinib as initial therapy for chronic phase CML had overall and event-free survivals of 89% and 83%, respectively. In terms of hematologic and cytogenetic responses, tolerability, and the likelihood of progression to accelerated-phase or blast-crisis CML, imatinib was superior to interferon alpha plus low-dose cytarabine as first-line therapy in newly diagnosed chronic-phase CML.

3. Ans. a. 5–9% blasts in the peripheral blood or bone marrow
Ref: WHO Classification of Tumours of Haematopoietic and Lymphoid Tissues. Lyon, France: IARC; 2017, NCCN guidelines for CML.

The WHO 2017 defines accelerated phase as patients with CML who show one or more of the following features: (1) 10–19% blasts in the peripheral blood or bone marrow, (2) Peripheral blood basophils ≥20%, (3) Platelets <100,000/μL, unrelated to therapy, (4) Platelets >1,000,000/μL, unresponsive to therapy, (5) Progressive splenomegaly and increasing white cell count, unresponsive to therapy, (6) Cytogenetic evolution (defined as the development of chromosomal abnormalities in addition to the Philadelphia chromosome). Though 5% blasts are considered as CML-CP, AP is defined as blasts equal to or more than 10% blasts (but less than 20%), so 5–9% blasts are probably in CML-CP. Sokal criteria identifies ≥5% blasts in peripheral smear as accelerated phase (*Ref: NCCN guidelines for CML*).

4. Ans. d. Allogeneic stem cell transplantation
Ref: Hoffbrand 7/e

There appears to be a significant relapse rate in patients in blast crisis or accelerated phase even after successful treatment with imatinib, dasatinib or nilotinib, and these patients are suitable candidate for allogeneic transplantation. The patient should be brought into second chronic phase and transplanted as remissions are short lived.

5. Ans. c. No basophils on differential
Ref: European Leukemia Network (LeukemiaNet). 2016

Complete hematologic response in CML is defined as—white blood cell count <10,000/μL with no immature granulocytes and <5% basophils on differential (not complete absence of basophils); platelet count <450,000/μL; and spleen not palpable.

6. Ans. e. All of the above
Ref: Baccarani M. European Leukemia Net recommendations for the management of chronic myeloid leukemia. Blood. 2013.

The ELN 2013 guidelines define optimal response as BCR-ABL less than 10% at 3 months, less than 1% at 6 months, and less than 0.1% at 12 months. It defines non-CHR at 3 months and BCR-ABL >10% at 6 months as failure to TKI. The optimal response with regards to Ph chromosome is less than 35% at 3 months and 0 at 6 months.

7. Ans. d. None of the above
Ref: Soverini S. Recommendations from an expert panel of ELN. Blood. 2011.

If after achieving a major molecular response, the single reading of BCR-ABL transcript is found to be more, then the test should be repeated and patient be continued on 400 mg imatinib. Transient or single changes in molecular findings alone should not be considered to change the therapy in individual patients. Changes in a single PCR result should not prompt changes in treatment because of variability in the reproducibility of the assay. A rising titer over a period of time should alert the hematologist to look for the reasons including compliance, mutational analysis, and disease progression.

8. Ans. d. Allogeneic stem cell transplantation
Ref: Hiwase DK. Expert Rev Hematol. 2011;4(3):285-99.

The T315I mutation occurs in about 15% of imatinib-resistant patients with ABL kinase domain mutation and may be more frequently detected in patients with advanced CML and Ph+ve ALL. Ponatinib is a potent pan-BCR–ABL inhibitor with activity against all tested imatinib-resistant mutants, including T315I. Homoharringtonine is also effective in T315I mutations. The T315I mutation has shown resistance to all other currently available TKIs and such patients are candidate for allogeneic stem cell transplantation.

9. Ans. c. Dasatinib

Ref: Branford S. Selecting optimal second-line tyrosine kinase inhibitor therapy for chronic myeloid leukemia patients after imatinib failure. Blood. 2009

The Y253H mutation is resistant to imatinib and nilotinib but sensitive to dasatinib. The current clinical data suggests that clinically relevant mutations are T315I for both inhibitors: F317L/I/C/V, V299L, and T315A for dasatinib and Y253H, E255K/V, and F359V/C for nilotinib.

10. Ans. c. Fusion protein p190 is most common though p210 is also seen in some cases

Absolute basophilia is the most common finding in the CML patients, and absolute eosinophilia is seen in about 90% of cases. Absolute monocytosis (>1,000/µL) is also common, although the percentage of monocytes is typically low (<3%). Occasional patients with CML can have an alternate breakpoint in chromosome 22, producing a p190 BCR-ABL1 fusion protein rather than the classic p210 BCR-ABL1 fusion protein seen in the majority of CML patients.

11. Ans. e. Needs further evaluation

The majority of CML patients (>95%) demonstrate the t(9;22)(q32;q11.2) reciprocal translocation that results in the classic Ph chromosome. Minority of patients can have variant translocations such as complex translocations involving other chromosome [e.g., t(9;14;22)]. The rest of the patients can have cryptic translocations of 9q34 and 22q11.2 that cannot be detected by routine cytogenetics. These are referred to as "Ph-negative" cases and require fluorescence in situ hybridization (FISH) analysis to identify the BCR-ABL1 fusion gene, or reverse transcription-polymerase chain reaction (RT-PCR) to identify the BCR-ABL1 fusion mRNA. So, this patient needs FISH or RT-PCR to confirm the diagnosis.

12. Ans. a. Trisomy 8 *Ref: Hoffbrand 6/e p486*

Though all of these abnormalities can be seen in accelerated phase and blast crises of CML including trisomy 8, trisomy 19, duplication of the Ph chromosome, and isochromosome 17q, the most common is trisomy 8.

13. Ans. e. All of the above *Ref: Williams 7/e Chap 88*

Juvenile myelomonocytic leukemia (JMML) is a rare disorder of infancy and early childhood characterized by lymphadenopathy, hepatosplenomegaly, fever, and skin rash and is highly fatal. Excess of monocytic lineage cells that are produced are hyper-responsive to granulocyte macrophage colony stimulating factor (GM-CSF). Infiltration of organs by monocytic cells leads to end organ damage. In contrast to CML, the karyotype in JMML is mostly normal, though sometimes monosomy 7 can be seen, and progression to acute leukemia is rare. Many patients with JMML have mutations in genes that encode elements of the GM-CSF signal transduction pathway, including *PTPN11*, *NRAS* and *KRAS2*, *CBL*, and *NF1*. Treatment of choice is bone marrow transplantation.

14. Ans. d. Prognosis is good

Ref: WHO Classification of Tumours of Haematopoietic and Lymphoid Tissues. Lyon, France: IARC; 2008 p80.

Atypical CML or BCR rearrangement-negative CML is a myelodysplastic/myeloproliferative neoplasm that is characterized by features of both dysplasia and myeloid proliferation. Patients are elderly and present with high neutrophil counts but with thrombocytopenia and/or anemia. It is BCR-ABL1-negative and Ph-negative. The major feature that characterizes atypical CML is dysgranulopoiesis, which is not a feature of Ph+ve CML. The prognosis is poor and transformation to AML can occur in 15–40% cases, the remainder die of marrow failure. It does not respond to imatinib.

15. Ans. c. Basophil percent

Ref: Sokal JE et al. Blood. 1984;63:789-99.

Sokal score is useful for predicting the survival of CML patients. The Sokal score for CML includes four clinical variables: Spleen size, percent blasts, age, and platelet count. Hasford score includes eosinophilia and basophilia. The Sokal score derives from a multivariate analysis of survival of 813 patients diagnosed with chronic phase CML between 1962 and 1981. Most patients were treated with single-agent chemotherapy, typically busulfan. Spleen size and percentage blasts were most strongly associated with survival. The EUTOS score is calculated as [7 × basophil (%)] + [4 × spleen (cm)]. Two risk groups are identified: Low-risk (EUTOS score <87, 79% of patients) and high-risk (EUTOS score ≥87, 21% of patients). The Hasford score includes basophils not the Sokal score. The EUTOS score (devised from imatinib-based regimens) has superior prognostic power when compared with the Sokal score.

16. Ans. d. All of the above

Ref: Gratwohl A. Chronic Leukemia Working Party of the European Group for Blood and Marrow Transplantation. Lancet. 1998;352(9134):1087-92.

The EBMT risk assessment score for allogeneic transplantation in CML include 5 parameters. These are: (1) type of donor (HLA identical/unrelated), (2) stage of disease (CP/AP/BC), (3) age of the recipient (less than 20 years, 20–40 years or more than 40 years), (4) time to HCT from diagnosis (less than or more than

12 months), and (5) sex matching. Scoring is from zero to a maximum of seven, with points scored for each of the five risk categories and 5 year survival probability is then calculated.

17. Ans. d. All of the above are true

Ref: Hehlmann R. How I treat CML blast crises. Blood. 2012.

Chronic myeloid blast crisis is refractory to chemotherapy, the preferred initial treatment is the use of tyrosine kinase inhibitors followed by an allogeneic HCT for eligible patients. Transplantation while the patient remains in blast crisis has poor results with less than 10% long-term survival. A reasonable approach is an attempt to convert the patient to an earlier phase of disease, with suitable patients subsequently undergoing allogeneic HCT. Imatinib treatment prior to transplantation has not been associated with an increase in transplant associated morbidity or mortality. Blast crises usually results from continued BCR-ABL activity leading to further genetic instability, DNA damage, and impaired DNA repair. Around 80% patients with blast crises develop additional multiple mutations. Treatment with tyrosine kinase inhibitors has improved survival in blast crises slightly, but most long-term survivors are those who have been transplanted.

18. Ans. d. All of the above   *Ref: Williams 7/e Chap 88*

Imatinib inhibits tyrosine kinases, c-kit, and platelet-derived growth factor receptor and can be used in treating malignancies in which these are overexpressed. The various disease in which imatinib has been used are chronic myeloid leukemia, gastrointestinal stromal tumors, dermatofibrosarcoma protuberans, Philadelphia chromosome positive ALL, hypereosinophilic syndromes, systemic mastocytosis, desmoid tumors, malignant melanoma, AIDS-related Kaposi sarcoma, chordomas, relapsed epithelial ovarian cancer, and steroid-refractory chronic graft-versus-host disease.

19. Ans. d. Interferon   *Ref: Williams 7/e Chap 88*

Treatment of chronic-phase CML during pregnancy is sometimes needed to prevent placental insufficiency from hyperleukocytosis. Imatinib use is not recommended during pregnancy. In preclinical studies, imatinib was found to be teratogenic in rats and impaired spermatogenesis was noted in rats, dogs, and monkeys. Continuation of imatinib may result in damage to the developing fetus. Interferon can be given safely during pregnancy. Treatment with interferon has been shown to offer a survival advantage compared to treatment with hydroxyurea or busulfan alone. A complete cytogenetic response with interferon is uncommon (13%), but 10-year survival rates are approximately 70% in low Sokal score patients. The dose of interferon is 3 million units/m^2 five times per week. The common toxicities are fatigue, low-grade fever, weight loss, liver function test abnormalities, hematologic changes, and neuropsychiatric symptoms.

20. Ans. d. Additional cytogenetic abnormalities

Ref: WHO Classification of Tumours of Haematopoietic and Lymphoid Tissues. Lyon, France: IARC; 2017 Revised edition.

WHO Criteria for CML blast crises include: (1) Blasts ≥20% of peripheral smear or bone marrow nucleated cells, (2) extramedullary blast proliferation, (3) large foci or clusters of blasts in the bone marrow biopsy. Additional cytogenetic abnormalities are seen in disease progression but are not criteria for diagnosis of blast crises.

21. Ans. d. Erythropoietin levels are raised

Ref: Williams 7/e; Hoffman 7/e

Erythropoietin (EPO) levels are normal or reduced in PV. EPO levels are raised in secondary erythrocytosis. Hypoxia causes increased EPO production which stimulates erythrocytes production. Secondary erythrocytosis generally develops from excessive production of EPO. Many conditions can physiologically increase the production of EPO. EPO overproduction occurs in hypoxia (e.g., pulmonary disease, high altitude, smoking due to carboxyhemoglobin, cyanotic cardiac disease, and methemoglobinemia), tumors (e.g., kidney, brain, hepatoma, uterine fibroid, and pheochromocytoma), renal artery stenosis, and renal cysts. Other causes include androgen therapy, congenital erythrocytosis, EPO receptor hypersensitivity, autotransfusion (blood doping), and self-injection of EPO. Serum EPO levels should be low to normal in patients with PV but high in patients with secondary polycythemia.

22. Ans. b. Myelofibrosis   *Ref: WHO 2017 Revised edition.*

Tear drop cells (dacrocytes) are characteristically seen in myelofibrosis. Idiopathic myelofibrosis is a chronic myeloproliferative neoplasm characterized by a stepwise evolution from an initial prefibrotic stage revealing a hypercellular bone marrow with absent or minimal reticulin fibrosis to an overt fibrotic stage with marked reticulin or collagen fibrosis that is often accompanied by osteosclerosis.

23. Ans. d. Essential thrombocytosis

Ref: Williams 7/e Chap 89

Disorders associated with secondary myelofibrosis include lymphoma, multiple myeloma, metastatic carcinoma, renal osteodystrophy, gray platelet syndrome, systemic lupus erythematosus, polyarteritis nodosa, hypereosinophilic syndrome, tuberculosis, leishmaniasis, HIV, vitamin D deficiency rickets, Langerhans cell histiocytosis, acute promyelocytic leukemia, Gaucher's disease, chemotherapy, and radiotherapy. Correction of the primary disorder can lead to disappearance of the marrow fibrosis. Some patients with idiopathic myelofibrosis may have platelet counts greater than 600,000/μL, mimicking primary thrombocythemia. The anisopoikilocytosis, nucleated red cells, and shift to left in the blood film is characteristic of myelofibrosis and is not present in patients with essential thrombocythemia. Marrow fibrosis usually is insignificant in essential thrombocythemia, and splenic enlargement often is absent or slight.

24. Ans. c. Essential thrombocytosis

Splenic enlargement is absent or minimal in ET. CML and MF can have massive splenomegaly. Spleen size increases when ET progresses to myelofibrosis.

25. Ans. c. Essential thrombocytosis
Ref: Tefferi A. How I work up the patient with thrombocytosis. ASCO Post. 2012.

In ET thrombocytosis is clonal not reactive. Thrombocytosis is defined as a platelet count greater than 450×10^9/L. In routine clinical practice, thrombocytosis is much more likely to be secondary or reactive (>80% of cases) than primary. Reactive thrombocytosis is usually associated with infections, inflammation, trauma, hemolysis, metastatic cancer, the postsplenectomy state, or iron-deficiency anemia. Causes of primary thrombocytosis include myeloproliferative neoplasms, myelodysplastic syndromes, myelodysplastic syndrome/myeloproliferative neoplasm overlap syndromes, and other myeloid malignancies.

26. Ans. c. May be associated with multiple myeloma
Ref: WHO Classification of Tumours of Haematopoietic and Lymphoid Tissues. Lyon, France: IARC; 2017 Revised edition.

Chronic neutrophilic leukemia (CNL) is characterized by sustained peripheral blood neutrophilia (>25 × 10^9/L) and hepatosplenomegaly. The bone marrow is hypercellular. No significant dysplasia is seen in any of the cell lineages, and bone marrow fibrosis is uncommon. There is no Philadelphia chromosome or BCR/ABL fusion gene. If BCR/ABL fusion gene is present then it is CML, not CNL. In up to 20% of cases, the neutrophilia is associated with a neoplastic disorder, usually multiple myeloma, so serum protein electrophoresis is an important workup in CNL. Cytogenetic studies are normal in about 90% of cases of CNL. *CSF3R* T618I is a highly specific molecular marker for CNL that is sensitive to inhibition in vitro and in vivo by currently approved protein kinase inhibitors. t(15;19) has been reported.

27. Ans. c. Chronic myeloid leukemia *Ref: See Q. No. 15*

Hasford, Sokal, and EUTOS scoring system are used for risk stratification in CML.

28. Ans. d. Chronic myeloid leukemia *Ref: Williams 8/e*

Donor lymphocyte infusion (DLI) is most effective in CML. DLI has been extremely effective and provides direct evidence for a GVL effect. Molecular remissions attained after DLI appear to be quite durable. The goal of donor lymphocyte infusion is to induce a remission in the CML by a process called the graft-versus-tumor (GVT) effect. Salvage therapy with DLI can restore remission in many patients with CML who have a relapse after allogeneic stem cell transplantation. The overall response rate to DLI is approximately 75%. The main toxicities of DLI are the development of GVHD and myelosuppression.

29. Ans. d. Renal dysfunction *Ref: Williams 7/e Chap 88*

The main side effects of imatinib are superficial edema, nausea, muscle cramps, rash, fatigue, diarrhea, elevated transaminases, and myelosuppression. Imatinib and its metabolites are not excreted via kidney and no dose modification is required in renal dysfunction.

30. Ans. c. p210 *Ref: Williams 7/e; Hoffman 5/e*

Three main breakpoint cluster regions are present on chromosome 22: (1) major (M-*bcr*), (2) minor (m-*bcr*), and (3) micro (μ-*bcr*). They encode a p210, p190, and p230 fusion protein, respectively. The majority of CML patients have a *BCR-ABL* fusion gene that encodes a fusion protein of 210 kDa. Ph positive ALL results in the production of a *BCR-ABL* protein of 190 kDa. The p230 encoded by μ-*bcr* is rarely expressed but has been associated with neutrophilic CML or thrombocytosis. The tyrosine kinase activity of the p210 has been linked to the development of Ph-chromosome positive leukemia.

31. Ans. d. All of the above

In CML patients, the Ph chromosome is present in all myeloid cell lineages, in some B cells and in a very small proportion of T cells. It is found in no other cells of the body. BCR-ABL fusion genes can also be found in the leukocytes of some normal individuals using a two-step reverse transcriptase polymerase chain reaction assay.

32. Ans. d. All of the above
Ref: Hoffbrand's 7/e; Williams 7/e

In CML patients serum potassium may be spuriously raised due to leakage of intracellular potassium from platelets and leukocytes after the blood is drawn. In such cases, the potassium level in freshly drawn citrated blood is usually normal, as is the electrocardiogram. The serum levels of vitamin B_{12} and B_{12}-binding capacity are greatly increased due to raised levels of transcobalamin I. The alkaline phosphatase content of the neutrophil cytoplasm is diminished or absent and LAP score may be as low as zero. The percentages of eosinophils and basophils are usually increased, and the absence of basophilia makes the diagnosis of CML doubtful.

33. Ans. b. Dephosphorylation

Ref: WHO Classification of Tumours of Haematopoietic and Lymphoid Tissues. Lyon, France: IARC; 2017 Revised edition.

Imatinib mesylate, a 2-phenylaminopyrimidine compound, is an ABL1 tyrosine kinase inhibitor. It binds to and occupies the ATP-binding pocket of the ABL1 kinase component of the BCR-ABL1 protein, thereby blocking the capacity of the enzyme to phosphorylate downstream effector molecules, thereby blocking the manifestations of CML. So imatinib acts as a synthetic ATP mimic which fits in the pocket for ATP in the BCR-ABL molecule thereby displacing it and preventing the ATP-mediated phosphorylation. The drug rapidly reverses the clinical and hematological abnormalities and induces major cytogenetic responses in over 80% of previously untreated CML chronic-phase patients.

34. Ans. b. Hair loss

Ref: Caldemeyer L. Long-term side effects of tyrosine kinase inhibitors in chronic myeloid leukemia. Curr Hematol Malig Rep. 2016

Side-effects of imatinib include nausea, headache, rashes, infraorbital edema, bone pains and, sometimes, more generalized fluid retention. Patients with black skin may sustain areas of depigmentation. Hepatotoxicity characterized by raised serum transaminases is occasionally seen and may necessitate stopping the drug. A significant minority of patients experience neutropenia and/or thrombocytopenia within the first few months of starting treatment with imatinib at standard dosage.

TKI can induce thyroid dysfunction leading to hypothyroidism.

35. Ans. c. Reduction in Ph-positive cells occurs after prolonged treatment

Hydroxycarbamide (also known as hydroxyurea) is a ribonucleotide-reductase inhibitor that targets relatively mature myeloid progenitors in proliferative cycle. Its pharmacological action is rapid and readily reversible. Treatment for patients in chronic phase usually starts with 1.0–2.0 g daily orally and continued indefinitely. The leukocyte count starts decreasing within days and the spleen reduces in size. It is usually possible to reverse all features of CML within 4–8 weeks of starting treatment with hydroxycarbamide. It rarely causes any degree of reduction in Ph-positive cells in the bone marrow, so cytogenetic responses are unlikely with the hydroxyurea, in contrast to imatinib.

36. Ans. d. 3-log reduction

Ref: Hughes T. Monitoring CML patients responding to treatment with tyrosine kinase inhibitors. Blood. 2006;108(1):28-37.

Complete cytogenetic response (CCyR) is considered equal to 1% BCR-ABL1 by reverse transcription quantitative polymerase chain reaction (RT-qPCR) [International Scale (IS)]. On the IS, patient results are expressed relative to the standardized baseline of 100% [for example, 0.1% BCR-ABL1 (IS) is a 3-log reduction equating to a major molecular response (MMR)].

Log reduction	Percentage	Times lesser
1-log reduction	90%	10 times lesser
2-log reduction	99%	100 times lesser
3-log reduction	99.9%	1,000 times lesser
4-log reduction	99.99%	10,000 times lesser
5-log reduction	99.999%	100,000 times lesser
6-log reduction	99.9999%	1,000,000 times lesser

1-log reduction corresponds to a reduction of 90% from the original concentration, and a 2-log reduction corresponds to a reduction of 99% from the original concentration.

So, a log reduction of 3 is a 99.9% reduction compared with a log reduction of 6 which is equivalent to a 99.9999% reduction.

37. Ans. a. Inflammatory

Ref: Gambacorti-Passerini C, Piazza R. How I treat newly diagnosed chronic myeloid leukemia in 2015. Am J Hematol. 2015;90:156-61.

Dasatinib-induced pleural effusion is supposed to be immune-mediated, based on reports of high lymphocyte counts, often of a natural killer cell phenotype, in pleural fluid and tissue. Dasatinib targets the SRC family of tyrosine kinase, which are involved in signal transduction in lymphoid cells, and results in natural killer cells expansion; this causes a dysregulation in the immune function by causing a "proinflammatory" phenotype in which specific responses are suppressed in favor of nonspecific ones, causing lymphocytosis and several inflammatory side effects such as serositis and panniculitis.

38. Ans. a. About 2–5% patients develop pleural effusion

Ref: Quintas-Cardama A. Pleural effusion in patients with chronic CML treated with dasatinib after imatinib failure. Clin Oncol. 2007;25:3908-14.

Pleural effusion is an adverse event that has been reported more commonly with dasatinib than with other TKIs. About 25% of CML patients on dasatinib can develop pleural effusion. Dasatinib-associated pleural effusions are usually exudative and show lymphocytosis. Common symptoms of pleural effusion include dyspnea, dry persistent cough, and chest tightness. It can develop years after treatment initiation, and can recur even at lower dosages. The role of diuretics and steroids in the management of dasatinib-related pleural effusions, although commonly used for this purpose is unclear, but have shown some benefits in mild-to-moderate effusions. For medium or large pleural effusions, dasatinib therapy should be temporarily stopped until the adverse event is resolved, and then resumed at lower doses. The occurrence of pleural effusion is significantly reduced with dasatinib, 100 mg once daily compared with 70 mg twice daily. A thorough medical history and physical examination remain crucial to investigate nondrug-related causes of the symptoms suggestive of pleural effusion (e.g., infections and cardiovascular conditions). In particular, when a patient has dyspnea without effusion or dyspnea out of proportion to effusion, the clinician should suspect pulmonary arterial hypertension. It may be useful to perform an echocardiogram on patients who develop pleural effusion. This can not only identify other conditions that may predispose to pleural effusion, but may also help identify pulmonary hypertension, a complication that has been reported in some patients treated with dasatinib.

39. Ans. d. Quantitative RT-PCR for BCR-ABL
Ref: Hochhaus A. ESMO Clinical Practice Guidelines for CML. Ann Oncol. 2017.

According to ESMO guidelines, CML diagnosis is confirmed by cytogenetics showing t(9;22)(q34;q11) and by multiplex RT-PCR showing BCR-ABL1 transcripts. In rare cases, BCR-ABL1 juxtaposition can be determined by interphase FISH (iFISH) of blood cells, using dual color dual fusion probes that allow the detection of BCR-ABL1 nuclei. Cytogenetic assessment is required because it is necessary to detect additional chromosome abnormalities. Qualitative multiplex RT-PCR is carried out on blood or marrow RNA. It identifies the transcript type, either typical e14a2 or e13a2 (also known as b3a2 and b2a2) or atypical variants. Determination of the transcript type is crucial for later monitoring, in particular for the accurate assessment of molecular response. Quantitative RT-PCR (qRT-PCR) measuring BCR-ABL1 transcripts level as BCR-ABL1 % on the IS and BCR-ABL1 mutation analysis are not required at baseline.

40. Ans. c. Complete cytogenetic response for >5 years
Ref: Hochhaus A. ESMO Clinical Practice Guidelines for CML. Ann Oncol. 2017.

Treatment discontinuation may be considered in individual CML patients on TKI, if proper, high-quality and certified monitoring can be ensured. Prerequisites for safe stopping are institutional requirements for safe supervision, identification of typical BCR-ABL1 transcripts at diagnosis which can be quantified over a 4.5 log dynamic range, at least 5 years of TKI therapy, achievement of 4.5 MR (4.5-log reduction, ≤0.0032% BCR-ABL1 IS) and a stability of deep molecular response (at least 4 or 4.5 MR) for at least 2 years. The likelihood of treatment-free remission after discontinuation would be similar irrespective of TKI in patients who have experienced and maintained deep molecular response. Approximately 40–60% of patients who discontinue TKI therapy after achieving deep molecular response experience recurrence within 6 months of treatment cessation.

41. Ans. e. All of the above
Ref: Müller MC. Ponatinib in chronic myeloid leukemia. Crit Rev Oncol Hematol. 2017;52-9.

Ponatinib is 500 times more potent than imatinib at inhibiting BCR-ABL1. Ponatinib has demonstrated marked antileukemic efficacy in heavily pretreated patients with CML and Philadelphia chromosome-positive (Ph+) acute lymphoblastic leukemia (ALL) and has been approved for treatment of these diseases. Ponatinib has also shown efficacy in patients with CP-CML who are resistant to dasatinib or nilotinib, without having the T315I mutation. Ponatinib should also be considered in patients with advanced CML (both AP-CML and BC-CML) as a second- or third-line treatment after dasatinib or nilotinib failure, regardless of the presence of the T315I mutation.

The potential risks of dasatinib include arterial hypertension, which can be sometimes severe, and serious arterial occlusive and venous thromboembolic events. It can also cause heart failure and hepatotoxicity.

42. Ans. e. All of the above
Ref: Hehlmann R. Management of CML-blast crisis. Best Prac Res Clin Haematol. 2016;29:295-307.

The best prognosis is observed in patients who achieve a second chronic phase. Allo-SCT probably further improves prognosis of patients in second CP. The choice of TKI should be directed by the mutation profile of the patient. Blast crises can be prevented. tBC is the consequence of continued BCR-ABL activity leading to genetic instability, DNA damage, and impaired DNA repair. Most patients with BC carry multiple mutations, and up to 80% show additional chromosomal aberrations in a nonrandom pattern. Patients in BC should be treated with a tyrosine kinase inhibitor according to mutation profile, with or without chemotherapy, with the goal of achieving a second chronic phase and proceeding to allogeneic stem cell transplantation as quickly as possible.

43. Ans. c. Micro-megakaryocytes are frequently seen in the CML-CP cases
Ref: Nowell & Hungerford. Science. 1960; 132:1497, WHO 2017 classification

The Philadelphia chromosome (Ph) is the truncated chromosome 22 generated by the reciprocal translocation t(9;22)(q34;q11) and was first identified in 1960 in a patient with CML. BCR-ABL1 fusion gene on the Ph chromosome. In 1960, Peter C. Nowell together with a graduate student, David Hungerford, described an unusual small chromosome present in leukocytes from patients with chronic myelogenous leukemia (CML). This chromosome was designated as the Philadelphia chromosome after the city in which it was discovered.

The site of breakpoints in chromosome 22 might vary and it may influence the presentation of the gene. In most cases break point results in p210 abnormal fusion protein. In some cases, a larger fusion protein, p230, is encoded. Patients with p230 protein may show prominent neutrophilic maturation and/or thrombocytosis. Rare cases might have p190 fusion protein and this fusion protein is associated with increase in monocytes, and these cases might resemble CMML.

Megakaryocyte morphology is key to differentiation between different types of myeloproliferative neoplasms. CML is characterized by small sized and hypolobated megakaryocytes, referred to as 'dwarf megakaryocytes' but are not true micro-megakaryocytes.

The presence of fibrosis was reported to be associated with a worse outcome in the pre-TKI era. It reportedly has no substantial impact on prognosis in patients treated with TKIs.

44. Ans. c. BCR-ABL1 levels ≤0.01%

Ref: Branford S. Molecular monitoring in chronic myeloid leukemia—how low can you go? Hematology, 2016)

BCR-ABL1 levels ≤10% at 3 months and ≤1% at 6 months represent the so-called early molecular response. Early molecular response has been shown to predict the rate and depth of any subsequent response and to correlate with significantly improved long-term outcomes (progression-free survival and overall survival). BCR-ABL1 ≤0.1% is MMR ($MR^{3.0}$ or 3 log reduction), the 'safe haven' for survival, to be achieved within 12 months of therapy. Finally, BCR-ABL1 ≤0.01% ($MR^{4.0}$ or 4 log reduction), down to 0.001% ($MR^{5.0}$ or 5 log reduction), defines the so-called deep molecular response (DMR) that has been shown to predict significantly better long-term outcomes (failure-free survival and overall survival).

45. Ans. a. Threonine 315

Ref: Azam M. Activation of tyrosine kinases by mutation of the gatekeeper threonine. Nat Struct Mol Biol, 2008)

Threonine 315 is a gatekeeper as it allows formation of hydrogen bonds with TKIs and thus allow their entry into the deep pocket. Its mutation leads to attachment of hydrophobic group rather than hydrophilic group thus inhibiting entry of TKIs. All 3 TKIs make a critical hydrogen bond with the side chain hydroxyl group of Thr315. A mutation of the threonine gatekeeper residue to isoleucine prevents the formation of this critical hydrogen bond. TKIs develop resistance through mutation of the 'gatekeeper' threonine residue.

CHAPTER 30

Hodgkin Lymphoma

1. **True about Hodgkin lymphoma (HL) is:**
   a. Most common age group affected is 50–60 years
   b. Incidence is increasing
   c. More common in females
   d. All of the above
   e. None of the above

2. **Popcorn appearance is seen in:**
   a. Nodular lymphocyte-predominant Hodgkin lymphoma (NLPHL)
   b. Nodular sclerosing HL
   c. Lymphocyte-rich HL
   d. Lymphocyte-depleted HL

3. **True regarding NLPHL is:**
   a. 80% of cases present with early stage disease
   b. Compared with classic Hodgkin lymphoma (cHL), mediastinal involvement and "B" symptoms are less common
   c. Positive for CD20
   d. All of the above

4. **Nodular lymphocyte-predominant Hodgkin lymphoma is included with HL because:**
   a. Positive for CD20
   b. Cells have B-cell morphology
   c. Presence of neoplastic Hodgkin and Reed-Sternberg (HRS) called lymphocyte-predominant cells in an inflammatory background of reactive T cells and eosinophils
   d. All of the above

5. **Lymphocyte-predominant cells in NLPHL express all, *except*:**
   a. CD15 and CD30
   b. CD20, CD45, CD75
   c. Epithelial membrane antigen
   d. All of the above

6. **Hasenclever index does not include:**
   a. Age >45 years
   b. Male gender
   c. Serum albumin 4 g/dL
   d. Hemoglobin 10.5 g/dL
   e. Neutropenia absolute neutrophil count (ANC) <1,500/μL

7. **Duration after which PET-CT (positron emission tomography-computed tomography) scan should be performed after chemotherapy is:**
   a. Within a week   b. After 1 week
   c. After 8 weeks   d. After 16 weeks

8. **Radiotherapy dose for stage IIA HL is:**
   a. 20 Gy   b. 30 Gy
   c. 36 Gy   d. 40 Gy

9. **Brentuximab vedotin (BV) is used for:**
   a. Frontline treatment for classic early stage HL
   b. Frontline treatment for classic advanced-stage HL
   c. Relapsed/refractory HL
   d. All of the above

10. **Bulky disease is defined as:**
    a. Mediastinal mass ratio >0.33
    b. Any single node or mass >10 cm
    c. Mediastinal mass exceeding more than one-third of the internal transverse diameter of thorax at T5-6 level in posteroanterior (PA) view chest radiograph
    d. All of the above

11. **Deauville criteria are used for:**
    a. Visual interpretation of PET-CT
    b. Histological grading of HL
    c. Prognostic scoring of HL by clinical markers
    d. Prognostic scoring of HL by laboratory markers

12. **The most valid indication for PET-CT scan in Hodgkin lymphoma is:**
    a. Diagnosis
    b. Interim treatment
    c. End of treatment
    d. Follow-up of treated lymphoma
    e. All of the above

13. **True regarding Hodgkin lymphoma in pregnancy is:**
    a. Chemotherapy can be delayed till delivery
    b. Initial management should include radiotherapy
    c. ABVD (adriamycin, bleomycin, vinblastine, dacarbazine) chemotherapy should be avoided
    d. None of the above

14. **Follow-up of a treated HL patient requires all, *except*:**
    a. Monitoring for second neoplasms
    b. Only irradiated blood product transfusion lifelong

c. Monitoring for hypothyroidism and diabetes
d. Yearly PET-CT scan
e. All of the above

15. The preferred treatment for unfavorable early stage Hodgkin lymphoma is:
a. Four cycles of ABVD plus 20 Gy RT
b. Four cycles of ABVD plus 30 Gy RT
c. Four cycles of BEACOPP plus 20 Gy RT
d. Four cycles of BEACOPP plus 30 Gy RT

16. Autologous stem cell transplant (ASCT) in Hodgkin lymphoma is indicated in all, *except*:
a. Relapsed patient who achieves an adequate response to salvage therapy
b. Primary resistant disease that achieves an adequate response to salvage therapy
c. Primary or relapsed disease failing to achieve an adequate response
d. Indicated in all of the above

17. In a young patient who has relapsed after autologous transplant for HL, the preferred treatment is:
a. Second autologous transplant after achieving remission
b. Allogenic stem cell transplant
c. Maintenance cytotoxic therapies post-ASCT
d. Radiotherapy

18. Which one of these is not true regarding treatment with the ABVD chemotherapy regimen?
a. It is the treatment of choice in most patients with stage III disease
b. It is associated with a risk of lung fibrosis
c. It leads to sterility in men
d. It is superior to MOPP [mechlorethamine hydrochloride, vincristine sulfate (Oncovin), procarbazine hydrochloride, and prednisone] regimen

19. Which of these is true regarding the appearance on the CT scan at the end of treatment for HL?
a. It is essential that all the lymph node masses have disappeared
b. Normal CT scan is associated with a 50% cure rate
c. Some residual tissue mass may remain and PET scan is valuable
d. The lymph node masses rarely disappear

20. Approximately what percentage of patients are cured of early stage HL?
a. 55–60   b. 65–70
c. 75–80   d. 85–90

21. Which of these is not true regarding the Reed-Sternberg cell?
a. It is thought to be of B-cell lineage
b. It is multinucleate
c. It represents the majority of cells in a lymph node of HL
d. It usually expresses CD15 and CD30

22. Which of the following is true about stage IA HL?
a. It is associated with a raised serum lactate dehydrogenase
b. It may present with weight loss
c. It is best left untreated with a "watch-and-wait" approach
d. It may be confined to the lymph nodes on one side of the neck

23. True regarding HL is:
a. May be associated with Epstein-Barr virus (EBV)
b. Family history increases the risk
c. Elderly patients are treated with 6–8 cycles of chemotherapy
d. Chemotherapy and antiretroviral therapy should be given simultaneously in an HIV patient with HL
e. All of the above

24. True regarding advanced-stage HL is:
a. For HL, the combination of doxorubicin, vinblastine, dacarbazine, and BV has emerged as a more effective primary chemotherapy than ABVD
b. A negative-interim PET is found in approximately 80% of patients, appears to be strongly predictive for a favorable outcome, and may largely override the prognostic impact of the international prognostic score
c. Patients with recurrent HL despite optimal primary chemotherapy should be offered treatment with high-dose chemotherapy followed by ASCT
d. All of the above

25. True regarding the mechanism of action of Brentuximab vedotin is:
a. It is an anti-CD30 monoclonal antibody that kills the HRS cells by ADCC
b. It is an anti-CD15 monoclonal antibody that kills the HRS cells by ADCC
c. The monomethyl auristatin E (MMAE) released binds to tubulin and causes apoptosis by antibody-drug conjugate
d. It binds to DNA and impairs cell division
e. All of the above

26. Brentuximab vedotin should not be given along with:
a. Doxorubicin   b. Vinblastine
c. Bleomycin   d. Dacarbazine

27. True regarding HL are all, *except*:
a. It represents 10% of all lymphomas
b. Disease has a bimodal distribution and affects both young adults and elderly patients
c. Epstein-Barr virus is a risk factor for the development of this malignancy
d. Subclassification is based on Reed-Sternberg cells
e. Immunosuppression is a risk factor for the development of this malignancy

28. **PD-1 (programmed death-1) stimulation causes:**
a. T-cell activation
b. T-cell inhibition
c. B-cell activation
d. B-cell inhibition

29. **The mechanism of action of nivolumab is:**
a. Inhibition of IKROS
b. Inhibition of PD-1
c. Inhibition of BCL2
d. Inhibition of cyclin D1

30. **Side effects of nivolumab include all, *except*:**
a. Flare of disease
b. Flare of graft-versus-host disease (GVHD)
c. Hair loss
d. Nephritis

31. **Which chromosome is involved in the pathogenesis of classical Hodgkin lymphoma?**
a. Chromosome 6
b. Chromosome 7
c. Chromosome 8
d. Chromosome 9

32. **Following are true regarding NLPHL, *except*:**
a. Comprises about 30% of HL patients
b. Is mostly EBV positive
c. The malignant cells are CD15 and CD30 negative
d. All of the above

33. **Least effect on fertility in women is seen with:**
a. ABVD
b. MOPP
c. BEACOPP
d. All have nearly equal effect

34. **Classic HL can be differentiated from anaplastic lymphoma kinase (ALK)-negative anaplastic large-cell lymphoma by:**
a. CD30
b. CD20
c. CD3
d. PAX5

35. **True about CD20 positivity in classical Hodgkin lymphoma is:**
a. Absent
b. <5%
c. 10–20%
d. 20–40%

ANSWERS WITH EXPLANATIONS

1. Ans. e. None of the above *Ref: Hoffman 5/e p1239*

Hodgkin lymphoma is a disease that affects young adults and is the third most commonly diagnosed cancer in people aged 15–29 years. The overall incidence is stable in comparison to that of non-HLs, which appears to be rising. The overall male-to-female ratio is 1.4:1.

2. Ans. a. Nodular lymphocyte predominant Hodgkin lymphoma (NLPHL)

Hodgkin lymphoma is named after Dr Thomas Hodgkin who first described the condition in 1832. NLPHL has a distinct histological appearance, with HRS cells having a lymphocytic and histiocytic (L&H) or "popcorn" appearance because of an increased number of nucleoli. Its proper name is a "lymphocyte-predominant cell" (or LP cell).

3. Ans. d. All of the above
Ref: Nogová L. Biology, clinical course and management of nodular lymphocyte-predominant Hodgkin lymphoma. ASH. 2006.

Nodular lymphocyte-predominant Hodgkin lymphoma tends to present with chronic asymptomatic lymphadenopathy; 70–80% of cases present with early stage disease and, compared with cHL, mediastinal involvement and "B" symptoms are less common. NLPHL tends to relapse as a large-cell lymphoma. NLPHL differs in histological and clinical presentation from cHL. The typical morphologic signs of NLPHL are atypical L&H cells, called popcorn cells, which are surrounded by a non-neoplastic nodular background of small lymphocytes of B-cell origin. The NLPHL cells are positive for CD45, CD19, CD20, CD22, and CD79a, but lack expression of CD15 and CD30, the typical markers for CHL. Treatment of NLPHL patients using standard HL protocols leads to complete remission (CR) in more than 95% of patients. Survival and freedom from treatment failure (FFTF) are worse in advanced-stage patients than in early stage patients. Thus, patients in advanced and in early stages with unfavorable risk factors are treated similarly to CHL patients. In contrast, patients with early stage NLPHL without risk factors can be sufficiently treated with reduced intensity programs having less severe adverse effects. As a result, treatment of early NLPHL is less clearly defined, including radiotherapy in extended field (EF) or involved field (IF) technique, combined modality treatment, and, more recently, monoclonal antibody rituximab. The European Society for Medical Oncology (ESMO) guidelines recommend radiotherapy alone for stage 1A NLPHL and chemotherapy (like cHL) for other stages. NLPHL can be difficult to distinguish from progressive transformation of germinal centers and T-cell-rich B-cell lymphoma.

4. Ans. c. Presence of neoplastic Hodgkin and Reed-Sternberg (HRS) called lymphocyte-predominant cells in an inflammatory background of reactive T cells and eosinophils *Ref: See Q. No. 1 and 3*

Hodgkin lymphoma is classified into two distinct entities: cHL and NLPHL. Both types are characterized by the histological appearance of neoplastic HRS and LP cells in an inflammatory background of reactive T cells and eosinophils. The REAL (Revised

European American Lymphoma) classification of lymphoid neoplasms proposed separating nodular LP HL (CD15–, CD20+, CD30–) from lymphocyte-rich cHL (CD15+, CD20–, CD30+), on the basis of these immunophenotypic differences. It has been shown that both NLPHL and cHL are malignant B-cell lymphomas of germinal center origin. NLPHL and lymphocyte-rich HL cannot be distinguished morphologically or clinically. However, the immunophenotypic profile of the neoplastic cells in lymphocyte-rich HL differs from that of the LP cells.

5. Ans. a. CD15 and CD30 *Ref: See Q. No. 1 and 3*

Immunophenotyping is critical for establishing a diagnosis of NLPHL. Unlike malignant Reed-Sternberg cells in cHL, LP cells lack expression of CD15 and CD30. A typical B-cell phenotype is seen, and cells express CD20, CD45, CD75, and often J-chain. Epithelial membrane antigen is present in 50% of cases.

6. Ans. e. Neutropenia absolute neutrophil count (ANC) <1,500/μL

Ref: Hasenclever D, Diehl V. A prognostic score for advanced Hodgkin's disease. International Prognostic Factors Project on Advanced Hodgkin's Disease. N Engl J Med. 1998;339(21):1506-14.

Hasenclever index was devised for patients with advanced-stage HL. Predicting the outcome in HL is important to avoid overtreating patients with low-risk HL and to identify others in whom standard treatment is likely to fail. Seven factors with similar independent prognostic effects were selected. The prognostic score was then defined as the number of adverse prognostic factors present at diagnosis. The prognostic score was used to predict rates of freedom from progression of disease and overall survival. It includes both clinical and laboratory features.

The seven factors which were found to have independent prognostic effects were: (1) a serum albumin level of <4 g/dL, (2) a hemoglobin level of <10.5 g/dL, (3) male sex, (4) an age of 45 years or older, (5) stage IV disease (according to the Ann Arbor classification), (6) leukocytosis (a white-cell count of at least 15,000/mm^3), and (7) lymphocytopenia (a lymphocyte count of <600/mm^3, a count that was less than 8% of the white-cell count, or both). The score predicted the rate of freedom from progression of disease as follows: 0, or no factors (7% of the patients), 84%; 1 (22% of the patients), 77%; 2 (29% of the patients), 67%; 3 (23% of the patients), 60%; 4 (12% of the patients), 51%; and 5 or higher (7% of the patients), 42%.

7. Ans. c. After 8 weeks

Ref: Hoffbrand 7/e; Follows GA, BCSH guidelines. BJH. 2014; PET Oncologic Imaging (Scott Williams).

The transport of glucose into a cell is mediated by a family of glucose transporter proteins. One of the biochemical characteristics of malignant cells is an enhanced rate of glucose metabolism due to an increased number of these cell surface glucose transporter proteins (primarily Glut-1 and Glut-3). This enhanced glycolytic rate of malignant cells facilitates their detection utilizing PET fluorodeoxyglucose (FDG) imaging. The most common glucose transport protein overexpressed on the tumor cell membranes is Glut-1, which is insulin independent. The appropriate timing of the PET-CT study for maximum accuracy is important. To avoid false-positive results, the best time to perform a PET-CT study is 8–12 weeks after completion of chemotherapy and radiotherapy. Postoperative inflammatory changes are seen till about 12 weeks or, at times, longer. The effect of colony-stimulating factor (administered to stimulate production of blood cells after chemotherapy) is seen as intense metabolic activity in the marrow of the bones. This effect is less pronounced after 3 weeks.

False-positive PET results can occur after treatment. Other causes of false-positive PET results include rebound thymic hyperplasia, infection, inflammation, brown fat, and extramedullary hemopoiesis. As per British Committee for the Standards in Haematology (BCSH) guidelines PET-CT is recommended at the end of treatment, a minimum of 10 days following chemotherapy, 2 weeks after granulocyte colony-stimulating factor (G-CSF) treatment, and 8–12 weeks after chemotherapy. FDG imaging is performed in the fasting state to minimize competitive inhibition of FDG uptake by glucose. FDG uptake is significantly influenced by plasma glucose levels and uptake will be decreased when plasma glucose levels are elevated (elevated serum glucose levels can result in decreased FDG accumulation within the tumors). The study should be delayed until the glucose level is <200 mg/dL. In patients with diabetes, blood sugar control should be achieved with oral hypoglycemic agents or insulin (not administered near the time of FDG administration).

The criteria have been developed for interpretation of FDG-PET at the end of treatment and not specifically for interim FDG-PET. Moreover, the aim of PET scan performed at the end of treatment is different from that of interim scan: the first is aimed at assessing the response and the second at assessing chemosensitivity. For the former, the gold standard reference is the biopsy to demonstrate CR or non-CR; for the second the gold standard does not exist, at the moment.

8. Ans. a. 20 Gy

Ref: NCCN 2019 guidelines and BCSH guidelines

A dose of 20 Gy following two cycles of ABVD is sufficient if the patient has stage I or IIA disease with erythrocyte sedimentation rate (ESR) <50 no extralymphatic lesion and only one or two lymph node regions involved (NCCN, 2019). The dose for favorable early stage disease should be 20 Gy and for all other patients 30 Gy (BCSH, 2014). The dose of radiotherapy is now well defined from the German Hodgkin Study Group (GHSG) trials

HD10 and HD11, which show that for favorable early HL 20 Gy is sufficient, and 30 Gy should be given to all other patients with early or advanced-stage disease, where radiotherapy is indicated.

9. Ans. d. All of the above

Ref: Connors JM. Brentuximab vedotin with chemotherapy for stage III or IV Hodgkin's Lymphoma. N Engl J Med. 2018;378(4):331-44.

Brentuximab vedotin is an antibody-drug conjugate directed to the protein CD30, which is expressed in cHL and systemic anaplastic large cell lymphoma (sALCL). The monoclonal antibody delivers MMAE to the CD30-positive cancer cells, and once inside the cancer cells, it stops them from dividing, which eventually kills the cancer cells.

The United States Food and Drug Administration (FDA) in 2011 approved BV for use in relapsed or refractory HL and relapsed or refractory sALCL. Brentuximab can also be used in combination with three other chemotherapy drugs as an initial, or first-line, treatment in patients with advanced disease. BV induces durable objective responses and results in tumor regression in most patients with relapsed or refractory CD30-positive lymphomas. The most common adverse reactions (≥20%) are chemotherapy-induced peripheral neuropathy, neutropenia, fatigue, nausea, anemia, upper respiratory tract infection, diarrhea, fever, rash, thrombocytopenia, cough, and vomiting.

10. Ans. d. All of the above

Ref: Das P. Hodgkin's lymphoma—unfavorable clinical stage I And II. ACR Appropriateness Criteria. 2010.

Numerous studies have evaluated the impact of prognostic factors in stage I–II Hodgkin's lymphoma in order to identify patients who benefit from more intensive therapy. Two factors that are important in stage I–II HL which influence management decisions are: (1) The first is constitutional (B) symptoms—unexplained fevers, drenching night sweats, or significant weight loss and (2) the second prognostic factor that influences treatment is the presence of large mediastinal adenopathy or bulky disease in nonmediastinal sites. The risk factor "large mediastinal tumor mass" is an internationally accepted unfavorable prognostic factor in the staging of Hodgkin's lymphoma and should be accurately measured by chest radiograph. It is required both for prognostication and for treatment/radiotherapy planning. A number of definitions of large mediastinal adenopathy have been reported. The most commonly used definition is based on a measurement of the maximum width of the mediastinal mass on standing posteroanterior (PA) chest radiograph, compared with the maximum intrathoracic diameter. A ratio of more than one-third is defined as "bulky." Other reports have used a ratio with the intrathoracic width at the T5–6 vertebral level. Bulky disease in nonmediastinal sites has similarly been classified with varying definitions. Some protocols define bulky as ≥10 cm while others use ≥5 cm or ≥6 cm. The standard of care for unfavorable stage I-II Hodgkin's lymphoma is combined-modality therapy, consisting of chemotherapy followed by radiation therapy. The most widely accepted chemotherapy regimen is ABVD. Other options, such as Stanford V and BEACOPP, can also be used. The recommended radiation dose is 30–36 Gy after ABVD, and the recommended radiation field is IFRT.

11. Ans. a. Visual interpretation of PET-CT

Ref: NCCN guidelines

PET-CT is the standard imaging modality for staging and determining remission status at the conclusion of therapy for the aggressive lymphomas. It is superior to CT alone when attempting to identify active disease after therapy completion. There needs to be standardization of reporting, specifically regarding criteria about what is positive and negative, as well as reproducibility among nuclear medicine physicians and machines. Deauville criteria are visual interpretation of the PET-CT scan uses a 5-point scale. PET scans are scored according to uptake in sites initially involved by lymphoma as: Score 1—no uptake, Score 2—uptake less than or equal to the mediastinum, Score 3—uptake greater than the mediastinum but less than the liver, Score 4—uptake moderately higher than the liver, and Score 5—uptake markedly higher than the liver. By Deauville criteria, scores 1 and 2 should be considered "negative" and 4, 5 considered "positive." Deauville score 3 should be interpreted according to the clinical context but in many HL patients it indicates a good prognosis with standard treatment. Biopsy is advised prior to second-line therapy to confirm residual disease with scores 4 and 5 where possible to exclude false-positive uptake with FDG. The Deauville criteria are recommended for reporting PET scans at interim and end-treatment assessment when using visual assessment of response.

12. Ans. c. End of treatment

Ref: NCCN guidelines and BCSH guidelines

Staging with contrast-enhanced CT neck to pelvis is required (BCSH, 2014), although PET-CT is preferable if clinically feasible. As pretreatment staging with PET-CT will upstage a minority of patients and aid the interpretation of subsequent PET-CT, it is recommended when clinically feasible. The optimal management of interim PET-positive patients remains uncertain. Therefore, at this time interim PET remains desirable for ABVD-treated patients but cannot be mandated as a standard of care. End-of-treatment PET-CT is recommended for all patients who have not achieved an interim PET-negative remission as this may directly affect radiotherapy planning, biopsy considerations, and follow-up strategy. There is no proven role for routine surveillance CT or PET-CT imaging in patients who are otherwise well following first-line therapy.

So, in summary PET-CT can be done at the time of diagnosis of HL; however, end-of-treatment PET-CT is must and interim and follow-up PET-CT scans are not recommended at present.

13. Ans. d. None of the above

Ref: Follows GA. BCSH guidelines. BJH. 2014

Pregnant patients with HL should be in a specialized obstetric/fetal medicine unit. Staging investigations and response evaluation should be tailored to the clinical presentation and radiation exposure should be minimized. Staging and response assessment with MRI scanning and ultrasound are preferred and may avoid the need for radiation-based imaging. ABVD is the regimen of choice unless specifically contraindicated. Delaying commencement of chemotherapy until postdelivery is not usually recommended. Wherever possible, RT should be delayed until postdelivery. While termination of pregnancy may be the most appropriate course of action for certain patients, for many cases, the fetal and maternal outcomes following HL treatment in pregnancy appear excellent, following ABVD treatment. Although ABVD has been used to treat patients in all three trimesters, the potential risk to fetal development from chemotherapy is likely to be higher in the first trimester and most clinicians would try and avoid exposure to chemotherapy at this time. Breast feeding should be avoided if the patient is getting chemotherapy.

14. Ans. d. Yearly PET-CT scan

Ref: Follows GA. BCSH guidelines. BJH. 2014

Hodgkin lymphoma patients who have been treated with chemotherapy/radiotherapy should be made aware that they are at an increased lifetime risk of second neoplasms, cardiovascular and pulmonary disease, and infertility. Apart from the current breast cancer screening program, there are no cancer screening programs tailored for HL survivors. Women treated with mediastinal radiotherapy before the age of 35 years should be offered the breast cancer screening measures. There should be complete avoidance of smoking and careful management of cardiovascular risks such as hypertension, diabetes mellitus, and hyperlipidemia. Patients who have had radiotherapy to the neck and upper mediastinum should have regular thyroid function tests. Hypothyroidism can occur up to 30 years after radiotherapy.

Patients should receive irradiated blood products for life. HL patients have been shown to have long-term anergic immunological responses and measurable defects in T-cell function. Cases of transfusion-associated GVHD have been reported. Consequently, all HL patients are recommended to receive lifelong irradiated blood products. There is no proven role for routine surveillance CT or PET-CT imaging in patients who are otherwise well following first-line therapy.

15. Ans. b. Four cycles of ABVD plus 30 Gy RT

Ref: NCCN guidelines and BCSH guidelines. 2019

Currently, four cycles of ABVD followed by 30 Gy RT are widely considered the standard of care for unfavorable early stage HL. There is no evidence to support the removal of RT from patients who present with bulky disease (BCSH, 2014). NCCN recommends four cycles of ABVD followed by 30 Gy RT or 2 more cycles of ABVD. The standard of care for patients with favorable early stage HL is 2× ABVD and 20 Gy RT. The standard of care for unfavorable early stage HL is 4× ABVD and 30 Gy. RT should not normally be omitted in patients presenting with bulky disease.

16. Ans. c. Primary or relapsed disease failing to achieve an adequate response

Ref: NCCN guidelines and BCSH guidelines

Autologous SCT is the standard treatment for patients with relapsed disease who achieve an adequate response to salvage therapy. ASCT is also the standard treatment for patients with primary resistant disease who achieve an adequate response to salvage therapy. Auto-SCT is not recommended in those failing to achieve an adequate response. Patients relapsing within 12–18 months of completing their first-line treatment should be considered for an allogeneic SCT (depending on age, stage of disease, and availability of a donor). In some patients, a reduced-intensity allograft may be preferable. Patients who are unable to undergo an auto-SCT (e.g., due to persistent bone marrow involvement or a failure to mobilize sufficient stem cells) may also be considered for an allogeneic transplant. Newer agents such as BV, checkpoint inhibitors (e.g., pembrolizumab, nivolumab), lenalidomide, and everolimus are also available for the treatment of patients relapsing after autologous hematopoietic cell transplantation (HCT).

17. Ans. b. Allogenic stem cell transplant

Ref: See Q. No. 16

Allogeneic transplantation using a reduced-intensity conditioning regimen is the treatment of choice for younger patients with a suitable donor and chemosensitive disease following failure of ASCT. An appropriately human leukocyte antigen (HLA)-matched unrelated donor should be considered when there is no HLA-matched sibling. A second autologous transplant is a reasonable clinical option in selected patients with late relapse following first ASCT. Current evidence does not support the use of maintenance cytotoxic therapies post ASCT. Tandem ASCT cannot currently be recommended outside of clinical trials.

18. Ans. c. It leads to sterility in men

Ref: Williams 7/e; Hoffman 7/e; Duggan BD. JCO. 2003

The acute toxicities of ABVD include a higher incidence of alopecia and vomiting compared with MOPP. Relative to MOPP, the neurotoxicity of ABVD is mild but the administration of dacarbazine often requires prolonged infusion in small peripheral vessels. Severe myelosuppression is rare when ABVD is administered alone, and the dose intensity of ABVD can often be maintained at >99% patients without the use of G-CSF. In contrast to MOPP, ABVD does not result in a high incidence of permanent azoospermia or amenorrhea. The incidence of myelodysplasia and secondary leukemia does not appear to be increased with ABVD. Use of ABVD may result in late bleomycin-related pulmonary toxicity, particularly in combination with mediastinal irradiation. Following ABVD, there may be a significant decline in median forced vital capacity and diffusing capacity [diffusing capacity for carbon monoxide (DLCO)]. Among patients treated with MOPP for HL, infertility and the development of secondary malignancy are of significant concern, which are less likely with ABVD.

19. Ans. c. Some residual tissue mass may remain and PET scan is valuable *Ref: See Q. No. 11 and 12*

PET-CT scan is the examination of choice for detecting disease activity after treatment. Compared with CT scan alone, PET-CT scanning is better able to distinguish between active tumor and necrosis or fibrosis in residual masses. A positive PET scan can be determined by visual assessment and does not require the use of the standardized uptake value (SUV). The negative predictive value of PET, or the ability of a negative scan to exclude persistent disease or future relapse, averages 90%. There is a 10–20% false-negative rate, which is likely due to the inability of imaging techniques to detect microscopic disease. The positive predictive value (PPV) of PET scans in response assessment is more variable with an average of 65%. Up to 40% of patients with a positive PET scan will not relapse. It is therefore imperative that positive PET scans be confirmed by tissue biopsy prior to giving more therapy. Causes of false-positive PET scans include postinflammatory changes after chemotherapy and radiation treatment, rebound thymic hyperplasia, infectious and inflammatory processes, and brown fat.

20. Ans. d. 85–90

Five-year survival rates for HL are very good, between 85 and 90% for those with early stage disease.

21. Ans. c. It represents the majority of cells in a lymph node of HL

Hodgkin lymphoma (formerly called Hodgkin's disease) is a neoplasm characterized by the presence of clonal malignant HRS cells in a reactive cellular background comprised of variable numbers of granulocytes, plasma cells, and lymphocytes. Polymerase chain reaction (PCR) studies have established a B-cell origin for HRS cells in the vast majority of cases of HL. Despite the clear molecular evidence in most cases of classic Hodgkin lymphoma (cHL) for a germinal center origin, HRS cells characteristically lose the phenotypic features of germinal center B cells. The peculiar absence of immunoglobulin (Ig) gene expression in HRS cells appears to be due to impaired activation of the immunoglobulin promoters and enhancers stemming from the lack of expression of the B-cell transcription factors OCT2, BOB-1, and PU.1, accompanied by epigenetic silencing of IgH promoters. In cHL, the RS cells typically express CD15 (85% of cases) and CD30 (virtually 100% of cases) and usually lack global expression of pan-B (CD19, CD20, CD79a) and pan-T (CD3, CD7) antigens. Failure to detect CD15 does not preclude a diagnosis of HL; however, absence of both CD15 and CD30 and expression of CD20 should prompt reexamination of the slides and consideration of either NLPHL, lymphocyte-rich HL, or an unusual variant of large B-cell NHL.

22. Ans. d. It may be confined to the lymph nodes on one side of the neck *Ref: NCCN guidelines and BCSH guidelines*

The treatment of early stage, favorable prognosis HL requires a careful balance between providing enough therapy to eradicate the tumor and avoiding unnecessary treatment that could result in excessive long-term treatment-related side effects. At this time, the preferred treatment option for early stage, favorable prognosis HL is the use of combination chemotherapy and involved field radiation therapy. For children with stage I and IIA (early) HL, the overall 5-year survival rate exceeds 90%, regardless of the therapeutic program chosen. The treatment regimen should consist of combination chemotherapy followed by involved field radiation. ABVD has demonstrated superior efficacy (i.e., freedom from progression) and less toxicity when compared with MOPP in patients with unfavorable prognosis, early stage and advanced-stage HL. Early results suggest that ABVD plus involved field irradiation in stage I-II HL may be more effective and less toxic than alkylating agent regimens and radiation therapy. For this reason, it is recommended that ABVD chemotherapy in combination with involved-field radiotherapy should be used for patients with favorable prognosis stage I-II HL. Night sweat, fever, and weight loss are B symptoms.

23. Ans. e. All of the above *Ref: BCSH guidelines; Hoffman 7/e*

The recognition that a proportion of HL harbors the EBV and that its genome is monoclonal in these tumors suggests that the virus contributes to the development of HL in some cases. The association of EBV with HL seems to depend on factors such as country of residence, histological subtype, sex, ethnicity, and age. EBV is more commonly associated with the mixed cellularity subtype of HL and less frequently with the other forms of this disease. HL is three times more common in the first-degree relatives of HL patients suggesting family history as a risk factor for HL. HL in elderly patients is a much more aggressive disease. The histology is more aggressive from the onset. It presents at an advanced stage, and there is an association with EBV. Fit elderly patients can be treated in the same way as young patients, though frail patients will have more toxicity with intensive chemotherapy. Age in general is not a contraindication for aggressive chemotherapy. HL in the HIV-seropositive population is more likely to have mixed cellularity or lymphocyte-depleted histology and is almost always EBV-associated. The majority of patients present with advanced-stage disease. Before the introduction of HAART (highly active antiretroviral therapy), treatment outcomes for HIV-HL were poor. Response rates and survival have improved significantly in patients treated with HAART and ABVD chemotherapy. The patient should be given PCP (*Pneumocystis carinii* pneumonia) prophylaxis and G-CSF support.

24. Ans. d. All of the above

Ref: Spinner MA, Advani RH, Connors JM, Azzi J, Diefenbach C. New treatment algorithms in Hodgkin lymphoma: too much or too little? Am Soc Clin Oncol Educ Book. 2018;38:626-36.

NCCN. (2019). NCCN guidelines for CML. Pennsylvania: NCCN.

The treatment of advanced-stage HL continues to evolve. Currently, the two best strategies that have emerged from clinical trials are either interim PET-guided escalation or de-escalation approaches or integration of the novel agent BV into primary chemotherapy.

25. Ans. c. The monomethyl auristatin E (MMAE) released binds to tubulin and causes apoptosis by antibody-drug conjugate

Ref: Younes A, Gopal AK, Smith SE, Ansell SM, Rosenblatt JD, Savage KJ, et al. Results of a pivotal phase II study of brentuximab vedotin for patients with relapsed or refractory Hodgkin's lymphoma. J Clin Oncol. 2012;30:2183-9.

Arming antibodies with highly potent toxic agents for selective intracellular release provide both targeting and delivery of doses of cytotoxic therapy that would not be possible if systemically given. BV is an antibody-drug conjugate containing the potent antimitotic drug monomethyl auristatin E (MMAE), which is linked to an anti-CD30 monoclonal antibody through a cleavable dipeptide linker. The linker undergoes proteolysis in lysosomes inside the CD30-positive cell, and free MMAE is released. HRS cells express CD30, a transmembrane glycoprotein that facilitates both cellular proliferation and survival. When anti-CD30 monoclonal antibodies alone were used, they showed only modest antitumor activity and were not very effective. So, to improve the antitumor activity of the CD30-specific antibody, an antibody-drug conjugate was created, where CD30 was used as a mode of attachment of the antibody by which the drug can be inserted into the cell to mediate the antitumor effect. In 2011, BV, an ADC that targets CD30 on the surface of Reed-Sternberg cells became the first US FDA-approved immunotherapy for the treatment of HL. BV is a chimeric CD30-specific IgG1 antibody conjugated to the microtubule disrupting agent, MMAE, by an enzyme-cleavable linker. Upon the binding of BV to CD30 on the HRS cell, the ADC is internalized and lysosomal enzymes cleave the linker allowing for the release of MMAE inside the cell. MMAE then binds to tubulin, resulting in cell cycle arrest and subsequent apoptosis of CD30-expressing cells.

26. Ans. c. Bleomycin

Ref: Tomassetti S, Herrera AF. Update on the role of brentuximab vedotin in classical Hodgkin lymphoma. Ther Adv Hematol. 2018;9(9):261-72.

A phase I trial that included 51 patients with newly diagnosed stage IIA bulky or stage IIB–IV HL compared BV added to standard ABVD (A-ABVD) and BV added to AVD without bleomycin (A-AVD). The CR rate was 95% in patients who received A-ABVD compared with 96% of patients who received A-AVD. However, in the A-ABVD cohort there was an unacceptably high rate of adverse pulmonary events (44%); therefore, it is recommended that BV not be given in combination with bleomycin. Neuropathy is the main nonhematologic toxicity of BV and is managed by dose reduction or drug holiday. A study of BV monotherapy in patients with HL over the age of 60 years resulted in an overall response rate of 92% and a CR rate of 73%. BV has drastically altered the management of relapsed and refractory Hodgkin lymphoma. It is currently being used as salvage treatment in the relapsed and refractory setting as well as maintenance therapy in the post-ASCT period. Given its efficacy in upfront, relapsed/refractory, and post-ASCT setting, BV is now being studied either alone or in combination with other drugs in the relapsed/refractory and in the upfront setting.

27. Ans. d. Subclassification is based on Reed-Sternberg cells

Hodgkin lymphoma is an uncommon malignancy involving B lymphocytes and represents approximately 10% of all lymphomas. The disease has a bimodal distribution and affects both young adults and elderly patients. Although there are no clearly defined risk factors for the development of this malignancy, factors associated with this disease include familiar factors, immunosuppression, and exposure to various viruses, including EBV. Typically, the malignant Reed-Sternberg cells present within the malignant tumor biopsy constitute <5% of the tumor cellularity. The predominant cells present within the tumor microenvironment include T cells, with variable numbers of macrophages, eosinophils, plasma cells, B cells, neutrophils, and fibroblasts being also present. The composition of the tumor microenvironment has led to the subclassification of cHL into nodular sclerosis, mixed cellularity, lymphocyte-depleted, and lymphocyte-rich HL. This subclassification is not based on the malignant Reed-Sternberg cells seen in the lymphoma.

28. Ans. b. T-cell inhibition

Ref: Ansell SM, Lesokhin AM, Borrello I, Halwani A, Scott EC, Gutierrez M, et al. PD-1 blockade with nivolumab in relapsed or refractory Hodgkin's lymphoma. N Engl J Med. 2015;372:311-9.

PD-1 is a negative regulator of T-cell activation and function. PD-1 expression typically increases as cells become activated and signaling through PD-1 by its ligands results in cells becoming senescent with an exhausted phenotype. A subset of cells subsequently becomes apoptotic.

29. Ans. b. Inhibition of PD-1

Ref: Ansell SM, Lesokhin AM, Borrello I, Halwani A, Scott EC, Gutierrez M, et al. PD-1 blockade with nivolumab in relapsed or refractory Hodgkin's lymphoma. N Engl J Med. 2015;372:311-9.

The discovery that HL is associated with 9p24.1 amplification and increased programmed death-ligand 1 (PD-L1) and programmed death-ligand 2 (PD-L2) expression led to clinical trials of immune checkpoint inhibitors for this disease. This led to the approval of nivolumab, an anti-PD-1 antibody, in HL. Nivolumab is a fully human monoclonal IgG4 antibody that targets PD-1. The ligands for this receptor, PD-L1 and PD-L2, are expressed on a variety of immune cells, and Reed-Sternberg cells express very high levels of PD-L1 and PD-L2. Incorporation of the EBV genome into Reed-Sternberg cells upregulates PD-L1 and PD-L2 expression. The presence of PD-1 ligands, predominantly on the Reed-Sternberg cells but also potentially expressed on macrophages present within the tumor and microenvironment, as well as the expression of PD-1 receptors on intratumoral T cells, suggests significant suppression of T-cell function due to PD-1/PD-L1/PD-L2 interactions. This provides the rationale for the use of PD-1 blockade to reverse the T-cell inhibition and allow for a more effective antitumor immune response in HL. PD-1 ligands are highly expressed on HRS cells due to chromosome 9p24.1 amplification or EBV infection. PD-L1 and PD-L2 signal through PD-1 expressed on intratumoral T cells and suppress T-cell function, resulting in an ineffective antitumor immune response. Blockade of PD-1 signaling by the anti-PD-1 mAb nivolumab prevents T-cell anergy and exhaustion. The 9p24.1 amplicon also contains JAK2, and translocation or amplification of this locus results in increased activation of JAK/STAT signaling with further upregulation of PD-L1 (CD274) and PPDL2/CD273, and genetic amplification appears to be the dominant mechanism for PD-1 ligand expression. Immunohistochemical studies have confirmed the upregulation of the expression of PD-L1 and PD-L2 specifically on Reed-Sternberg cells.

EBV infection also induces PD-L1 expression in cHL. Most cHL specimens show chromosome 9p24.1 alterations (56% show copy gain, 5% polysomy, and 36% amplification), which result in overexpression of the PD-1 ligands and promote their induction.

30. Ans. c. Hair loss

Checkpoint inhibition is not associated with the toxicities of traditional cytotoxic therapy, such as nausea, vomiting, and hair loss, but comes with a risk of several autoimmune side effects. These adverse reactions are related to a hyperactive T-cell response, resulting in the generation of high levels of CD4 T-helper cell cytokines or increased migration of cytolytic CD8T cells within normal tissues. Skin rash is the most common immune-mediated side effect of checkpoint inhibition and presents most commonly with a maculopapular rash. Other immune-mediated adverse reactions include pneumonitis, colitis, hepatitis, endocrinopathies, nephritis and renal dysfunction, rash, and encephalitis.

Immune activation by PD-1 blockade may increase the risk of worsening of GVHD after subsequent allogeneic stem cell transplant. Therefore, checkpoint inhibition might act as an alternative to donor lymphocyte infusion for select patients with relapsed/refractory HL after allogeneic-HSCT who need a tumor response, but such treatment is complicated by high rates of GVHD. Furthermore, PD-1 blockade can induce tumor flares with increased positivity on PET scan despite clinical improvement, and such patients should continue the therapy.

31. Ans. d. Chromosome 9

Ref: Ansell SM, Lesokhin AM, Borrello I, Halwani A, Scott EC, Gutierrez M, et al. PD-1 blockade with nivolumab in relapsed or refractory Hodgkin's lymphoma. N Engl J Med. 2015;372:311-9.

Most classic Hodgkin lymphoma cases show chromosome 9p24.1 alterations (56% show copy gain; 5% polysomy and 36% amplification), which result in overexpression of the PD-1 ligands and promote their induction through Janus kinase-signal transducer and activator of transcription signaling.

32. Ans. c. The malignant cells are CD15 and CD30 negative

Nodular lymphocyte-predominant Hodgkin lymphoma comprises a small percentage (about 5%) of the total number of patients diagnosed with HL. It is generally a much more indolent lymphoma, is usually asymptomatic, and is always negative for EBV. Unlike classic Hodgkin lymphoma, in which HRS cells are CD15-positive, CD30-positive, and CD45-negative, the malignant cells in NLPHL are CD15-negative, CD30-negative, and CD45-positive germinal center B cells and invariably express CD20. The malignant cells exhibit a nodular growth pattern and popcorn-like, lymphocytic-histiocytic malignant cells without much fibrosis. The natural history of both diseases is very different.

33. Ans. a. ABVD

ABVD carries a little to no excess risk of premature ovarian failure compared with alkylating chemotherapy like MOPP and BEACOPP, which can impair gonadal function and fertility recovery postchemotherapy.

The dose-escalated BEACOPP (bleomycin, etoposide, doxorubicin, cyclophosphamide, vincristine, procarbazine, and prednisone, where the alkylating agents are cyclophosphamide and procarbazine) regimen has been linked to a higher incidence of secondary amenorrhea than the ABVD regimen (doxorubicin, vinblastine, dacarbazine, and bleomycin, where an alkylating agent is dacarbazine).

The BEACOPP regimen has been reported to be superior to ABVD in advanced-stage HL, despite increased rates of hematologic toxicity, secondary malignancy, and infertility in patients who receive the BEACOPP regimen.

34. Ans. d. PAX5

Ref: Chan JKC, Kwong YL. Common misdiagnoses in lymphomas and avoidance strategies. Lancet Oncol. 2010;11:579-88.

Differentiating tumor-cell-rich classic Hodgkin lymphoma from ALK-negative anaplastic large-cell lymphoma can be difficult, because both are characterized by abundant large neoplastic cells with CD30 expression, but do not have expression of conventional B-cell (CD20 or CD79a) and T-cell (CD3) lineage markers, or ALK. cHL tends to have more prominent coagulative necrosis and eosinophilic infiltration than does ALK-negative ALCL, and diagnosis can be confirmed by positive staining for the B-cell transcription factor Pax-5 in the large cells. ALK-negative anaplastic large-cell lymphoma is favored if Pax-5 is negative, especially when other T-lineage markers (such as CD2, CD4, CD5, and CD7) are positive.

35. Ans. d. 20–40%

Hodgkin's lymphoma (HL) is a tumor comprising non-malignant and malignant B-cells. Classical HL expresses CD15+ and CD30+ antigens, and 20–40% of patients are CD20+. This antigen is a ligand free protein present in B lymphocyte cells and its function is not well known. Some studies suggest that expression of CD20 may play a major role in Hodgkin's disease pathophysiology and may affect the patients' treatment prognosis, as well as relapse and refractory response.

CHAPTER 31

Non-Hodgkin Lymphoma

1. **BCL2 translocation and t(14;18) are seen in:**
   a. Germinal center B cell-diffuse large B cell lymphoma (B-cell-DLBCL)
   b. Activated B-cell-DLBCL
   c. Primary mediastinal B-cell lymphoma
   d. All of the above

2. **International Prognostic Index for non-Hodgkin lymphoma (NHL) include all, *except*:**
   a. Age
   b. Sex
   c. Nodal sites
   d. Extranodal sites

3. **Follicular Lymphoma International Prognostic Index (FLIPI) include all, *except*:**
   a. Hemoglobin level
   b. Performance status
   c. Nodal sites
   d. Extranodal sites
   e. All except b and d

4. **True regarding PET-CT scan in lymphoma is:**
   a. Preferred for follicular lymphoma staging
   b. Better for monitoring remission status
   c. Can be done after 1 week of chemotherapy
   d. None of the above

5. **The following viruses are implicated in the pathogenesis of non-Hodgkin lymphoma, *except*:**
   a. Epstein-Barr virus
   b. Human T-cell lymphotropic virus 1
   c. Human Herpesvirus-8
   d. Hepatitis B virus

6. **Addition of rituximab to CHOP-based regimen increases the response rate by:**
   a. 5%
   b. 10%
   c. 20%
   d. 25%

7. **Preferred treatment for stage IA diffuse large B-cell lymphoma is:**
   a. R-CHOP × 3 cycles followed by PET-CT and RT in PET negative
   b. R-CHOP × 2 cycles followed by PET-CT and 2 more cycles for PET negative
   c. Radiotherapy
   d. R-CHOP × 6 cycles followed by PET-CT and 2 more cycles for PET negative

8. **Treatment for DLBCL patient with poor left ventricular function include all, *except*:**
   a. R-CVP (cyclophosphamide, vincristine, prednisone)
   b. R-CEPP (cyclophosphamide, etoposide, prednisone, procarbazine)
   c. R-CNOP (cyclophosphamide, mitoxantrone, etoposide, vincristine, prednisone)
   d. R-CEOP (cyclophosphamide, etoposide, vincristine, prednisone)

9. **True regarding testicular lymphoma are all, *except*:**
   a. Common in elderly
   b. DLBCL is the most common type
   c. Central nervous system involvement is common
   d. Orchiectomy is the treatment of choice

10. **True regarding primary mediastinal large B-cell lymphoma is, *except*:**
    a. Female predominance
    b. Median age third to fourth decade
    c. Bone marrow is commonly involved
    d. Thymus is commonly involved
    e. Hodgkin lymphoma is common differential

11. **Most common site for extranodal marginal zone B-cell lymphoma is:**
    a. Lungs
    b. Thyroid
    c. Airway sinuses
    d. Stomach

12. **True regarding secondary involvement of the central nervous system by non-Hodgkin lymphoma is:**
    a. Median survival without treatment is in the range of 3–13 months
    b. Risk is increased with lymphomatous involvement of bone marrow
    c. Common with high-grade lymphomas
    d. All of the above

13. **Intravascular large cell lymphoma most commonly involves:**
    a. Bone marrow
    b. Peripheral blood
    c. Lymph node
    d. Central nervous system

14. The most common cytogenetic finding in follicular lymphoma is:
   a. t(14;18)
   b. t(4;14)
   c. t(14;16)
   d. t(14;20)

15. Treatment for stage I follicular lymphoma is:
   a. Radiotherapy
   b. Chemotherapy
   c. Radiotherapy + chemotherapy
   d. Only rituximab
   e. Wait and watch

16. Treatment of symptomatic advanced stage follicular lymphoma is:
   a. Radiotherapy
   b. Chemotherapy
   c. Chemoimmunotherapy
   d. Autologous transplant

17. Which of the following is the treatment option for relapsed follicular lymphoma?
   a. Wait and watch
   b. Rituximab alone
   c. Radioimmunotherapy
   d. Autologous stem cell transplant
   e. All of the above

18. Tumor in which lymphocytes are small and have a characteristic folded, cerebriform nucleus is:
   a. Mycosis fungoides
   b. Burkitt lymphoma
   c. Follicular lymphoma
   d. Histiocytosis

19. Which one of these is not true regarding the epidemiology of non-Hodgkin lymphoma?
   a. It is more frequent after solid organ transplantation
   b. It is associated with hepatitis C infection
   c. The incidence is decreasing
   d. It may be associated with malaria

20. A 60-year-old man presents with headaches and anemia. Investigations reveal an IgM paraprotein of 30 g/L. What is the most likely diagnosis?
   a. Burkitt's lymphoma
   b. Mycosis fungoides
   c. Follicular lymphoma
   d. Lymphoplasmacytic lymphoma

21. Cold agglutinin disease is most commonly seen with:
   a. Chronic lymphocytic leukemia
   b. Large granular lymphocytic leukemia
   c. Splenic marginal zone lymphoma
   d. Lymphoplasmacytic lymphoma

22. Absolute indications for treatment in lymphoplasmacytic lymphoma are all, *except*:
   a. Thrombocytopenia
   b. Presence of M protein
   c. Progressive splenomegaly
   d. All of the above

23. A patient presents with abdominal lymphadenopathy and peripheral blood lymphocytosis. The immunophenotype is CD22+, CD5+, and CD23−. Cytogenetic analysis shows a t(11:14) translocation. What is the diagnosis?
   a. Mantle cell lymphoma
   b. Marginal zone lymphoma
   c. Follicular lymphoma
   d. Chronic lymphocytic lymphoma variant

24. Which of these infectious agents has not been associated with development of non-Hodgkin lymphoma?
   a. *Helicobacter pylori*
   b. Cytomegalovirus
   c. Epstein–Barr virus
   d. HTLV1

25. All are true regarding the diagnosis of chronic lymphocytic leukemia, *except*:
   a. Mature small B-cell lymphocytes
   b. Dim expression of surface IgM/IgD
   c. The presence of more than 1,000/μL monoclonal B lymphocytes
   d. Can transform into Hodgkin lymphoma

26. True regarding B-cell prolymphocytic leukemia (B-PLL) is:
   a. More than 20% prolymphocytes in the blood
   b. B-PLL is usually transformed from CLL
   c. Strongly express surface IgM
   d. All of the above

27. True about follicular lymphoma are all, *except*:
   a. BCL6 positive
   b. BCL2 positive
   c. IRF4/MUM1 positive
   d. All of the above

28. True regarding pediatric follicular lymphoma is:
   a. Involves the head and neck region
   b. BCL-2 negative
   c. Negative for t(14;18) translocation
   d. Usually high grade 3
   e. All of the above

29. Primary central nervous system lymphoma is staged as:
   a. Stage IE
   b. Stage IIE
   c. Stage IIIE
   d. Stage IVE

30. True about primary central nervous system lymphoma is:
   a. Whole brain radiotherapy is the treatment of choice
   b. Rituximab–CHOP is equally affective
   c. High-dose methotrexate is preferred treatment
   d. High-dose chemotherapy and autologous stem cell transplant should be considered upfront

31. True regarding Burkitt lymphoma is:
   a. Associated with c-myc translocation
   b. Has highest proliferation index
   c. Good response to chemotherapy
   d. Upfront transplant is not required
   e. All of the above

32. The following are EBV-associated lymphomas in HIV-positive patients, *except*:
   a. Burkitt lymphoma
   b. Diffuse large B-cell lymphoma
   c. Primary CNS lymphoma
   d. Marginal zone lymphoma

33. Treatment of HIV-associated lymphoma is:
   a. CHOP
   b. R-CHOP
   c. HAART plus R-CHOP
   d. HAART plus CVP

34. BCL1 positive lymphoma is:
   a. Follicular lymphoma
   b. Burkitt lymphoma
   c. DLBCL
   d. Mantle cell lymphoma

35. Treatment of stage IVA follicular lymphoma is:
   a. Wait and watch
   b. Radiotherapy
   c. R-CHOP
   d. R-CHOP followed by radiotherapy

36. Treatment of stage III B follicular lymphoma is:
   a. Wait and watch
   b. Radiotherapy
   c. R-CHOP followed by maintenance rituximab
   d. R-CHOP followed by radiotherapy

37. Treatment of asymptomatic stage IV relapsed follicular lymphoma is:
   a. Wait and watch
   b. Radiotherapy
   c. R-CHOP
   d. R-CHOP followed by radiotherapy

38. Treatment of symptomatic stage IV relapsed follicular lymphoma is:
   a. Wait and watch
   b. Radiotherapy
   c. R-CHOP
   d. Clinical trials

39. Treatment for stage 1A diffuse large B-cell lymphoma is:
   a. Wait and watch
   b. Radiotherapy
   c. R-CHOP
   d. R-CHOP followed by radiotherapy

40. Treatment of stage IVA diffuse large B-cell lymphoma is:
   a. Wait and watch
   b. Radiotherapy
   c. R-CHOP
   d. R-CHOP followed by radiotherapy

41. Treatment of asymptomatic stage IV relapsed diffuse large B-cell lymphoma is:
   a. Wait and watch
   b. Radiotherapy
   c. R-CHOP
   d. R-CHOP followed by radiotherapy
   e. Autologous stem cell transplant in CR2

42. Treatment of symptomatic stage IV relapsed diffuse large B-cell lymphoma is:
   a. Wait and watch
   b. Radiotherapy
   c. R-CHOP
   d. R-CHOP followed by radiotherapy
   e. Autologous SCT in CR2

43. Follicular lymphoma-specific International Prognostic Index (FLIPI) includes all, *except*:
   a. >4 involved extranodal sites
   b. Elevated LDH
   c. Age >60 years
   d. Advanced stage III/IV
   e. Hemoglobin <12 g/dL

44. Treatment of choice for splenic marginal zone lymphoma is:
   a. Splenectomy
   b. R-CHOP
   c. Rituximab
   d. Radiotherapy

45. True regarding adult T-cell leukemia/lymphoma is:
   a. Caused by a virus
   b. Prognosis is good
   c. Autologous transplant is the preferred treatment
   d. All of the above

46. True regarding angioimmunoblastic lymphoma are all, *except*:
   a. Elderly population is affected
   b. Caused by virus
   c. Autoimmune features are present
   d. Autologous transplant should be considered early
   e. All of the above

47. True about ALK positive anaplastic large cell lymphoma is:
   a. ALK positivity has prognostic significance
   b. Presents at younger age
   c. Good survival
   d. All of the above

48. Most common pediatric T cell lymphoma is:
   a. Anaplastic large cell lymphoma
   b. Angioimmunoblastic lymphoma
   c. T-cell lymphoblastic leukemia/lymphoma
   d. Cutaneous T cell lymphoma

49. **True about extranodal NK/T cell lymphoma is:**
    a. Midline structures are most commonly involved
    b. EBV has prognostic significance
    c. Prognosis is poor
    d. All of the above

50. **Diffuse large B-cell lymphoma associated with chronic inflammation is seen in all, *except*:**
    a. Pyothorax
    b. Rheumatoid arthritis
    c. Metallic implants in bone
    d. Chronic venous ulcers
    e. Seen in all of the above

51. **Double-hit lymphomas consist of all, *except*:**
    a. MYC and BCL2
    b. BCL2 and BCL6
    c. MYC and BCL6
    d. All of the above

52. **True regarding double-hit lymphomas is:**
    a. Are same as double expressor lymphoma
    b. Have prognosis better than double expressor lymphoma
    c. Are less common than double expressor lymphoma
    d. All of the above

53. **Which of the following combination is correct?**
    a. The Epstein-Barr virus is closely associated with nasal NK-T-cell lymphoma
    b. *Helicobacter pylori* causes gastric mucosa-associated lymphoid tissue (MALT) lymphomas.
    c. Hepatitis C virus is associated with splenic marginal zone lymphoma
    d. *Borrelia burgdorferi* and *Chlamydia psittacosis* are associated with the development of marginal zone lymphomas
    e. All are correct

54. **True regarding follicular lymphoma with translocation t(14;18)(q32;q21) is:**
    a. This translocation places BCL2 under control of the immunoglobulin heavy chain enhancer element
    b. This translocation places BCL6 under control of the immunoglobulin heavy chain enhancer element
    c. This translocation places immunoglobulin heavy chain enhancer element under control of BCL2
    d. This translocation places immunoglobulin heavy chain enhancer element under control of BCL6
    e. Any of the above

55. **True about hepatosplenic T-cell lymphoma is:**
    a. Gamma-delta T-cell lymphoma is more common than alpha-beta T-cell lymphoma
    b. Occurs most commonly in young men
    c. Common in immunocompromised
    d. The neoplastic cells are CD4 and CD8 negative
    e. All of the above

56. **MYD88 mutation is useful in the diagnosis of:**
    a. Lymphoplasmacytic lymphoma
    b. Splenic marginal zone lymphoma
    c. Mantle cell lymphoma
    d. Hairy cell leukemia

57. **Bing-Neel syndrome is:**
    a. Cutaneous involvement by mantle cell lymphoma
    b. Ocular involvement by extranodal marginal zone lymphoma
    c. Cutaneous involvement by diffuse large B-cell lymphoma
    d. Central nervous system involvement by Waldenström macroglobulinemia

58. **Waldenström macroglobulinemia can present with:**
    a. Neuropathy
    b. Diarrhea
    c. Hyperviscosity
    d. Coagulopathy
    e. All of the above

59. **Features of BCL2 in follicular lymphoma include:**
    a. It is expressed more in low-grade follicular lymphoma than high-grade follicular lymphoma
    b. It is helpful in distinguishing neoplastic from reactive follicles
    c. Both are true
    d. Both are false

60. **Multiple lymphomatous polyposes are seen in:**
    a. Mantle cell lymphoma
    b. Gastric marginal zone lymphoma
    c. Gastric DLBCL
    d. Follicular lymphoma

61. **Histological transformation to a typical diffuse large B-cell lymphoma does not occur in:**
    a. Follicular lymphoma
    b. Mantle cell lymphoma
    c. Marginal zone lymphoma
    d. Chronic lymphocytic leukemia

62. **True about primary diffuse large B-cell lymphoma of central nervous system is:**
    a. Can arise from leptomeninges
    b. Can arise from duramater
    c. Can manifest as intravascular large B-cell lymphomas
    d. Can be seen in immunodeficiency states
    e. All of the above

63. **True about primary diffuse large B-cell lymphoma of CNS are all, *except*:**
    a. A single lesion is present in 60–70% of cases
    b. About 20% of patients present with or develop intraocular lesions
    c. Cognitive dysfunction is more common than headache at presentation
    d. With steroid therapy, lesions may vanish within hours
    e. Majority are CD10 positive

64. True about primary mediastinal large B-cell lymphoma are all, *except*:
  a. Dissemination to liver and CNS is relatively common
  b. Bone marrow involvement is usually absent
  c. CD20 is positive
  d. CD30 is positive
  e. All are true

65. False about plasmablastic lymphoma is:
  a. Common in immunocompromised patients
  b. CD38 positive
  c. CD30 positive
  d. Poor prognosis
  e. All are true

66. Burkitt lymphoma is negative for:
  a. BCL2
  b. BCL6
  c. MYC
  d. PAX5

67. The most preferred treatment for double-hit lymphoma is:
  a. DA-EPOCH-R (Dose adjusted etoposide, prednisone, vincristine, cyclophosphamide, doxorubicin, and rituximab)
  b. R-Hyper CVAD (rituximab and cyclophosphamide/doxorubicin/vincristine/dexa-methasone)
  c. R-CODOX-M/R-IVAC (rituximab and cyclo-phosphamide/doxorubicin/vincristine/metho-trexate/cytarabine)/(rituximab/etoposide/cytarabine/ifosfamide)
  d. R-CHOP

68. True about T-cell histiocyte-rich large B-cell lymphoma is:
  a. Nodular lymphocyte predominant Hodgkin lymphoma is the most common differential
  b. PET CT is a useful investigation
  c. It is an aggressive lymphoma
  d. All of the above are true

69. According to WHO 2016 lymphoma classification, high-grade B-cell lymphomas include:
  a. Burkitt lymphoma
  b. DLBCL NOS
  c. Double-hit lymphoma
  d. All of the above

70. Which of the following is a double-hit lymphoma?
  a. BCL2 with BCL6 translocation
  b. MYC with BCL2 translocation
  c. MYC with CCND1 translocation
  d. All of the above

71. Morphologically double hit lymphomas look-like:
  a. Diffuse large B-cell lymphoma
  b. Burkitt lymphoma
  c. Blastoid variant of mantle cell lymphoma
  d. Morphological features intermediate between diffuse large B-cell lymphoma and Burkitt lymphoma
  e. All of the above

72. Which is not a feature of EBV-positive T and NK-cell lymphoproliferative disorders?
  a. Most common in childhood
  b. Severe mosquito bite allergy
  c. Associated with a hemophagocytic syndrome
  d. Good prognosis

73. True about hepatosplenic T-cell lymphoma are all, *except*:
  a. Occurs in elderly
  b. Proliferation of gamma delta T
  c. Not associated with lymphadenopathy
  d. Bone marrow is mostly involved

74. The least common type of peripheral T-cell lymphoma is:
  a. Peripheral T-cell lymphoma, not otherwise specified (NOS)
  b. Anaplastic large cell lymphoma, primary systemic type
  c. Angioimmunoblastic T-cell lymphoma
  d. Hepatosplenic T-cell lymphoma

75. Cell of origin of angioimmunoblastic T-cell lymphoma is:
  a. Mature CD4+ T follicular helper cells
  b. Activated mature CD4+ T cells
  c. Activated mature CD8+ T cells
  d. CD4+, CD25+, FOXP3+ Treg cells

76. Cell of origin of adult T-cell leukemia/lymphoma:
  a. Mature CD4+ T follicular helper cells
  b. Central memory T cells
  c. Activated mature CD8+ T cells
  d. CD4+, CD25+, FOXP3+ Treg cells

77. Silicone breast implants are associated with:
  a. Peripheral T-cell lymphoma, not otherwise specified
  b. Anaplastic large cell lymphoma
  c. Angioimmunoblastic T-cell lymphoma
  d. Subcutaneous panniculitis like T-cell lymphoma

78. True about Sézary syndrome is:
  a. It is the systemic manifestation of mycosis fungoides
  b. Its cell of origin is skin-homing memory CD4+ T cells
  c. Express CD279
  d. All of the above

79. True regarding mantle cell lymphoma:
  a. SOX11 expression is highly specific
  b. Autologous stem cell transplant upfront is indicated
  c. Rituximab maintenance following autologous SCT is indicated
  d. All of the above

80. The CD5-ve/CD10-ve lymphomas include all, *except*:
  a. Marginal zone lymphoma
  b. Lymphoplasmacytic lymphoma
  c. Hairy cell leukemia
  d. Mantle cell lymphoma

81. Which of the following lymphoma is CD10 positive?
   a. Follicular lymphoma
   b. Burkitt lymphoma
   c. Diffuse large B-cell lymphoma
   d. All of the above

82. A 48-year-old woman presented with an increasing swelling on the left side of the neck for 2 years. There were no constitutional symptoms and no organomegaly. HIV test was negative. The mass was removed and surgical biopsy of the lymph node revealed hyaline-vascular type Castleman's disease.

How would you proceed further?
   a. Surgery is enough, no further treatment is required
   b. Radiotherapy is needed
   c. Start CHOP chemotherapy (cyclophosphamide, doxorubicin, vincristine, prednisone)
   d. Observation alone, no treatment required

83. True about mycosis fungoides and Sézary syndrome is:
   a. Both originate from same T cell
   b. Sézary syndrome is the leukemic spread of mycosis fungoides
   c. Both of the above
   d. None of the above

84. Criteria for the diagnosis of Sézary syndrome include all, *except:*
   a. Absolute Sézary cell count ≥100/mL
   b. A CD4/CD8 ratio ≥10 (due to the clonal expansion of CD4+ cells)
   c. Demonstration of T-cell clonality
   d. All of the above

ANSWERS WITH EXPLANATIONS

1. Ans. a. Germinal center B-DLBCL

Ref: WHO Classification of Tumors of Hematopoietic and Lymphoid Tissues, 2008, Table 10.16

By gene expression profiling (GEP) DLBCL can be divided into three distinct subtypes: Germinal center B (GCB)-cell-like, activated B-cell (ABC)-like, and primary mediastinal B-cell lymphoma (PMBL). The t(14;18) is present in 35% of germinal center B-cell (GCB) type DLBCL, but not in activated B-cell (ABC) type and PMBL-DLBCL. The t(14;18) seen in >90% of cases of follicular lymphomas. GCB has better prognosis than ABC DLBCL.

2. Ans. b. Sex

Ref: A predictive model for aggressive non-Hodgkin's lymphoma. NEJM. 1993.

Researchers in the United States, Canada, and Europe participated in an International non-Hodgkin lymphoma Prognostic Factors Project. Patients with aggressive NHL were evaluated for pretreatment features which predicted for survival following treatment with doxorubicin-containing chemotherapy regimens. The following factors were found to correlate significantly with shorter overall or relapse-free survival: (1) Age >60, (2) Serum lactate dehydrogenase (LDH) concentration greater than normal, (3) ECOG performance status ≥2, (4) Ann Arbor clinical stage III or IV, (5) Number of involved extranodal disease sites >1. In aggressive NHL treated patients with anthracycline-based regimens that did not include rituximab, 5-year overall survival rates for patients with scores (according to IPI) of 0–1, 2, 3, and 4–5 were 73%, 51%, 43%, and 26%, respectively. Given the improved results when patients with diffuse large B-cell lymphoma (DLBCL) are treated with CHOP plus rituximab (R-CHOP), as compared with CHOP alone, a revised IPI has been developed, using the same five factors from the IPI.

3. Ans. e. All *except* b and d

Ref: Solal-Céligny. Follicular Lymphoma International Prognostic Index. Blood. 2004.

The IPI was originally developed in patients with aggressive NHL; its application to patients with indolent lymphomas has resulted in conflicting results due to a low number of patients belonging to the higher risk groups. Five adverse prognostic factors in FLIPI include: (1) Age >60 years, (2) Ann Arbor stage III or IV, (3) Hemoglobin level <12.0 g/dL, (4) Number of involved nodal areas >4, and (5) Serum lactate dehydrogenase level greater than the upper limit of normal. Since FL is an indolent lymphoma and mostly localized to nodal areas, performance status, and extranodal sites are not included in FLIPI. Similarly, because of frequent bone marrow involvement in FL compared to DLBCL, hemoglobin level reflects extent of disease. The FLIPI index divides FL into 3 risk groups: Low (0–1 risk factor), intermediate (2 risk factors), high (≥3 risk factors). The FLIPI may be used for selecting treatment in individual patients. In patients with a good prognosis (0–1 adverse factor), the 10-year overall survival is 71%. This indicates that optimal treatment in these patients has to avoid toxicity and to preserve quality of life. Involved-field radiation therapy for patients with limited disease and an initial "no treatment policy," for patients with disseminated disease may be recommended outside clinical trials.

4. Ans. d. None of the above

Ref: Williams 9/e; Hoffman 7/e

PET scanning before treatment is recommended only for those lymphomas that are routinely avid for labelled glucose (e.g., DLBCL, Hodgkin lymphoma). There is not sufficient evidence in support of the use of PET scanning for other lymphoma subtypes. Use of PET for treatment monitoring during a course of therapy should only be done as part of a clinical trial. PET scanning after completion of therapy should be performed at least 3 weeks and preferably at 6–8 weeks after chemotherapy or chemoimmunotherapy and 8–12 weeks after radiation or chemoradiotherapy. A smaller residual mass or a normal sized lymph node (i.e., ≤1 × 1 cm in diameter) should be considered positive if its activity is above that of the surrounding background. There is no role for the use of PET to follow patients in remission.

5. Ans. d. Hepatitis B virus

Ref: Engels EA. Infectious agents as causes of non-Hodgkin lymphoma. Cancer Epidemiol Biomarkers Prev. 2007;16(3):401-4.

Various viruses have been implicated in the causation of lymphomas. Infectious agents causing NHL have been classified, according to mechanism, into three broad groups: (1) Some viruses can directly transform lymphocytes. Lymphocyte-transforming viruses include Epstein-Barr virus (linked to Burkitt's lymphoma, NHLs in immunosuppressed individuals, and extranodal natural killer/T-cell NHL), human herpesvirus 8 (primary effusion lymphoma), and human T-lymphotropic virus type I (adult T-cell leukemia/lymphoma). (2) Human immunodeficiency virus is unique in causing profound depletion of $CD4^+$ T-lymphocytes, leading to acquired immunodeficiency syndrome and an associated high-risk for some NHL subtypes. (3) Some infections increase NHL risk through chronic immune stimulation. These infections include hepatitis C virus as well as certain bacteria that cause chronic site-specific inflammation and seem to increase risk for localized mucosa-associated lymphoid tissue NHLs. EBV is found in cases of endemic Burkitt's lymphoma from Africa. It has also been found in sporadic forms of Burkitt's lymphoma and of AIDS-associated lymphomas. Other lymphomas associated with EBV infection include those occurring in the setting of immunosuppressive therapy after organ transplantation and those related to chronic low-dose methotrexate therapy, usually used in the treatment of rheumatic diseases. Infection with HTLV-I has been implicated in adult T-cell lymphoma/leukemia (ATLL) seen in the Caribbean and Japan. ATLL is associated with HTLV-I infection of the tumor clone in 100% of the cases. Among lymphomas, HHV-8 infection is selectively restricted to body-cavity-based lymphomas (primary effusion lymphoma), where the viral genome is found within the tumor cells in virtually 100% of cases. HBV has not been linked to any lymphoma.

6. Ans. b. 10%

Ref: Coiffier B. CHOP chemotherapy plus rituximab compared with CHOP alone in elderly patients with diffuse large-B-cell lymphoma. N Engl J Med. 2002;346:235-42.

Rituximab is a chimeric human murine antihuman antigen CD20 monoclonal antibody. It binds specifically to the antigen CD20, a hydrophobic transmembrane protein located on normal, malignant pre-B and mature B-lymphocytes. Treatment with rituximab depletes the pool of circulating B-cells. B-cell recovery begins approximately 6 months following the completion of treatment and median B-cell levels return to normal by 12 months. Rituximab was approved by the US FDA in 1997. With the advent of combination chemotherapy with cyclophosphamide, doxorubicin, vincristine, and prednisone (CHOP) disease-free survival rates in DLBCL of 35–45% at 5 years were achieved. Survival has been further improved with the addition of rituximab to standard CHOP-based therapy (R-CHOP). The addition of rituximab results in an approximately 10% overall increase in survival beginning at 1 year from initiation of therapy in patients of all ages with almost no to mild increase in toxicity. Rituximab therapy does impose a risk of hepatitis B reactivation among patients positive for HBsAg or anti-HBc. In MInT trial, after a median follow-up of 34 months, patients assigned to R-CHOP had significantly higher rates of 3-year event-free (79% vs. 59%) and overall (93% vs. 84%) survival.

7. Ans. a. R-CHOP × 3 cycles followed by PET-CT and RT in PET negative

Ref: NCCN guidelines 2019

Limited disease (stage I or II) is defined as the disease which can be contained within one irradiation field. These patients accounts for less than 30% of patients with DLBCL. Limited stage DLBCL is treated primarily with combined modality therapy consisting of abbreviated systemic chemotherapy (3 cycles of R-CHOP), and involved field radiation therapy. An alternative, yet less desirable approach is the administration of full course systemic chemotherapy plus rituximab (6–8 cycles of R-CHOP) without radiation therapy. According to NCCN 2012 NHL treatment guidelines treatment for patients with limited disease include a combined modality approach, consisting of 3 cycles of R-CHOP (cyclophosphamide, doxorubicin, vincristine, and prednisone plus rituximab) chemotherapy followed by locoregional radiation therapy (IFRT). The studies have demonstrated that combination therapy consisting of abbreviated chemotherapy (CHOP × 3) plus radiation therapy results in at least equivalent if not improved survival when compared with 8 cycles of chemotherapy alone in patients with nonbulky limited stage disease over the first 10 years of follow-up. As combined modality therapy results in less toxicity than chemotherapy alone, this approach is preferred. Thus, for patients with limited DLBCL treatment is with three cycles of R-CHOP followed by involved-field radiation rather than six to eight cycles of R-CHOP alone.

8. Ans. c. R-CNOP regimen

Ref: NCCN guidelines 2019

Cardiotoxicity is a well-recognized complication of anthracycline therapy. The reported incidence of doxorubicin-induced cardiac dysfunction varies from 4%, at a cumulative dose of 500–550 mg/m^2, to >36% in patients receiving 600 mg/m^2 or more. The prognosis of anthracycline-induced cardiotoxicity is poor. Although anthracycline-based therapy, such as CHOP, is recommended for patients with DLBCL, patients with underlying cardiac disease may not be able to tolerate the use of an anthracycline since this agent is toxic to cardiac cells. Doxorubicin or other anthracyclines should not be administered to patients with a baseline ejection fraction below 30%. For patients who are unable to receive an anthracycline, the use of cyclophosphamide, etoposide, prednisone, procarbazine (CEPP) plus rituximab is advised. NCCN 2019 recommends CEPP (cyclophosphamide, etoposide, prednisone, procarbazine), CDOP (cyclophosphamide, liposomal doxorubicin, vincristine, prednisone), CVP (cyclophosphamide, vincristine, prednisone), CEOP (cyclophosphamide, etoposide, vincristine, prednisone), and dose-adjusted EPOCH (cyclophosphamide, etoposide, prednisone, vincristine, doxorubicin at lowest dose). Rituximab is given with all regimens. ECOG poor performance state is not a contraindication to anthracyclines if cardiac function is normal. NCCN 2019 does not mention R-CNOP in DLBCL.

9. Ans. d. Orchiectomy is the treatment of choice
Ref: NCCN Guidelines 2019

Testicular lymphoma is the most common malignant testicular tumor in men over 60 years and accounts for approximately 1% of lymphomas overall. DLBCL is the most common subtype and the median age of presentation is in the sixth to seventh decade. The prognosis is poor. Orchiectomy alone is not sufficient treatment even in the case of localized disease. Even with systemic chemotherapy, relapse is often systemic and frequently involves the central nervous system (CNS) or contralateral testis. Given the high rates of relapse at sites protected from the effects of systemic chemotherapy, prophylactic therapy directed at the testes and central nervous system should be given. Retrospective and/or nonrandomized studies have suggested that CNS prophylaxis with either intrathecal chemotherapy or high dose systemic methotrexate may decrease the rate of CNS relapse in those with primary testicular involvement.

10. Ans. c. Bone marrow is commonly involved

Primary mediastinal large B-cell lymphoma (PMBL) is considered to arise from the B-cells within the thymus. In PMBL, there is a female predominance and a median age at diagnosis is the third to fourth decade. Patients present with anterior mediastinal mass originating in the thymus, which can compress the superior vena cava causing SVC syndrome. Up to 50% of patients may have a pleural effusion. While PMBL may spread to local lymph nodes, by definition, there is no evidence of tumor spread to bone marrow or more distant lymph nodes. Approximately 75% of patients present in stage I or II disease, with masses greater than 10 cm (i.e., bulky disease) present in the majority. Diagnosis of PMBL may be difficult because obtaining an adequate biopsy specimen may be a problem. Staining for pan-B-cell markers, such as CD20 and CD79a is sufficient to establish the diagnosis in many cases. Hodgkin lymphoma (nodular sclerosing) which is a differential of PMBL, share many clinical and pathologic features. They are both more common in young women and present with a large mediastinal mass. On biopsy, PMBL may have cells that resemble the neoplastic Reed–Sternberg cells of Hodgkin lymphoma (HL). Immunophenotype can help to distinguish PMBL from HL in most cases. In classical HL, the neoplastic Reed–Sternberg cells typically express CD15 (85% of cases) and CD30 (>95% of cases, usually bright), and lack pan-B and pan-T antigens. In contrast, PMBL cells typically express pan-B-cell antigens, have weak expression of CD30, and only rarely express CD15. The optimal first-line therapy for PMBCL is unclear. DA-EPOCH-R without using radiotherapy has been preferred by some over R-CHOP.

11. Ans. d. Stomach
Ref: Kahl B, Yang D. Marginal zone lymphomas: management of nodal, splenic, and MALT NHL. Hematology Am Soc Hematol Educ Program. 2008.

Extranodal marginal zone B-cell lymphoma (MALT) is an extranodal lymphoma that arises in a number of epithelial tissues, including the stomach, salivary gland, lung, small bowel, etc. Paradoxically, they arise in sites normally devoid of lymphoid tissues and are often preceded by chronic inflammation of the affected sites leading to chronic immune stimulation, often due to bacterial or autoimmune stimuli, for example, the association of *H. pylori* infection with chronic gastritis and the development of gastric MALT. Chronic inflammation leads to the local infiltration and proliferation of antigen-dependent B-cells and T-cells. The stomach is the most frequent site of involvement. Gastric MALT lymphoma comprises about 30% of all MALT lymphomas. Most patients with gastric MALT lymphoma present with symptoms of dyspepsia, reflux, pain, nausea, and weight loss. Patients harboring t(11;18) are more likely to have widely disseminated disease, are more likely to be *H. pylori* negative. Treatment involves eradication of *H. pylori* for early stage disease and chemotherapy for advanced stage disease (single-agent rituximab, R-CVP, R-CHOP, R-fludarabine, etc.)

12. Ans. d. All of the above

Non-Hodgkin lymphoma can involve the central nervous system either as the sole area of disease (i.e., primary CNS lymphoma) or as secondary spread of systemic disease. Median survival following the diagnosis of neurologic involvement by NHL is in the range of 3-13 months. Risk of brain involvement is higher with lymphomatous involvement of bone marrow, testes, paranasal sinuses, and retroperitoneal lymph nodes. Advanced and high-risk disease, as determined by staging and the International Prognostic Index, appear to be the most important risk factors for nervous system involvement. Standard treatment regimens for CNS NHL include radiation therapy in addition to intrathecal chemotherapy with cytarabine or methotrexate. Some centers have also used high-dose intravenous cytarabine or MTX to provide drug to meningeal sites, nodular disease, and systemic burden. Patients can also be considered for autologous stem cell transplantation and has been shown to prolong survival.

13. Ans. d. Central nervous system

Ref: Ponzoni M, Ferreri AJ, Campo E, Facchetti F, Mazzucchelli L, Yoshino T, et al. Definition, diagnosis, and management of intravascular large B-cell lymphoma: proposals and perspectives from an international consensus meeting.
J Clin Oncol. 2007;25(21):3168-73.

Intravascular large cell lymphoma (ILCL) is a rare subtype of large cell lymphoma that is characterized by the proliferation of lymphoma cells within the lumina of small blood vessels, particularly capillaries and postcapillary venules, without an obvious extravascular tumor mass or detectable circulating tumor cells in the peripheral blood. According to WHO, the diagnosis of ILCL is made by demonstrating large B-cell lymphoma cells within small to medium blood vessels and capillaries. Due to the presence of lymphoma cells within the blood vessels, all cases of ILCL are considered disseminated and are therefore treated as advanced disease. CNS and skin involvement is commonly seen. Treatment is with combination chemotherapy. Anthracycline-based chemotherapy is associated with nearly a 60% response rate and a 3-year overall survival rate higher than 30%. The use of high-dose chemotherapy supported by autologous stem-cell transplantation, an important strategy to intensify treatment against NHL, may improve current outcomes.

14. Ans. a. t(14;18)

Ref: Ott G, Rosenwald A. Molecular pathogenesis of follicular lymphoma. Haematologica. 2008;93(12):1773-6.

The t(14;18)(q32;q21) chromosome translocation is considered the cytogenetic hallmark of follicular lymphoma and is encountered in 85-90% of cases. This translocation leads to the juxtaposition of the B-cell lymphoma/leukemia 2 (*BCL2*) protooncogene with enhancer sequences of the immunoglobulin heavy chain gene (*IGH*) promoter region, thereby destabilizing its expression and resulting in an overexpression of the BCL2 protein in the neoplastic follicles. The constitutive overexpression of BCL2 in germinal center B-cells caused by the t(14;18)(q32;q21) leads to an accumulation of inappropriately rescued B cells with decreased apoptosis resulting in prolonged life span, allowing for the development of additional genetic hits to occur, that finally results in overt follicular lymphoma.

15. Ans. a. Radiotherapy

Ref: NCCN, 2019; Hoffman 7/e

Approximately 15-30% of patients with follicular lymphoma (FL) will present with clinical stage I/II disease. Radiation (involved site RT, 30-36 Gy) therapy is the treatment of choice for limited stage FL and results in 10-year overall survival rates of 60-80%. However, if significant morbidity is expected from radiotherapy based on the location of the tumor or if the patient chooses against radiotherapy, initial observation may be a reasonable alternative. Chemotherapy without radiation has rarely been used in early stage disease due to the extreme radio-responsiveness of these tumors. Therefore, for most patients with stage I or II FL, initial treatment with radiation therapy rather than treatment with chemotherapy or an initial period of observation is suggested. This is principally based upon the observation that some patients may be cured with radiation therapy. No evidence indicates adjuvant chemotherapy in this setting improves survival or diminishes the risk for recurrent disease.

16. Ans. c. Chemoimmunotherapy

Ref: NCCN, 2019; ESMO Clinical Practice Guidelines, 2015

Advanced stage follicular lymphoma includes disease on both sides of the diaphragm (stage III) or diffuse involvement of one or more extralymphatic tissues (stage IV). Seventy to 85% of patients present with advanced stage disease. Patients with advanced stage disease are usually not cured with conventional treatment. While remissions can be attained, repeated relapses are common. There is no standard of care for patients with advanced stage FL. Asymptomatic patients can be observed initially. Therapy should be initiated only upon the occurrence of symptoms including B-symptoms, hematopoietic impairment, bulky disease, vital organ compression, ascites, pleural effusion, or rapid lymphoma progression. Once therapy is indicated, immunotherapy-based treatment (e.g., chemotherapy plus rituximab) is preferred because it results in superior response rates, progression-free survival, and overall survival. For asymptomatic, stable patients with advanced stage FL initial observation rather than chemotherapy at the time of diagnosis is suggested.

Chemotherapy is reserved for disease progression. This preference is largely based upon the prospective trials that have demonstrated no difference in overall survival with deferred therapy. The benefit of adding rituximab to combination chemotherapy has been demonstrated in several randomized trials of chemotherapy with or without rituximab. All of these trials have demonstrated improved response rates and time to progression when rituximab was added; many also showed an improvement in overall survival with rituximab. Progression-free survival rates at 3 years were increased approximately 15–30%.

If complete remission and long PFS are to be achieved, rituximab in combination with chemotherapy [such as CHOP (cyclophosphamide, doxorubicin, vincristine and prednisone), CVP (cyclophosphamide, vincristine and prednisone), purine analog-based therapy: FC (fludarabine and cyclophosphamide) or FM (fludarabine and mitoxantrone) or bendamustine should be used. Patients assigned to R-CHOP had significantly higher overall response rates (96% vs. 90%) and superior rates of 2-year progression-free survival (approximately 85% vs. 65%) and overall survival (95% vs. 90%) compared to CHOP without rituximab. The role of radiation therapy in advanced stage FL is limited to the use of local palliative radiation for the treatment of locally symptomatic disease.

Allogeneic hematopoietic cell transplantation (HCT) may cure a percentage of patients with advanced-stage disease, but is associated with a treatment-related mortality rate of approximately 30%. Given this high mortality rate, allogeneic HCT is reserved for young, highly motivated patients with relapsed or resistant FL. Few randomized trials utilizing autologous HCT in the treatment of newly diagnosed FL have demonstrated improvements in progression-free survival, though none have shown an overall survival benefit.

17. Ans. e. All of the above

Ref: NCCN, 2019; ESMO Clinical Practice Guidelines, 2015; Williams 9/e

Majority of patients treated for follicular lymphoma (FL) will have an initial response to therapy, but nearly all of these patients will develop progressive disease requiring subsequent treatment. Patients with recurrent FL without any symptoms do not necessarily require immediate treatment, but should be followed closely for the development of symptomatic disease. Immunotherapy either with rituximab alone or rituximab plus chemotherapy is a treatment option for most patients with relapsed or refractory disease. Single agent rituximab has response rates as high as 40% with minimal toxicity. Radioimmunotherapy with radiolabeled antibodies (ibritumomab and tositumomab) has demonstrated response rates of approximately 60–80%. Autologous HCT may prolong progression-free and overall survival rates in a subset of patients who are in complete remission or have minimal disease at the time of HCT. Myeloablative allogeneic HCT has a treatment-related mortality rate that approaches 40%, but may be curative in a highly selected cohort of patients. In contrast, reduced-intensity allogeneic HCT appears to have a lower treatment-related mortality (approximately 10–20%) with an approximately 60% long-term progression-free survival rate. FL is extremely responsive to radiation therapy (RT); low-dose RT (e.g., total dose of 4 Gy) can be used for the palliation of patients who have symptoms related to a single disease site.

18. Ans. a. Mycosis Fungoides

Ref: WHO 2017 Revised edition; Prince HM, Whittaker S, Hoppe RT. How I treat mycosis fungoides and Sézary syndrome. Blood. 2009.

Sézary syndrome (SS) and mycosis fungoides (MF) are T-cell lymphomas whose primary manifestation is in the skin. Mycosis fungoides is the most common form of cutaneous T-cell lymphoma. It generally affects the skin, but may progress internally over time. The name mycosis fungoides is somewhat misleading—it loosely means "mushroom-like fungal disease." It was so named because the skin tumors of a severe case as having a mushroom-like appearance. SS is defined by the triad of erythroderma, generalized lymphadenopathy and the presence of clonally related neoplastic T-cells with cerebriform nuclei (Sézary cells) in skin, lymph nodes, and peripheral blood. The average age of onset is between 45 and 55 years for patients with patch and plaque disease only, but is over 60 for patients who present with tumors, erythroderma (red skin) or a leukemic form (the SS). The malignant cells are small to medium in size with irregular (cerebriform) nuclei, a minority of larger cells may be present (classical Sézary cells) but only in minority. T-cell receptor genes are clonally rearranged in most cases. Complex karyotypes are present in many cases in advanced stages.

The majority of patients have slowly progressing, indolent disease; and since the disease is incurable, management is directed on improving symptoms while limiting toxicity. Management of MF/SS is based on the stage of the disease: (1) treatment of early-stage disease (IA-IIA) typically involves local skin directed therapies including topical corticosteroids, phototherapy (psoralen plus ultraviolet A radiation or ultraviolet B radiation), topical chemotherapy, topical or systemic bexarotene (retinoids), and radiotherapy, (2) Systemic approaches are used for recurrent early-stage disease and advanced-stage disease (IIB-IV) and include retinoids, such as bexarotene, interferon-α, histone deacetylase inhibitors, denileukin diftitox, extracorporeal photopheresis, systemic chemotherapy, and transplantation.

Response rates to PUVA therapy in patients with patchy disease are high with CR rates of approximately 58–83% and overall response rates of up to 95%. Cutaneous lymphomas are also highly radiosensitive.

19. Ans. c. The incidence is decreasing

Non-Hodgkin lymphomas represent about 2.4% of all cancers registered in England and Wales, and 2.6% of all cancer deaths. Prevalence rises with age and is about 50% higher in men than women. Prevalence is highest in North America and Western Europe and lower in Eastern Europe and Asia. For the past 20 years, the incidence has been rising steadily across all age groups and in both sexes, by about 3–5% per year. In most cases of non-Hodgkin lymphoma, cause is unknown. Some subtypes are associated with infection, for example, Epstein–Barr virus in Burkitt's lymphoma or postorgan-transplant immune deficiencies, and human T-lymphotropic virus in adult T-cell leukemia and lymphoma. Immunosuppression is the most clearly defined risk factor, leading to 50–100-fold excess risk. Hypertrophic splenomegaly syndrome seen in malaria endemic areas is also a risk factor B cell lymphoproliferative disorders where there is heightened B cell immune response to malarial antigen.

20. Ans. d. Lymphoplasmacytic lymphoma
Ref: Treon SP. How I treat Waldenström macroglobulinemia. Blood. 2009; Buske C. How to manage Waldenström's macroglobulinemia. Leukemia. 2013.

The immunoproliferative (plasmacytic) manifestations of LPL/Waldenström's macroglobulinemia include an IgM paraprotein in the blood and plasmacytoid differentiation in lesional cells, while the lymphoproliferative manifestations are reflected by lymphoid histologic features, lymphadenopathy, and splenomegaly. In the World Health Organization (WHO) Classification, essential features of LPL/WM include elevated monoclonal serum IgM levels in the blood of a patient with a lymphoma composed of small cells and lacking in histologic or immunophenotypic features characteristic of another specific type of lymphoma, it remains a diagnosis of exclusion. The phenotype of lymphoplasmacytic cells in WM cell suggests that the clone is a postgerminal center B-cell. Bone marrow examination is required for the diagnosis of WM and it shows bone marrow infiltration by a lymphoplasmacytic cell population consisting of small lymphocytes with evidence of plasmacytoid/plasma cell differentiation. Waldenström's macroglobulinemia typically presents as an indolent disease. The hyperviscosity associated with WM results in the characteristic manifestations of headache, blurring of vision, and cryoglobulinemia.

21. Ans. d. Lymphoplasmacytic lymphoma

The morbidity associated with Waldenström's macroglobulinemia is caused by the concurrence of two main components: Tissue infiltration by neoplastic cells and, more importantly, the physicochemical and immunological properties of the monoclonal IgM. Blood hyperviscosity is affected by increased serum IgM levels leading to hyperviscosity-related complications. Monoclonal IgM may present with cold agglutinin activity, i.e., it can recognize specific red cell antigens at temperatures below physiological, producing chronic hemolytic anemia. This disorder occurs in <10% of WM patients and is associated with cold agglutinin titers >1:1,000 in most cases. Because of its large size (almost 1,000,000 Daltons), most IgM molecules are retained within the intravascular compartment and can exert an undue effect on serum viscosity. The bone marrow is always involved in WM.

22. Ans. b. Presence of M protein
Ref: Treon SP. How I treat Waldenström macroglobulinemia. Blood, 2009; Buske C. How to manage Waldenström's macroglobulinemia. Leukemia. 2013.

The median survival of patients with WM reported in several large series has ranged from 8 to 10 years. Though IgM is implicated in the hyperviscosity, the initiation of therapy should not be based on the IgM level per se, since this may not correlate with the clinical manifestations of WM. The initiation of therapy is appropriate for patients with constitutional symptoms, such as recurrent fever, night sweats, fatigue due to anemia, or weight loss. The presence of progressive symptomatic lymphadenopathy or splenomegaly provides additional reasons to begin therapy. Anemia and thrombocytopenia owing to marrow infiltration also justifies treatment. Certain complications, such as hyperviscosity syndrome, symptomatic sensorimotor peripheral neuropathy, systemic amyloidosis, renal insufficiency, or symptomatic cryoglobulinemia, may also be indications for therapy.

An International Scoring System for Waldenström's Macroglobulinemia (ISSWM) has been developed. It divides the patients into low-, intermediate, and high-risk groups with 5 years survival of 87%, 68%, and 36% respectively. The ISSWM includes five parameters: (1) Age more than 65 years, (2) Hemoglobin less than 11.5 g/dL, (3) Platelet count less than 100,000/μL, (4) beta-2 microglobulin more than 3 mg/L, and (5) IgM more than 7 g/dL. Each parameter is given 1 point.

23. Ans. a. Mantle cell lymphoma
Ref: McKay P. Guidelines for the investigation and management of mantle cell lymphoma. BJH. 2012.

Mantle cell lymphoma is included in the WHO classification as distinct lymphoma subtype characterized by the t(11;14) (q13;q32) translocation, which results in overexpression of Cyclin D1. The clinical presentation often includes extranodal involvement, particularly of the bone marrow and gut. The prognosis of patients with mantle cell lymphoma (median overall survival, 3–5 years) is poorest among B-cell lymphoma patients.

The classic cytologic appearance of MCL is a monomorphic proliferation of small- to medium-sized lymphoid cells with irregular nuclear contours and inconspicuous nucleoli. Four cytologic variants of MCL can be recognized, including the small cell variant, the marginal zone-like variant, the blastoid variant, and the pleomorphic variant. The blastoid and pleomorphic variants are considered to be associated with a poorer prognosis. The majority of MCL cases express CD20, CD5, BCL2, and cyclin D1. The cells are usually negative for CD10, BCL6, and CD23. Although MCL, such as chronic lymphocytic leukemia, often shows CD5 positivity, these two entities must be clearly distinguished: CLL is normally FMC7 negative, CD79b negative/weak, CD23 positive, CD20 weak positive with weak surface light chain expression. At times, it may be difficult to diagnose MCL as a result of omission of immunostaining for cyclin D1 in the standard lymphoma panel, especially when CD5 is negative or weakly expressed. Moreover, cyclin D1 is also weakly expressed by hairy cell leukemia and may be detected in up to 25% of multiple myeloma cases, which may create confusion in diagnosis by bone marrow trephine biopsy assessment. Ki67 Proliferation Index should also be recorded at baseline, because index of >30% is suggestive of poorer outcome.

Though microscopic gastrointestinal tract involvement may be seen in as much as 90% of MCL cases, routine endoscopy and colonoscopy are not recommended unless patient has GIT-related symptoms. Treatment is not clear-cut though R-CHOP is widely used. R-hyper-CVAD is also the preferred first-line treatment. Fit patients in CR should be considered for autologous stem cell transplant. Relapsed patients should be taken up for reduced intensity conditioning-allogeneic stem cell transplant (RIC-allo SCT) in CR2.

24. Ans. b. Cytomegalovirus

Ref: Engels EA. Infectious Agents as Causes of Non-Hodgkin Lymphoma. Cancer Epidemiol Biomarkers Prev. 2007.

CMV does not cause NHL, all other are associated with NHL.

25. Ans. c. The presence of more than 1,000/µL monoclonal B lymphocytes

Ref: Gribben JG. How I treat CLL up front. Blood. 2010; Hoffman 6/e

Chronic lymphocytic leukemia/small lymphocytic lymphoma (CLL/SLL) is a neoplasm of mature small B-cell lymphocytes that commonly express CD5 and CD23 and have dim expression of surface IgM/IgD. For CLL diagnosis International Workshop on CLL (IWCLL) requires, in the absence of extramedullary tissue involvement, the presence of 5,000/µL monoclonal B lymphocytes with a CLL phenotype in the blood. The diagnosis of CLL may be established with lower cell counts when the patient has cytopenias or disease-related symptoms. Transformation into a more aggressive tumor occurs in 2-10% of patients (Richter syndrome). The two most common forms of transformation are DLBCL and, less frequently, Hodgkin lymphoma (HL). DLBCL arising in unmutated CLL usually corresponds to the clonal evolution of the preceding CLL, whereas in mutated CLL it frequently corresponds to a different lymphoid neoplasm.

26. Ans. c. Strongly express surface IgM

B-cell prolymphocytic leukemia is a malignancy of B prolymphocytes that affects the blood, bone marrow, and spleen and is characterized by more than 55% prolymphocytes in the blood. B-PLL does not include transformed CLL. B-PLL is an uncommon disease of old patients (median age 65-69 years) and similar male/female distribution. Patients have "B" symptoms, massive splenomegaly, absent or minimal lymphadenopathy, and a rapidly rising lymphocyte count. Anemia and thrombocytopenia are seen in 50%. The cells strongly express surface IgM with or without IgD and mature B-cell antigens. CD5 and CD23 are only positive in 20-30% and 10-20% of cases, respectively.

27. Ans. c. IRF4/MUM1 positive

Follicular lymphoma has a mature B-cell phenotype with coexpression of the germinal-center markers CD10 and BCL-6. CD5, CD43, and CD23 are negative. IRF4/MUM1, an antigen related to plasma cell differentiation, is also usually negative. BCL-2 is positive in 85-90% of FL grade 1-2 but only in 50% of grade 3. BCL-2 staining is very useful because reactive germinal centers are negative. This expression reflects the presence of the t(14;18) translocation that is the genetic hallmark of follicular lymphoma. Expression of BCL-6 also is found in most Burkitt lymphomas and DLBCLs. So, follicular lymphoma is both BCL-2 and BCL-6 positive. The MUM1 (multiple myeloma oncogene 1)/IRF4 (interferon regulatory factor 4) gene has been identified as a myeloma-associated oncogene which is activated at the transcriptional level as a result of t(6;14)(p25;q32) chromosomal translocation. Some high grade lymphomas also show MUM 1 positivity. MUM1 provides a marker for the identification of transition from BCL-6 positivity (germinal center B cells) to CD138 expression (immunoblasts and plasma cells).

28. Ans. e. All of the above

Ref: Oschlies I. Pediatric follicular lymphoma. Haematologica. 2010.

The majority of B-cell non-Hodgkin lymphomas in children and adolescents are aggressive lymphomas, predominantly Burkitt lymphomas and DLBCL. Follicular lymphomas (FL), although frequent in adults, are rare in children and account for not more than 2% of non-Hodgkin's lymphomas in this age group. Moreover, pediatric follicular lymphoma is a disease that differs from its adult counterpart both genetically and clinically. The genetic hallmark of adult follicular lymphoma, t(14;18)(q32;q21), is usually not detectable in the pediatric cases. Pediatric follicular lymphoma usually involves the head and neck region but also the testis with localized disease. The lymphomas are usually BCL-2 negative and do not carry the t(14;18) translocation. The outcome of pediatric FL is very good and, in contrast to adult FL, the clinical course is not dominated by frequent relapses, if the pediatric FL are treated according to NHL-BFM protocols.

29. **Ans. a. Stage IE**

Ref: DeAngelis LM. JCO. 2002;20:4643-8.

There is no standard staging system for primary CNS lymphoma. Using the clinical staging criteria applied to systemic non-Hodgkin's lymphoma (Ann Arbor Staging), primary CNS lymphoma is classified as a stage IE lymphoma; that is, it involves a single extranodal site, the brain. Memorial Sloan Kettering (MSKCC) group has found only two factors, age and performance status, as predictive markers of PCNSL outcome. These factors were able to differentiate patients into three very different prognostic groups. Patients with Class I prognosis (age under 60) experienced a median overall survival of 50.4 months whereas patients who were Class III (age over 60 and poor functional status) had overall survival of 13 months.

30. **Ans. c. High dose methotrexate is preferred treatment**

Ref: Marcus R. BCSH Guidelines on the diagnosis and management of adult patients with primary CNS lymphoma. 2009.

When primary CNS lymphoma is suspected, stereotactic biopsy is the preferred surgical procedure. Dexamethasone is the treatment of choice for short-term palliation but should be avoided before biopsy. Whole brain radiotherapy can provide effective palliation but is not be used as first-line therapy in patients who are sufficiently fit to receive chemotherapy. The utility of whole-brain radiotherapy in the treatment of CNS lymphoma is limited by at least three factors: (1) Insufficient local control of lymphoma; (2) dissemination of lymphoma cells within the CSF circulation, outside of the radiation field; and (3) detrimental effects of radiation on brain function. There is no role for CHOP-like chemotherapy in the treatment of primary CNS lymphoma. All patients should be offered chemotherapy as first-line treatment if they are sufficiently fit. Chemotherapy should consist of a regimen that includes high–dose methotrexate (3–5 doses of ≥ 3 g/m^2). There is no evidence supporting a role for intrathecal chemotherapy as an adjunct to high-dose intravenous MTX in patients with PCNSL. First-line treatment with high-dose chemotherapy and autologous stem cell transplantation remains experimental and should not be conducted outside clinical trials.

31. **Ans. e. All of the above** *Ref: Williams 8/e; Hoffman 6/e*

Burkitt Lymphomas carry a translocation of the c-myc oncogene from chromosome 8 to either the immunoglobulin (Ig) heavy-chain region on chromosome 14 [t(8;14)] or one of the light-chain loci on chromosome 2 (kappa light chain) [t(8;2)], or chromosome 22 (lambda light chain) [t(8;22)]. Histologically, BL is characterized by the presence of a "starry sky" appearance. Patients with limited (i.e., Stage A) disease have an excellent prognosis, with a survival rate greater than 90%. Patients with more extensive disease, especially bone marrow and CNS involvement, have a worse prognosis, but long-term survival rates as high as 80% can be achieved with more aggressive chemotherapy regimens. Murphy staging system is used for staging Burkitt lymphoma. Given the excellent results in Burkitt lymphoma of intensive regimens without allogeneic transplantation, and the high morbidity and mortality associated with this procedure, allogeneic transplantation is reserved for the setting of relapsed disease. CNS prophylaxis is given in almost all patients with BL. Radiation therapy does not play a role in the treatment of BL.

32. **Ans. d. Marginal zone lymphoma**

Ref: Williams 8/e; Hoffman 6/e

EBV-associated lymphomas in AIDS include Burkitt lymphoma, DLBCL with immunoblastic (IB) morphology, primary central nervous system lymphoma (PCNSL), Kaposi sarcoma, and primary effusion lymphoma.

33. **Ans. c. HAART plus R-CHOP**

Ref: Williams 8/e; Hoffman 6/e

Before the introduction of highly active antiretroviral therapy (HAART), the use of aggressive chemotherapy regimens in HIV patients leads to high mortality rate because of the incidence of opportunistic infections. The introduction of rituximab has significantly improved survival from NHL in this population also. So, the preferred treatment for HIV-associated NHL is HAART plus R-CHOP.

34. **Ans. d. Mantle cell lymphoma**

Mantle cell lymphoma (MCL) is characterized by a t(11;14)(q13;q32) translocation. This juxtaposes the CCND1 (BCL-1) locus to the immunoglobulin (IgH) gene sequences and leads to deregulation of cyclin D1. BCL1 is cyclin D1. Follicular lymphoma is BCL2 positive.

35. **Ans. a. Wait and watch**

Ref: Williams 8/e; NCCN guidelines, 2014

"Watch and Wait" remains a valid option in patients with asymptomatic stage III or IV follicular lymphoma. Involved field radiotherapy may also be an option in certain clinical instances. In the majority of patients with asymptomatic advanced stage III and IV disease, no curative therapy is yet established. Since the natural course of the disease is characterized by spontaneous regressions in up to 25% of cases and varies significantly from case to case, therapy should be initiated only upon the occurrence of symptoms including B-symptoms, hematopoietic impairment, bulky disease, vital organ compression, ascites, pleural effusion, or rapid lymphoma progression. In four randomized trials, an early initiation of therapy in asymptomatic patients did not result in any improvement of disease-specific survival or overall survival (OS).

36. **Ans. c. R-CHOP followed by maintenance rituximab**

Ref: Dreyling M. Newly diagnosed and relapsed follicular lymphoma: ESMO Clinical Practice Guidelines for diagnosis, treatment and follow-up. Ann Oncol. 2011.

In the majority of patients with advanced stage III and IV disease, no curative therapy is yet established. If complete remission and long PFS are to be achieved, rituximab in combination with chemotherapy [such as CHOP (cyclophosphamide, doxorubicin, vincristine and prednisone), CVP (cyclophosphamide, vincristine and prednisone), purine analog-based therapy: FC (fludarabine and cyclophosphamide) or FM (fludarabine and mitoxantrone) or bendamustine] should be used. In cases with (histologically or clinically) suspected transformation to aggressive lymphoma, an anthracycline-based regimen should be preferred. Four prospective first-line trials and two salvage trials as well as a systematic meta-analysis confirmed an improved overall response, PFS, and OS when rituximab was added to chemotherapy. The PRIMA study shows that the addition of maintenance rituximab in FL after first-line therapy improves outcomes. R-CVP or R-CHOP (mainly indicated in presence of bulky disease, raised LDH or other clinical suspicion high-grade transformation) are recommended in accordance with NICE guidance.

37. **Ans. a. Wait and watch**

Ref: Gribben JG. How I treat indolent lymphoma. Blood. 2007;109(11):4617-26.

Relapsed asymptomatic disease is not necessarily an indication for treatment, and patients can again be managed expectantly.

38. **Ans. d. Clinical trials**

Ref: Dreyling M. Newly diagnosed and relapsed follicular lymphoma: ESMO Clinical Practice Guidelines for diagnosis, treatment and follow-up. Ann Oncol. 2011.

A repeated biopsy is strongly recommended to rule out a secondary transformation into aggressive lymphoma. In early relapses (<12 months), a noncross-resistant scheme should be preferred (e.g., bendamustine after CHOP or vice versa). Rituximab should be added if the previous antibody-containing scheme achieved >6–12 months duration of remission. High-dose chemotherapy with autologous stem cell transplantation prolongs PFS and OS and should be especially considered in patients with short-lived first remissions after R-containing regimens.

Patient can be enrolled into clinical trial or can be given auto SCT after 2nd remission. If refractory to first-line therapy or early relapse postfirst-line therapy, offer the following options: (1) Fludarabine containing regimen and consider autologous or allogeneic transplantation in suitable patients; (2) dose intensified treatment as for high-grade transformation and consider autologous or allogeneic transplantation in suitable patients; (3) radioimmunotherapy if not suitable for intensive chemotherapy, or failure of stem cell harvest. Myeloablative radiochemotherapy followed by autologous stem cell transplantation prolongs PFS but not OS when used as frontline treatment for FL in four randomized trials. High-dose chemotherapy with autologous stem cell transplantation prolongs PFS and OS only in relapsed FL and should be especially considered in patients with short-lived first remissions after R-containing regimens.

39. **Ans. d. R-CHOP followed by radiotherapy**

Ref: Guideline for the Management of Non-Hodgkin's Lymphomas (NHL) in Adults, NHS 2011; NCCN guidelines 2019

Patients with nonbulky disease and no adverse risk factors (elevated LDH, PS <2) should receive combined modality therapy of 3–4 cycles of R-CHOP followed by involved site radiotherapy (ISRT). Patients with bulky disease should receive 6–8 cycles of R-CHOP. Radiotherapy (ISRT or IFRT) should be considered for residual mass at the completion of treatment.

40. **Ans. c. R-CHOP**

Ref: Guideline for the Management of Non-Hodgkin's Lymphomas (NHL) in Adults, NHS 2011; NCCN guidelines 2019.

The GELA study, NCCN and NICE guidance suggests that the patients with CD20 positive DLCBL stage II–IV disease should be offered 6–8 cycles of R-CHOP as first-line treatment. Patients with high/intermediate and high-risk disease have a higher (>50%) risk of relapse. There is, however, currently no evidence to support the use of up-front high-dose therapy (HDT) and autologous stem cell rescue.

41. **Ans. e. Autologous SCT in CR2**

Ref: Friedberg JW. Relapsed/refractory diffuse large B-cell lymphoma. ASH. 2011.

Despite overall improvements in outcomes of DLBCL, approximately 30% of patients develop relapsed/refractory disease which remains a major cause of morbidity and mortality. The standard approach to relapsing DLBCL is high-dose therapy and autologous stem cell transplantation (HD/ASCT). Prior to the rituximab era, results from the PARMA trial demonstrated improved event-free survival (EFS) and OS in chemosensitive patients who received a platinum and cytarabine-based chemotherapy regimen (DHAP) in combination with autologous SCT, compared to those who received DHAP treatment alone. In CORAL trial, a total of 396 relapsing DLBCL patients were randomized to receive three courses of either R-ICE or R-DHAP salvage therapy; responders were given HDT and autologous SCT. No significant differences were seen between R-ICE and R-DHAP in terms of overall response rates, 3-year PFS and OS. The best outcomes of HD/ASCT have been reported in patients who are negative on FDG-PET imaging before HD/ASCT. There is no standard conditioning regimen for HD/ASCT. Commonly used myeloablative regimens include BEAM, cyclophosphamide, carmustine, etoposide (CBV), and cyclophosphamide/total body irradiation (TBI).

42. Ans. e. Autologous SCT in CR2

Ref: See Q. No. 40 and 41

Overall, >30% of DLBCL will ultimately relapse. Salvage chemotherapy followed by high-dose chemotherapy (BEAM) and autologous stem cell rescue is now the standard of care in patients considered suitable. Allogeneic transplantation (reduced intensity) may be considered in suitably fit candidates who relapse after HDT and autologous stem cell rescue or who fail to mobilize sufficient autologous stem cells or who have had extensive marrow involvement. Radiotherapy (ISRT or IFRT) should be considered after these procedures to sites of residual disease or initial bulky disease. In suitable patients with adequate performance status (no major organ dysfunction, age <65–70 years), salvage regimen with association of rituximab and chemotherapy followed in responsive patients by high-dose treatment with stem-cell support is recommended. Salvage regimens such as R-DHAP (rituximab, cisplatin, cytosine arabinoside, and dexamethasone) or R-ICE (rituximab, ifosfamide, carboplatin, and etoposide) did not exhibit different outcome. BEAM (carmustine, etoposide, cytosine-arabinoside, and melphalan) is the more frequently used high-dose regimen. Maintenance with rituximab in responding patients is not recommended in DLBCL. Allogeneic transplantation following chemotherapy should probably be considered in patients with refractory disease, early relapse or relapse after ASCT.

43. Ans. a. >4 involved extranodal sites

Ref: Solal-Celigny P. Follicular Lymphoma International Prognostic Index. Blood. 2004;104:1258-65; Pastore A. Integration of gene mutations in risk prognostication for patients receiving first line immunochemotherapy for follicular lymphoma: a retrospective clinical trial and validation in a population based registry. Lancet Oncol. 2015;16:1111-22.

The Follicular Lymphoma International Prognostic Index (FLIPI) includes parameters related to patient characteristics (age), tumor burden (Ann Arbor stage, number of nodal sites), tumor aggressiveness (serum LDH level), and consequences of the lymphoma on the host (hemoglobin level). Because of contiguous spread and less involvement of extranodal sites, more than 4 involved nodal (not extranodal) sites are included. FLIPI was developed prior to the routine use of rituximab. A clinicogenetic model, termed M7FLIPI, consisting of the FLIPI risk factors, Eastern Cooperative Oncology Group performance status, and mutations in seven genes (i.e., *EZH2, ARID1A, EP300, FOXO1, MEF2B, CREBBP, and CARD11*) have been constructed and is more closely associated with outcome compared to the clinical or genetic predictors alone. The M7FLIPI is the first prognostic score in lymphoma to incorporate both genetic and clinical factors, resulting in the identification of a high-risk group in patients treated with standard chemoimmunotherapy. The high- and low-risk M7FLIPI patients have 5-year overall survival of 65% and 90%, respectively.

44. Ans. c. Rituximab

Ref: Kalpadakis C. Treatment of splenic marginal zone lymphoma with rituximab monotherapy: progress report and comparison with splenectomy. Oncologist. 2013.

Splenic marginal zone lymphoma (SMZL) is an uncommon indolent B-cell lymphoma causing marked splenic enlargement with CD20-rich lymphoma cells infiltrating blood and bone marrow. SMZL expresses B-cell antigens (CD19, CD20, CD22) and is typically CD5-negative, CD10-negative, CD43-negative, CD103-negative, and CD25-negative. The lack of CD5 distinguishes SMZL from chronic lymphocytic leukemia and mantle cell lymphoma, and the lack of CD103 and CD25 distinguishes SMZL from hairy cell leukemia.

Because splenic marginal zone lymphoma may often follow an indolent course with an overall 5-year survival rate of 80%, asymptomatic patients can be followed with a conservative "watch and wait" approach. In those patients requiring treatment, there are several different treatment approaches, including single-agent rituximab, splenectomy, and traditional chemotherapy. In the prerituximab era, the treatment of choice for patients with symptomatic splenomegaly or threatening cytopenia was splenectomy, since chemotherapy had limited efficacy. Responses to splenectomy occurred in approximately 90% of patients. Now, in rituximab era, splenectomy should no longer be considered as initial therapy for SMZL but rather as palliative therapy for patients not responsive to immunotherapy with or without chemotherapy. Rituximab is a very effective and well-tolerated therapy and may be substituted for splenectomy as the first-line treatment of choice for patients with SMZL. Patient should be given weekly rituximab for 4–6 weeks followed by maintenance rituximab every 2 monthly for 2 years.

45. Ans. a. Caused by a virus
Ref: Dearden C. Guidelines for the Management of Mature T-cell and NK-cell Neoplasm; BCSH guidelines; NCCN guidelines. 2019.

Adult T-cell leukemia/lymphoma (ATLL) is caused by the retrovirus, human T-cell lymphotropic virus I (HTLV-I), which is endemic in Japan, the Caribbean, Africa, South America, and parts of the south eastern USA. ATLL is divided into four different clinical subtypes: acute (leukemic; 57%), lymphoma (19%), chronic (19%), and smoldering (5%). The acute form is the highly aggressive form and is characterized by a rapidly proliferating white cell count and hypercalcemia. ATLL cells on morphology show characteristic "flower cells" and phenotype is invariably CD4 positive and CD25 positive. The diagnosis is based on the presence of morphologically and immunophenotypically characteristic cells together with serological evidence of HTLV-I antibodies. The prognosis for acute and lymphoma subtypes is poor with a median survival of only 6.2 and 10.2 months, respectively. The results of treatment for ATLL remain disappointing. Initial treatment involves CHOP-like chemotherapy. All patients should be given antiretroviral drug zidovudine. There appears to be minimal long-term benefit in autologous SCT in patients with ATLL with the majority of patients relapsing or dying of transplant complications within 1 year. Allogeneic transplant should be considered in 1st CR for eligible patients.

46. Ans. b. Caused by virus
Ref: Dearden C. Guidelines for the Management of Mature T-cell and NK-cell Neoplasm; BCSH guidelines; NCCN guidelines. 2019.

Angioimmunoblastic lymphoma (AITL) is difficult to diagnose and treat because of the presence of both B- and T-cell clones. It has a variable clinical course and patients present with fever, hepatosplenomegaly, lymphadenopathy, and autoimmune features. AITL is a disease of the elderly, with most patients presenting within the sixth and seventh decades. A significant proportion of patients have circulating autoantibodies (66–77%), including a positive direct antiglobulin test (DAT), cold agglutinins, cryoglobulins and circulating immune complexes resulting in autoimmune hemolytic anemia, vasculitis, polyarthritis, rheumatoid arthritis, and autoimmune thyroiditis. Histologically, AITL shows prominent vascularization by arborizing venules, expansion of CD21+ follicular dendritic cells and the malignant T-cell population expresses CD4, CD10, BCL6, and CXCL13. The CHOP or fludarabine-cyclophosphamide are considered as standard initial therapies. Consolidation with autologous stem cell transplant for patients in first complete remission should be considered in patients eligible for transplant.

47. Ans. D. All of the above
Ref: Dearden C. Guidelines for the Management of Mature T-cell and NK-cell Neoplasm; BCSH guidelines; NCCN guidelines. 2019.

In anaplastic large cell lymphoma (ALCL), the characteristic feature is the chromosome translocation t(2;5)(p23;q25) resulting in the formation of a fusion gene of nucleophosmin 1-anaplastic lymphoma kinase (NPM1-ALK). ALK-positive ALCL occurs at a younger age, compared to other T-cell lymphomas. The majority of patients present with B symptoms (75%) and 75% have stage IV disease at presentation. Inspite of stage IV at presentation and the involvement of multiple extranodal sites, the majority of patients fall into a low/low-intermediate IPI risk category because of good performance status, younger age, and a normal LDH. ALCL is a chemosensitive malignancy and has outcomes comparable to, or better than IPI adjusted DLBCL following anthracycline-based chemotherapy. In contrast to ALK positive ALCL, it is difficult to diagnose ALK-negative ALCL since, unlike ALK-positive ALCL, there is no specific marker, and histologically there is overlap with PTCL-NOS and with Hodgkin lymphoma. The IPI has predictive value in ALCL but ALK positivity is the most important prognostic factor. Patients with limited stage ALK positive ALCL and no adverse prognostic features by IPI should be treated with 3–4 cycles of CHOP chemotherapy and involved field radiotherapy, whereas advanced stage requires 6–8 cycles of CHOP. Prognosis of ALK positive ALCL is better than ALK negative ALCL.

48. Ans. c. T-cell lymphoblastic lymphoma/leukemia
Ref: NK El-Mallawany. Pediatric T- and NK-cell lymphomas: new biologic insights and treatment strategies. Blood Cancer Journal; 2012, WHO 2017, Revised Edition.

Among the various T- and natural killer (NK)-cell neoplasms comprising over 20 distinct entities in WHO classification, the most common types in pediatric patients are T-cell lymphoblastic lymphoma (T-LBL) and anaplastic large cell lymphoma (ALCL). In 80–90% of LBL, disease is T-cell lineage, unlike acute lymphoblastic leukemia (ALL) where precursor B-cell is most common. CD3 is positive along with frequent coexpression of CD4 and CD8. Thus, T-LBL is the most common pediatric T-cell lymphoma. T-LBL and T-ALL are considered having variant clinical manifestations of the same disease T-LBL is often advanced at diagnosis (stage III–IV), unlike B-cell LBL, which primarily is a localized disease. Accordingly, stage I and II T-LBLs are relatively rare. As no molecular features can yet reliably differentiate T-LBL from T-ALL, the clinical finding of 25% of marrow infiltration by malignant lymphoblasts continues to define ALL, while 5–25% marrow involvement is regarded as stage IV LBL. T-LBL is treated as T-ALL. Among mature T-cell neoplasms in pediatric population, ALK positive ALCL is most prevalent.

49. Ans. d. All of the above

Ref: WHO 2017, Revised Edition.

Extranodal NK/T-cell lymphoma of the nasal type is also known as lethal midline granuloma. It is common in Asian population. The disease most commonly affects men, with a median age of 50 years. Extranodal NK/T-cell lymphoma is EBV positive and expresses CD56. Absence of EBV makes diagnosis less likely. The disease activity can be monitored by measuring circulating EBV DNA, a high titer is correlated with extensive disease, unfavorable response to therapy and poor survival. Other T-cell markers, including CD3, are absent. Nasal symptoms with obstruction, bleeding, and a nasal mass are characteristic presenting features. It involves midline facial structures. Primary disease is treated with combined local radiation therapy and a chemotherapy regimen that includes doxorubicin. Prognosis is poor.

50. Ans. b. Rheumatoid arthritis

Ref: WHO 2017, Revised Edition

Diffuse large B-cell lymphoma that develops in the setting of long-standing chronic inflammation is typically associated with Epstein–Barr virus, and usually presents as tumor mass involving body cavities, as in pyothorax-associated lymphoma. Lymphomas with similar features are also recognized to develop in other chronic inflammatory conditions, such as use of metallic implants in bones and joints, chronic osteomyelitis, chronic venous ulcer, and use of surgical mesh implant. The patient usually presents with pain or mass lesion. The WHO has classified "DLBCL associated with chronic inflammation" as a distinct entity. It is an aggressive lymphoma. Patients with rheumatoid arthritis may also develop DLBCL around chronically inflamed joints, but these cases are EBV negative and are not considered in this category.

51. Ans. b. BCL2 and BCL6

Ref: WHO 2017, Revised edition

Double-hit lymphomas (DHL) represent a subset of highly aggressive B-cell malignancies characterized by the presence of recurrent cytogenetic rearrangements affecting MYC and either BCL2 and/or BCL6. When MYC rearrangements occur simultaneously with other translocation partners, such as BCL2 or BCL6, the resultant lymphomas have distinctive biology and highly aggressive clinical behavior and have been termed DHL. Presence of MYC/BCL2/BCL6 constitutes "triple hit" lymphomas. Patients found to have MYC rearrangements should have subsequent FISH for BCL2 and BCL6 rearrangements.

52. Ans. c. Are less common than double expressor lymphoma

Ref: Friedberg JW. How I treat double-hit lymphoma. Blood. 2017;130(5):590-6.

Lymphomas with mutations involving both MYC and either BCL2 or BCL6 have been referred to as double-hit lymphomas. Lymphomas that overexpress the proteins BCL-2 and MYC but do not have translocations in the respective genes have been referred to as double expressors. Patients with DLBCL whose tumors express both MYC/BCL2 are more common than cytogenetic double-hit lymphomas. MYC/BCL2 coexpressing lymphomas account for 21–34% of DLBCL; their outcomes appear inferior to nonoverexpressing cases but not as poor as cytogenetic MYC/BCL2 double-hit lymphomas. Patients with cytogenetic MYC/BCL2 double-hit lymphomas have an aggressive course with poorer responses to standard therapies. All patients with DLBCL should be tested for MYC and BCL2 by IHC, as their presence defines protein coexpressing lymphoma. The prognosis of double expressor lymphoma is between DLDCL and double-hit lymphoma.

53. Ans. e. All are correct

Ref: Armitage JO. Non-Hodgkin lymphoma. Lancet. 2017;390:298-310.

Both viral and bacterial infections have been closely associated with the development of non-Hodgkin lymphomas. *Helicobacter pylori* causes most gastric mucosa-associated lymphoid tissue (MALT) lymphomas. The Epstein-Barr virus is closely associated with both Burkitt lymphoma and nasal NK–T-cell lymphoma. Hepatitis C virus has been associated with splenic marginal zone lymphoma and DLBCL. *Borrelia burgdorferi* and *Chlamydia psittacosis* are thought to be associated with the development of marginal zone lymphomas, and *Coxiella burnetii* has been proposed as a risk factor for DLBCL and follicular lymphoma.

54. Ans. a. This translocation places BCL2 under control of the immunoglobulin heavy chain enhancer element

Ref: Hoffman 7/e

The immunoglobulin heavy chain (IGH) locus on chromosome 14q32 is actively transcribed in B-cells because these cells require the expression of a B-cell receptor on the cell surface for their survival. Follicular lymphoma most commonly results from the t(14;18)(q32;q21) translocation; this translocation places BCL2 (which encodes B-cell CLL/lymphoma 2) directly under control of the IGH enhancer element, leading to constitutive BCL2 expression. BCL-2 is an antiapoptotic protein, and the t(14;18)(q32;q21) translocation results in markedly elevated expression of BCL-2, which blocks the healthy germinal center default program of apoptotic cell death and represents a defining pathogenic feature of follicular lymphoma.

55. Ans. e. All of the above

Hepatosplenic T-cell lymphoma is a sinusoid gamma-delta T-cell lymphoma found in the splenic red pulp and liver sinusoids and infiltrating the bone marrow. It occurs most commonly in young, immunosuppressed men, most with either a history of organ transplant or

Crohn disease and on treatment with tumor necrosis factor alpha inhibitors. The neoplastic cells are positive for CD56 and cytotoxic markers. CD4 and CD8 are negative.

56. Ans. a. Lymphoplasmacytic lymphoma

Ref: Swerdlow SH. Lymphoplasmacytic lymphoma; WHO, 2017.

The great majority (>90%) of lymphoplasmacytic lymphoma have myeloid differentiation factor 88 (MYDBB L265P) mutation. MYD88 L265P may therefore be useful in distinguishing LPL from marginal-zone lymphoma and multiple myeloma—an often difficult task owing to overlapping morphologic, immunophenotypic, cytogenetic, and clinical features.

57. Ans. d. Central nervous system involvement by Waldenström macroglobulinemia

Ref: Minnema MC. Guideline for the diagnosis, treatment and response criteria for Bing-Neel syndrome. Hematologica. 2017;102(1):43-51.

Bing–Neel syndrome is a rare disease manifestation of Waldenström's macroglobulinemia that results from infiltration of the central nervous system by malignant lymphoplasmacytic cells. Diagnostic work-up should include cerebral spinal fluid analysis with multiparameter flow cytometry to establish B-cell clonality, protein electrophoresis, and immunofixation for the detection and classification of a monoclonal protein as well as molecular diagnostic testing for immunoglobulin gene rearrangement and mutated *MYD88*. MRI of the brain and spinal cord is also essential. The symptoms are gradually progressive in nature, usually developing over the course of weeks or months. The differential diagnosis of Bing–Neel syndrome includes hyperviscosity syndrome with neurological symptoms such as new-onset headaches, visual impairment, and spontaneous nosebleeds. Confirmation of hyperviscosity syndrome with appropriately increased IgM or serum viscosity measurements can aid in differentiating hyperviscosity syndrome-related CNS symptoms from Bing–Neel syndrome. Chemotherapy regimens commonly used for the treatment for Bing–Neel syndrome are mainly adapted from treatment schedules used in the treatment of PCNSL. These treatments include high-dose methotrexate and high-dose cytarabine for several cycles. Fludarabine, cladribine, bendamustine, and Ibrutinib have also been used.

58. Ans. e. All of the above *Ref: Hoffman 7/e*

Most patients with Waldenström macroglobulinemia have IgM serum paraprotein. Hyperviscosity occurs in as many as 30% of cases. Neuropathies occur in a minority of patients and may result from reactivity of the IgM paraprotein with myelin sheath antigens, or paraprotein deposition. Deposits of IgM may occur in the gastrointestinal tract, where they may cause diarrhea. Coagulopathies may be caused by IgM binding to clotting factors, platelets, and fibrin.

59. Ans. c. Both are true

Ref: Follicular Lymphoma. WHO, 2017.

BCL2 distinguishes follicular hyperplasia of lymph node (germinal centers are BCL2 negative) from follicular lymphoma (germinal centers are BCL2+). BCL2 is overexpressed in follicular lymphoma due to t(14,18)(q32;q21), which brings *BCL2 gene* adjacent to active immunoglobulin heavy chain (IgH) gene; however, some follicular lymphomas are BCL2 negative. The function of the BCL-2 protein is to block apoptosis. The inhibition of apoptosis leads to accumulation of B lymphocytes, which might later acquire additional mutations that eventually result in the development of follicular lymphoma. BCL2 overexpression increases lifespan of B-cells. BCL2 overexpression is the hallmark of follicular lymphoma, and BCL2 protein is expressed by a variable proportion of the neoplastic cells in 85–90% of cases of grade 1–2 follicular lymphoma, but in <50% of grade 3 follicular lymphomas. BCL2 protein can be useful in distinguishing neoplastic from reactive follicles, although absence of BCL2 protein does not exclude the diagnosis of a follicular lymphoma. BCL2 protein is not useful in distinguishing follicular lymphoma from other types of low-grade B-cell lymphomas, most of which also express BCL2. Grade 3B follicular lymphoma is biologically more closely related to DLBCL than to other follicular lymphomas. Translocations involving BCL2 are relatively rare in such cases. BCL2 is a target for BCL2 inhibitors venetoclax and navitoclax.

60. Ans. a. Mantle cell lymphoma

Most cases of multiple lymphomatous polyposis of large bowel constitute mantle cell lymphoma.

61. Ans. b. Mantle cell lymphoma

In contrast to chronic lymphocytic lymphoma and low-grade follicular lymphomas, mantle cell lymphoma, formerly known as intermediate lymphocytic lymphoma, rarely transforms histologically into large cell lymphoma.

62. Ans. a. Can arise from leptomeninges

Ref: Kluin PM. Primary diffuse large B-cell lymphoma of CNS. WHO 2017, p300-02.

Primary DLBCL of the CNS is defined as DLBCL arising within the brain, spinal cord, leptomeninges, or eye. Excluded are lymphomas of the duramater, intravascular large B-cell lymphomas, lymphomas with evidence of systemic disease, or secondary lymphomas, and all immunodeficiency-associated lymphomas. The most widely accepted prognostic markers for patients with PCNSL are age and performance status.

63. Ans. e. Majority are CD10 positive

Ref: Kluin PM. Primary diffuse large B-cell lymphoma of CNS. WHO 2017, p300-02.

About 60% of CNS DLBCLs involve the supratentorial space. A single tumor is present in 60–70% of cases, with the remainder presenting as multifocal disease. Approximately 20% of patients present with or develop intraocular lesions. Patients more frequent present with cognitive dysfunction, psychomotor slowing, and focal neurological symptoms than with headache, seizures, and cranial nerve palsies. With steroid therapy, lesions may vanish within hours. Corticosteroids have been shown to prevent diagnosis in as many as 50% of patients. CD10 positivity in a CNS lymphoma with DLBCL should prompt an intense search for systemic DLBCL that has disseminated to the CNS as CD10 positivity is rare in primary CNS lymphoma.

64. Ans. e. All are true

Ref: Gaulard P. Primary mediastinal large B-cell lymphoma. WHO 2017, p314-6.

Primary mediastinal large B-cell lymphoma frequently invades adjacent structures, such as the lungs, pleura, and pericardium. Regional involvement of supraclavicular and cervical lymph nodes can occur. At progression, dissemination to distant extranodal sites, such as the kidneys, adrenal glands, liver, and CNS, is relatively common; however, bone marrow involvement is usually absent. The absence of distant lymph node and bone marrow involvement is important to help exclude systemic DLBCL with secondary mediastinal involvement. Pleural or pericardial effusion is present in one-third of cases and is associated with inferior outcome. PMBL expresses B-cell-lineage antigens, such as CD19, CD20, CD22, and CD79a, About 80% of cases are stage I-II at the time of diagnosis. CD30 is present in >80% of cases.

65. Ans. e. All are true

Ref: Campo E. Plasmablastic lymphoma. WHO 2017, p321-2.

Plasmablastic lymphoma occurs predominantly in adults with immunodeficiency, most commonly due to HIV infection but also in the setting of iatrogenic immunosuppression (transplantation and autoimmune diseases). The neoplastic cells express a plasma cell phenotype, including positivity for CD138, CD38, and IRF4/MUM1. CD30 is frequently expressed. CD45, CD20, and PAX5 are usually negative. The prognosis is generally poor.

66. Ans a. BCL2

Ref: Leoncini L. Burkitt lymphoma. WHO 2017, p329-33.

The Burkitt lymphoma cells typically express moderate to strong membrane IgM with light chain restriction, B-cell antigens (CD19, CD20, CD22, CD79a, and PAX5), and germinal center markers (CD10 and BCL6). CD38, CD77, and CD43 are also frequently positive. Almost all Burkitt lymphomas have strong expression of MYC protein in most cells. The neoplastic cells are usually negative for CD5, CD23, CD138, BCL2, and TdT.

Diffuse large B-cell lymphomas with expression—but not rearrangements—of MYC and BCL2: These are double-expressor lymphomas, and their prognosis is better than double-hit lymphomas. Approximately 25% of DLBCLs are the high-risk subset of double-expressors, without translocations but with immunohistochemical expression of the MYC and BCL2 proteins. Without translocations, their prognosis is worse than that of routine DLBLC—about a 50% overall survival rate—but better than that of double-hit lymphomas. With R-CHOP, their 3-year overall survival is approximately 50%.

67. Ans. a. DA-EPOCH-R

Ref: Friedberg JW. How I treat double-hit lymphoma. Blood. 2017;130:590-6.

Patients with double-hit lymphomas have a poor prognosis when treated with standard chemo-immunotherapy and have increased risk of central nervous system involvement and progression. R-CHOP is not sufficient induction therapy for this group. In a study from MD Anderson cancer center, 2-year event-free survival rates in patients who received R-CHOP, R-EPOCH, and R-Hyper CVAD/MA were 25%, 67%, and 32%, respectively. Double-hit lymphoma is associated with advanced age, therefore, regimens such as CODOX-M/IVAC and Hyper CVAD/MA, which are poorly tolerated in elderly patients, are not appropriate for the majority of these patients; however, DA-R-EPOCH is better tolerated by elderly and is therefore preferred among all these regimens.

68. Ans. d. All of the above are true

T-cell/histiocyte-rich large B-cell lymphoma (THRLBCL) is characterized by a scattered, large B-cells embedded in a background of abundant T cells and histiocytes. THRLBCL may arise de novo; however, progression from nodular lymphocyte predominant Hodgkin lymphoma (NLPHL) can also result in THRLBCL, indicating that NLPHL may proceed to or contain areas indistinguishable from THRLBCL. Because THRLBCL is more PET-avid than is NLPHL, staging procedures such as FDG-PET and CT may facilitate the differential diagnosis. THRLBCL is considered an aggressive lymphoma.

69. Ans. c. Double-hit lymphoma

Ref: Kluin PM. High-grade B-cell lymphoma. Geneva: WHO; 2017. p335-41.

According to WHO, high-grade B-cell lymphoma (HGBL) is a group of aggressive, mature B-cell lymphomas that for biological and clinical reasons should not be classified as DLBCL, NOS, or as Burkitt lymphoma. There are two categories of HGBL. The first category, HGBL with MYC and BCL2 and/or BCL6 rearrangements, i.e., the so-called double-hit and triple-hit lymphomas, which have been referred to in the 2008 WHO as B-cell lymphoma, unclassifiable, with features intermediate between DLBCL and Burkitt lymphoma, is no longer recommended. The second category, HGBL-NOS, encompasses cases that either have features intermediate between DLBCL and BL or appear blastoid, but by definition do not harbor a genetic double hit as defined above.

70. Ans. b. MYC with BCL2 translocation

Ref: Kluin PM. High-grade B-cell lymphoma. WHO 2017, p335-41.

According to WHO 2016, the term double-hit lymphoma has been defined only with the co-occurrence of MYC and BCL2 and/or BCL6 translocations. Lymphomas with two oncogenic translocations other than MYC (e.g., concomitant BCL2 and BCL6 translocations without a MYC breakpoint) or other gene translocations associated with MYC translocations (e.g., CCND1 translocations) are not included in this category. The presence of only copy-number increase/amplification or somatic mutations, without an underlying rearrangement, is insufficient to qualify a case for this category.

Although so-called double-expresser DLBCLs that show immunohistochemical overexpression of MYC and BCL2 protein also have a relatively poor prognosis, overexpression is not used as a surrogate marker for double-hit cytogenetic status. Most double-hit lymphomas are also double-expressers, but most double-expressers are not double-hit lymphomas; the majority are the activated B-cell subtype of DLBCL, and do not harbor translocations. Specifically, it is important to distinguish DLBCL with MYC and BCL2 coexpression, which is not a diagnostic category, from high grade B-cell lymphomas with MYC and BCL2 and/or BCL6 rearrangements that also often show this double-expression.

71. Ans. e. All of the above

Ref: Kluin PM. High-grade B-cell lymphoma. WHO 2017, p335-41.

Double-hit high-grade B-cell lymphomas have variable morphology. Approximately half of the cases have the morphology of a DLBCL, NOS. Another subset (also accounting for about 50% of cases) shows a morphology that mimics that of Burkitt lymphoma, or has features intermediate between DLBCL and BL. Other cases may have a blastoid cytomorphology, with medium-sized cells resembling small centroblasts. Because the blastoid variant of mantle cell lymphoma shares many of these features, cyclin D1 staining should also be performed.

72. Ans. d. Good prognosis

Ref: WHO 2017, Revised Edition

Chronic active EBV infection of T- and NK-cell type shows a broad range of clinical manifestations, from indolent, localized forms such as hydroa vacciniforme-like lymphoproliferative disorder and severe mosquito bite allergy to more systemic disease characterized by fever, hepatosplenomegaly, and lymphadenopathy, with or without cutaneous manifestations diseases. Most cases have a fulminant clinical course resulting in death, usually within days to weeks of diagnosis. The disease is usually complicated by hemophagocytic syndrome.

73. Ans. a. Occurs in elderly

Ref: Gaulard P. Hepatosplenic T-cell lymphoma. WHO 2017, p381-3.

Peak incidence of hepatosplenic T-cell lymphoma is in adolescents and young adults (median patient age at diagnosis about 35 years). The neoplasm results from a proliferation of cytotoxic T cells, usually of gamma delta T-cell receptor type. There is no lymphadenopathy but bone marrow is almost always involved. Platinum-cytarabine-based chemotherapy is effective, but prognosis is poor.

74. Ans. d. Hepatosplenic T-cell lymphoma

Hepatosplenic T-cell lymphoma (HSTCL) is an uncommon neoplasm that comprises 5% of peripheral T-cell lymphomas. The majority of cases express the γδ T-cell receptor, however, recently, a small number of cases have been reported to express the αβ T-cell receptor. Typical clinical features of this lymphoma include a predominance of young male patients, an aggressive clinical course, massive hepatosplenomegaly with sinusoidal infiltration of the liver, spleen, and bone marrow, minimal lymphadenopathy, expression or rearrangement of the γδ T-cell receptor, and frequent presence of an isochromosome 7q and trisomy 8.

75. Ans. a. Mature CD4+ T follicular helper cells

Ref: WHO 2017, Revised Edition

Angioimmunoblastic (AITL) T-cell lymphoma is a neoplasm of mature T follicular helper (TFH) cells characterized by systemic disease and a polymorphous infiltrate involving lymph nodes, with a prominent proliferation of high endothelial venules (HEVs) and follicular dendritic cells (FDCs). EBV-positive B cells are nearly always present, and in some cases constitute a significant part of the cellular infiltrate.

76. Ans. d. CD4+, CD25+, FOXP3+ Treg cells
Ref: WHO 2017, Revised Edition

The postulated normal counterpart is a peripheral CD4+T cell with CD4+, CD25+, FOXP3+ Treg cell immunophenotype which is consistent with the disease's characteristic association with immunodeficiency. The disease is usually widely disseminated and is caused by the human retrovirus HTLV-1.

77. Ans. b. Anaplastic large cell lymphoma
Ref: WHO 2017, Revised Edition

Breast implant can cause anaplastic large-cell lymphoma. These lymphomas are CD30 positive and ALK negative. Patients usually present with swelling associated with a seroma and discomfort in a breast containing a silicone-coated implant. Therapy has usually included removal of the implant and associated fibrous capsule along with any associated mass. Adjuvant treatments have included various chemotherapy regimens and radiotherapy. Most patients with this entity have a good treatment outcome.

78. Ans. c. Express CD279
Ref: WHO guidelines, 2017 Revised Edition

Sézary syndrome is the "leukemic" form (i.e., involving blood) of cutaneous T-cell lymphoma, in which the dominant CD4+ T-cell population also circulates in the peripheral blood as Sézary cells and may affect internal organs. Even though SS and mycosis fungoides are closely related neoplasms, they are considered separate entities on the basis of differences in clinical behavior and cell of origin. The cell of origin of Sézary cells are circulating central memory CD4+ T cells (CD27+, CD45RA-, CD45RO+); this is in contrast to the tumor cells of mycosis fungoides, which are derived from skin-homing memory CD4+ T cells. The neoplastic T cells have a CD3+, CD4+, CD8-phenotype; characteristically lack CD7 and CD26; and express PD1 (also known as CD279) in almost all cases.

79. Ans. d. All of the above
Ref: Jain P. Mantle cell lymphoma: 2019 update on the diagnosis, pathogenesis, prognostication, and management. Am J Hematol. 2019;94:710-25.

SOX11 expression is highly specific for mantle cell lymphoma (MCL). The diagnostic significance of SOX11 is that it is helpful in the diagnosis of MCL cases, particularly those which are cyclin D1 negative. MCL is usually an aggressive lymphoma which behaves slightly different from other aggressive lymphomas in that it is difficult to cure, less sensitive to chemotherapies, higher rates of relapse, and thus needs consolidation with autologous SCT upfront. Therefore, in transplant eligible young patients auto SCT should be done upfront in first CR. Induction therapy should include high-dose cytarabine. Rituximab maintenance following auto SCT is indicated. The therapeutic options in MCL are constantly evolving, with dramatic responses from nonchemotherapeutic agents (ibrutinib, acalabrutinib, and venetoclax).

80. Ans. d. Mantle cell lymphoma
Ref: Wang HY. Diagnostic algorithm of common mature B-cell lymphomas by immunohistochemistry. Arch Pathol Lab Med. 2017;141:1236-46.

Mantle cell lymphoma is CD5+ve and CD10-ve, all other mentioned lymphomas are CD5 and CD10 negative. The classic prototypes of CD5+ve/CD10-ve lymphomas are small lymphocytic lymphoma (SLL) and mantle cell lymphoma. Mantle cell lymphoma is usually, but not always, negative for BCL6, CD10, and CD23. The three prototypic CD5-ve/CD10-ve mature B-cell lymphomas of small cell size are marginal zone lymphoma (splenic, nodal, and extranodal MZL), LPL, and HCL. Most DLBCL NOS are also negative for both CD5 and CD10.

81. Ans. d. All of the above
Ref: Wang HY. Diagnostic algorithm of common mature B-cell lymphomas by immunohistochemistry. Arch Pathol Lab Med. 2017;141:1236-46.

Follicular lymphoma and Burkitt's lymphoma are the two prototypical B-cell lymphomas expressing CD10, and the third, DLBCL is CD10+ve in approximately 10–40% patients. Assessing CD10 expression in DLBCL NOS by IHC has dual benefits. First, positive expression of CD10 in DLBCLs NOS should alert the pathologist to exclude a secondary DLBCL transformed from an underlying FL. Secondly, in the absence of transformation, positive CD10 makes DLBCL a de-novo CD10+ve DLBCL.

82. Ans. a. Surgery is enough, no further treatment is required
Ref: Talat N. Surgery in Castleman's disease: a systematic review. Ann Surg. 2012

Castleman's disease (CD) is a lymphoproliferative disorder. It is a type of angiofollicular lymph node hyperplasia. CD is classified into 3 distinct types: unicentric CD, HHV-8 associated multicentric CD, HHV-8 negative multicentric CD. Unicentric CD affects just one lymph node region. Morphologically it can be either hyaline vascular, plasma cell type or mixed type on histopathological evaluation. Complete surgical resection of the involved lymph nodes is almost always curative and is considered the gold standard for treatment of resectable unicentric CD.

83. Ans. d. None of the above
Ref: WHO Book, 2017

Mycosis fungoides subtypes and SS originate from different T-cell subsets and are genetically distinct. Clonal T cells in mycosis fungoides are derived from tissue resident memory cells, thus explaining their tendency to remain confined to the skin. The difference in the cell of origin between SS (central memory derived T cells) and mycosis fungoides (tissue resident derived memory T cells) is the reason for their distinct clinical behavior, as central memory derived T cells may be found in both the peripheral blood, lymph node and skin and are long-lived cells resistant to apoptosis, while skin-resident T cells fail to circulate in peripheral blood, remaining confined within the skin.

84. Ans. a. Absolute Sézary cell count ≥100/mL

Ref: WHO Book 2017, Hoffman

Criteria recommended for the diagnosis of SS include the following: absolute Sézary cell count ≥1,000/mL, a CD4/CD8 ratio ≥10 (due to the clonal expansion of CD4+ cells), aberrant expression of pan-T-cell antigens, demonstration of T-cell clonality (Sézary cells in the skin, peripheral blood, and lymph nodes) by Southern blot or PCR-based methods, or cytogenetic demonstration of an abnormal clone. Expression of the antigen PD-1 (programmed death-1) is reported as a reliable marker of Sézary cells.

CHAPTER 32

Multiple Myeloma and Amyloidosis

1. **Staging of multiple myeloma includes all, *except*:**
   a. Globulin
   b. Albumin
   c. Beta-2 microglobulin
   d. None

2. **Waldenström macroglobulinemia (WM) is characterized by all, *except*:**
   a. Lymphadenopathy
   b. Organomegaly
   c. Hypercalcemia
   d. Hyperviscosity

3. **Seligmann disease is:**
   a. Gamma-heavy chain disease (gamma-HCD)
   b. Alpha-HCD
   c. Mu-HCD
   d. Light-chain disease

4. **Plasma cell leukemia (PCL), on peripheral smear, should have:**
   a. <1000/µL plasma cells
   b. 1,000–2,000/µL plasma cells
   c. >2,000/µL plasma cells
   d. None of the above

5. **Hyperviscosity is commonly seen with which paraprotein:**
   a. IgM (immunoglobulin M)
   b. IgG
   c. IgA
   d. IgD

6. **True about multiple myeloma are:**
   a. Microcytic anemia may be the presenting complaint
   b. Lytic lesions are common in forearm and leg bones
   c. 20% of patients are <40 years of age
   d. It accounts for 1% of all cancers
   e. All of the above

7. **What percent of myeloma is nonsecretory?**
   a. <1%
   b. 2–3%
   c. 5–7%
   d. 7–10%

8. **Myeloma cells express the following antigens, *except*:**
   a. CD79a
   b. CD138
   c. CD56
   d. CD19
   e. All of the above

9. **Monoclonal gammopathy of undetermined significance (MGUS) is characterized by the following, *except*:**
   a. Clonal bone marrow plasma cells <10%
   b. Absence of lytic lesions, anemia, hypercalcemia, and renal insufficiency
   c. Absence of M band on immunofixation
   d. All of the above

10. **Diagnosis of solitary plasmacytoma includes all of the following, *except*:**
    a. Biopsy-proven solitary lesion that demonstrates clonal plasma cells
    b. Normal bone marrow with no evidence of clonal plasma cells
    c. Skeletal survey and magnetic resonance imaging (MRI) of the spine and pelvis are normal except for the primary solitary lesion
    d. Absence of lytic lesions, anemia, hypercalcemia, and renal insufficiency
    e. Absence of M band on serum protein electrophoresis (SPEP)

11. **Lytic lesions are seen in:**
    a. Multiple myeloma
    b. Renal carcinoma
    c. Breast cancer
    d. All of the above

12. **Indications for treatment in multiple myeloma are all, *except*:**
    a. Anemia
    b. Lytic bone lesions
    c. Extramedullary plasmacytoma
    d. M band >3 g/L
    e. All of the above

13. **The most appropriate regimen for autologous transplantation in multiple myeloma is:**
    a. Melphalan 140 mg/m^2 plus 8 Gy total body irradiation
    b. Melphalan 200 mg/m^2 plus 8 Gy total body irradiation
    c. Melphalan 200 mg/m^2
    d. Any of the above

14. **Treatment for myeloma patient relapsed 6 months after autologous stem cell transplant is:**
    a. Second autologous stem cell transplant
    b. Allogeneic stem cell transplant
    c. Matched unrelated stem cell transplant
    d. Clinical trials

15. Poor prognosis in multiple myeloma is associated with the following, *except*:
   a. deletion 13q
   b. t(4;14)
   c. deletion 17p
   d. t(11;14)

16. Side effects from thalidomide include:
   a. Somnolence
   b. Peripheral neuropathy
   c. Thrombosis
   d. All of the above

17. True regarding lenalidomide are all, *except*:
   a. Increases overall response rate and time to disease progression
   b. Causes significantly more cytopenias
   c. Safe in renal failure
   d. Can cause stem cell damage

18. Side effects of bortezomib are all, *except*:
   a. Peripheral neuropathy
   b. Thrombosis
   c. Cutaneous reactions
   d. Increased risk of herpes zoster

19. The most common site of extramedullary plasmacytoma is:
   a. Head and neck region
   b. Urinary bladder
   c. Central nervous system
   d. Lymph nodes
   e. Skin

20. POEMS (Polyneuropathy, Organomegaly, Endocrinopathy, Monoclonal gammopathy, and Skin changes) syndrome is characterized by all, *except*:
   a. Neuropathy
   b. Osteolytic lesions
   c. Endocrinopathy
   d. Myopathy
   e. All of the above

21. Cause of amyloidosis is:
   a. Production of an acquired or inherited variant protein with an abnormal structure
   b. Normal concentration of amyloidogenic protein
   c. Sustained abnormally high concentration of certain normal proteins
   d. All of the above

22. Bendamustine can be used in:
   a. Chronic lymphocytic leukemia (CLL)
   b. Follicular lymphoma
   c. Multiple myeloma
   d. All of the above

23. Radiological finding of multiple myeloma is:
   a. Bony mass
   b. Lytic lesions
   c. Osteoporosis
   d. All of the above

24. Systemic amyloidosis involves all, *except*:
   a. Eyes
   b. Peripheral nervous system
   c. Central nervous system
   d. Tongue
   e. All of the above

25. True about diagnosis of amyloid light-chain (AL) amyloidosis are all, *except*:
   a. Abdominal fat by needle aspiration is diagnostic in 50–80% of cases
   b. The appearance on hematoxylin and eosin-stained tissue of pink amorphous material should raise suspicion of amyloid
   c. Congo red stain is generally accepted to be the diagnostic gold standard in amyloidosis.
   d. Serum amyloid P (SAP) scintigraphy is must for diagnosis

26. True about cardiac amyloidosis are all, *except*:
   a. Symptomatic cardiac amyloid is associated with a survival of 4–6 years
   b. NT-proBNP (N-terminal pro b-type natriuretic peptide) concentration has prognostic significance
   c. Cardiac amyloidosis is a restrictive cardiomyopathy
   d. All of the above

27. Treatment of AL amyloidosis is:
   a. Autologous stem cell transplantation
   b. Melphalan and dexamethasone
   c. Cyclophosphamide, thalidomide, and dexamethasone (CTD)
   d. Bortezomib
   e. All of the above

28. Indications for serum-free light-chain assessment are:
   a. Screening for the presence of myeloma or related disorders
   b. Prognostic value
   c. Monitoring of patients with oligosecretory plasma-cell disorders
   d. Documenting stringent complete response
   e. All of the above

29. Mechanism of action of denosumab is:
   a. Inhibition of RANKL
   b. Inhibition of osteoprotegerin (OPG)
   c. Inhibition of Dickkopf-1 (DKK1)
   d. Inhibition of MUM1
   e. All of the above

30. Denosumab differs from zoledronic acid in that it does not cause:
   a. Hypocalcemia
   b. Osteonecrosis of jaw
   c. Hypophosphatemia
   d. Both cause all of the above

31. Daratumumab acts on:
 a. Natural killer (NK) cells b. Platelets
 c. Plasma cells d. Red blood cells (RBCs)
 e. All of the above

32. False regarding daratumumab is:
 a. It is an IgG1kappa human monoclonal antibody
 b. Interferes with the SPEP
 c. Interferes with the indirect Coomb's test
 d. Interferes with blood grouping
 e. None of the above

33. True regarding bortezomib and carfilzomib is:
 a. Both are reversible inhibitors of proteasome
 b. Both contain boronic acid
 c. Both are structurally and mechanistically similar
 d. Both have nearly similar cytotoxic responses and tolerability profile
 e. None of the above   f. All of the above

34. How bortezomib works?
 a. It inhibits protein synthesis.
 b. It augments protein synthesis.
 c. It inhibits protein degradation.
 d. It augments protein degradation.

35. Most sensitive method for assessment of minimal residual disease (MRD) in multiple myeloma is:
 a. Serum-free light-chain assay and immunofixation
 b. 4-6-color flowcytometry
 c. Next-generation sequencing (NGS)
 d. All have equal sensitivity

36. True regarding maintenance therapy in myeloma is:
 a. Maintenance therapy should be offered to all patients after transplant
 b. Lenalidomide maintenance confers a significant overall survival gain for low-risk patients
 c. Bortezomib-based therapy as a single agent for maintenance therapy has been shown to overcome the negative impact of del17p
 d. Both a and b
 e. All of the above

37. The organ which is not involved by amyloid light-chain (AL) amyloidosis is:
 a. Spleen b. Joints
 c. Liver d. Brain

38. The pathophysiology of AL amyloidosis involves:
 a. Deposition of normally produced beta pleated sheets
 b. Defective configuration of alpha-helical light-chains
 c. Excessive deposition of alpha-helical light-chains
 d. All of the above

39. Which of the following is true about AL amyloidosis?
 a. Around 20% of patients with light-chain amyloidosis also have a concurrent diagnosis of MM
 b. All patients with AL amyloid have clonal light-chain production
 c. There is clonal population of plasma cells in the bone marrow
 d. All of the above

40. Not true about AL amyloidosis is:
 a. The prognosis is poor
 b. Subcutaneous fat aspirate demonstrates amyloid deposits in 75% of patients
 c. Staining of the bone marrow biopsy for amyloid deposition in blood vessels is positive in 50% cases
 d. Amyloid is highly resistant to solubilization
 e. Congo staining is diagnostic of AL amyloidosis

41. All are used in treatment of AL amyloid, *except*:
 a. Dezamizumab b. Doxycycline
 c. Miridesap d. Diflunisal

42. Most common structural cytogenetic abnormality in AL amyloidosis associated with poor prognosis is:
 a. t(11;14) b. gain of 1q
 c. del13q d. t(14;16)

43. Prognostic markers for cardiac AL amyloidosis involve all of the following parameters, *except*:
 a. Difference in free light chains >18 mg/dL
 b. Trop T >0.025 µg/L c. NT-Pro-BNP >1,800 ng/L
 d. Cardiac MRI

44. True about cardiac involvement in AL amyloidosis is:
 a. Diagnosis should be suspected in a patient with heart failure with severely reduced ejection fraction
 b. Echocardiography can diagnose most of the cases of cardiac amyloidosis and is the investigation of choice
 c. NT-Pro-BNP levels increase only when patient develops symptomatic left ventricular dysfunction
 d. All of the above e. None of the above

45. Risk stratification of smouldering multiple myeloma includes all, *except*:
 a. Bone marrow plasma cells > 20%
 b. Serum free light chain ratio > 20
 c. Serum creatinine > 2 mg/dL
 d. Serum M band >2 g/dL

46. A 58 years old male presented with fever, palpable lymphadenopathy, hepatosplenomegaly and chronic urticaria for 3 months duration. Investigations revealed leucocytosis with IgM paraprotein. Patient likely has:
 a. Schnitzler syndrome b. C1 esterase deficiency
 c. Stills disease d. Acute leukemia

47. Belantamab mafodotin is an approved for:
 a. ETP ALL b. Multiple myeloma
 c. TTP d. DLBCL

ANSWERS WITH EXPLANATIONS

1. Ans. a. Globulin *Ref: Williams 7/e*

The International Staging System (ISS) includes only albumin and beta-2-microglobulin and divides multiple myeloma into three stages. Stage I—b_2m <3.5 mg/L and serum albumin ≥3.5 g/dL. Stage III—b_2m ≥5.5 mg/L. Patients with b_2m < 3.5 mg/L and albumin < 3.5 g/dL were classified as stage II. The median overall survival for patients with ISS stages I, II, and III are 62, 44, and 29 months, respectively. The ISS should be used only in patients with symptomatic, overt myeloma; it should not be used in patients with smoldering myeloma or MGUS since its value in such populations is not known.

2. Ans. c. Hypercalcemia
Ref: Treon SP. How I treat Waldenstrom macroglobulinemia. Blood. 2009.

Waldenström macroglobulinemia demonstrates lymphoplasmacytic lymphoma (LPL) in the bone marrow with an IgM monoclonal gammopathy in the blood. Patients may present with symptoms related to the infiltration of the hematopoietic tissues or the effects of monoclonal IgM in the blood. A diagnosis of IgM multiple myeloma is preferred over a diagnosis of WM if bone lesions are present. Symptoms of hyperviscosity and the presence of lymphadenopathy and/or splenomegaly favor a diagnosis of WM. Easy bruisability, cold agglutinin disease, and peripheral neuropathy may also be present. Hypercalcemia is usually a feature of multiple myeloma where there is significant bone involvement. To establish the diagnosis of WM, it is necessary to demonstrate an IgM monoclonal protein, along with histologic evidence of infiltration of the bone marrow by lymphoplasmacytic cells. Whereas IgM levels will be elevated in almost all WM patients, IgA and IgG levels are subnormal and may contribute to recurring sinus and bronchial infections.

3. Ans. b. Alpha-HCD
Ref: Seligmann M. Alpha-chain disease. J Clin Pathol. 1975.

Alpha-HCD is a type of HCD characterized by the production of incomplete monoclonal alpha-heavy chains without associated light chains. Alpha-HCD is considered to be a subtype of immunoproliferative small intestinal disease (IPSID). Alpha-HCD appears to be a condition affecting the secretory IgA system and mainly the digestive tract. Its age distribution is in sharp contrast to that of multiple myeloma since it occurs mainly in the second and third decades of life (20–30 years). Patients present with symptoms of malabsorption. Diarrhea, weight loss, and abdominal pain are common. Infiltration of the jejunal mucosa with plasmacytoid cells is the most frequent pathologic feature. The diagnosis of alpha-HCD is based on identification of free alpha-heavy chains without associated light chains. Truncated alpha-heavy chains can be detected in biological fluids (serum, urine, jejunal secretions) by immunoelectrophoresis or immunofixation. Alpha-HCD disease must be differentiated from non-Hodgkin lymphoma (NHL) and needs exclusion of celiac disease. For patients with symptomatic disease not responding adequately to antibiotics, chemotherapy similar to that used to treat NHL is recommended.

4. Ans. c. >2,000/µL plasma cells
Ref: van de Donk. How I treat plasma cell leukemia. Blood. 2012.

Primary PCL is the most aggressive form of the plasma-cell disorders. It is defined by the presence of >2,000/µL peripheral blood plasma cells or plasmacytosis accounting for 20% of the differential white cell count and does not arise from pre-existing MM. Circulating monoclonal plasma cells can also be detected using a slide-based immunofluorescence assay, a two-color immunoassay technique (ELISPOT), or flow cytometry by gating on CD38+/CD45 cells. When PCL develops from MM, then it is referred to as secondary PCL. Compared with classic MM, PCL has both a different biologic background and distinct clinical and laboratory features. The prognosis of PCL is very poor, with a median overall survival of only 7–8 months with standard chemotherapy. In contrast to MM, the dissemination of tumor cells out of the bone marrow in PCL is related not only to changes in expression of adhesion molecules and chemokine receptors on plasma cell but also to the presence of several molecular aberrations, which contribute to bone marrow microenvironment-independent tumor growth, inhibition of apoptosis, and escape from immune surveillance.

5. Ans. a. IgM (immunoglobulin M)
Ref: Stone MJ. Evidence-based focused review of management of hyperviscosity syndrome. Blood. 2012.

IgM, which is a giant molecule and 80% of it remains intravascular, is the most common cause of hyperviscosity. The most common condition in which IgM is raised is WM. The serum viscosity is measured by the Ostwald viscometer (capillary tube method). It is a simple, cheap, and reliable method for measuring relative serum viscosity in patients. The viscosity of water at 20°C is 1.0 centipoise. Viscosity is measured by the time required for a serum or plasma sample to flow through a tube under the influence of gravity. Viscous samples flow more slowly and hence have high viscosity. The most common automated viscometers used is the cone/plate type. Normal viscosity measured with an Ostwald tube is 1.4–1.8 relative to water. Hyperviscosity is unlikely unless the serum viscosity is >4. For IgM paraproteins, relative viscosity can rise exponentially above a concentration of 3 g/dL. Plasmapheresis is a safe and effective short-term treatment for hyperviscosity in WM because it can easily remove IgM as most of it remains in vessels (80% intravascular). A relatively small reduction in IgM concentration has a significant effect on lowering serum viscosity and hence reduction in clinical manifestations. Urgent plasmapheresis should be carried out for patients having visual or central nervous symptoms in WM to reduce the likelihood of blindness from retinal hemorrhages or CNS manifestations. Plasma exchange has transient effects only and does not affect the underlying disease process, and so chemotherapy should be started concomitantly. Plasma exchange reduces plasma viscosity approximately 20–30% per cycle. Patients started on Rituximab can have a flare due to transient increases in IgM levels. Therefore, it is recommended that plasmapheresis be carried out before starting rituximab if serum viscosity is more or IgM level is >5 g/dL or omitting the rituximab for the first one or two cycles of combination chemotherapy [such as R-CVP (rituximab plus cyclophosphamide, vincristine, and prednisone) or BR (bendamustine plus rituximab)].

6. Ans. d. It accounts for 1% of all cancers

Ref: Williams 7/e; Hoffman 5/e

Multiple myeloma (MM) accounts for approximately 1% of all cancers and slightly more than 10% of hematologic malignancies. MM is a disease of elder patients. The median age at diagnosis is 66 years; only 2% of patients are younger than 40 years. A normocytic, normochromic anemia (hemoglobin ≤12 g/dL) is present in 73% at diagnosis (not microcytic hypochromic). This anemia can be related to bone marrow replacement, kidney damage, or can be due to dilution in the case of a large M-protein. The skeletal survey for patients with MM includes a posteroanterior view of the chest, anteroposterior and lateral views of the cervical spine (including an open mouth view), thoracic spine, lumbar spine, humeri and femora, anteroposterior and lateral views of the skull and anteroposterior view of the pelvis. The most frequent sites of lytic lesions include areas with active hematopoiesis, such as the vertebral bodies, skull, thoracic cage, pelvis, and proximal humeri and femora. Distal limbs and hands and feet bones are rarely involved.

7. Ans. b. 2–3%

Ref: WHO classification of tumors of hematopoietic and lymphoid tissues. 2008.

Symptomatic myeloma without detectable monoclonal immunoglobulin levels on serum or urine immunofixation electrophoresis characterizes non-secretory myeloma by the World Health Organization (WHO) definition. SPEP demonstrates a localized band or peak in 82% of patients with multiple myeloma. Addition of serum protein immunofixation increases the sensitivity to 93%. If, in addition, a urine protein electrophoresis and urine immunofixation are done, the sensitivity increases to 97%. The remaining 3% of patients who lack detectable M protein by any of these tests are considered to have "nonsecretory myeloma." Up to 20% of myeloma is characterized by only a light chain in the serum or urine, lacking expression of the immunoglobulin heavy chain. These patients can be detected by urine protein electrophoresis and urine immunofixation. Of the nonsecretory myeloma, the majority (approximately 85%) will have M-protein that can be detected in the cytoplasm of the neoplastic plasma cells by immunochemistry but have impaired secretion of this protein (i.e., nonsecretory myeloma). The other 15% do not have immunoglobulin detectable in the plasma cells (i.e., nonproducer myeloma). The proposed pathophysiology of nonsecretory myeloma includes the diminished capacity to synthesize immunoglobulins, defects in secretion, and rapid degradation of immunoglobulins. The manifestations and overall survival of secretory and nonsecretory myeloma are comparable, though nonsecretory myeloma is less aggressive.

8. Ans. d. CD19

Ref: Kumar S. Immunophenotyping in multiple myeloma and related plasma cell disorders. Best Pract Res Clin Haematol. 2010.

Non-neoplastic polyclonal plasma cells are normal components of a bone marrow aspirate and increase in many benign inflammatory conditions, and need to be distinguished from neoplastic, clonal plasma cells of plasma-cell dyscrasias. Like normal plasma cells, myeloma cells also express CD79a, CD138, and CD38. However, in contrast to normal plasma cells, myeloma cells infrequently express CD19. Identification of the plasma cells has typically been based on the demonstration of high CD38 and CD138 expression. In addition to CD38 and CD138, normal plasma cells are generally positive for CD19 and CD45 whereas abnormal plasma cells characteristically lack CD19 and variably express CD45. Further the clonality of plasma cells can be confirmed based on the light-chain restriction pattern, i.e., presence of either kappa or lambda cytoplasmic immunoglobulin light chains. Expression of CD56 (neural cell adhesion molecule) is also commonly used to identify abnormal plasma cells, since normal plasma cells typically lack CD56. WM is typically associated with lymphoplasmacytoid cells which are typically CD19 and CD38 positive and variably express CD138. In contrast to typical plasma-cell neoplasms, however, the plasma cells in LPL are almost always CD19 and CD45 positive. CD20 is not expressed by normal plasma cells. The most important findings that characterize malignant versus normal plasma cells are Absent or low expression of CD27, CD19, and/or CD45; increased expression of CD28, CD33, CD117, and/or CD56; and monoclonal light-chain restriction.

9. Ans. c. Absence of M band on immunofixation

Ref: Landgren O. Monoclonal Gammopathy of Undetermined Significance and Smoldering Myeloma. ASH. 2010.

Robert Kyle coined the term "monoclonal gammopathy of undetermined significance" (MGUS) in 1978. Screening studies have found MGUS to be present in approximately 3.2% of Caucasians above the age of 50 years. MGUS has three features: (1) Serum monoclonal protein (whether IgA, IgG, or IgM) <3 g/100 mL, (2) clonal bone marrow plasma cells <10%, and (3) absence of end-organ damage (lytic lesions, anemia, hypercalcemia, and renal insufficiency). MGUS carries a risk of progression to multiple myeloma of approximately 1% per year. MGUS can be divided into two types—the first is on the basis of the cell type (plasma-cell or lymphoid cell MGUS) and the second is on the risk of progression (low-risk or high-risk MGUS). Plasma-cell MGUS tumors can progress to multiple myeloma or related plasma-cell disorders, whereas lymphoid MGUS tumors progress to WM, lymphoma, or other malignant lymphoproliferative disorders. MGUS can be divided into low risk and high risk based on (1) quantity of M band (< or >1.5 g/dL), (2) type of M band (IgG or non-IgG), and serum-free light-chain ratio (normal or abnormal). High-risk MGUS has a high risk of progression to myeloma compared to low-risk MGUS but requires no treatment at present.

10. Ans. e. Absence of M band on serum protein electrophoresis (SPEP)

Ref: Williams 7/e; Hoffman 5/e

The diagnosis of solitary plasmacytoma requires the following four criteria: (1) Biopsy-proven solitary lesion of the bone or soft tissue that demonstrates clonal plasma cells, (2) normal bone marrow with no evidence of clonal plasma cells, (3) skeletal survey and MRI of the spine and pelvis are normal except for the primary solitary lesion, and (4) absence of lytic lesions, anemia, hypercalcemia, and renal insufficiency [no CRAB (hypercalcemia, renal insufficiency, anemia, and bone lesions)]. M band may be present in plasmacytoma which disappears after treatment. Radiotherapy is the treatment of choice. The patient should receive a dose of 40–50 Gy over approximately 4 weeks. Radiotherapy localized to the tumor site should be given even if the plasmacytoma appears to have been completely excised for diagnostic purposes. Overt multiple myeloma ultimately develops in 50–60% of patients with solitary plasmacytoma of bone. The presence or absence of an M protein at the time of diagnosis of solitary plasmacytoma does not appear to have a major effect on long-term outcome, although persistence of a serum M-protein after radiation therapy appears to be a significant predictor of subsequent progression to multiple myeloma.

11. Ans. d. All of the above

Metastatic carcinoma (e.g., kidney, breast, nonsmall cell lung cancer) can produce lytic lesions, and few patients presenting in this way may have metastatic cancer with an associated, unrelated monoclonal gammopathy. Patients presenting with lytic bone lesions, constitutional symptoms, a small M component, and fewer than 10% clonal plasma cells in the bone marrow are more likely to have metastatic carcinoma with an unrelated MGUS rather than multiple myeloma. Other conditions such as hyperparathyroidism, fibrous dysplasia, eosinophilic granuloma, and histiocytosis can also produce lytic lesions.

12. Ans. d. M band >3 g/L

Ref: Haehle M. Smoldering myeloma and MGUS: ASH 2013 preview.

Smoldering myeloma is a precursor for multiple myeloma. The disease is characterized by an excess of monoclonal protein in the blood and urine, but, by definition, smoldering myeloma patients do not have any myeloma-related symptoms. The following are indications for treatment in plasma-cell dyscrasia: Anemia (i.e., hemoglobin <10 g/dL or 2 g/dL below normal), hypercalcemia (i.e., serum calcium >11.5 mg/dL), renal insufficiency (i.e., serum creatinine >2 mg/dL), lytic bone lesions or severe osteopenia, and extramedullary plasmacytoma. M band without symptoms is not an indication for treatment. A diagnosis of smoldering multiple myeloma is made when a patient's monoclonal protein level (M-spike) is at least 3 g/dL or the proportion of plasma cells in the bone marrow is at least 10%. The risk of progression from smoldering myeloma to symptomatic myeloma is estimated to be about 10% per year. The current standard of care for smoldering myeloma is a "watch and wait" approach, which involves monitoring the patient regularly and beginning treatment only after the disease progresses to symptomatic myeloma.

13. Ans. c. Melphalan 200 mg/m^2

Ref: Moreau P. The Intergroupe Francophone du Myélome 9502 randomized trial. Blood. 2002.

The study [Intergroupe Francophone du Myélome (IFM) 9502 trial] compared the two most widely used conditioning regimens before autologous stem cell transplantation: 8 Gy total body irradiation plus 140 mg/m^2 melphalan versus 200 mg/m^2 melphalan. The study showed that melphalan 200 mg/m^2 had significantly faster hematologic recovery, less transfusion requirements, shorter hospitalizations, and a lower incidence of severe mucositis (30% vs. 50%). While the median duration of event-free survival was similar in both arms (21 months), survival at 45 months was significantly better in patients receiving melphalan 200 mg/m^2 (66% vs. 46%). Total body irradiation increased toxicity.

14. Ans. d. Clinical trials

Treatment options for relapsed multiple myeloma after an autologous HCT include a second autologous HCT, allogeneic HCT as part of a clinical trial, or treatment with salvage chemotherapy regimens. Patients who relapse within the first 12 months have a shorter median overall survival when compared with those who relapse after 12 months. A second autologous HCT is not recommended for patients who relapse within 12 months of the first, since the progression-free survival following the second HCT will most likely be even shorter than the benefit seen with the first transplant. These patients are best treated with active agents that they have not received before or have had good responses to in the past as well as clinical trials investigating novel therapies. The agents with novel mechanisms of action useful in myeloma are monoclonal antibodies (anti-CD38 MoAb, such as daratumumab), cell cycle-specific drugs, deacetylase inhibitors, agents acting on the unfolded protein response, signaling transduction pathway inhibitors, and kinase inhibitors. Marizomib is an irreversible proteasome inhibitor administered intravenously. Ixazomib is an orally administered reversible proteasome inhibitor. Pomalidomide, like lenalidomide, is an immunomodulatory compound with pleiotropic properties shown to be beneficial in treating multiple myeloma.

15. Ans. d. t(11;14)

Ref: Fonseca R. Genetics and cytogenetics of multiple myeloma. Cancer Res. 2004
WHO 2008 (Table 10.09)

Understanding the biology of multiple myeloma genetics lagged behind other hematological malignancies because of the low yield for karyotype abnormalities from multiple myeloma bone marrow samples. Multiple myeloma has been successfully studied by interphase FISH (fluorescence in situ hybridization), because this assay can be done in nondividing cells. Cytogenetic evaluation is mandatory in all patients with newly diagnosed multiple myeloma and should always include interphase FISH in isolated plasma cells. According to the International Myeloma Working Group, the term high-risk multiple myeloma includes patients with one of the following features: deletion of 17p, t(4;14) or t(14;16), detected by FISH analysis. Hypodiploidy and t(14;20) are also considered high-risk factors. Monosomy 13/13q deletions are also considered as high risk. When detected by conventional cytogenetics, the presence of a chromosome 13 deletion signifies a more pronounced poor outcome. The adverse prognosis of chromosome 13 deletion has been independent of the treatment approach using chemotherapy, autotransplantation, or miniallogeneic transplantation. Deletions of 17p13, the p53 locus, are also associated with a shorter survival after both conventional and hematopoietic cell transplantation. This deletion is highly associated with disease progression, advanced disease stages, PCL, and central nervous system multiple myeloma. The t(4;14) is also associated with poor prognosis. The t(11;14), t(6;14) and hyperdiploidy are associated with a favorable prognosis.

16. Ans. d. All of the above

Thalidomide is a derivative of glutamic acid, an oral agent with antiangiogenic and immunomodulatory properties. Thalidomide is poorly soluble in water and thus no parenteral preparation is available. Cereblon has been identified as a primary target of thalidomide activity, which is also required for its antimyeloma activity. Thalidomide binds to and inactivates cereblon, which leads to an antiproliferative effect on myeloma cells.

Thalidomide can cause constipation, weakness, fatigue, or somnolence in about 25% patients. A dose-dependent peripheral neuropathy (sensory more than motor axonal neuropathy) occurs in up to 30–80% of patients with prolonged therapy and may not be reversible. Thrombotic complications can occur with thalidomide therapy and incidence increases up to 25% of patients when thalidomide plus dexamethasone are used. The severity of sedation appears to decrease with continued administration at a constant dose and can be minimized by taking the drug in the evening before going to bed. Constipation is a common side effect and its severity may be dose-related. The most serious adverse effects associated with thalidomide are deep vein thrombosis and peripheral neuropathy.

17. Ans. c. Safe in renal failure

Lenalidomide is a synthetic compound derived by modifying the chemical structure of thalidomide to improve its potency and reduce its side effects. Lenalidomide is a 4-amino-glutamyl analog of thalidomide that lacks the neurologic side effects of sedation and neuropathy. It is approved by FDA for clinical use in myelodysplastic syndromes with deletion of chromosome 5q and multiple myeloma. The immune system has two major components: one is cellular (mediated by macrophages, dendritic cells, NK cells, T cells, and B cells) and the second is humoral (mediated by antibodies and cytokines). Lenalidomide is an immunomodulator, affecting both cellular and humoral components of the immune system. It also has antiangiogenic properties. The immune system can prevent development of cancers by multiple ways including suppressing oncogenic agents, altering the local milieu conducive to tumor growth, and by immune surveillance by identifying and destroying cancer cells. Lenalidomide has been shown to inhibit production of proinflammatory cytokines TNF-α, interleukin-1 (IL-1), IL-6, IL-12 and elevate the production of anti-inflammatory cytokine IL-10. Reduction in IL-6 and TNF-α levels leads to its antimyeloma activity. IL-6 inhibits the apoptosis of myeloma cells and helps in their proliferation. Lenalidomide downregulates the production of IL-6 and is thus effective in myeloma.

The most common severe (grade 3/4) toxicities seen in patients treated with lenalidomide plus dexamethasone include neutropenia (30-40%), anemia (9-13%), thrombocytopenia (12-15%), and venous thromboembolism (11%). Lenalidomide is secreted via the kidneys and should be used with caution in patients with renal impairment. For multiple myeloma patients, the normal starting dose of lenalidomide is 25 mg/day on days 1-21 of repeated 28-day cycles. According to new recommendations, patients with moderate kidney impairment should only receive 10 mg/day and patients with severe kidney impairment should only receive 15 mg every other day.

Prolonged treatment can lead to difficulty in harvesting stem cells. With the prolonged use of lenalidomide, (1) the number of CD34+ cells collected is reduced, (2) the number of collections to obtain a target number of cells increased, and (3) the number of failed collections is increased in patients whose initial therapy contained lenalidomide when mobilized with granulocyte-colony stimulating factor (G-CSF) alone. However, up to four cycles of lenalidomide exposure have minimal negative impact on peripheral blood stem cell (PBSC) collection.

Other reported long-term complications with the use of lenalidomide are risk of second malignancies. Tumor flare reaction has also occurred during the use of lenalidomide for CLL and lymphoma and is characterized by tender lymph node swelling, low-grade fever, pain, and rash.

18. Ans. b. Thrombosis

Bortezomib is a novel proteasome inhibitor. It functions in myeloma via the inhibition of the breakdown of inhibitory kappa B (IκB) and consequently stabilization of the nuclear factor kappa B (NF-κB) complex. This prevents NF-κB translocation to the nucleus with consequent inactivation of multiple downstream pathways known to be important in myeloma cell signaling. Other effects in myeloma include inhibition of angiogenesis, inhibition of DNA repair, and impairment of osteoclast activity. Peripheral neuropathy is the most common dose-limiting toxicity. Peripheral neuropathy, often painful, develops in approximately 35% of patients. It is more frequent and severe in those who have previously received neurotoxic therapy and those with preexisting neuropathy. Thrombocytopenia occurs in 43% of patients but is rarely severe enough to postpone subsequent cycles. Platelet count nadir typically occurs at day 11 and drops to approximately 40% of baseline. Bortezomib therapy may be associated with an increased risk of herpes zoster (varicella zoster reactivation). Antiviral prophylaxis should be given to all patients receiving bortezomib therapy with acyclovir 400 mg twice daily or valacyclovir 500 mg once daily. Lenalidomide and thalidomide along with steroids cause thrombosis and should be given aspirin prophylaxis.

19. Ans. a. Head and neck region

Ref: Hughes M. Guidelines on the diagnosis and management of solitary plasmacytoma of bone, extramedullary plasmacytoma and multiple solitary plasmacytomas. 2009 update.

Extramedullary plasmacytomas are plasma-cell tumors that arise outside of the bone marrow. They are most often located in the head and neck region, mainly in the upper aerodigestive tract, but may also occur in the gastrointestinal tract, urinary bladder, central nervous system, thyroid, breast, testes, parotid gland, lymph nodes, and skin. Approximately 80% involve the upper respiratory tract (i.e., oronasopharynx and paranasal sinuses), producing epistaxis, nasal discharge, or nasal obstruction. The treatment of choice for extramedullary plasmacytoma is tumoricidal radiation in a dosage of 50-54 Gy over a 4-week period.

20. Ans. d. Myopathy

Ref: Dispenzieri1 A. How I treat POEMS syndrome. Blood. 2012.

POEMS syndrome is a rare paraneoplastic syndrome resulting from an underlying plasma-cell disorder. POEMS syndrome is characterized by polyneuropathy, organomegaly, endocrinopathy, M-protein, and skin changes. The clinical picture consists of a chronic inflammatory demyelinating polyneuropathy, motor more than sensory, and the bone marrow contains <5% plasma cells. Thrombocytosis is common and vascular endothelial growth factor (VEGF) levels are elevated. The best choice of therapy has not been derived through clinical trials, and autologous transplant is the preferred therapy. Treatment of the POEMS syndrome can be broken down into two major categories: Targeting the underlying clone and targeting the rest of the syndrome. Cyclophosphamide, corticosteroid, bortezomib, and lenalidomide can also be used as in multiple myeloma. VEGF response appears to correlate with disease activity better than serum M-spike and can be used to follow-up the treatment response.

21. Ans. d. All of the above

Ref: Leung N. How I treat amyloidosis: the importance of accurate diagnosis and amyloid typing. Blood. 2012.
Hoffman 5/e

Amyloidosis is a rare disorder in which there is change in protein's conformation and aggregation leading to fibril formation that infiltrate tissues, leading to end-organ damage, and death.

Amyloid deposition can occur (1) when there is an abnormally high concentration of certain normal proteins, such as serum amyloid A (SAA) protein in chronic inflammation and b2-microglobulin in renal failure, which underlie susceptibility to AA and b2-microglobulin amyloidosis, respectively; (2) when there is a normal, but inherently amyloidogenic, protein produced over a very prolonged period, such as transthyretin, or (3) when there is production of an acquired or inherited variant protein with an abnormal structure, such as amyloidogenic monoclonal immunoglobulin light chains in AL amyloidosis or the hereditary amyloidogenic variants of transthyretin (TTR), lysozyme, and apolipoprotein A-I.

The clinical presentation of amyloidosis can be highly variable. Proteinuria is present in 73% of the AL amyloidosis patients, with 30% exhibiting nephrotic syndrome. Heart is the next most common organ involved in AL amyloidosis with abnormal echocardiographic findings noted in 65% of patients. Low voltage on ECG and concentric thickened ventricles on echocardiogram are classic signs of cardiac involvement by amyloidosis. Peripheral nerve involvement can present with paresthesia or carpel tunnel syndrome. Automatic nervous system involvement can present with syncope, erectile dysfunction, gastroparesis, and diarrhea. Gastrointestinal manifestations can be macroglossia, nausea, vomiting, and pseudo-obstruction, which accounts for <10% of AL amyloidosis cases. Bruising is common and often occurs after minor trauma or procedure, especially around the eyes. In AL amyloidosis, which is almost always the result of a plasma-cell dyscrasia, antimyeloma therapies have been effective.

Congo red stain and electron microscopy are helpful to discriminate between amyloid and other pathologic fibrils. Screening for amyloidosis should be performed in all patients presenting with unexplained heart failure, neuropathy, and nephrotic syndrome. In addition to serum and urine protein electrophoresis and immunofixation, serum-free light-chain test can increase the sensitivity. Abdominal fat biopsy has a sensitivity of ~80%. Bone marrow biopsy may also contain amyloid deposits, but sensitivity is only 56%. The gold standard for diagnosis of amyloid is the Congo red stain which gives an apple-green birefringence under polarized light. AL amyloid can be typed by immunofluorescence using FITC-labeled antibodies to IgA, IgM, IgG, κ, and λ light chain, and only one of the immunoglobulin light chains should stain positive in the amyloid deposits.

22. Ans. d. All of the above

Combination of bendamustine/bortezomib/dexamethasone is an effective treatment for patients with relapsed/refractory myeloma. The regimen induces responses in two-thirds of patients and produces a progression-free survival of 9 and overall survival of 25.6 months in patients with a median of 2 prior treatment lines frequently containing bortezomib and/or lenalidomide and is active in patients with FISH-defined high-risk cytogenetics. Bendamustine has been considered as first-line treatment along with rituximab for CLL and follicular lymphoma. Though the FDA approval is for CLL and FL only, it has been used in relapsed multiple myeloma also.

23. Ans. d. All of the above

Ref: Williams 7/e; Hoffman 7/e

Bone involvement is the most frequent clinical complication in patients with multiple myeloma. About 70% of patients have lytic bone lesions with or without osteoporosis and another 20% have severe osteoporosis without lytic lesions. The existence of a solitary bone mass (plasmacytoma) has been recognized in up to 3% of patients with a plasma-cell dyscrasia, usually on the vertebral column. Extramedullary plasmacytoma is a plasma-cell tumor that arises outside the bone marrow, most frequently in the upper respiratory tract (nose, paranasal sinuses, nasopharynx, and tonsils).

24. Ans. c. Central nervous system

Ref: Vaxman I. When to suspect a diagnosis of amyloidosis? Acta Haematol 2020;143:304–11.

Amyloid light-chain amyloidosis must always be confirmed histologically. A biopsy specimen should stain positively with Congo red and demonstrate apple-green birefringence under polarized light. In systemic amyloidosis, virtually any organ of the body other than the brain may be directly affected. The kidneys, heart, liver, skin, and peripheral nervous system are the organs most often involved and most often associated with clinical consequences. Macroglossia (large tongue) occurs in 5–10% but is almost pathognomonic of AL amyloidosis. The heart is affected in more than 50% of patients and in 30% a restrictive cardiomyopathy is a presenting feature. Painful sensory polyneuropathy with changes in pain and temperature sensation followed later by motor deficits occurs in 10–20% of cases and carpal tunnel syndrome occurs in 20% of patients. Autonomic neuropathy leading to impotence, postural hypotension, and gastrointestinal disturbances may occur alone or together with peripheral neuropathy and has a poor prognosis. Involvement of dermal blood vessels is common and may cause purpura, most distinctively in a periorbital distribution ("raccoon eyes"). Direct skin involvement takes the form of papules, nodules, and plaques. So, any patient presenting with multisystem disease needs to be considered for AL amyloidosis as a potential diagnosis, and the need for prompt appropriate investigations, such as biopsy of the affected organ or abdominal fat pad biopsy and serum-free light chain (SFLC) analysis. An uncommon but serious manifestation of AL amyloidosis is an acquired bleeding diathesis that may be associated with deficiency of factor X and sometimes also factor IX.

25. Ans. d. Serum amyloid P (SAP) scintigraphy is must for diagnosis

Biopsy of the rectum by flexible sigmoidoscopy or of abdominal fat by needle aspiration is diagnostic in 50–80% of cases. Bone marrow trephine biopsies performed to differentiate MGUS from myeloma in a newly diagnosed plasma-cell dyscrasia can also be used to diagnose amyloidosis and are almost pathognomonic of the AL type; hence, routine Congo red staining should be considered in these instances. Diffuse parenchymal amyloid deposits may occur in few or many organs, and biopsy of a clinically affected organ, for example the kidney, heart, liver or gastrointestinal tract, is likely to give positive results in >95% of cases. The appearance on hematoxylin and eosin—stained tissue of pink amorphous material should raise suspicion of amyloid and prompt furthermore specific stains. Many cotton dyes, fluorochromes, and metachromatic stains are used, but Congo red stains that produce green birefringence under cross—polarized light is generally accepted to be the diagnostic gold standard in amyloidosis. Radiolabeled SAP scintigraphy is a specific nuclear medicine imaging technique that demonstrates the presence and distribution of amyloid deposits in vivo in a quantitative manner. ^{123}I-labeled SAP localizes rapidly and specifically to amyloid deposits of all fibril types, in proportion to the amount of amyloid present. SAP scintigraphy confirms the presence of amyloid in most patients with AL type and virtually all with AA type, as well as most hereditary forms, but is not a routine investigation for evaluation.

26. Ans. a. Symptomatic cardiac amyloid is associated with a survival of 4–6 years

Cardiac amyloidosis is a restrictive cardiomyopathy. Echocardiography reveals concentrically thickened and echogenic heart valves. Cardiac MRI is a useful tool for identifying cardiac amyloidosis and distinguishing it from other restrictive cardiomyopathies. Elevation of NT-pro-BNP and cardiac troponin concentrations occur in a wide variety of cardiac conditions and in chronic kidney disease. However, significant cardiac AL amyloidosis is excluded by NT-pro-BNP concentrations <30 pmol/L. Cardiac troponin and NT-pro-BNP concentrations appear to be powerful predictors of prognosis and survival after chemotherapy. NT-pro-BNP concentration has been introduced as a prognostic marker, with raised values at diagnosis associated 30% after chemotherapy with a poorer prognosis and a fall in concentration associated with improved survival. Symptomatic or substantial echocardiographic evidence of cardiac amyloid has a very poor prognosis and is associated with a survival of only 6–12 months.

27. Ans. e. All of the above

Autologous stem cell transplant with melphalan 200 mg/m^2 is often recommended as first-line therapy without induction chemotherapy except in those with underlying myeloma. Lower doses of melphalan appear to compromise the efficacy of transplantation. Melphalan and dexamethasone have been found to be well-tolerated and effective oral chemotherapy agents, with clonal response rates of 67% including complete responses in 37%, organ response rates of 50%, and median overall survival of about 5 years. The CTD regimen has been used extensively in the treatment of AL amyloidosis and incorporates the addition of weekly oral cyclophosphamide 500 mg to low-dose thalidomide (100–200 mg) and dexamethasone over a 21-day cycle. The proteasome inhibitor bortezomib is also emerging as one of the most effective and rapidly acting therapies in the treatment of AL amyloidosis.

28. Ans. e. All of the above

Ref: Dispenzieri A. International Myeloma Working Group guidelines for serum-free light chain analysis in multiple myeloma and related disorders. Leukemia. 2009.

The serum immunoglobulin-free light chain (FLC) assay measures levels of free kappa and lambda immunoglobulin light chains. Serum concentrations of FLC are dependent on the balance between production of light chains by plasma cells and renal clearance. Serum FLC are cleared rapidly through the renal glomeruli with a serum half-life of 2–4 hours and are then metabolized in the proximal tubules of the nephrons. According to International Myeloma Working Group (IMWG) guidelines, there are four major indications for the FLC assay in the evaluation and management of plasma-cell disorders: (1) For screening for the presence of myeloma or related disorders, the serum FLC assay in combination with SPEP and immunofixation yields high sensitivity and negates the need for 24-hour urine studies when screening for multiple myeloma. (2) The FLC assay has prognostic value in plasma-cell disorder, including MGUS, smoldering myeloma, active myeloma, immunoglobulin light-chain amyloidosis, and solitary plasmacytoma. (3) The FLC assay allows for quantitative monitoring of patients with oligosecretory plasma-cell disorders, including patients with AL amyloidosis and oligosecretory myeloma. Increasing FLC may be the first indicator of relapse. (4) The ratio of FLC is required for documenting stringent complete response according to the International Response Criteria.

29. Ans. a. Inhibition of RANKL

Ref: Hanley DA. Denosumab: mechanism of action and clinical outcomes. Int J Clin Pract. 2012;66:1139-46.

Denosumab binds to RANKL (receptor activator of nuclear factor kappa-B ligand), a transmembrane or soluble protein essential for the formation, function, and survival of osteoclasts, the cells responsible for bone resorption. Denosumab is an inhibitor of RANKL. Increased osteoclast activity, stimulated by RANKL, is a mediator of bone pathology in many malignancies. Stromal cells expressing RANK (receptor activator of NF-kappa B) receptor, and signaling through the RANKL contribute to osteolysis and tumor growth. Denosumab prevents RANKL from activating its receptor, RANK, on the surface of osteoclasts, their precursors, and osteoclast-like giant cells, thus inhibiting osteoclast. OPG is a soluble RANKL decoy receptor which binds RANKL and is the key regulator of the RANKL-RANK pathway. Denosumab binds to RANKL, thus blocking the interaction of RANKL with RANK, mimicking the endogenous effects of OPG. The essential difference between bisphosphonates and denosumab is that bisphosphonates inhibit mature osteoclasts while denosumab inhibits osteoclastic precursors.

30. **Ans. d. Both cause all of the above**
Ref: Hanley DA. Denosumab: mechanism of action and clinical outcomes. Int J Clin Pract. 2012;66:1139-46.

The most common adverse reactions in patients receiving denosumab are fatigue/asthenia, hypophosphatemia, nausea osteonecrosis of jaw, and hypocalcemia. Osteonecrosis of jaw and hypocalcemia are more common with denosumab than with zoledronic acid. Oral examination should be performed prior to starting denosumab and invasive dental procedures should be avoided during treatment with denosumab. Calcium levels should be monitored and adequately supplemented in all patients with low calcium and vitamin D levels. There is some convenience from using denosumab. First, denosumab can be given subcutaneously which may be preferable to the intravenous administration of zoledronic acid. Second, denosumab is dosed the same for all patients, and no adjustment is needed according to renal function, whereas dose adjustments are necessary for zoledronic acid.

31. **Ans. e. All of the above**
Ref: Plesner T. Daratumumab for the treatment of multiple myeloma. Front Immunol. 2018;9:1228.

Daratumumab binds to CD38 on RBCs and results in a positive indirect antiglobulin test (indirect Coombs test). NK cells express CD38 and are susceptible to daratumumab-mediated cell lysis. Daratumumab binds CD38-expressing malignant plasma cells with high affinity and induces tumor cell death. In addition to being expressed by leukocytes, erythrocytes, platelets, and immature cells of the bone marrow, CD38 is also expressed by neuronal cells and glial cells of the central nervous system, peripheral nerves, pancreas islet cells, osteoclasts, skeletal muscle cells, cardiac muscle cells, and bronchial epithelium. The reason for using daratumumab for the treatment of multiple myeloma is the very high level of expression of CD38 by myeloma cells. Immunoregulatory cells belonging to the T cell, B cell, and monocyte-macrophage system also express CD38 and are eliminated during treatment with daratumumab.

32. **Ans. d. Interferes with blood grouping**
Ref: Hoffman 7/e p1415

Daratumumab is an IgG1κ human monoclonal antibody that binds to CD38 and inhibits the growth of CD38 expressing tumor cells by inducing apoptosis directly through Fc-mediated cross linking as well as by immune-mediated tumor cell lysis through complement-dependent cytotoxicity (CDC), antibody-dependent cell-mediated cytotoxicity (ADCC), and antibody-dependent cellular phagocytosis (ADCP). Daratumumab interferes with the indirect Coombs test by binding to CD38 on RBCs. Daratumumab-mediated positive indirect Coombs test may persist for up to 6 months after treatment completion. The patient's blood should be typed and screened prior to initiating treatment. Daratumumab is a human IgG kappa monoclonal antibody that can be detected on both the SPEP and immunofixation (IFE) assays used for the clinical monitoring of endogenous M-protein. This can affect the monitoring of response and disease progression in some patients with IgG kappa myeloma protein. This can lead to false-positive SPE and IFE assay results for patients with IgG kappa myeloma protein impacting initial assessment of complete responses. The determination of a patient's ABO and Rh blood type are not impacted by daratumumab.

33. **Ans. e. None of the above**

Carfilzomib differs structurally and mechanistically from bortezomib. Carfilzomib is an irreversible, epoxyketone proteasome inhibitor, whereas bortezomib is a reversible, boronic acid-based proteasome inhibitor. Carfilzomib is a more advanced next generation proteasome inhibitor that differs structurally and mechanistically from bortezomib. It is thought that the selectivity of carfilzomib for the β5 subunit contributes to its greater cytotoxic response and improved tolerability profile relative to bortezomib.

34. **Ans. c. It inhibits protein degradation**
Ref: Meister S. Extensive immunoglobulin production sensitizes myeloma cells for proteasome inhibition. Cancer Res. 2007;67.

Myeloma cells produce enormous numbers of immunoglobulin and accumulate deleterious amounts of unfolded proteins under the condition of proteasome inhibition. Extensive protein synthesis in myeloma cells is accompanied by unfolded proteins, including defective ribosomal products, which need to be degraded by the ubiquitin-proteasome system. Therefore, the proapoptotic effect of bortezomib in multiple myeloma is mainly due to the accumulation of unfolded proteins in cells with high-protein biosynthesis. Proteasome inhibition prevents the clearance of unfolded proteins resulting in an endoplasmic reticulum stress response. Reactive oxygen species are involved in the process of bortezomib-induced apoptotic cell death. Reactive oxygen species, produced by misfolded proteins (oxidation and reduction of disulfide bonds), contribute to cell death.

35. Ans. c. Next-generation sequencing (NGS)
Ref: Davies FE. Hematology. 2017;205-11.

The most widely used methods for the assessment of MRD are bone marrow flow cytometry or the use of clonality detection with NGS technologies. The sensitivity of serum-free light-chain assay is about 1 in 10^2 to 1 in 10^3 whereas the sensitivity of 4–6-color flowcytometry is 1 in 10^4 to 1 in 10^5 and that of NGS is 1 in 10^5 to 1 in 10^6. The patients achieving an MRD-negative state have improved progression-free survival and overall survival.

36. Ans. e. All of the above
Ref: Ludwig H. Hematology. 2017;212-7.

Maintenance therapy should be offered to all patients after transplant. Lenalidomide maintenance confers a significant overall survival gain for low-risk patients. Bortezomib-based therapy as a single agent for maintenance therapy has been shown to overcome the negative impact of del17p and partly that of t(4;14).

37. Ans. d. Brain

All vascular organs including liver, kidney, spleen, heart, joints, muscles, and gastrointestinal tract are often involved in the systemic forms of amyloidosis. The brain, however, is usually not involved, except for vascular structures, because of the presumed blood-brain barrier to plasma proteins.

38. Ans. b. Defective configuration of alpha-helical light-chains

AL amyloidosis is characterized by deposition of a misfolded monoclonal light-chain that is secreted from a malignant plasma cell clone, because the defective protein does not conform to the alpha-helical configuration of most proteins but rather forms beta pleated sheets. This structure is insoluble and deposits in tissues and interferes with an organ's normal function.

39. Ans. d. All of the above *Ref: Hoffman 7/e p1392*

Around 20% of patients with light-chain (AL) amyloidosis also have a concurrent diagnosis of multiple myeloma (MM), and all patients with AL amyloid have clonal light-chain production. Amyloidosis and MM both share the presence in the bone marrow of a clonal population of plasma cells.

40. Ans. e. Congo staining is diagnostic of AL amyloidosis
Ref: Hoffman 7/e p1432-35

Patients with advanced amyloid have a poor overall outcome. Therapeutic interventions are the same in patients with myeloma and amyloidosis. Amyloid is highly resistant to solubilization unless it is subjected to the harshest denaturation conditions. This insolubility in physiologic solution likely contributes to amyloid's ability to disrupt normal organ function and leads to the clinical disease amyloidosis. Subcutaneous fat aspirate demonstrates amyloid deposits in 75% of patients tested. In a patient with light-chain amyloidosis, staining of the bone marrow biopsy for amyloid deposition in blood vessels is positive in 50% cases. Congo staining is diagnostic of amyloidosis but it cannot differentiate primary amyloidosis form secondary amyloidosis, so it is not diagnostic of AL amyloidosis.

41. Ans. d. Diflunisal

Systemic AL amyloidosis is characterized by deposition of beta pleated fibrils in association with serum amyloid P component. Newer strategies to treat systemic AL amyloid involve pretreatment with Miridesap (inhibitor of SAP protein), followed by treatment with Dezamizumab that acts by dissolving amyloid protein deposits. Doxycycline has also shown to be effective in dissolution of deposited amyloid protein. Diflunisal is salicylic acid derivative that has been shown to be useful in treatment of transthyretin related hereditary amyloidosis, but not in AL amyloidosis.

42. Ans. a. t(11;14)
Ref: Gertz MA. Immunoglobulin light chain amyloidosis diagnosis and treatment algorithm. Blood Can J. 2018;8:44.

The t(11;14) is the most common abnormality in AL amyloidosis, followed by del13q, and gain of 1q. t(14;16) is rarely described in AL amyloidosis. t(11;14) is associated with poor prognosis, with poor response to even bortezomib based therapy. Patients with this abnormality may be benefitted by upfront autologous stem cell transplant or by use of venetoclax.

43. Ans. d. Cardiac MRI
Ref: Gertz MA. Immunoglobulin light chain amyloidosis diagnosis and treatment algorithm. Blood Can J. 2018;8:44.

Staging of AL amyloidosis is based on a four-point system where one point is assigned for a differential free light chains > 18 mg/dL, a cardiac troponin T > 0.025 μg/L, or an NT pro-BNP ≥1,800 ng/L, and if none of these parameters are present then 0 point is given. This provides a staging system of I, II, III, IV based on the number of points assigned (0, 1, 2 or 3).

44. Ans. e. None of the above
Ref: Gertz MA. Immunoglobulin light chain amyloidosis diagnosis and treatment algorithm. Blood Can J. 2018;8:44.

Diagnosis of AL amyloidosis should be suspected when patient presents with heart failure and preserved ejection fraction. NT-Pro-BNP is released from myocardial cells in response to increased wall stress, and levels increase with both asymptomatic and symptomatic left ventricular dysfunction, making it a useful tool in the diagnosis of cardiac failure and a strong prognostic factor in congestive heart failure. Although cardiac magnetic resonance imaging with gadolinium can be quite specific, this test is often not ordered unless the diagnosis is suspected. Heart failure with preserved ejection fraction, one of the most common manifestations of AL amyloidosis, can be misdiagnosed because the echocardiogram has nonspecific findings.

45. Ans. c. Serum creatinine > 2 mg/dL

Ref: Malik S. Update on Risk Stratification Model of Smoldering Multiple Myeloma: A Systematic Review. Blood. 2019

Smouldering multiple myeloma (SMM) is defined as an asymptomatic disease with an increased clonal burden. It is characterized by presence of Serum monoclonal protein IgG or IgA ≥3 g/dL, or Urinary monoclonal (M) protein ≥500 mg per 24 hours, or Clonal BPMC of 10–60% and no CRAB features. The Mayo Clinic's revised risk stratification for SMM is based on the 20/2/20 criteria; bone marrow plasma cells >20%, M spike >2 g/dL and serum free light chain ratio >20. Patients are stratified as low-risk (absence of any of these 3 factors), intermediate-risk (one factor present) or high-risk (two or more factors present). Risk of progression of smouldering multiple myeloma to symptomatic multiple myeloma at 10 years is 50%, 65% and 84% respectively for low, intermediated and high risk groups.

46. Ans. a. Schnitzler syndrome

Ref: Lipsker D. The Schnitzler syndrome. Orphanet. 2010

The Schnitzler syndrome is a rare entity considered part of monoclonal gammopathy of clinical significance. It is associated with chronic urticarial skin rash, a monoclonal IgM component and at least 2 of the following signs: fever, joint and/or bone pain, enlarged lymph nodes, spleen and/or liver, increased ESR, increased neutrophil count, abnormal bone imaging findings. It is a chronic disease. About 20% of patients will develop a lymphoproliferative disorder, mainly Waldenström disease and lymphoma, a percentage close to other patients with IgM MGUS.

47. Ans. b. Multiple myeloma

Ref: Lonial S. Belantamab mafodotin for relapsed or refractory multiple myeloma (DREAMM-2): a two-arm, randomised, open-label, phase 2 study. Lancet Oncol. 2020

Belantamab mafodotin-blmf is approved as a monotherapy treatment for adult patients with relapsed or refractory multiple myeloma who have received at least four prior therapies including an anti-CD38 monoclonal antibody, a proteasome inhibitor and an immunomodulatory agent. It employs a multi-faceted mechanism of action and is directed toward BCMA, a cell-surface protein that plays an important role in the survival of plasma cells and is expressed on multiple myeloma cells. The most commonly reported adverse events (≥20%) were keratopathy, decreased visual acuity, nausea, blurred vision, pyrexia, infusion-related reactions, and fatigue.

CHAPTER 33

Hairy Cell Leukemia

1. Most specific marker for the diagnosis of hairy cell leukemia (HCL) is:
    a. TRAP
    b. DBA 44
    c. Annexin A1
    d. CD11c

2. Which is the most useful immunohistochemical stain to use when assessing remission status post-treatment in HCL?
    a. CD20
    b. CD11c
    c. CD25
    d. CD123
    e. Annexin 1

3. Indications for treatment in HCL are:
    a. Symptomatic cytopenias
    b. Painful splenomegaly
    c. Recurrent infections
    d. All of the above

4. True regarding treatment for HCL are all, *except*:
    a. Cladribine is more efficacious than pentostatin in the treatment of HCL
    b. Subcutaneous cladribine administration is likely to be the most cost-effective option
    c. Patients who have received cladribine or pentostatin should be transfused only with irradiated blood products
    d. Patients who have received cladribine or pentostatin should receive acyclovir and co-trimoxazole prophylaxis

5. Response to purine analog therapy by bone marrow examination should be assessed after:
    a. 7 days
    b. 28 days
    c. 45 days
    d. 60 days
    e. 120 days

6. Cladribine can be given as:
    a. 0.1 mg/kg/day as a continuous IV infusion for 7 days
    b. 0.14 mg/kg/day as an IV infusion over 2 hours for 5 consecutive days
    c. 0.14 mg/kg/day as an IV infusion once weekly for 6 consecutive weeks
    d. 0.14 mg/kg/day as a SC bolus injection for 5 consecutive days
    e. All of the above

7. Hairy cell leukemia-variant (HCL-v) differs from HCL by:
    a. It is resistant to interferon alpha and rarely responds to cladribine
    b. There is lack of monocytopenia and leukocyte count is elevated
    c. CD25 and HC2 are not expressed
    d. All of the above

8. Patient with hairy cell leukemia can develop:
    a. Vasculitis
    b. Autoimmune hemolytic anemia
    c. Lytic bone disease
    d. All of the above

9. True regarding HCL are all, *except*:
    a. Male:female ratio is 5:1
    b. Median age at diagnosis is 55 years
    c. Majority of patients present with pancytopenia
    d. Hairy cells are present in nearly all patients
    e. All of the above

10. Hairy cell leukemia patient with active infection should be treated with:
    a. Cladribine
    b. Pentostatin
    c. Rituximab
    d. Vemurafenib

11. Treatment of variant HCL is:
    a. Cladribine
    b. Pentostatin
    c. Cladribine plus rituximab
    d. Vemurafenib

12. True regarding variant HCL is:
    a. BRAF V600E negative
    b. CD200 negative
    c. TRAP negative
    d. Annexin 1 negative
    e. All of the above

13. True about BRAF V600E mutation in HCL is:
    a. BARF mutation can be diagnosed by PCR
    b. BARF mutation can be diagnosed by immunohistochemistry
    c. Its inhibition can reverse the hairy morphology to normal
    d. All of the above

ANSWERS WITH EXPLANATIONS

1. Ans. c. Annexin A1

Ref: WHO classification of tumors of hematopoietic and lymphoid tissues, Revised Edition.

Annexin A1 is the most specific hairy cell leukemia marker since it is not expressed in any other small B-cell lymphomas other than HCL. Expression of annexin A1 can be used to distinguish HCL from SMZL and HCL variant as both are annexin 1 negative. Despite its specificity, annexin A1 is not useful for detecting minimal involvement at diagnosis or low levels of residual HCL after treatment as it also expressed by myeloid cells and some T cells. Hairy cells are CD5 and CD23 negative, express surface membrane immunoglobulin (SmIg) strongly with either κ (kappa) chain or λ (lambda) chain and are FMC7 positive. Expression of both TRAP and CD72 (the antigen reactive with DBA.44) has been shown to have high sensitivity for HCL and a high specificity for the disease; combined TRAP/DBA.44 positivity was found in only 3% of cases of non-HCL lymphoproliferative diseases. CD11c, CD25 and CD123 also show bright expression. The BRAF V600E mutation is now recognized as the causal genetic event of HCL because it is somatic, present in the entire tumor clone, detectable in almost all cases at diagnosis and stable at relapse.

2. Ans. a. CD20

Ref: Jones G. BCSH Revised Guidelines for the Diagnosis and Management of Hairy Cell Leukaemia and Hairy cell Leukaemia Variant. 2012.

Flow cytometric evaluation should be undertaken when liquid material is available. CD11c, CD25, CD103 and CD123 are advised if HCL is suspected or for monitoring minimal residual disease. Immunohistochemistry on bone marrow trephine specimens should include CD20 and CD72 (DBA.44). Use of DBA.44 and other more HCL-specific antibodies is not recommended unless as part of a wider panel including CD20 since their performance is inferior in MRD detection. Clusters of positively stained cells or widely dispersed CD20-positive lymphocytes are taken as evidence of residual disease. CD20 is the most useful immunohistochemical stain to use when assessing remission status post-treatment.

3. Ans. d. All of the above

Ref: See Q. No. 2; and Grever MR. How I treat hairy cell leukemia. Blood. 2010.

The majority of patients will require therapy to correct the cytopenias and associated problems of anemia, infections, and bleeding. If the patient is asymptomatic and cytopenias are minimal, however, it is reasonable to adopt a watch-and-wait policy. It should be noted that the risk of opportunistic infection in patients with monocytopenia and/or neutropenia is high; even asymptomatic patients may be considered for early treatment.

4. Ans. a. Cladribine is more efficacious than pentostatin in the treatment of HCL

Ref: See Q. No. 2 and 3

Purine analogs (cladribine or pentostatin) are the most appropriate agents for first-line therapy. No difference in efficacy between these has been demonstrated. Subcutaneous cladribine administration is likely to be the most cost-effective option. Patients who have received cladribine or pentostatin should be transfused only with irradiated blood products for the rest of their lives in order to minimize the risk of transfusion-associated graft-versus-host disease. They should also receive acyclovir and co-trimoxazole prophylaxis for herpes infections and *Pneumocystis jiroveci* infection respectively until the lymphocyte count is $\geq 1 \times 10^9$/L. In administering either pentostatin or cladribine, careful attention should be directed to renal function, as these agents are excreted through a renal route. Some prefer to use pentostatin because it permits titration of dose and schedule, cladribine has generally been regarded as the treatment of choice, with pentostatin being recommended for those in relapse.

5. Ans. e. 120 days

Ref: Jones G, Parry-Jones N, Wilkins B, Else M, Catovsky D. BCSH Revised Guidelines for the Diagnosis and Management of Hairy Cell Leukaemia and Hairy cell Leukaemia Variant. Br J Haematol. 2012;156(2):186-95.

Response to purine analog therapy should be assessed by bone marrow examination once the blood count has recovered, typically 4–6 months after cladribine therapy or after 8–9 courses of pentostatin. Eradication of minimal residual disease (MRD), in contrast to overtly persistent disease, should not be the aim of therapy except as part of a clinical trial. CR is defined as the absence of hairy cells from the peripheral blood and bone marrow along with resolution of organomegaly and cytopenias. In CR, immunohistochemistry reveals no clustering (≥3 cells) of CD20-positive or DBA.44-positive cells.

6. Ans. e. All of the above

Ref: Grever MR. How I treat hairy cell leukemia. Blood. 2010;115(1):21-8.

Cladribine can be given with either of the routes and dosages. The experience from Scripps Clinic with a 7-day administration of this agent at 0.1 mg/kg per day by continuous intravenous infusion showed that 91% of patients achieved a complete remission. If the agent is administered at 0.14 mg/kg per day by a 1- or 2-hour intravenous infusion for 5 doses, the results are reported to be similar. Subcutaneous administration for 5 or 7 days or weekly administration by intravenous route for 5 or 6 weeks produces comparable rates of complete remission.

7. Ans. d. All of the above
Ref: See Q. No. 2 and 3

Hairy cell leukemia-variant is considered different from HCL and is categorized separately in the WHO classification. It also responds differently to standard HCL treatment, being generally resistant to interferon alpha and rarely achieving complete response with either pentostatin or cladribine. HCL-variant differs from HCL in the lack of monocytopenia and the elevated white blood cell count, in the region of 40–60 × 10^9/L. Cells in most cases of HCL-v are villous and large, as in HCL, but have a distinct nucleolus and round nucleus resembling B-cell prolymphocytic leukemia (B-PLL). Bone marrow is often easy to aspirate in HCL-v because the reticulin fiber content is low. The immunophenotype of HCL-v cells differs from that of HCL in that Annexin 1, CD25 and HC2 are not expressed. CD103 is expressed infrequently and CD11c is nearly always positive. There is no adequate treatment for this condition. Splenectomy has shown good partial remission in two-thirds patients. Purine analogs combined with rituximab have also been used.

8. Ans. d. All of the above

Patients with HCL may develop disease-related autoimmune complications, including vasculitis and autoimmune hemolytic anemia. Lytic bone disease has also been observed, and extramedullary HCL has involved many tissues within the body.

9. Ans. d. Hairy cells are present in nearly all patients
Ref: Troussard X. Hairy cell leukemia 2018: update on diagnosis, risk-stratification, and treatment. Am J Hematol. 2017;92:1382-90.

Hairy cell leukemia has a striking male predominance, with a male:female ratio of approximately 5:1. The median age at diagnosis is approximately 50-60 years. The majority of patients present with pancytopenia. Monocytopenia is characteristic. Circulating hairy cells in the blood are generally sparse and may be absent.

10. Ans. d. Vemurafenib
Ref: Tiacci E. Targeting mutant BRAF with vemurafenib in relapsed or refractory hairy cell leukemia. NEJM. 2015;373:1733-47.

One of the most challenging clinical situations involves the patient with HCL who requires treatment but has an active infection. Attempts to control the infection should be pursued before beginning treatment with the purine nucleoside analog. Vemurafenib has no myelotoxicity. Vemurafenib increases peripheral blood counts and thus enhances the control of infection. Both cladribine and pentostatin cause profound and prolonged T-cell depletion and increase the risk of infections.

11. Ans. c. Cladribine plus rituximab
Ref: Thompson PA. How I manage patients with hairy cell leukemia. Br J Haematol. 2017;177:543-56.

Hairy cell leukemia variant responds poorly to cladribine monotherapy. It also responds poorly to therapy with pentostatin. The combination of cladribine and rituximab achieves the maximum response in HCL variant. It is BARF negative so BARF inhibitor vemurafenib is not effective. Patients with multiply relapsed HCL variant are appropriate candidates for moxetumomab pasudotox because HCL variant retains a high level of expression of CD22, and bendamustine with rituximab or pentostatin is also appropriate for HCL variant.

12. Ans. e. All of the above
Ref: Troussard X. Hairy cell leukemia 2018: update on diagnosis, risk-stratification, and treatment. Am J Hematol. 2017;92:1382-90.

A more aggressive variant of HCL lacking CD25, Annexin 1, TRAP, and BRAF V600E, called HCL variant, has been classified as a separate disease by the WHO. HCL variant has more lymphocytosis and less severe cytopenias compared with classic HCL. BRAF V600E mutation is considered as the molecular hallmark of the classic HCL.

13. Ans. d. All of the above
Ref: Falini B. BRAF V600E mutation in hairy cell leukemia: from bench to bedside. Blood. 2016;128(15):1918-27.

The BRAF V600E mutation causes constitutive activation of the RAS-RAF-MEK-ERK signaling pathway leading to HCL. The BRAF V600E mutation can be detected in BM or peripheral blood samples by Sanger sequencing or other more sensitive polymerase chain reaction (PCR)-based techniques. An alternative approach for detecting BRAF V600E in routine paraffin sections is based on immunostaining with the monoclonal antibody (VE1) specifically directed against the BRAF V600E mutant. This antibody has the potential to represent a reliable surrogate for molecular PCR assays. BRAF inhibition dramatically reversed the characteristic phenotypic and molecular signature of classic HCL cells. These changes coincided with loss of the hairy cytoplasmic projections seen by light microscopy. Subsequently, cells undergo apoptosis. So, exposure of primary HCL cells to BRAF and MEK inhibitors result in conversion of their morphology from "hairy" to "smooth".

CHAPTER 34

Myeloproliferative Neoplasms

1. True about myelofibrosis is:
   a. Males and females are equally affected
   b. Occurs most commonly in the sixth to seventh decades of life
   c. The blood and bone marrow are always involved
   d. About 30% of cases are asymptomatic at the time of diagnosis
   e. All of the above

2. True about extramedullary hematopoiesis in myelofibrosis are all, *except*:
   a. The frequency of bone marrow CD34+ cells is directly related to the number of circulating CD34+ cells
   b. It is not seen in polycythemia vera or essential thrombocythemia
   c. Spleen is most commonly affected
   d. Any organ can be affected
   e. All of the above are true

3. True about the mutational status of primary myelofibrosis (PMF) are all, *except*:
   a. JAK2 V617F mutation is found in 50–60% cases
   b. CALR mutations are found in about 24% cases
   c. MPL mutations are found in 8% cases
   d. About 30% of cases are triple-negative

4. Which cytogenetic abnormality can be seen in myelofibrosis?
   a. del(13)(q12-22)   b. t(1;6)(q21-23)
   c. del(20q)   d. Partial trisomy 1q
   e. All of the above

5. The DIPSS plus scoring system includes all, *except*:
   a. Weight loss
   b. Age > 65 years
   c. Transfusion dependency
   d. Triple negative mutational status
   e. All of the above are included

6. MIPSS70 plus scoring system for primary myelofibrosis includes:
   a. Cytogenetic mutations   b. Molecular mutations
   c. Clinical features   d. All of the above
   e. Only a and b

7. True about ruxolitinib is:
   a. It is a selective JAK2 inhibitor
   b. Should be stopped immediately in case of toxicity
   c. Can eradicate the disease
   d. All of the above
   e. None of the above

8. The most important differentiating feature between prefibrotic myelofibrosis and overt-myelofibrosis is:
   a. Degree of fibrosis
   b. Molecular analysis
   c. Clinical parameters
   d. All of the above

9. The most common mutation in essential thrombocythemia is:
   a. JAK2-V617F   b. MPL
   c. CALR   d. Triple negative
   e. Triple positive

10. True about polycythemia vera (PV) is:
   a. Bone marrow biopsy is not needed for all patients
   b. Detection of JAK2-V617F mutation in the presence of raised hemoglobin/hematocrit is specific for PV
   c. In 15% of patients with JAK2-mutated PV, the serum EPO levels may fall within the normal range
   d. All of the above

11. True about ruxolitinib are all, *except*:
   a. It delays progression to post PV-myelofibrosis
   b. Patients have improvements of intractable pruritus
   c. The incidence of new or worsening anemia or thrombocytopenia is generally highest in the first 6 months of treatment and decreases thereafter
   d. The discontinuation rate can be as high as 50% at 3 years

12. False about bone marrow biopsy in polycythemia vera is:
   a. Included in the major diagnostic criteria
   b. Can distinguish PV from ET and MF
   c. Can prognosticate the disease
   d. Bone marrow iron is increased
   e. All of the above

13. High risk features in polycythemia vera include:
   a. Age more than 50 years   b. History of thrombosis
   c. JAK-2 negativity   d. Splenomegaly
   e. All of the above

14. Treatment of high risk polycythemia vera includes:
a. Phlebotomy
b. Aspirin
c. Hydroxyurea
d. All of the above

15. The following statements are true regarding polycythemia vera:
a. Essential thrombocythemia can transform to polycythemia vera
b. JAK2 exon 12 mutations only cause polycythemia vera
c. MPL mutations do not cause polycythemia vera
d. All of the above

16. In revised IPS-ET criteria for essential thrombocythemia, the high-risk factors are all, *except*:
a. Previous history of thrombosis
b. Triple negative mutational status
c. JAK2 mutational status
d. CALR positivity

17. CD123, CD203c, and CD63 are the markers for:
a. Eosinophils
b. Mast cells
c. Basophils
d. Dendritic cells
e. Sezary cells

ANSWERS WITH EXPLANATIONS

1. Ans. e. All of the above

Ref: Thiele J. Primary myelofibrosis. Geneva: WHO; 2017. p44-50

Primary myelofibrosis affects men and women nearly equally. It occurs most commonly in the sixth to seventh decades of life, and only about 10% of overt PMF cases are diagnosed in patients aged < 40 years. The blood and bone marrow are always involved. As many as 30% of cases are asymptomatic at the time of diagnosis and are discovered by detection of splenomegaly during a routine physical examination or when a routine blood count reveals anemia, leukocytosis, and/or thrombocytosis.

2. Ans. a. The frequency of bone marrow CD34+ cells is directly related to the number of circulating CD34+ cells

Ref: Thiele J. Primary myelofibrosis. Geneva: WHO; 2017. p44-50

The frequency of bone marrow CD34+ cells is inversely related to the number of circulating CD34+ cells. This increase in the number of circulating CD34+ cells is a phenomenon largely restricted to overt PMF; it is not seen in non-fibrotic polycythemia vera or essential thrombocythemia. Extramedullary hematopoiesis is a consequence of the unique ability of the spleen to sequester the numerous circulating CD34+ cells. Other possible sites of extramedullary hematopoiesis are the liver, lymph nodes, kidneys, adrenal glands, dura mater, gastrointestinal tract, lungs and pleura, breasts, skin, and soft tissue. The grade of bone marrow fibrosis has been shown to negatively influence prognosis in primary myelofibrosis.

3. Ans. d. About 30% of cases are triple-negative

Ref: Thiele J. Primary myelofibrosis. Geneva: WHO; 2017. p44-50

In WHO-defined PMF, JAK2-V617F mutation is found in 50–60% of early-stage cases, as well as in advanced stages. CALR mutations are found in about 24% of PMF cases and MPL mutations in 8%. About 12% of cases are triple-negative for mutations in JAK2, CALR, and MPL. The triple negative mutation status is associated with poor prognosis. Mutations in ASXL1, EZH2, IDH1/2, and SFSF2 are associated with poorer outcome.

4. Ans. e. All of the above

Cytogenetic abnormalities occur in as many as 30% of primary myelofibrosis patients. The presence of either del(13)(q12-22) or der(6)t(1;6)(q21-23;p21.3) is strongly suggestive (but not diagnostic) of PMF. The most common recurrent abnormalities are del(20q) and partial trisomy 1q.

5. Ans. d. Triple negative mutational status

Ref: Gangat N. DIPSS plus: a refined Dynamic International Prognostic Scoring System for primary myelofibrosis that incorporates prognostic information from karyotype, platelet count, and transfusion status. JCO. 2011;29:392-7.

The widely used refined Dynamic International Prognostic Scoring System (DIPSS Plus) includes eight predictors of inferior survival: patient age >65 years, hemoglobin concentration <10 g/dL, leukocytes >25 × 10^9/L, circulating blasts more than or equal to 1%, constitutional symptoms, red blood cell transfusion dependency, platelet count <100 × 10^9/L, and unfavorable karyotype (i.e., a complex karyotype or 1–2 of the following abnormalities: gain of chromosome 8, loss of chromosome 7/7q, isochromosome 17q, inv(3), loss of chromosome 5/5q or 12p, or 11q23 rearrangement).

6. Ans. d. All of the above

Ref: Guglielmelli P. MIPSS70: Mutation-enhanced International Prognostic Score System for transplantation-age patients with primary myelofibrosis. J Clin Oncol. 2018;36;310-8.

MIPSS70 plus includes cytogenetic information, in addition to mutations and some of the clinical risk variables included in MIPSS70. The seven inter-independent risk variables for MIPSS70 plus include four genetic (absence of CALR type 1/like mutation; presence of high molecular risk mutations, specifically ASXL1, SRSF2, EZH2, IDH1, or IDH2; presence of ≥2 high molecular risk mutations; and "unfavorable" karyotype) and three clinical risk factors (hemoglobin <10 g/dL; circulating blast ≥2%; and constitutional symptoms).

7. Ans. e. None of the above

Ruxolitinib is an oral JAK1/JAK2 inhibitor. Unlike the BCR-ABL1 inhibitors, the JAK inhibitors are not selective for mutated JAK2, which explains their efficacy in JAK2-positive and JAK2-negative MF. Sudden ruxolitinib withdrawal has been reported to provoke a shock-like syndrome due to reemergence of the suppressed cytokines (ruxolitinib withdrawal syndrome), so it should be tapered slowly. Despite the efficacy of JAK inhibitors in controlling signs and symptoms of MF, they do not eradicate the disease. The drug is generally contraindicated in individuals with platelet counts <50 × 10^9/L, making this a subgroup of patients with high unmet need.

8. Ans. a. Degree of fibrosis

Ref: Curto-Garcia N. What is prefibrotic myelofibrosis and how should it be managed in 2018? Br J Haematol. 2018:183;23-34.

The inclusion within the 2016 WHO classification of the entity, pre-MF, characterized by low grade bone marrow fibrosis, particular features of megakaryocytes, and variably elevated LDH, leukocytosis, splenomegaly, mild anemia and thrombocytosis poses difficult problems in clinical practice. These problems arise from significant overlapping features with the classical MPN making the diagnosis sometimes challenging. Histopathological features may be helpful in discriminating prefibrotic-MF from fibrotic MF. Leukoerythroblastosis is not usually seen in pre-MF compared to overt MF. Prognosis of pre-MF is better compared to overt MF, so differentiating these two entities is important.

9. Ans. a. JAK2-V617F

Ref: Vannucchi AM, Guglielmelli P. What are the current treatment approaches for patients with polycythemia vera and essential thrombocythemia? Hematology Am Soc Hematol Educ Program. 2017;2017(1):480-8.

About 60% of ET patients have JAK2-V617F mutation. About 3–5% of the patients present with MPL gene mutations. CALR mutation can be detected in 20–25% cases. The remaining 10–15% of patients with ET who lack any of the above mutated "driver" genes are usually referred to as "triple negative". In contrast to triple negative ET, patients with triple negative MF exhibit a more aggressive disease course with poorer outcomes, including a higher incidence of leukemic transformation and shortened overall survival.

10. Ans. d. All of the above

Ref: WHO Book, 2017 Revised Edition.

Detection of JAK2-V617F mutation in the presence of raised hemoglobin/hematocrit is virtually specific for PV. In up to 15% of patients with JAK2-mutated PV, the serum EPO levels may fall within the normal range. Patients meeting 2 major criteria and 1 minor criterion may not need bone marrow biopsy, though it can help in knowing the degree of marrow fibrosis.

11. Ans. a. It delays progression to post PV-myelofibrosis

Ruxolitinib can induce complete hematologic responses, i.e., normalization of leukocytosis and thrombocytosis in 24% of the patients. Most patients have impressive improvements of their intractable pruritus with ruxolitinib. The incidence of new or worsening grade 3/4 anemia (38%) or thrombocytopenia (12%) is generally highest in the first 6 months of ruxolitinib treatment and decreases thereafter. The discontinuation rate in COMFORT-I and COMFORT-II trials was about 50% at 3 years and 75% at 5 years. In the COMFORT trials, 25% to 35% of patients discontinued ruxolitinib due to treatment-related adverse events. The most common nonhematological adverse events are diarrhea (36%) and peripheral edema (33%). Infections of special interest among ruxolitinib-treated patients have included urinary tract infection (25%), pneumonia (13%), herpes zoster infection (12%), sepsis (8%), and tuberculosis (1%). Ruxolitinib does not delay progression to post PV-myelofibrosis.

12. Ans. d. Bone marrow iron is increased

Ref: Thiele J. Polycythemia vera. Geneva: WHO; 2017. p39-43

It is usually possible to distinguish polycythemia vera from essential thrombocythemia, primary myelofibrosis, and reactive erythrocytosis and thrombocytosis on the basis of the characteristic histological pattern of polycythemia vera, in biopsy examination. Therefore, WHO has adopted bone marrow morphology as one of the major diagnostic criteria for polycythemia vera. Determination of JAK2 and CALR mutation status alone (without morphological examination) is not sufficient to differentiate PV from JAK2-mutated essential thrombocythemia. Initial fibrosis seen in polycythemia vera (present in as many as 20% of patients) can only be detected by bone marrow biopsy, and this finding may predict a more rapid progression to overt myelofibrosis (post-PV myelofibrosis). Endogenous erythroid colony growth is no longer included as a minor diagnostic criterion because of the factors like its limited practicality, time-consuming, unstandardized, restricted to specialized institutions, and costly. In > 95% of cases, stainable iron is absent in bone marrow aspirate and biopsy specimens.

13. Ans. b. History of thrombosis

The two strongest variables associated with thrombosis risk in PV and ET are older age (>60 years) and history of cardiovascular events (arterial or venous thrombosis). High-risk patients present either of the two variables, whereas low-risk patients are younger and have not suffered from thrombosis.

14. Ans. d. All of the above

There are two evidence-based recommendations for patients with PV. The first recommendation is to achieve a steady hematocrit level < 45%. The second is the use of low-dose aspirin which can reduce the combined risk of cardiovascular events. Hydroxyurea is used for high risk patients.

15. Ans. d. All of the above

Ref: Spivak JL. Polycythemia Vera. Curr Treat Opt Oncol. 2018;19:12.

The ET to PV transformation, particularly in woman occurs in approximately 20–30% of JAK2 V617F-positive ET patients. In contrast to JAK2 V617F, which can cause ET or PMF, JAK2 exon 12 mutations only cause PV. CALR mutations can rarely cause PV but MPL mutations apparently cannot. Neither JAK2-V617F nor CALR mutations are specific for PV, ET, or PMF and only the presence of erythrocytosis can distinguish PV from its companion MPN. Since PV is the most common MPN and the one with the highest morbidity and mortality rates due to thrombotic events, it should be the first disorder considered when an MPN is a diagnostic possibility. When a patient has an elevation of the hematocrit, hemoglobin level or red cell count in conjunction with a neutrophilic leukocytosis and thrombocytosis, with or without splenomegaly, the diagnosis of polycythemia vera is established. The presence of myelofibrosis does not change the diagnosis.

16. Ans. d. CALR positivity

Ref: Barbui T. Development and validation of an International Prognostic Score of thrombosis in World Health Organization—essential thrombocythemia (IPSET-thrombosis). Blood. 2012;120:5128-33.

In patients with essential thrombocythemia, the revised International Prognostics Score System (IPSET)-thrombosis, which incorporates the JAK2-V617F mutation status, allows more accurate prediction of thrombosis risk compared with the 2-tiered score of age and thrombosis history only. In ET patients, JAK2 mutational status is considered as a high-risk factor. Patients with ET harboring CALR mutation are at a reduced risk of thrombotic events when compared with JAK2-V617F mutation. Triple negative myelofibrosis is a high-risk disease, not triple negative ET.

17. Ans. c. Basophils

For basophil identification markers, a combination of CD123 and CCR3 is recommended, while CD123 alone may be used as an alternative. For basophil activation markers, either CD203c alone on unprimed basophils or CD203c and CD63 on primed basophils are recommended, while CD63 alone on primed basophils may be used as an alternative.

CHAPTER 35 Myelodysplastic Syndrome

1. Myelodysplastic syndrome with multilineage dysplasia (MDS-MLD) includes all, *except*:
   a. Cytopenia(s)
   b. Dysplasia in >10% of cells of any one of the myeloid lineages
   c. <5% blasts
   d. <15% ring sideroblasts

2. True about myelodysplastic syndrome with 5q deletion are, *except*:
   a. More common in elderly women
   b. Macrocytic anemia
   c. Thrombocytopenia
   d. Minimal dysplasia in bone marrow

3. Pathophysiology of myelodysplastic syndrome involves:
   a. Maturation arrest
   b. Ineffective hematopoiesis
   c. Increased apoptosis
   d. Immunological abnormalities
   e. All of the above

4. Compared to primary myelodysplastic syndrome, secondary myelodysplastic syndrome is associated with increased frequency of following cytogenetic abnormalities, *except*:
   a. Complex karyotype
   b. del(5q)/monosomy 5
   c. del(7q)/monosomy 7
   d. del(20q)
   e. All of the above

5. Pseudo-Pelger-Huët anomaly is seen in:
   a. Monocytes
   b. Neutrophils
   c. Basophils
   d. Platelets

6. International Prognostic Scoring System (IPSS) includes all, *except*:
   a. Cytopenias
   b. Dysplasia
   c. Karyotype
   d. Blast count
   e. All of the above

7. The median survival for high-risk myelodysplastic syndrome is:
   a. 4–8 months
   b. 1–2 years
   c. 2–4 years
   d. 4–6 years

8. Cytopenias are defined in MDS-IPSS as, *except*:
   a. Hemoglobin less than 10 g/dL
   b. Neutrophils less than 1,500/µL
   c. Platelets less than 100,000/µL
   d. All of the above

9. Preferred treatment for elderly myelodysplastic syndrome patient with del7q is:
   a. Supportive care
   b. Lenalidomide
   c. Azacitidine
   d. 3+7 induction

10. Treatment for young patient with refractory high-risk myelodysplastic syndrome is:
    a. Reduced intensity conditioning–allogeneic SCT
    b. Standard myeloablative SCT
    c. FLAMSA based sequential SCT
    d. Supportive care

11. Response to myelodysplastic syndrome treatment is assessed by:
    a. Hematological improvement
    b. Cytogenetic improvement
    c. Alteration of disease progression
    d. Quality-of-life
    e. All of the above

12. Treatment for low-risk myelodysplastic syndrome include all, *except*:
    a. Erythropoietin
    b. G-CSF
    c. Lenalidomide
    d. Reduced intensity allogeneic-SCT

13. Treatment for young IPSS intermediate risk-1 MDS patient is:
    a. Erythropoietin
    b. G-CSF
    c. Lenalidomide
    d. Reduced intensity allogeneic-SCT
    e. All of the above

14. True about chronic myelomonocytic leukemia (CMML) is:
    a. Constitutes about 1% of MDS cases
    b. Therapy related causes are most common
    c. Promonocytes and monoblasts are more than 20%
    d. Dysplasia is common
    e. All of the above

15. Neutrophil hyposegmentation and MDS-like changes can be seen by:
 a. Cotrimoxazole
 b. Tacrolimus
 c. Mycophenolate mofetil
 d. All of the above

16. Which mutation in MDS is associated with ring sideroblasts?
 a. SF3B1 mutation
 b. ASXL1 mutation
 c. RUNX1 mutation
 d. SRSF2 mutation

17. Myelodysplastic syndrome with ring sideroblasts is characterized by:
 a. Cytopenias
 b. Dysplasia
 c. Ring sideroblasts usually constituting >15% of the bone marrow erythroid precursors
 d. In the presence of SF3B1 mutation the diagnosis can be made with >5% marrow ring sideroblasts
 e. All of the above

18. Presence of auer rods in a patient with MDS indicates:
 a. MDS-EB 1
 b. MDS-EB 2
 c. Progressing to AML
 d. All of the above

19. True about myelodysplastic syndrome with excess blasts and fibrosis:
 a. Develops from myelofibrosis
 b. Is same as acute panmyelosis with myelofibrosis
 c. Is a rare entity among MDS
 d. All of the above
 e. None of the above

20. True about refractory cytopenia of childhood is:
 a. It is the most common subtype of MDS in childhood
 b. There are <2% blasts in the peripheral blood
 c. Presence of dysplasia is required for the diagnosis
 d. Monosomy 7 is the most common cytogenetic abnormality
 e. All of the above

21. Myeloid neoplasms with germline predisposition and preexisting platelet disorders include the following, *except*:
 a. Myeloid neoplasms with germline RUNX1 mutation
 b. Myeloid neoplasms with germline ANKRD26 mutation
 c. Myeloid neoplasms with germline ETV6 mutation
 d. Myeloid neoplasms with germline FLT3 mutation

22. True about thrombocytopenia 2 platelet defect is:
 a. Autosomal dominant disorder
 b. Moderate thrombocytopenia is present
 c. Increased risk of developing MDS/AML
 d. All of the above

23. Inherited bone failure syndromes with predisposition to acute myeloid leukemia is maximum in:
 a. Fanconi anemia
 b. Severe congenital neutropenia
 c. Diamond-Blackfan anemia
 d. Shwachman-Diamond syndrome

24. The drug associated with sideroblastic anemia is:
 a. Isoniazid
 b. Chloramphenicol
 c. Cycloserine
 d. Pyrazinamide
 e. All of the above

25. True regarding pediatric MDS is:
 a. Refractory anemia with ringed sideroblasts is more common in pediatrics patients than in adults
 b. Del7q is more common in pediatrics than in adults
 c. Del5q is more common in pediatrics than in adults
 d. All of the above

26. Luspatercept acts by:
 a. Activating JAK-STAT pathway
 b. Activating hypoxia inducible genes
 c. Activating endogenous erythropoietin synthesis
 d. Inhibiting transforming growth factor-beta

27. MDS, unclassifiable (MDS-U) include all, *except*:
 a. MDS with 1% blood blasts
 b. MDS with single lineage dysplasia and pancytopenia
 c. MDS based on defining cytogenetic abnormality
 d. Refractory cytopenia with multilineage dysplasia

28. Clonal somatic mutations without definitive diagnosis of MDS is termed as:
 a. Idiopathic cytopenia of undetermined significance
 b. Clonal cytopenia of undetermined significance
 c. Clonal hematopoiesis of indeterminate potential
 d. Evolving MDS/AML

29. The efficacy of hypomethylating agents in MDS can be improved by adding:
 a. Histone deacetylase inhibitors
 b. Lenalidomide
 c. Etoposide
 d. Any of the above
 e. None of the above

ANSWERS WITH EXPLANATIONS

1. Ans. b. Dysplasia in >10% of cells of any one of the myeloid lineages

Ref: WHO Classification of Tumors of Hematopoietic and Lymphoid Tissues, 2017 Revised Edition

In myelodysplastic syndrome, the cytopenias are defined as a hemoglobin level of less than 10 g/dL, an absolute neutrophil count of less than 1,800/μL, and a platelet count of less than 100,000/μL. A diagnosis of MDS with multilineage dysplasia requires that dysplastic features be present in more than 10% of cells in each of the affected cell lineages. There are less than 1% blasts in the peripheral blood and less than 5% blasts in the bone marrow. It was found that patients with RA but less than 5% marrow blasts had a poorer clinical prognosis if there was evidence of multilineage dysplasia as opposed to unilineage erythroid dysplasia. If MDS-MLD patients have more than 15% ring sideroblasts then it becomes MDS-RS.

2. Ans. c. Thrombocytopenia

Ref: WHO Classification of Tumors of Hematopoietic and Lymphoid Tissues, 2017 Revised Edition

MDS with 5q deletion occurs more usually in elderly women and is characterized by marked macrocytic anemia and thrombocytosis that is commonly referred to as 5q-syndrome. The bone marrow is typically hypercellular with prominent megakaryocytes that are slightly decreased in size with conspicuously nonlobated or hypolobated nuclei. Erythroid activity is often reduced but dysplasia is generally minimal and myeloblasts comprise less than 5% of cells. Thrombocytosis and megakaryocyte hyperplasia with nuclear hypolobation are classic associated features of the 5q-syndrome. Lenalidomide has pronounced therapeutic effects in MDS patients with del(5q).

3. Ans. e. All of the above

Immunological abnormalities are commonly encountered in MDS, suggesting that they may play a role in the pathogenesis of the disease. This is particularly apparent in cases of hypoplastic MDS that share a number of features in common with aplastic anemia, notably clinical presentation with macrocytosis and varying levels of dyserythropoietic features of MDS is the presence of cytopenias. For those patients undergoing leukemic transformation, the cytopenias arise due to maturation block of the malignant cells. However, in cases of MDS that lack an excess of blasts, the cytopenias are a reflection of the ineffective hemopoiesis. The mechanism appears to be one of increased apoptosis of hemopoietic precursors in the marrow, as demonstrated using in situ end-labeling of fragmented DNA to reveal cells undergoing programmed cell death.

4. Ans. d. del(20q) *Ref: Williams 8/e; Hoffman 7/e*

Clonal abnormalities are observed in approximately half of all primary MDS cases and in up to 90% of cases of secondary therapy-related MDS. The common chromosomal abnormalities found in MDS include loss of Y, 5q- or monosomy 5, 7q- or monosomy 7, trisomy 8, 20q-, abnormalities of 11q23, and deletions of 17p, 12p, 13q and 11q among others.

Cytogenetic abnormalities	Primary MDS (%)	Therapy-related MDS (%)
del(20q)	10	—
del(5q)/monosomy 5	20	40
del(7q)/monosomy 7	15	50
Complex karyotype	20	80

Cytogenetic analysis is required for calculating a risk score according to established prognostic scoring systems, with normal, –Y, del(5q) and del(20q) recognized as good-risk karyotypes while chromosome 7 anomalies, complex (more than three abnormalities) and very complex (more than five abnormalities) are recognized as poor-risk karyotypes. Monosomy 7 confers a poor prognosis that ranges from 14 months as an isolated abnormality down to 7 months if the karyotype is complex and involves other abnormalities.

5. Ans. b. Neutrophils

The pseudo-Pelger-Huët neutrophil is one that exhibits dense clumping of the chromatin and hypolobulation the nucleus that is classically bilobed (resembling a pair of spectacles) or even nonlobed (resembling a dumb-bell). Neutropenia is common and neutrophils often exhibit reduced granulation and the acquired Pelger-Huët anomaly hypogranular neutrophils arise due to defective formation of secondary granules, with the agranular ones being highly specific for MDS. The pseudo-Pelger-Huët is pathognomonic of MDS.

6. Ans. b. Dysplasia

Ref: WHO Classification of Tumors of Hematopoietic and Lymphoid Tissues, 2017 Revised Edition

International Prognostic Scoring System (IPSS) includes three variables—bone marrow blasts, cytogenetics and cytopenias. It is for prognostication. Dysplasia is required for diagnosis not for prognosis. The WPSS incorporates the WHO-based morphologic categories, the IPSS cytogenetic categories and the patient's RBC transfusion dependence.

Variable	Score value				
	0	0.5	1.0	1.5	2.0
Blasts (BM) (%)	<5	5–10	—	11–20	21–30
Karyotype	Good	Intermediate	Poor	—	—
Cytopenias	0/1	2/3	—	—	—

7. Ans. a. 4–8 months

Survival and risk of AML transformation are predicted by the IPSS. According to IPSS risk stratification, the median survival for the risk groups ranges from 4 to 12 years for low-risk, 2 to 4 years for intermediate-1, 1 to 2 years for intermediate-2, and to <1 year for high-risk across all age groups.

8. Ans. b. Neutrophils less than 1500/μL

Ref: WHO Classification of Tumors of Hematopoietic and Lymphoid Tissues, 2017 Revised Edition

Cytopenias are defined in MDS-IPSS as hemoglobin less than 10 g/dL, neutrophils less than 1,800/μL (not 1500/μL) and platelets less than 100,000/μL.

9. Ans. c. Azacitidine

Treatment of MDS patients with intensive chemotherapy regimens generally yields low remission rates and high relapse rates. AML induction regimens (3+7) often result in prolonged chemotherapy related hypoplasia with remission rates that are considerably lower than for de novo AML. Studies with intensive chemotherapy have reported remission rates for high-risk MDS of 38–79% but these were generally short-lived, lasting 5–15 months. The karyotype appears to be the major determinant of response to intensive chemotherapy in MDS, with normal karyotype associated with high complete remission (CR) rate and longer remissions while complex karyotypes, particularly loss of chromosome 5 or 7, are associated with low CR rate and shorter remissions.

Standard myeloablative allotransplant is reserved for younger patients with good performance status and high-risk disease whose prognosis is otherwise very poor. Compared with standard conditioning, reduced intensity conditioning (RIC) regimens are characterized by reduced myelosuppression aimed at decreasing toxicity and related mortality. A Phase III trial in MDS patients with intermediate-2 or high-risk disease, the AZA-001 study compared azacitidine with conventional care regimens (best supportive care, low-dose cytarabine or intensive chemotherapy) and demonstrated that azacitidine confers a median survival benefit of over 9 months (24.5 vs. 15 months), with almost doubling of the survival at 2 years (51% vs. 26%). In addition, subgroup analysis demonstrated that azacitidine is associated with significant benefit in patients with adverse cytogenetics involving chromosome 7, with a 67% reduction in deaths and a survival advantage at 2 years of 33% compared with 8%. This latter finding has been confirmed by another study that found a significant survival advantage in high-risk patients, with median survival of 24.8 months for patients with monosomy 7 or 7q– and 17.3 months for patients with complex cytogenetics. Lenalidomide is used mostly in lower-risk MDS; 63% of patients who were transfusion-dependent became independent of transfusion, with the most marked responses observed in those patients with del(5q) compared with normal karyotype or other cytogenetic abnormalities (83% vs. 57% vs. 12%, respectively).

10. Ans. c. FLAMSA based sequential SCT

Ref: Saure C. BBMT. 2012;18:466-72.

Patient should be brought into remission before transplants for better results post-transplant, but if the patient fails to achieve at least a good partial remission following intensive chemotherapy, then the prospects of successful outcome from allogeneic transplantation are minimal and palliative treatment with supportive care may be a preferable option. A FLAMSA-conditioned RIC transplant could be considered in these cases. It is a more intensive conditioning regimen comprising fludarabine, cytarabine and amsacrine (FLAMSA) combined with ATG, cyclophosphamide and 4–Gy total body irradiation which has recently been pioneered by a German group in patients with refractory disease at time of transplantation, with impressive 2–year survival rates of 40%. Patient undergoes sequential SCT after conditioning.

11. Ans. e. All of the above

The International Working Group criteria define four specific aspects of responses based on treatment goals: hematological improvement, cytogenetic improvement, alteration of disease progression, and quality of life. Hematological improvement is scored for each lineage according to whether there is a major or minor response, while cytogenetic improvement is scored according to whether there is a partial or complete response. Alteration of the natural course of the disease is determined according to various measures of disease progression and survival.

12. Ans. d. Reduced intensity allogeneic-SCT

Ref: Williams 8/e; Hoffman 7/e

The median survival for low-risk MDS is 4.8 years for those aged over 60 years to 11.8 years for those under 60 years. For this reason, intensive chemotherapy and SCT cannot be justified given their potential for morbidity and mortality. Individuals should be monitored for disease progression and supported as necessary. Where possible, a trial of erythropoietin with or without G-CSF should be undertaken in patients with symptomatic anemia, while those with del(5q) should ideally receive lenalidomide.

13. Ans. d. Reduced intensity allogeneic-SCT

For older patients above the age less than 65 years, if there are significant comorbidities, supportive care should be offered as for low-risk patients. Immunosuppression with ATG and ciclosporin should be considered for cytopenic patients who are otherwise deemed unfit for intensive chemotherapy, particularly if the marrow is hypocellular with no excess of blasts or adverse cytogenetics. For younger patients below the age of 50 who have either a sibling or unrelated donor available, allogeneic transplantation should be offered as a potentially curative procedure. Conditioning regimen could be myeloablative or nonmyeloablative. The impressive data emerging for patients treated with RIC transplantation makes this an attractive treatment option, especially when a sibling donor is available, although unrelated donor transplants are also feasible.

14. Ans. d. Dysplasia is common

Chronic myelomonocytic leukemia (CMML) constitutes 20–30% of cases of MDS. The hallmark feature is peripheral blood monocytosis accompanied by morphological dysplasia of other lineages. CMML is a clonal malignancy that has a male predominance and a median age of presentation of approximately 70 years; only 10% of CMML cases occur in individuals less than 60 years. While the etiology is largely unknown, therapy-related cases of CMML are very rare. By definition, the monocyte count must be greater than 1000/μL. The monocytes generally appear mature and morphologically unremarkable but may have agranular cytoplasm and/or abnormal nuclear lobulation. Promonocytes and monoblasts may also be seen but if they comprise more than 20%, then the diagnosis is AML rather than CMML. The number of blast cells plus promonocytes should account for less than 5% of peripheral blood leucocytes and less than 10% of nucleated marrow cells to give a diagnosis of CMML-1. If the blast/promonocyte count is higher than this but less than 20% in either the peripheral blood or bone marrow, or if Auer rods are present, then the diagnosis is CMML-2. CMML-0 has <2% blasts in the blood and <5% in the bone marrow. Typical features of dysplasia can be identified in all three lineages in over 80% of patients. Cytogenetic analysis is important for confirming clonality, although abnormalities are only found in 30–40% of cases, notably +8, 7/del(7q) and del(12p). CMML shows poor long-term outcomes. In younger patients, particularly with adverse features, intensive treatment and allogeneic transplantation represent the only possibility of cure.

15. Ans d. All of the above

The antibiotic cotrimoxazole and the immuno-suppressants tacrolimus and mycophenolate mofetil can cause marked neutrophil hyposegmentation, often indistinguishable from the changes seen in MDS.

16. Ans. a. SF3B1 mutation

Ref: Hasserjian RP. Myelodysplastic syndromes: Overview. WHO 2017

SF3B1 mutation is associated with ring sideroblasts and mutations in ASXL1, RUNX1, TP53 and SRSF2 are associated with severe granulocytic dysplasia. The close association between *SF3B1* mutation and the ring sideroblast phenotype is consistent with a causal link; *SF3B1* is the first gene to be strongly associated with a specific feature of MDS. Up to 28% of all patients with MDS harbor *SF3B1* mutations making *SF3B1* the most commonly mutated gene found in MDS.

17. Ans. e. All of the above

Ref: Hasserjian RP. Myelodysplastic syndrome with ring sideroblasts. WHO 2017 p109

MDS with ring sideroblasts is an MDS characterized by cytopenias, morphological dysplasia and ring sideroblasts usually constituting >15% of the bone marrow erythroid precursors. There is associated SF381 mutation in most cases, and in the presence of such mutation, the diagnosis can be made with >5% marrow ring sideroblasts.

18. Ans. b. MDS-EB 2

The presence of Auer rods in blasts designates any MDS case as MDS-EB-2 irrespective of the blast percentage.

19. Ans. e. None of the above

Ref: Orazi A. Myelodysplastic syndrome with excess blasts and fibrosis. WHO 2017 p114

In about 15% of cases of MDS, the bone marrow shows a significant degree of reticulin fibrosis (grade 2 or 3 according to the WHO grading system). Such cases have been termed MDS with fibrosis (MDS-F), and most belong to the MDS-EB category (MDS-EB-F). The presence of fibrosis is an independent prognostic parameter in MDS. MDS-EB-F may overlap morphologically with acute panmyelosis with myelofibrosis; however, acute panmyelosis with myelofibrosis is distinguished by its abrupt onset with fever and bone pain, as well as by its higher blast count.

20. Ans. e. All of the above

Ref: Refractory cytopenia of childhood. WHO 2017 p116

Refractory cytopenia of childhood (RCC) is the most common subtype of MDS in childhood, accounting for about 50% of all cases. RCC is characterized by persistent cytopenia, with <5% blasts in the bone marrow and <2% blasts in the peripheral blood. On bone marrow aspirate smears, dysplastic changes should be present in two myeloid cell lineages or account for at least 10% in one cell line. Monosomy 7 is the most common cytogenetic abnormality in RCC. Hematopoietic stem cell transplantation is the only curative therapy available, and is the treatment of choice.

21. Ans. d. Myeloid neoplasms with germline FLT3 mutation

Ref: Peterson LC. Myeloid neoplasms with germline predisposition. WHO 2017 p122

Patients with germline RUNX1, ANKRD26, or ETV6 mutations can bleed out of proportion to their platelet counts and may require anticipatory transfusion of normal platelets prior to invasive procedures or childbirth. Because the clinical management of patients with malignant myeloid disorders often involves allogeneic hematopoietic stem cell transplantation, careful donor selection is critical in these families, to avoid reintroduction of the deleterious mutation. Inadvertent use of affected donor stem cells has resulted in poor or failed stem cell engraftment, poor graft function, and donor-derived leukemias. Therefore, it is critical to distinguish myeloid neoplasms that arise as a consequence of germline predisposition from those that arise spontaneously or are secondary to environmental or chemical exposures.

22. Ans. d. All of the above

Ref: Peterson LC. Myeloid neoplasms with germline predisposition. WHO 2017 p122

Thrombocytopenia-2-platelet defect is an autosomal dominant disorder characterized by moderate thrombocytopenia and increased risk of developing MDS/AML. This disorder is characterized by germline mutations in ANKRD26, located on chromosome band 10p12. Bleeding tendencies in affected patients are usually mild.

23. Ans. b. Severe congenital neutropenia

Ref: Peterson LC. Myeloid neoplasms with germline predisposition. WHO 2017 p127

Severe congenital neutropenia should be regarded as a preleukemic condition whereby a substantial proportion of patients develop leukemia.

24. Ans. e. All of the above

Ref: Hoffman 7/e p955

Isoniazid and chloramphenicol, and to a lesser extent cycloserine and pyrazinamide, have been associated with modest sideroblastic anemia. The anemia associated with isoniazid, in particular, can often be reversed with high doses of vitamin B6 (pyridoxine).

25. Ans. b. Del7q is more common in pediatrics than in adults

Ref: Locatelli F. How I treat myelodysplastic syndromes of childhood. Blood. 2018;131:1406-14.

Significant differences in MDS between children and adults are evident for morphology, cytogenetics, and therapy approaches. The somatic mutation landscape also differs between children and adults with myelodysplasia. Monosomy 7 is the most frequent cytogenetic lesion, occurring in about 11% of patients and being more frequently detected in patients with normocellular or hypercellular bone marrow than in children with marrow hypocellularity. In patients with refractory cytopenias of childhood, the presence of monosomy 7 is correlated with a high-risk of progression to more advanced MDS as well as to frank AML, and therefore these patients should receive a transplant as soon as possible.

26. Ans. d. Inhibiting transforming growth factor-beta

Ref: Fenaux P. Luspatercept for the treatment of anemia in MDS. Blood. 2019;133:790-4.

TGF-beta signaling normally inhibits terminal erythroid differentiation by induction of apoptosis and cell-cycle arrest in erythroblasts. During early erythroid maturation, parallel suppression of TGF-b signaling through reduced growth differentiation factors (GDF) expression and stimulation by erythropoietin occurs. In MDS patients increased TGF-b signaling, plasma GDF11, and phosphorylated Smad2/3 lead to constitutive activation of TGF-b signaling which inturn lead to ineffective erythropoiesis, iron overload, and erythroid hyperplasia. Luspatercept inhibits the TGF-b pathway and has been used to treat anemia of lower-risk MDS. By reducing the expression of GDF11 and ActRIIB, luspatercept particularly promotes differentiation of cells already committed to the erythroid lineage, correct erythroid hyperplasia and ineffective erythropoiesis, and increase the number of erythrocytes without acceleration of leukemic progression.

27. Ans. d. Refractory cytopenia with multilineage dysplasia

Ref: WHO Revised Edition, 2017

Refractory cytopenia with multilineage dysplasia was included in WHO 2008 but has been removed from WHO 2017 revised classification of MDS.

28. Ans. c. Clonal hematopoiesis of indeterminate potential

Clonal somatic mutations involving MDS-associated genes are detectable in individuals who otherwise do not meet the criteria for a definitive diagnosis of MDS or other myeloid neoplasms. Their presence has been associated with an increased risk of mortality and development of hematologic malignancies. The condition describing the presence of such mutations has been termed clonal hematopoiesis of indeterminate potential (CHIP). On the other hand, patients who have unexplained persistent cytopenias without detectable MDS-defining chromosomal abnormalities are labeled as having idiopathic cytopenia of undetermined significance (ICUS). Furthermore, the term clonal cytopenia of undetermined significance (CCUS) has been used to denote the presence of cytopenias as well as evidence of clonality in the absence of morphologic features of MDS.

29. Ans. e. None of the above

Empirical addition of other agents to hypomethylating agents in frontline therapy, such as histone deacetylase inhibitors, lenalidomide, or even cytotoxic agents, do not substantially improve the outcomes.

Chapter 36

Tumor Lysis Syndrome

1. **Metabolic abnormalities seen in tumor lysis syndrome (TLS) include all, *except*:**
   a. Hyperphosphatemia
   b. Hyperkalemia
   c. Hyperuricemia
   d. Hypercalcemia

2. **True regarding rasburicase is:**
   a. Recombinant urate oxidase
   b. Recombinant urate oxidase inhibitor
   c. Not recommended for children
   d. Hemolysis does not occur

3. **True about rasburicase is:**
   a. Converts existing uric acid to allantoin
   b. Dose is 0.15 mg/kg
   c. Allantoin is 5-10 times more soluble in urine than uric acid
   d. Decreases in uric acid levels occur within 4 hours after administration of rasburicase
   e. All of the above

4. **True regarding hyperkalemia in tumor lysis syndrome is:**
   a. Pseudohyperkalemia precedes true hyperkalemia
   b. ECG shows T wave inversion
   c. Metabolic alkalosis can aggravate the hyperkalemia
   d. None of the above

5. **Clinical tumor lysis syndrome includes all of the following, *except*:**
   a. Renal failure
   b. Seizures
   c. Arrhythmias
   d. Respiratory failure

6. **True regarding hyperphosphatemia in tumor lysis syndrome is, *except*:**
   a. The phosphorus concentration in malignant cells is up to four times higher than in normal cells
   b. When the calcium concentration times phosphate concentration (the calcium phosphate product) exceeds 60 mg^2/dL^2, there is an increased risk of calcium phosphate precipitation
   c. Hyperphosphatemia is more common with chemotherapy associated tumor lysis syndrome than with spontaneous tumor lysis syndrome
   d. Rasburicase decreases the risk of hyperphosphatemia
   e. All of the above

7. **Tumor lysis syndrome is least common with:**
   a. Acute lymphoblastic leukemia
   b. Acute myeloid leukemia
   c. Burkitt lymphoma
   d. Chronic myeloid leukemia (CML)

8. **The most important step in the management of tumor lysis syndrome is:**
   a. Hydration
   b. Alkalization of the urine
   c. Use of diuretics
   d. All of the above

9. **True about allopurinol is:**
   a. It is used for the treatment of tumor lysis syndrome
   b. Safe in renal failure
   c. It is a competitive xanthine oxidase inhibitor
   d. Does not cause serious adverse effects
   e. All of the above

10. **The cause of renal failure in tumor lysis syndrome is:**
    a. Precipitation of uric acid in the renal tubules
    b. Renal vasoconstriction
    c. Decreased renal blood flow
    d. Calcium phosphate deposition in the renal tubules
    e. All of the above

11. **A child with Burkitt lymphoma has large cervical lymph nodes and uric acid of 7.5 mg/dL. True about the use of allopurinol in this patient is:**
    a. Allopurinol does not reduce the pre-existing serum uric acid concentration
    b. Allopurinol can cause kidney damage
    c. Dose of mercaptopurine should be reduced by 75%
    d. If he is unable to take oral medications, intravenous allopurinol can be administered
    e. All of the above

ANSWERS WITH EXPLANATIONS

1. Ans. d. Hypercalcemia

Ref: Cairo MS, Bishop M. Tumour lysis syndrome: new therapeutic strategies and classification. Br J Haematol. 2004;127:3-11.

Tumor lysis syndrome describes the clinical and laboratory sequelae that result from the rapid release of intracellular contents of dying cancer cells. Rapid turnover of tumor cells results in a massive release of various intracellular contents (potassium, phosphate, nucleic acids, lactate dehydrogenase, etc.) into the systemic circulation. Metabolic abnormalities in tumor lysis syndrome include hyperphosphatemia, hyperkalemia, hyperuricemia and/or hypocalcemia, and renal, cardiac and neurologic dysfunction. Cairo and Bishop devised a classification system to help standardize the definition of tumor lysis syndrome. Clinical tumor lysis syndrome requires the presence of laboratory tumor lysis syndrome in addition to evidence of renal, cardiac, or neurologic dysfunction.

2. Ans. a. Recombinant urate oxidase

Ref: Wilson PF, Berns JS. Onconephrology: tumor lysis syndrome. Clin J Am Soc Nephrol. 2012;7:1730-9.

Rasburicase is a recombinant urate oxidase enzyme approved for use by the US Food and Drug Administration in patients who are at risk of developing tumor lysis syndrome or for the management of elevated uric acid levels. Urate oxidase metabolizes uric acid to the much more soluble allantoin, carbon dioxide, and hydrogen peroxide. The former is readily excreted by the kidneys. Clinical trials have demonstrated rasburicase to be effective in both pediatric and adult population. Adverse effects associated with rasburicase can be significant, ranging from anaphylactic reactions to methemoglobinemia. Rasburicase is contraindicated in patients who are glucose-6-phosphate dehydrogenase deficient because these patients cannot break down hydrogen peroxide, a byproduct of rasburicase, which can lead to hemolysis. To overcome the hypersensitivity related risk of rasburicase, PEG-uricase is being tested in trials. Rasburicase will continue to be active in blood samples ex vivo, and thus inappropriately handled laboratory specimens may manifest spuriously low uric acid levels. Samples for uric acid should be placed on ice immediately after phlebotomy and run as quickly as possible to maximize reliable approximation of in vivo uric acid concentration.

3. Ans. e. All of the above

Ref: Ueng S. Rasburicase: a novel agent for tumor lysis syndrome. Proc (Bayl Univ Med Cent). 2005;18(3):275-9.

Rasburicase is derived by a recombinant DNA from a modified *Aspergillus flavus* strain and expressed in a modified yeast strain of *Saccharomyces cerevisiae*. A recombinant urate oxidase enzyme, rasburicase converts existing uric acid to allantoin, which is 5-10 times more soluble in urine than uric acid. Rasburicase differs from allopurinol since it can affect existing plasma uric acid; allopurinol affects only the future production of uric acid by inhibiting xanthine oxidase. Rasburicase is contraindicated in patients who are glucose-6-phosphate dehydrogenase deficient because these patients cannot breakdown hydrogen peroxide, a byproduct of rasburicase, which can lead to hemolysis.

4. Ans. d. None of the above *Ref: See Q No. 1 and 2*

In the case of hematologic malignancies, much of the 2.5 kg of bone marrow in the average human may be replaced by malignant cells. The rapid liberation of potassium into the extracellular fluid will lead to severe hyperkalemia if it exceeds the normal homeostatic uptake of potassium into liver and muscle cells. Potassium is the main intracellular cation regulated through the Na-K ATPase system. Its normal regulation is critical in maintaining the normal resting membrane potential of various cells: skeletal muscle, neural and cardiac muscle. Hyperkalemia is defined as serum potassium level >6.0 mEq/L or 25% increase from baseline. Neuromuscular and cardiac tissues are most susceptible to changes in potassium level. Neuromuscular symptoms may include fatigue, muscle cramps, anorexia, paresthesias, and irritability. In the cardiac tissue, depending on the degree of hyperkalemia, a variety of electrocardiographic changes can occur, including peaked T wave (>5 mm) with serum potassium level of 6-7 mEq/L, QRS complex widening and smaller amplitude of P wave with serum potassium of 7-8 mEq/L, fusion of QRS complex with T wave forming sine waves with serum potassium of 8-9 mEq/L, and ultimately atrioventricular dissociation, ventricular tachycardia, or ventricular fibrillation and death when the serum potassium level increases above 9 mEq/L. Most symptoms appear when serum potassium level are >6.0 mEq/L. Coexisting renal failure, metabolic acidosis, and potassium sparing medications can worsen hyperkalemia and must be observed closely and corrected. Pseudohyperkalemia can also sometimes occur in patients with AML and ALL exhibiting hyperleukocytosis (>100,000/mL). The falsely elevated potassium level occurs as a result of mechanical lysis of white blood cells (WBCs) during phlebotomy or ionic shifts following coagulation of blood in the vial.

5. Ans. d. Respiratory failure *Ref: See Q No. 1 and 2*

Clinical tumor lysis syndrome is defined as laboratory tumor lysis syndrome plus one or more of the following:

increased serum creatinine concentration (≥ 1.5 times the upper limit of normal), cardiac arrhythmia/sudden death, or a seizure. Rapid lysis of tumor cells releases massive quantities of intracellular contents (potassium, phosphate, and nucleic acids that can be metabolized to uric acid) into the systemic circulation, causing clinical manifestations.

6. Ans. d. Rasburicase decreases the risk of hyperphosphatemia

With the development of effective hypouricemic agents (rasburicase and allopurinol), hyperphosphatemia has become the major metabolic complication associated with tumor lysis syndrome. The phosphorus concentration in malignant cells is up to four times higher than in normal cells. Thus, rapid tumor breakdown often leads to hyperphosphatemia which can cause secondary hypocalcemia. When the calcium concentration times phosphate concentration (the calcium phosphate product) exceeds 60 mg^2/dL^2, there is an increased risk of calcium phosphate precipitation in the renal tubules, which can lead to renal failure. In addition, precipitation in the heart may lead to cardiac arrhythmias. Spontaneous tumor lysis syndrome is associated with hyperuricemia but frequently not with hyperphosphatemia. It has been postulated that rapidly growing neoplasms with high cell turnover rates produce high serum uric acid levels through rapid nucleoprotein turnover but that the tumor is able to reutilize released phosphorus for resynthesis of new tumor cells. In contrast, tumor lysis syndrome after chemotherapy is due to cell destruction in the absence of reuptake of phosphorus. The primary toxicity of hyperphosphatemia is the secondary hypocalcemia that results from chelation of calcium by phosphate anions. Hypocalcemia can lead to cardiac arrhythmias, seizures, tetany, and death.

7. Ans. d. Chronic myeloid leukemia (CML)

High-risk group for tumor lysis syndrome include Burkitt lymphoma, ALL with a WBC ≥ 100,000/μL, and AML (especially of the monoblastic type) with WBC ≥ 50,000/μL.

8. Ans. a. Hydration

Ref: Wilson PF, Berns JS. Onconephrology: tumor lysis syndrome. Clin J Am Soc Nephrol. 2012;7:1730-9.

Fluid resuscitation is a mainstay of therapy in tumor lysis syndrome and is recommended as prophylaxis in any patient at risk of developing tumor lysis syndrome. Crystalloid volume expansion increases renal clearance of the electrolytes including potassium, phosphate, and uric acid. In addition, distal delivery of sodium and chloride augment potassium secretion. Increased urine flow in the setting of volume expansion decreases both the calcium-phosphate product in the urine as well as the urine concentration of uric acid, potentially reducing obstructive crystal formation. Diuretics do not have a proven role in reducing the incidence or severity of tumor lysis syndrome, their routine use is not recommended unless there are clinical signs or symptoms of volume overload, and their use can lead to excessive volume depletion. Alkalinization of the urine favors conversion of uric acid to the more soluble urate salt, decreasing the potential for intratubular crystal formation. However, administering exogenous alkali decreases the solubility of calcium-phosphate salts, leading to increased soft-tissue and renal tubular deposition of calcium-phosphate crystals. Further, alkalemia favors calcium binding to albumin, decreasing ionized calcium concentration, which may precipitate tetany or arrhythmia in these patients who are already prone to hypocalcemia. Therefore, urinary alkalinization for the prevention or treatment of tumor lysis syndrome is not generally recommended and may be harmful.

9. Ans. c. It is a competitive xanthine oxidase inhibitor

Ref: Wilson PF, Berns JS. Onconephrology: tumor lysis syndrome. Clin J Am Soc Nephrol. 2012;7:1730-9.

Allopurinol is a competitive xanthine oxidase inhibitor. Oxypurinol, a metabolite of Allopurinol is excreted by the kidneys with a long half-life of up to 24 hours in normal individuals, making dosing complex in patients with acute or chronic renal failure. Allopurinol decreases the generation of uric acid from xanthine but does not have a direct effect on uric acid levels. As such, initiation of allopurinol therapy after marked hyperuricemia has already occurred and tumor lysis syndrome has progressed significantly is unlikely to alter the clinical course of tumor lysis syndrome. However, prophylactic use of allopurinol is generally recommended in patients with high- or intermediate-risk tumors. Allopurinol is associated with several potentially severe adverse effects, including Stevens-Johnson syndrome, toxic epidermal necrolysis, hepatitis, bone marrow suppression, and the allopurinol hypersensitivity syndrome. Febuxostat, a novel xanthine oxidase inhibitor that does not have the hypersensitivity profile of allopurinol and does not require dosing adjustments for reduced GFR, is an attractive consideration for prophylaxis in patients at risk for tumor lysis syndrome with impaired kidney function. So allopurinol is used as a prophylactic drug for tumor lysis syndrome and not for the treatment of tumor lysis syndrome for which rasburicase is used. Moreover, its dose modification is required in renal failure.

10. Ans. e. All of the above *Ref: Hoffbrand 7/e p415*

Catabolism of the nucleic acids to uric acid leads to hyperuricemia, and the marked increase in uric acid excretion can result in the precipitation of uric acid in the renal tubules and can also induce renal vasoconstriction, decreased renal blood flow and inflammation, resulting in acute kidney injury. Hyperphosphatemia with calcium phosphate deposition in the renal tubules can also cause acute kidney injury.

11. Ans. e. All of the above *Ref: Hoffbrand 7/e p415*

There are several limitations to the use of allopurinol. Because it acts by decreasing uric acid formation, allopurinol does not reduce the serum uric acid concentration before treatment is initiated. Thus, for patients with preexisting hyperuricemia (serum uric acid ≥7.5 mg/dL), rasburicase is the preferred hypouricemic agent. Allopurinol increases serum levels of the purine precursors hypoxanthine and xanthine, which may lead to xanthinuria, deposition of xanthine crystals in the renal tubules, and acute kidney injury. Since allopurinol also reduces the degradation of other purines, dose reductions of 65–75% are needed in patients being treated with mercaptopurine or azathioprine. Allopurinol has the potential to interact with a number of other drugs, including cyclophosphamide, high-dose methotrexate, ampicillin, and thiazide diuretics. Among patients who are unable to take oral medications, IV allopurinol can be administered at a dose of 200–400 mg/m^2 per day, in one to three divided doses.

SECTION 4
Hematopoietic Stem Cell Transplantation and GVHD

37. Stem Cell Transplantation
38. Graft versus Host Disease

CHAPTER 37

Stem Cell Transplantation

1. **The risk of graft-versus-host disease (GVHD) in 10/10 matched unrelated donor compared to 6/6 sibling matched donor will be:**
   a. More
   b. Less
   c. Same
   d. Varies

2. **Acute GVHD is mediated by:**
   a. Host T cells
   b. Donor T cells
   c. Host B cells
   d. Donor B cells

3. **True regarding immune reconstitution post-transplant are all, *except*:**
   a. Can be evaluated in the clinic by monitoring the absolute numbers of T cells
   b. Thymus plays an important role
   c. GVHD delays immune reconstitution
   d. B cell recovery is the first to occur
   e. All of the above are true

4. **The number of CD34 positive cells required for successful engraftment in autologous transplant are:**
   a. 1×10^6/kg
   b. 2×10^6/kg
   c. 3×10^6/kg
   d. 4×10^6/kg

5. **True about cyclophosphamide is:**
   a. Has both immunosuppressive and antileukemic properties
   b. It is a prodrug
   c. Produces interstrand DNA links
   d. Major complications are hemorrhagic cystitis and cardiac toxicity
   e. All of the above

6. **True regarding cytomegalovirus (CMV) reactivation following allogeneic stem cell transplant are:**
   a. Highest risk of CMV reactivation is in seropositive recipients
   b. Increased risk in those who receive T-cell depleted graft
   c. Reduced risk in those who develop GVHD
   d. Can be reduced by transfusing irradiated blood products

7. **Treatment of CMV pneumonia is:**
   a. High-dose acyclovir
   b. Ganciclovir
   c. Valganciclovir
   d. Foscarnet

8. **Engraftment is defined as:**
   a. Absolute neutrophil count greater than 500/µL and a platelet count greater than 20,000/µL
   b. Absolute neutrophil count greater than 1,000/µL and a platelet count greater than 50,000/µL
   c. Absolute neutrophil count greater than 500/µL and a platelet count greater than 50,000/µL
   d. Absolute neutrophil count greater than 1,500/µL and a platelet count greater than 20,000/µL

9. **The following are more common during the first month of transplant, *except*:**
   a. Pulmonary edema
   b. Diffuse alveolar hemorrhage
   c. Aspergillosis
   d. CMV pneumonia

10. **A patient developed headache, blurred vision followed by seizures on day 20 postallogeneic stem cell transplant for acute myeloid leukemia (AML) in second complete remission. He had engrafted on day 14 and was on cyclosporine as GVHD prophylaxis. His blood pressure was 170/100 mm Hg. The most likely cause is:**
    a. Leukemic meningoencephalitis
    b. Bacterial meningitis
    c. Cerebral aspergillosis
    d. Posterior reversible encephalopathy syndrome
    e. Cerebral sinus thrombosis

11. **The basic requirement for the development of GVHD is:**
    a. The graft must contain immunologically competent cells
    b. The host must possess transplantation antigens that are lacking in the graft, thereby appearing foreign to the graft; host cells subsequently stimulate donor cells via these specific antigenic determinants
    c. The host must be incapable of mounting a reaction against the graft for a period of time sufficient to allow graft cells to attack the host
    d. All of the above

12. **The most important HLA loci determining a graft-versus-host reaction are:**
    a. HLA-A, -B, -C
    b. HLA-DQ, -DR, -DP
    c. HLA-A, -B, -DR
    d. All of the above

13. True regarding total body irradiation (TBI)-based regimens are, *except*:
   a. Can be combined with cyclophosphamide or etoposide
   b. Given as fraction doses
   c. Mucositis is the major dose limiting factor
   d. Maximum dose recommended is 15 Gy
   e. All of the above

14. Busulfan/cyclophosphamide when compared to with total body irradiation/cyclophosphamide as myeloablative regimen has the following advantages, *except*:
   a. Similar risk of hepatic sinusoidal obstruction syndrome (SOS) in both groups
   b. Similar acute GVHD in both groups
   c. Similar chronic GVHD in both groups
   d. Increased interstitial pneumonitis with busulfan/cyclophosphamide
   e. Overall survival same in both groups

15. Which of the following is monoclonal anti-CD-20 antibody?
   a. Rituximab   b. Tositumomab
   c. Ibritumomab
   d. Ofatumumab
   e. All of the above

16. The usual volume of fresh frozen plasma (FFP) required for management of bleeding is:
   a. 5–10 mL/kg   b. 10–15 mL/kg
   c. 15–20 mL/kg   d. 20–25 mL/kg

17. Prognostic factors for transplant in thalassemia include all of the following, *except*:
   a. Hepatomegaly
   b. Splenomegaly
   c. Liver fibrosis
   d. Iron chelation therapy

18. Compared to the use of filgrastim (G-CSF)-mobilized autologous peripheral blood stem cells (PBSCs) versus autologous bone marrow, the filgrastim-mobilized PBSCs is associated with the following significant benefits, *except*:
   a. A shorter time to platelet recovery
   b. A shorter time to neutrophil recovery
   c. A shorter time in hospital
   d. A cost saving
   e. All of the above

19. Risk factors for the development of acute GVHD include:
   a. Degree of HLA disparity
   b. Increasing age of host
   c. Donor and recipient gender disparity
   d. CMV status of donor and host
   e. All of the above

20. True regarding skin GVHD are all, *except*:
   a. The first clinical manifestation of acute GVHD is a maculopapular rash, usually occurring at or near the time of the white blood cell engraftment
   b. The palms and the soles are spared
   c. Dermal and epidermal layers are involved
   d. The most consistent histologic feature is individual cell death at the base of crypts
   e. All of the above

21. The pathophysiology of liver GVHD involves:
   a. Damage to hepatocytes
   b. Damage to the bile canaliculi, leading to cholestasis
   c. Damage to sinusoids
   d. Damage to interstitium

22. Mycophenolate mofetil has following properties:
   a. Antibacterial   b. Antifungal
   c. Antitumor   d. Immunosuppressive
   e. All of the above

23. The following are used in the treatment of acute GVHD, *except*:
   a. Antithymocyte globulin
   b. Daclizumab
   c. Extracorporeal photochemotherapy
   d. Etanercept
   e. All of the above

24. True regarding acute GVHD are, *except*:
   a. Development of moderate (grade II) acute GVHD after marrow transplantation is associated with a significant decrease in survival
   b. Severe (grade III or IV) acute GVHD after marrow transplantation is associated with a significant decrease in survival
   c. Once GVHD occurs, it may not be treatable
   d. It is mediated by activated T cells from the recipient
   e. All of the above

25. The most common prophylaxis for prevention of acute GVHD is:
   a. Methotrexate and prednisolone
   b. Methotrexate and cyclosporine
   c. Cyclosporine and prednisolone
   d. Cyclosporine and methylprednisolone

26. Mycophenolate mofetil acts by inhibiting:
   a. Calcineurin pathway
   b. Cyclooxygenase pathway
   c. Inosine monophosphate dehydrogenase
   d. All of the above

27. Treatment of choice for acute GVHD is:
   a. Methotrexate   b. Prednisolone
   c. Cyclosporine   d. Methylprednisolone
   e. Combination of all of the above

28. Limited chronic GVHD is treated with all of the following, *except*:
   a. Topical steroids
   b. Topical cyclosporine
   c. Pilocarpine
   d. Extracorporeal photopheresis

29. True about regulatory T cells is:
   a. CD4+/CD25+   b. FoxP3+
   c. Decrease acute GVHD
   d. All of the above

30. True regarding second malignancy following stem cell transplantation is:
   a. Chronic GVHD is a predisposing factor
   b. Squamous cell cancers primarily of the skin and buccal cavity are common
   c. Have aggressive behavior and poor prognosis
   d. Azathioprine use for GVHD increases the risk
   e. All of the above

31. Risk factors for post-transplant lymphoproliferative disease include all, *except*:
   a. Unrelated or HLA-mismatched related donor
   b. T cell depletion of donor marrow
   c. Administration of antithymocyte globulin
   d. Chronic GVHD
   e. All of the above

32. Which one of these approaches would be most suitable for mobilization of donor stem cells into the peripheral blood for allogeneic stem cell transplantation?
   a. Administration of subcutaneous granulocyte colony stimulating factor (GCSF)
   b. Administration of subcutaneous GCSF and plerixafor
   c. Administration of subcutaneous GCSF, plerixafor, and intravenous cyclophosphamide
   d. Administration of granulocyte-macrophage colony stimulating factor (GMCSF)

33. Which of these individuals might be considered as the optimal stem cell donor for an adult patient with acute myeloid leukemia in first remission?
   a. An identical twin
   b. A cord blood stem cell donation
   c. An HLA-matched unrelated donor
   d. An HLA-matched sibling donor
   e. Any of the above

34. Which viral infection is most likely to be responsible for a clinical picture of fever and pulmonary infiltration 6 weeks after an allogeneic stem cell transplant?
   a. Cytomegalovirus
   b. Varicella zoster virus
   c. Herpes simplex virus
   d. *Pneumocystis jiroveci*

35. Which of these is not suitable for donation of stem cells for allogeneic stem cell transplantation?
   a. A sibling of the same blood group without further genetic testing
   b. An unrelated donor who is matched for HLA alleles
   c. A syngeneic donor (identical twin)
   d. Cord blood cells from donor with 5/6 match at major HLA alleles

36. Which of these is most useful in evaluating that a stem cell donation has an adequate number of stem cells prior to transplantation?
   a. The relative depletion of T cells
   b. The number of CD34+ cells in the graft
   c. The number of CD33+ myeloid cells in the graft
   d. The total nucleated cell count

37. Which of these is true regarding donor leukocyte infusions (DLI)?
   a. The dose that is given is calculated by the number of T cells in the infusion
   b. The patient is given conditioning therapy before DLI
   c. Donor is given growth factor for 4–5 days before procedure
   d. DLI given after the transplant has a reduced risk of causing GVHD
   e. All of the above

38. Best donor for haploidentical stem cell transplant is:
   a. Son   b. Brother
   c. Mother d. Father

39. Allogeneic stem cell transplantation is indicated in the following, *except* in:
   a. AML with monosomy 7 in CR1
   b. Philadelphia positive ALL in CR1
   c. High-risk APML in CR1
   d. Low-risk AML in CR2
   e. Indicated in all of the above

40. Recovery of T cell reconstitution by post-transplant cyclophosphamide (PT-Cy) post-haploidentical transplant is:
   a. Similar to that in matched sibling donor (MSD) transplant without PT-Cy
   b. Earlier than MSD transplant without PT-Cy
   c. Delayed than that in MSD transplant without PT-Cy
   d. Depends upon T cell dose in the graft

41. True regarding the major risk for graft rejection following haploidentical transplant is:
   a. 5/10 match has more chances of rejection compared to 7/10 match
   b. Presence of donor-specific antibodies (DSA) against HLA molecules are a major risk factor for graft failure
   c. B cells and NK cells do not participate in the immune response to HLA-mismatched tissues
   d. Pregnancy and blood transfusions have no effect on haplotransplant
   e. All of the above

42. The benefit of treatment of bone marrow donors with G-CSF before donation is:
   a. Increases marrow CD34+ cells
   b. Reduces total lymphocytes
   c. Reverses the CD4+/CD8+ T-cell ratio
   d. All of the above
   e. None of the above

43. True about engraftment syndrome are all, *except*:
   a. Mediated by T cells
   b. There is increased cytokine production
   c. More common in autologous than allogeneic transplant
   d. Steroids are effective
   e. All of the above are true

44. Which of the following is not a risk factor for sinusoidal obstruction syndrome (SOS) of liver post-HSCT?
   a. TBI-based conditioning
   b. Busulfan-cyclophosphamide conditioning
   c. Nonmyeloablative conditioning
   d. Alcoholic hepatitis

45. Risk factors for sinusoidal obstruction syndrome is:
   a. Total body irradiation   b. Busulfan
   c. Gemtuzumab ozogamicin
   d. Sirolimus
   e. All of the above

46. True about post-transplant lymphoproliferative disorders (PTLD) is:
   a. Seen almost equally in autologous and allogeneic HCT recipients
   b. Develop mostly after the first year of HCT
   c. ATG serotherapy reduces the risk
   d. Incidence is 5–10%
   e. None of the above

47. A 25-year-old girl with AML with inv16 is in second complete remission. She is planned for an allogeneic stem cell transplant. Her blood group is B positive. She has a 21-year-old sister (O positive) who is 5/10 match with her. Her parents are aged 52 years (father, A positive) and 50 years (mother, B positive) and both have well-controlled hypertension. Mother is 6/10 and father is 7/10 match. She does not have any anti-HLA antibodies. There are no 10/10 matches in unrelated donor searches and the best unrelated match is 7/10. Who is the most suitable donor for her?
   a. 21 years old sister   b. 50 years old mother
   c. 52 years old father
   d. 7/10 MUD

48. The following is an indication for autologous stem cell transplant:
   a. Mantle cell lymphoma
   b. Plasma cell dyscrasia
   c. T-cell lymphoma
   d. Relapsed Burkitt lymphoma
   e. All of the above

49. Which of the following is true about palifermin?
   a. The dose of palifermin is 60 µg/kg/day for 3 days prior to high-dose chemotherapy
   b. Grade III–IV mucositis can be effectively treated with palifermin
   c. Side effects of palifermin include hepatotoxicity
   d. Palifermin is naturally produced in epithelial cells and acts on a wide variety of cells

50. The following group of drugs have a role in treating CMV reactivation post-HSCT:
   a. High dose acyclovir, Valganciclovir, Ganciclovir, Foscarnet, IVIG
   b. Valganciclovir, Ganciclovir, Foscarnet, Cidofovir, Maribavir, CMX001, Leflunomide
   c. Valganciclovir, Ganciclovir, Foscarnet, IVIG
   d. Low dose acyclovir, Valganciclovir, Ganciclovir, Foscarnet, Cidofovir
   e. All of the above

51. The following are risk factors for acute GVHD post-HSCT:
   a. CMV reactivation
   b. Development of engraftment syndrome during transplant
   c. Matched unrelated donor
   d. Myeloablative conditioning regimen
   e. All of the above

52. Which of the following statements is false?
   a. Acute GVHD is a risk factor for chronic GVHD
   b. Sirolimus is used for acute GVHD prophylaxis
   c. Etanercept is used for the treatment of acute GVHD
   d. Isolated acute liver GVHD is commonly seen
   e. All of the above

53. Which of the following statement is true about post-transplant thrombotic thrombocytopenic purpura?
   a. Plasma exchange is the proven treatment
   b. Rituximab is an effective drug
   c. IVIG and high-dose steroids are effective if started immediately
   d. Replacing calcineurin inhibitor is curative
   e. Eculizumab is a very effective drug

54. Which of the following is false about HSCT in JMML?
   a. HSCT is the only curative treatment for all patients with JMML
   b. Cytoreductive therapy consisting of fludarabine and high-dose cytarabine concomitantly with 13-*cis*-retinoic acid prior to HSCT may be given
   c. Relapse is the major cause of treatment failure in patients with JMML undergoing HSCT especially within the first year

d. Splenectomy pre transplant does not help to improve engraftment, survival and reduces relapse
e. None of the above

55. Which of the following are rare indications for a HSCT?
a. Sézary syndrome
b. Subcutaneous panniculitic T cell lymphoma
c. Hypereosinophilic syndrome
d. None of the above
e. All of the above

56. The following are cryoprotectant solutions used for cryopreservation of hematopoietic stem cells:
a. Glycerol
b. Hydroxy ethyl starch (HES)
c. Di methyl sulfoxide (DMSO)
d. Propylene glycol
e. All of the above

57. The following is false about HSCT in Fanconi anemia:
a. The optimum time for HCT is when the patient is young and has received few red cell and/or platelet transfusion
b. Worse outcomes to be expected if the patient has progressed to MDS or leukemia
c. Choose conditioning for these patients keeping in mind hypersensitivity to alkylating agents and radiation
d. Poor outcome is primarily due to excessive regimen-related toxicity, including severe acute GVHD
e. None of the above

58. Which of the following statements is false about VZV reactivation in HSCT recipients?
a. Serious VZV disease after transplantation is related to the compromise of B-lymphocyte function
b. VZV prophylaxis in HSCT recipients with risk factors, such as those with T-cell depletion, ATG therapy, anti-CD3 antibody therapy, or unrelated or HLA-mismatched transplantation is recommended
c. Prophylaxis with acyclovir in general delays but does not prevent VZV reactivation
d. Immunization with inactivated varicella vaccine has the potential to reduce the morbidity of VZV reactivation after HSCT
e. The rationale for avoiding routine use of prolonged prophylaxis is that prolonged administration of antiviral enhances the emergence of VZV strains that are resistant to the drug

59. Which of the following is false about HSV infection post-HSCT?
a. The drug of choice for the treatment of HSV mucocutaneous infection post-HSCT is acyclovir
b. There is no decrease in CMV infection/disease and improved survival in HSCT recipients after high doses of acyclovir prophylactically
c. For acyclovir-resistant HSV the drug of choice is foscarnet
d. For foscarnet/acyclovir-resistant cases cidofovir is the drug of choice
e. Acyclovir, valcyclovir, famciclovir, foscarnet or cidofovir can be used for HSV treatment

60. Which viral reactivation occurs first in HSCT recipient?
a. CMV reactivation
b. HSV infection
c. VZV infection
d. EBV infection
e. None of the above

61. Which of the following is not a risk factor for idiopathic pneumonia syndrome post-HSCT?
a. Use of TBI 200 cGy in conditioning
b. Longer duration from diagnosis to transplant
c. Use of methotrexate as GVHD prophylaxis
d. HLA mismatch between donor and recipient

62. Which of the following is false regarding stem cell doses in adult patients?
a. The generally accepted minimal cell dose is 2×10^6 CD 34+ cells/kg.
b. Higher doses result in faster engraftment and reduced rates of infection and non relapse mortality
c. Higher doses are associated with lower rates of GVHD
d. Cell dose of $4\text{-}5 \times 10^6$ CD 34+ cells/kg seems most reasonable

63. Miracle mouth wash consists of:
a. 2% viscous lidocaine + diphenhydramine + antacid
b. Chlrohexidine mouth wash + dexamethasone + morphine
c. tetracycline + lidocaine + agar
d. activated charcoal + antacid

ANSWERS WITH EXPLANATIONS

1. Ans. a. More

Even with a complete 10/10 match, the risk of GVHD is higher than for an HLA—identical sibling, presumably because the number of polymorphic minor H antigen differences are likely to be greater.

2. Ans. b. Donor T cells

Ref: Thomas' Hematopoietic Cell Transplantation 4/e

GVHD is a complex immunological disorder in which donor T cells with specificity for recipient antigens not expressed in the donor initiate tissue damage. Induction of GVHD requires the interaction of donor T cells with host antigen-presenting cells (APCs), most probably dendritic cells within secondary lymphoid organs such as lymph nodes and gut-associated lymphoid tissue. Donor CD4 and CD8 T cells with antihost-specificity, activated on interaction with host APCs, proliferate and develop effector functions that, lead to the secretion of effector cytokines (e.g., TNF, interferons, IL-17) or the induction of perforin/granzyme B pathways required for cellular cytotoxicity. In acute GVHD, CD8 cells are regarded as the most relevant effectors, whereas CD4 cells are thought to be more important for the development of chronic GVHD.

3. Ans. d. B cell recovery is the first to occur

Allogeneic stem cell transplantation (SCT) is followed by a prolonged period of cellular and humoral immunodeficiency while donor-derived immune recovery occurs. Reconstitution of an immune response after transplantation can be evaluated in the clinic by monitoring the absolute numbers of T (CD4, CD8), B and NK cell numbers. NK cell numbers recover most rapidly while other subsets (especially CD4 cells and B cells) recover more slowly. Thymus plays an important role in immune reconstitution. Thymic function is reduced in adults and may be further compromised by the effects of chemoradiotherapy and GVHD. Quantitative B-cell deficiency is present in virtually all patients in the first months after transplantation and may persist for a number of years post-transplantation as a consequence of reductions in the number of marrow B-cell precursors, particularly in patients with chronic GVHD.

4. Ans. b. 2×10^6/kg

Ref: Thomas' Hematopoietic Cell Transplantation 4/e p1210

The sole determinant of durable engraftment after an autologous or syngeneic transplant is stem cell number and graft failure is exceedingly rare providing at least 2×10^6 cells are transplanted. The lowest CD34 acceptable stem cell dose to secure engraftment in an allogeneic setting is considered to be 2×10^6 cells (2×10^8/kg mononuclear cells if bone marrow is used), although in practice the majority of patients transplanted using in excess of 1×10^6/kg will engraft.

5. Ans. e. All of the above

Ref: Thomas' Hematopoietic Cell Transplantation 4/e p299

Cyclophosphamide is an alkylating agent that, when administered in the doses routinely used in myeloablative conditioning regimens (120–200 mg/kg), has both immunosuppressive and antileukemic properties. It is a prodrug that must be metabolized by the cytochrome P450 system in the liver to produce metabolically active derivatives, principally phosphoramide mustard, which exert their cytotoxic activity through the production of interstrand DNA links. The two major complications of cyclophosphamide at the doses employed in allogeneic transplantation are hemorrhagic cystitis and cardiac toxicity. Hemorrhagic cystitis results from the toxic effects of a cyclophosphamide metabolite, acrolein, on the uroepithelium and can be reduced by use of sodium 2-mercaptoethane sulfonate (MESNA), while cardiac toxicity is very rare at doses of cyclophosphamide below 150 mg/kg.

6. Ans. b. Increased risk in those who receive T-cell depleted graft

Ref: Boeckh M, Ljungman P. How I treat cytomegalovirus in hematopoietic cell transplant recipients. Blood. 2009; Thomas' Hematopoietic Cell Transplantation 4/e

Patients at the highest risk of CMV reactivation are seropositive recipients, especially those who receive T cell depleted (TCD) or unrelated donor grafts, and patients who develop GVHD requiring steroid therapy. CMV reactivation occurs in 40–80% of at-risk patients and until recently a substantial number of such patients developed CMV disease. Low levels of CMV infection can be detected after transplantation, using either polymerase chain reaction (PCR)-based detection of CMV or detection of pp65 antigen in peripheral blood leucocytes (CMV antigenemia). Primary infection of seronegative patients may occur as a result of the infusion of stem cell or blood products from a CMV-positive donor but is rare. For this reason seronegative transplant recipients should receive CMV-negative or leukodepleted blood products to limit the possibility of primary infection. Irradiation prevents transfusion associated GVHD not CMV infection. So, post-transplant, patient should receive both irradiated and leukodepleted blood products. If only a CMV-seropositive donor is available for a CMV-seronegative patient, the risk of transmission of CMV by the stem cell product to the recipient is approximately 20–30%.

7. Ans. b. Ganciclovir

Ref: Thomas' Hematopoietic Cell Transplantation 4/e

CMV pneumonia remains the most feared complication of CMV in hematopoietic cell transplantation (HCT) recipients because its attributable mortality continues to be high. Treatment is with ganciclovir in combination with intravenous immunoglobulin. The diagnosis of CMV pneumonia is established by detection of CMV in bronchoalveolar lavage (BAL) or lung biopsy in the presence of clinical signs and symptoms.

8. Ans. a. Absolute neutrophil count greater than 500/μL and a platelet count greater than 20,000/μL

Ref: Thomas' Hematopoietic Cell Transplantation, 4/e, p1204

Engraftment is defined as an absolute neutrophil count that is greater than 500/μL and a sustained platelet count that is greater than 20,000/μL that lasts for three consecutive days without transfusions.

9. Ans. d. CMV pneumonia

Ref: Sharma SK, Kumar S, et al. Diffuse alveolar hemorrhage following allogeneic peripheral blood stem cell transplantation: a case report and a short review. Indian J Hematol Blood Transfus. 2014

Pulmonary edema typically occurs in the second or third week after the transplant pulmonary edema may be due to increased capillary hydrostatic pressure or increased pulmonary capillary permeability. DAH is a form of noninfectious pneumonitis that is characterized by the sudden onset of dyspnea, nonproductive cough, fever, and hypoxemia; hemoptysis is rare. DAH is typically diagnosed with bronchoalveolar lavage (BAL). The diagnosis of DAH is considered when successive aliquots of BAL fluid become increasingly hemorrhagic; the diagnosis is established if all cytologic, pathologic, and microbiologic studies exclude the presence of pulmonary infection. The onset of Aspergillus infection occurs in a bimodal distribution, with the first peak at a median of 16 days and the second peak at a median of 96 days after BMT. The clinical features of invasive pulmonary aspergillosis include fever, dyspnea, dry cough, wheezing, pleuritic chest pain, and hemoptysis. Localized infiltrates that are nodular or cavitary on CT of the chest are likely to be Aspergillus infection. CMV pneumonitis usually occurs 6–12 weeks after BMT and affects 10–40% of patients. Ninety percent of CMV pneumonitis cases occur within the first 100 days after BMT.

10. Ans. d. Posterior reversible encephalopathy syndrome

Ref: Bartynski WS. Posterior reversible encephalopathy syndrome. AJNR. 2008

Posterior reversible encephalopathy syndrome (PRES) is a clinicoradiological abnormality that can develop in patients receiving chemotherapy or after stem cell transplant. The most common clinical symptoms and signs included headache, altered alertness and confusion, vomiting, seizures, and visual disturbance ranging from blurred vision to cortical blindness. Neuroimaging typically shows white matter edema in the posterior portions of the cerebral hemispheres, particularly in the parieto-occipital regions. MRI is the best modality of investigation. The presumed etiologies include hypertension, cyclosporine, tacrolimus, chemotherapeutic agents. and infections. With control of blood pressure and withdrawal or reduction of the immunosuppressive agent, patients have resolution of symptoms within 2 weeks and neuroimaging usually normalizes. Toxic levels of the immunosuppressive medications do not appear to be required for the development of PRES. Although PRES is usually reversible with prompt withdrawal or reduction of the immunosuppressive agent and blood pressure control, it can be associated with permanent neurologic deficits and death.

Table 1: Causes of pulmonary involvement during early post-transplant period.

S. No	Differential diagnosis	Clinical features	Signs	Predisposing factors	Radiology	Usual treatment
1.	Pulmonary edema	Breathlessness, orthopnea	Basal fine crackles	Fluid overload	Bilateral pulmonary infiltrates, Kerley B lines	Fluid restriction, diuretics
2.	TRALI	Breathlessness	Hypoxia, cytopenias	Anti-bodies to HLA	Bilateral pulmonary infiltrates	Supportive care
3.	Engraftment syndrome	Fever, skin rash, breathlessness	Rash, effusions	Cytokine release, capillary leakage	Pleural effusions, pulmonary infiltrates	Glucocorticoids
4.	Diffuse alveolar hemorrhage	Breathlessness, cough	Hypoxia, tachypnea	Not known	Bilateral diffuse ground glass and patchy consolidation	Supportive, steroids
5.	CMV pneumonia	Fever, breathlessness, cough	Hypoxia, tachypnea	Immuno-compromised state, steroids use, T-cell depletion	Diffuse GGO and nodules, mainly in the mid and lower zones	Ganciclovir, immunoglobulins
6.	Pneumocystis jirovecii pneumonia	Fever, non-productive cough	Hypoxia, tachypnea, chest signs less	Immuno-compromised state, steroids use, T-cell depletion	Bilateral interstitial-alveolar infiltrates	Trimethoprim and sulfamethoxazole
7.	Other infections (bacterial and fungal, viz. Aspergillus)	Fever, chest pain, cough	Bronchial breath sounds	Neutropenia, mucosal injury	Consolidations, Halo sign	Antibacterials, antifungals
8.	Drug toxicity	Breathlessness	Occasional crackles	Low FEV1/VC	Nonspecific	Supportive

11. Ans. d. All of the above
Ref: Ferrara JLM. The immunopathophysiology of acute graft-versus-host-disease. Stem Cells. 1996

In 1966, observations following splenic cell infusion into irradiated mice, led Billingham to formulate the requirements for the develoment of GVHD. First, the graft must contain immunologically competent cells.

Second, the recipient must be incapable of mounting an effective response to destroy the transplanted cell and third, the recipient must express tissue antigens that are not present in the transplant donor. According to these criteria, GVHD can develop in various clinical settings when tissues containing immunocompetent cells (blood products, bone marrow, solid organs) are transferred between individuals. Although the mice recovered from the radiation injury and marrow aplasia, they died of a wasting syndrome characterised by diarrhea, weight loss, skin changes and liver abnormalities, later termed GVHD.

12. Ans. c. HLA-A, -B, -DR
Ref: Thomas' Hematopoietic Cell Transplantation 4/e

The genes of the HLA locus encode two distinct classes of cell surface molecules, classes I and II. Class I molecules are expressed on the surfaces of virtually all nucleated cells at varying densities, while class II molecules are more restricted to cells of the immune system, primarily B lymphocytes and monocytes. There are three different class I (HLA-A, -B, -C) and class II (HLA-DQ, -DR, -DP) antigens. HLA-A, -B and -DR antigens appear to be the most important loci determining whether transplanted cells initiate a graft-versus-host reaction. In hematopoietic cell transplantation, the principal antigenic targets of the T cells of the graft are the host major histocompatibility complex (MHC) molecules if the patient and donor MHC molecules differ. However, for grafts matched at the MHC, mismatching of other antigens, termed minor histocompatibility antigens, appear to underlie the development of GVHD. CD4 positive cells interact with the MHC class II molecules of antigen presenting cells (APCs), and CD8 positive cells interact with MHC class I antigens. In most centers, a complete match at the HLA-A, -B (both class I) and -DR loci (class II) is required for that individual to be used as a transplant donor, since mismatches at these loci are associated with a higher risk of severe GVHD and death.

13. Ans. e. All of the above

TBI-based regimens typically fractionate the radiation and administer the total dose over several days which help decrease toxicity and increase tolerability. TBI is combined with cyclophosphamide. Cyclophosphamide is usually given at a dose of 60 mg/kg of for 2 successive days. The maximally tolerated dose of TBI is approximately 15 Gy. Higher doses produce excessive nonhematologic toxicity, primarily to the lungs and heart. Decreased relapse rates were observed with the higher TBI dose (e.g., 12 vs. 35% at 3 years in patients with acute myeloid leukemia), but overall survival was similar due primarily to increased transplant-related mortality at the higher doses (e.g., 32 vs. 12% at 3 years) Etoposide (VP16) has also been given with fractionated TBI at a maximally tolerated dose of 60 mg/kg, with excellent results having been obtained in large numbers of patients. The major limitations of fractionated TBI include mucositis, lung toxicity, infertility, and the relatively sophisticated instrumentation required to effectively administer this treatment. Fractionated TBI has been relatively difficult to standardize due to differences in dose rates, shielding, and center-specific techniques.

14. Ans. a. Similar risk of hepatic sinusoidal obstruction syndrome (SOS) in both groups
Ref: Hartman AR. Survival, disease-free survival and adverse effects of conditioning for allogeneic bone marrow transplantation with busulfan/cyclophosphamide vs total body irradiation: a meta-analysis. Bone Marrow Transplant. 1998

A meta-analysis of five prospective randomized studies compared Bu/Cy with TBI/Cy. It was concluded that Bu/Cy increased risk of hepatic SOS but there was no significant differences in acute or chronic GVHD, interstitial pneumonitis, disease-free survival, or overall survival.

15. Ans. e. All of the above *See Chapter 43, Tables, S No. 4*

Tositumomab (Bexxar), an Iodine-131 conjugated anti-CD20 antibody, and ibritumomab (Zevalin), an Yttrium-90 conjugated anti-CD20 antibody are being used as preparative regiments in the autologous setting for the treatment of patients with B-cell NHL.

16. Ans. b. 10–15 mL/kg
Ref: O'Shaughnessy. Guidelines for the use of fresh-frozen plasma, cryoprecipitate and cryosupernatant. BJH. 2004

Hemostasis can be achieved when the activity of coagulation factors is at least 25–30% of normal, since the plasma volume in adults is approximately 40 mL/kg, this requires a dose of FFP of approximately 10–15 mL/kg (25–30%). This dose represents approximately 3–5 units of FFP for most adult patients.

17. Ans. b. Splenomegaly
Ref: Lucarelli G, et al. Bone marrow transplantation in patients with thalassemia. N Engl J Med. 1990

Splenomegaly is not the risk factor for poor outcome in thalassemic transplants.

18. Ans. e. All of the above

A study by Schmitz N et al. (Lancet 1996) compared the use of filgrastim (G-CSF)-mobilized autologous PBPCs versus autologous bone marrow in 58 patients with relapsed Hodgkin's disease and non-Hodgkin lymphoma treated with carmustine, etoposide, cytarabine and melphalan. Early post-transplant morbidity and mortality and overall survival were similar in both groups, but use of filgrastim-mobilized PBPCs was associated with the following significant benefits: (1) A shorter time to platelet recovery above 20,000/μL (16 vs. 23 days), (2) A shorter time to neutrophil recovery (11 vs. 14 days), (3) A shorter time in hospital (17 vs. 23 days), (4) A cost saving of 23% due to lower autograft collection costs and shorter hospitalizations with less supportive care.

19. Ans. e. All of the above

Ref: Thomas' Hematopoietic Cell Transplantation 4/e

Risk factors for the development of acute GVHD include: degree of HLA disparity, intensity of the transplant conditioning regimen, peripheral blood stem cell versus bone marrow transplantation, acute GVHD prophylactic regimen used, increasing age of host, donor and recipient gender disparity and CMV status of donor and host.

20. Ans. b. The palms and the soles are spared

Ref: Thomas' Hematopoietic Cell Transplantation 4/e

The first and most common clinical manifestation of acute GVHD is a maculopapular rash, usually occurring at or near the time of the white blood cell engraftment. The rash initially involves the nape of the neck, ears, shoulders, the palms of the hands, and the soles of the feet. It appears as a sunburn and may be pruritic or painful. In severe GVHD, the maculopapular rash forms bullous lesions with toxic epidermal necrolysis. Histologic examination of acute GVHD of the skin reveals changes in the dermal and epidermal layers. Characteristic findings include exocytosed lymphocytes, dyskeratotic epidermal keratinocytes, follicular involvement, satellite lymphocytes adjacent to or surrounding dyskeratotic epidermal keratinocytes, and dermal perivascular lymphocytic infiltration. The most consistent histologic feature is individual cell death (apoptosis) at the base of crypts. Skin GVHD is divided into four stages.

21. Ans. b. Damage to the bile canaliculi, leading to cholestasis

Ref: Thomas' Hematopoietic Cell Transplantation 4/e

The primary histologic finding in liver GVHD is extensive bile duct damage (e.g., bile duct atypia and degeneration, epithelial cell dropout, lymphocytic infiltration of small bile ducts), leading to occasionally severe cholestasis. In veno-occlusive disease (VOD), there is sinusoidal obstruction due to endothelial cell destruction. In viral hepatitis, there is destruction of hepatocytes. In Budd-Chiari syndrome, there is obstruction of hepatic veins.

22. Ans. e. All of the above

Mycophenolate mofetil has antibacterial, antifungal, antiviral, antitumor, and immunosuppressive properties. Several other agents have been studied in small phase I/II studies to assess potential use for the treatment of acute GVHD. These include thalidomide, photochemotherapy, and anti-TNF receptor (etanercept). With mycophenolate mofetil, an overall grade improvement was found in 65% patients and a lower dose of prednisolone was required. Mild leukopenia, anemia, and thrombocytopenia occurred but did not require discontinuation of therapy. Diarrhea can also occur with MMF.

23. Ans. e. All of the above

The primary role of T cells in the pathogenesis of GVHD provides the rationale for the use of antithymocyte globulin (ATG) and other anti-T cell antibodies. The monoclonal antibody OKT3 is directed against the CD3 antigen that is closely associated with the T cell receptor. Another approach to the treatment of steroid-resistant grade II-IV acute GVHD is the administration of monoclonal antibodies directed against the IL-2 receptor (B-B10, anti-CD25, Daclizumab). Daclizumab has been utilized in steroid refractory GvHD. The presumed contribution of tumor necrosis factor-alpha (TNF-alpha) to acute GVHD and the association of higher serum levels with worse outcome provide the rationale for the use of anti-TNF-alpha antibodies in this disorder. Etanercept, a recombinant human TNF-alpha receptor fusion protein, has been used alone or in combination with steroids to treat chronic and acute GVHD. Extracorporeal phototherapy (ECP) consists of infusion of ultraviolet-A irradiated autologous peripheral lymphocytes, which have been collected by apheresis and incubated with 8-methoxypsoralen. This approach appears to be effective in the treatment of cutaneous T-cell lymphoma and several autoimmune diseases and has been used to treat rejection after organ transplantation and bone marrow transplant. ECP appears to downregulate activated T cell clones. It has a role in the treatment of both acute and chronic GVHD.

24. Ans. d. It is mediated by activated T cells from the recipient

Ref: Dignan FL, et al. BCSH/BSBMT Guideline: Diagnosis and management of acute graft versus-host disease. BJH. 2012

The presence of GVHD remains the most important post-transplant factor influencing outcome following allogeneic HCT. Development of moderate (grade II) or severe (grade III or IV) acute GVHD after marrow transplantation is associated with a significant decrease in survival. Furthermore, once GVHD occurs, it may not be treatable. It is mediated by activated T cells from the donor (not recipient).

25. Ans. b. Methotrexate and cyclosporine

The most widely used regimen is the combination of methotrexate and cyclosporine. Cyclosporine is started from day minus 2. Methotrexate is given on day +1, +3, +6, and +11 of transplant. Dose adjustments are made according to the serum creatinine and bilirubin concentrations. The dose of methotrexate is usually reduced in patients who have hyperbilirubinemia, severe mucositis, or renal insufficiency. Prednisone is not part of the standard prophylactic regimen but can be used if there are concerns about administering methotrexate, in patients who do not tolerate methotrexate, and in those at high risk of veno-occlusive disease. The efficacy of the addition of glucocorticoids to standard prevention with cyclosporine/methotrexate is uncertain.

26. Ans. c. Inosine monophosphate dehydrogenase

MMF inhibits the proliferation of T and B cells and the production of antibodies through the inhibition of inosine monophosphate dehydrogenase (IMPDH). This enzyme catalyzes oxidation of inosine monophosphate to xanthine monophosphate, a required intermediate in the synthesis of guanosine triphosphate and a critical enzyme for the de novo biosynthesis of purine nucleotides, specifically guanosine monophosphate (GMP). Blockade of GMP synthesis leads to a negative feedback inhibition of 5-phosphoribosyl-1-pyrophosphate and prevention of T-cell activation. Purines are essential for the growth and survival of cells. Cells have two pathways to produce purines, a de novo and a salvage pathway. Lymphocytes are highly dependent on de novo synthesis, while other cells can utilize both pathways. The therapeutic index of MMF depends on the lymphocyte's reliance on de novo synthesis of purines, allowing for greater immunosuppressive activity with less toxicity. Depletion of guanosines would lead to a decrease in 5-phosphoribosyl-1-pyrophosphate synthetase and inhibition of the purine synthesis which is required for T-cell activation.

27. Ans. d. Methylprednisolone

Ref: Dignan FL, et al. BCSH/BSBMT Guideline: Diagnosis and management of acute graft versus-host disease. BJH. 2012; Thomas Hematopoietic Cell Transplantation 4/e

If the patient develops acute GVHD, the first and most effective treatment option is the use of glucocorticoids. The most commonly used glucocorticoid is methylprednisolone, which differs from prednisolone and prednisone only by the addition of 6 alpha-methyl group. The 6-alpha-methyl group blocks the specific binding of this corticosteroid to transcortin, the protein that transports steroids in the plasma. Instead, methylprednisolone is primarily bound to albumin. The lack of transcortin-binding leads to a larger partition coefficient, resulting in a significantly greater penetration of this agent into bronchial alveolar fluids, which may provide a therapeutic advantage for treatment of pulmonary inflammatory states. If the patient has not received glucocorticoids for GVHD prophylaxis, methylprednisolone (2 mg/kg per day in divided doses) is begun. Initial treatment with low-dose glucocorticoids for patients with grades I-II acute GVHD did not compromise disease control or mortality and was associated with decreased length of hospitalization, as well as reductions in the incidence of invasive fungal infection and gram-negative bacteremia. Nonresponders to the above treatment at day 5 are treated with higher dose steroids (e.g., 5 mg/kg per day). If they respond within 3-5 days, the dose is lowered to 2 mg/kg per day and the subsequent course is similar to that in responders to low-dose therapy. If higher doses of steroids are not successful in controlling GVHD by 3-5 days, second-line treatments are required, but are generally less successful than steroids. These include cyclosporine, tacrolimus, antithymocyte globulin, and mycophenolate mofetil.

28. Ans. d. Extracorporeal photopheresis

Ref: Thomas' Hematopoietic Cell Transplantation 4/e

Patients with limited chronic GVHD and without any significant morbidity may not need any specific systemic therapy. As examples, patients with limited skin involvement may only require the administration of topical steroids (such as a fluorinated topical steroid), those with chronic GVHD involving the eye may respond to topical cyclosporine eyedrops, and those with localized disease of the mouth (e.g., xerostomia) may improve with agents such as pilocarpine, gargled oral dexamethasone, or use of a nonabsorbable steroid mouthwash. PUVA therapy and extracorporeal photopheresis are used for extensive chronic GVHD. Patients with limited chronic GVHD have a favorable prognosis even without therapy, while those who have extensive GVHD, particularly with multiorgan involvement, have poor long-term outcomes.

29. Ans. d. All of the above

Regulatory T cells (Treg), defined as CD4+/CD25 high, CD3+, L-Selectin-high, FoxP3+, and CD103+, are useful in the prevention of GVHD. Naturally arising Treg cells can influence most immune responses including autoimmunity, transplantation tolerance, antitumor immunity, and anti-infectious responses. These cells appear to be central control elements of immunoregulation, and will be important for therapeutically manipulating post-transplant immune responses.

30. Ans. e. All of the above

The presence of chronic GVHD is a predisposing factor for the development of solid tumors, particularly squamous cell cancers, primarily of the skin and buccal cavity, often with an aggressive behavior, poor prognosis, and an association with prior chronic lichenoid lesions of the oral mucosa. The predominant underlying primary diseases for patients in whom squamous cell carcinoma developed were leukemia and severe aplastic anemia, with a median time from HCT to the diagnosis of a solid tumor of 7.0 years. Azathioprine use for GVHD increases the risk.

31. Ans. e. All of the above

Ref: Loren AW, Porter DL, Stadtmauer EA, Tsai DE. Post-transplant lymphoproliferative disorder: a review. BMT. 2003;31(3):145-55.

Post-transplant lymphoproliferative disorder (PTLD) represents a heterogeneous group of abnormal lymphoid proliferations, generally of B cells that occur in the setting of ineffective T-cell function because of pharmacologic immunosuppression after organ/stem cell transplantation. Unlike most other forms of non-Hodgkin's lymphoma, nearly all PTLDs are associated with Epstein-Barr virus (EBV) infection, as manifested by the presence of EBV within the malignant cells. The major risk factors for early PTLD are an unrelated or HLA-mismatched related donor, T cell depletion of donor marrow, particularly if natural killer cells are also removed, and the administration of antithymocyte globulin or anti-CD3 antibodies for prophylaxis or treatment of acute GVHD. Chronic GVHD is a risk factor for late onset PTLD. The mainstay of therapy for PTLD is reduction of immunosuppression and PTLD carries a high risk of mortality.

32. Ans. a. Administration of subcutaneous granulocyte colony stimulating factor (GCSF)

Autologous HSC transplantation is used to facilitate hematopoietic recovery after administration of high-dose chemotherapy in patients with Hodgkin's disease, non-Hodgkin's lymphoma, multiple myeloma, leukemia, and some solid tumors. There are limitations to the existing methods of mobilizing CD34+ HSC with chemotherapy and/or granulocyte colony-stimulating factor (G-CSF). Plerixafor, a bicyclam molecule that acts as a pure antagonist of chemokine receptor-4, is approved by the US Food and Drug Administration for use in combination with G-CSF for mobilization of CD34+ HSC in patients undergoing autologous stem cell transplant. After administration of plerixafor, HSC migrate from the bone marrow into the peripheral blood, permitting collection by apheresis. The combination of G-CSF+ plerixafor facilitates mobilization of HSC. In patients with MM without extensive previous treatment who were undergoing a first mobilization, the use of G-CSF+ plerixafor was reported to double counts of circulating peripheral CD34+ HSC and thus double the number of CD34+ HSC collected in half as many apheresis procedures. Rescue plerixafor to assist peripheral blood stem cell harvest in healthy allogeneic donors has been found to be effective, but not routinely used, as it has not been approved for it yet.

GM-CSF-based mobilization is usually well-tolerated in normal healthy donors, but for mobilizing PBSC, higher doses more than 250 µg/m^2 that might be more effective, in some cases, are not that well-tolerated, and this has somewhat limited the utility of this drug. A sequential combination regimen with GM-CSF and G-CSF appears to have synergistic effect. Chemotherapy obviously is not indicated for allogeneic donors.

33. Ans. d. An HLA-matched sibling donor

Ref: Cornelissen J, Löwenberg B. Role of allogeneic stem cell transplantation in current treatment of acute myeloid leukemia. Hematology Am Soc Hematol Educ Program. 2005:151-5.

Allogeneic HSC transplantation is an established and effective consolidation therapy in acute myeloid leukemia in first (high-risk patients) or subsequent remission. The risk of GVHD, graft failure, and mortality increases progressively with the number of HLA disparities, emphasizing the need of high-resolution HLA typing and the selection of donors with, preferably, no more than one mismatched allele out of ten. An HLA-matched sibling donor would offer the optimal degree of alloreactive mismatch to allow development of a degree of graft versus leukemia effect which is likely to be required to cure cases of relapsed acute leukemia. Treatment-related mortality will be higher with unrelated compared to related donor. Due to the smaller number of stem cells in the cord blood unit, cord blood stem cell transplants engraft more slowly than stem cells from marrow or peripheral blood and until engraftment occurs, patients are at risk of developing life-threatening infections.

34. Ans. a. Cytomegalovirus *Ref: See Q. No. 6 and 7*

Cytomegalovirus remains an important complication postallogeneic-SCT. Its reactivation is common in the first 3 months after transplant. CMV infection post-transplant can manifest as pneumonia, hepatitis, gastroenteritis, retinitis, or encephalitis. Seronegative patients with seropositive stem cell donors develop primary CMV infection in about 30%. Other identified risk factors include acute and chronic GVHD and the use of mismatched or unrelated donors. The lack of specific immunity to CMV both regarding cytotoxic T cell response and helper T-cell response to CMV has been associated with a high risk for CMV disease. *Pneumocystis jiroveci* pneumonia (PCP) has become a rare opportunistic infection due to the use of prophylactic regimens. *Pneumocystis jiroveci* is an atypical fungus causing severe pneumonia in immunocompromised patients, particularly among allogeneic HSC transplant recipients. Before the use of prophylaxis, 5–16% of patients who received allogeneic marrow transplants developed PCP with a median onset at 9 weeks post-transplantation and a mortality rate of up to 76%. Since the use of effective prophylaxis with trimethoprim-sulfamethoxazole, less than 5% of HSCT recipients still develop PCP. PCP prophylaxis should be given for at least 6 months after engraftment for all patients, but should be continued for patients still receiving immunosuppressive drugs, having chronic

GVHD, relapse of hematological malignancy, or CD4+ cell counts less than 200/μL.

35. Ans. a. A sibling of the same blood group without further genetic testing

In an allogeneic stem cell transplant, the most suitable donor is usually a family member, often a brother or sister whose stem cells are as close a genetic match (tissue type) as possible to the patient's. This is called a related or matched sibling donor transplant. However, only about 1 in 4 patients has such a donor, so the donor may be an unrelated, but matched volunteer. This is called a matched, or voluntary unrelated donor transplant (MUD or URD). If an exact match with the patient's tissue type cannot be found, a partially matched donor can sometimes be used.

36. Ans. b. The number of CD34+ cells in the graft

Progenitor cells expressing the surface antigen CD34+ are capable of long-term engraftment. Within this CD34+ population resides a subset of multipotent (lineage-nonspecific) stem cells capable of myeloid, lymphoid, erythroid, or megakaryocyte commitment. CD34 is also found on progenitor cells that have already committed toward lineage specificity. Characterization of CD34+ cells by flow cytometry allows identification of these cells. The earliest multilineage stem cell is CD34+, MDR-1+, c-kit+, and CD45RO+, but CD38–, HLA-DR–, and lineage-differentiation marker negative. In contrast, lineage-specific progenitor cells coexpress CD34 antigens associated with myeloid (CD33 and CD13), megakaryocytic (CD41 and CD61), erythroid (CD71), B-lymphoid (CD19), or T-lymphoid (CD7) differentiation. In autologous transplants, the most important factors affecting neutrophil recovery are CD34+ cells. A dose-response relationship exists between the number of CD34+ cells infused and both neutrophil and platelet recovery. The median time to an absolute neutrophil count (ANC) $>0.5 \times 10^9$/L (for three consecutive days) decreased with increasing CD34+ stem cell dose: 11 days for $<2.5 \times 10^6$ CD34+ cells/kg; 10 days for 2.5 to 7.5×10^6 CD34+ cells/kg; 9 days for 7.5 to 12.5×10^6 CD34+ cells/kg; and 8 days for $>12.5 \times 10^6$ CD34+ cells/kg. Therefore, for autologous transplantations, a higher CD34+ cell dose appears to correlate with improved long-term hematopoiesis. Beyond the larger number of CD34+ cells infused, the relative proportions of CD34+ lineage-specific subsets may be important. For example, platelet recovery correlated with the number of CD34+/CD41+ cells infused. Patients receiving $<0.5 \times 10^8$ CD34+/CD41+ cells/kg had a median platelet recovery of 19 days versus 11 days for patients who received $>0.5 \times 10^6$ cells/kg. Maximizing the number of infused autologous CD34+ progenitor cells results in fewer complications, fewer blood product requirements, more rapid hospital discharge, and better long-term peripheral blood counts. In contrast, allogeneic peripheral blood transplantations are complicated by an increased risk of chronic GVHD with increased number of stem cells infused. Therefore, the short-term favorable engraftment kinetics of allogeneic peripheral blood stem cells appear to be offset by an increase in morbidity and mortality from chronic GVHD.

37. Ans. a. The dose that is given is calculated by the number of T cells in the infusion

Major difference between donor lymphocyte infusion (DLI) and a stem cell transplant is that only lymphocytes (not stem cells) are collected from the donor. Usually the patient does not require any conditioning therapy before receiving the donor lymphocytes, but if there are a large number of blasts still present further chemotherapy may be given prior to the DLI infusion. There are two main reasons for using DLI. The first is to destroy any residual disease. DLI may be considered if there is any residual disease after a transplant or if there are signs of relapse of the disease. The donor lymphocytes recognize the patient's cells as "foreign" and can attack them causing GVHD, which may be severe and even life-threatening. However, there is also a beneficial aspect to this immune response by the donor cells because the same process can kill any residual leukemia cells very effectively, i.e., graft versus leukemia effect (GvL). The second reason to use DLI is to treat mixed chimerism, particularly in transplants using reduced intensity conditioning regimens. Donor lymphocytes are easy to collect from the blood of a donor as they are present in considerable numbers in blood, and do not require growth factors. DLI can suppress the bone marrow (myelosuppression). Approximately 8 weeks after the dose of donor lymphocytes has been given, the response is assessed in terms of the disease or chimerism status. If there is still evidence of disease being present or if there is still mixed chimerism, and there has been no significant GVHD, then another slightly higher dose of donor lymphocytes may be given. Further doses are usually given at 3 monthly intervals. Sometimes several doses of donor lymphocytes are given until the desired effect is reached or until significant GVHD develops.

38. Ans. a. Son

Ref: Wang U, Chang YJ, Xu LP, Liu KY, Liu DH, Zhang XH, et al. Who is the best donor for a related HLA haplotype-mismatched transplant? Blood. 2014;124(6):843-50.

According to the study by Wang et al., child is the best donor for haploidentical transplant and mother should be avoided as a donor as far as possible. Use of young, male, noninherited maternal antigen (NIMA) mismatched donors results in the best survival after HLA haploidentical mismatched related donor transplants. This study confirms that degree of HLA disparity on the HLA-mismatched haplotype is not significantly correlated with transplant outcomes among recipients of T-cell–replete HLA-haplotype-mismatched transplants. The older donors are associated with more acute GVHD than donors less than 30 years. The study showed lower nonrelapse mortality and better survival with younger sibling donors than parent donors. Mother donors were associated with more acute GVHD.

39. Ans. c. High-risk APML in CR1

Ref: Milligan DW, Grimwade D, Cullis JO, Bond L, Swirsky D, Craddock C, et al. BCSH, Guidelines on the management of acute myeloid leukaemia in adults. Br J Haematol. 2006;135(4):450-749; Williams 8/e

Hematopoietic stem cell transplantation has two main mechanisms of action. First, it replaces an abnormal hematopoietic system with one from a healthy donor. Second, it allows the delivery of myeloablative doses of radiation and/or chemotherapy to cure hematologic malignancies. Moreover, allogenic graft also has third function of alloreactivity which provides the immunological attack on malignant cells by graft-versus-leukemia effect.

Allogeneic transplantation should be offered to patients with high-risk AML in first remission who have a human leucocyte antigen identical donor. Allogeneic transplantation may be the preferred treatment for younger AML patients who are in second remission. Older patients with high-risk disease or beyond first remission may be offered a reduced-intensity conditioned transplant. Intensive consolidation chemotherapy treatment during CR1 should be offered as the preferred treatment to patients with favorable cytogenetics (low-risk group). For intermediate risk group, some studies have shown benefit of allo-SCT in CR1.

In APML, treatment of relapse, with respect to use of autologous or allogeneic SCT as consolidation should be guided by minimal residual disease assessment. If patient is PML-RARA positive then allo-SCT is the treatment of choice but if patient is PML-RARA negative then auto-SCT is preferred. Transplantation using autologous or allogeneic stem cells performed in first CR (CR1) confers no overall survival advantage in patients with APL, and patients should not routinely undergo transplant in CR1. So, stem cell transplantation is not recommended for patients with APL in first complete remission, even if it is high risk as per Sanz criteria.

Allogeneic stem cell transplantation is an option for patients with ALL with poor prognostic features such as Philadelphia chromosome or t(4;11) positivity or delayed time to first complete remission. Allogeneic transplantation is the recommended treatment option for eligible patients with ALL who achieve a second remission. Allogeneic stem cell transplantation is also an option for patients with CML for whom medical therapy has failed, as well as those in accelerated phase or blast crisis.

40. Ans. a. Similar to that in matched sibling donor (MSD) transplant without PT-Cy

Ref: Shabbir-Moosajee M. An overview of conditioning regimens for haploidentical stem cell transplantation with post-transplantation cyclophosphamide. Am J Hematol. 2015;90:541-8.

Reconstitution of CD3+, CD4+, and CD8+ T-cell subsets to normal levels usually occurs by 6 months post-transplantation. Several studies have suggested that the T-cell recovery for Haplo-SCT treated with PT-Cy is similar to matched donor transplants, which could, in part, explain comparable outcomes.

41. Ans. b. Presence of DSA against HLA molecules are a major risk factor for graft failure

Ref: Hoffman 7/e p1620

B cells and NK cells also participate in the immune response to HLA-mismatched tissues. Allogeneic HLA molecules can elicit the formation of alloantibody. Pre-existing DSA against HLA molecules are a major risk factor for graft failure after HLA-haploidentical SCT. Pregnancy and blood transfusions are sensitizing events that can lead to the formation of antibodies against HLA molecules.

42. Ans. d. All of the above *Ref: Hoffman 7/e p1624*

Treatment of bone marrow donors with G-CSF before donation increases marrow CD34+ cells and granulocyte-macrophage colony-forming units, reduces total lymphocytes, and reverses the CD4+/CD8+ T-cell ratio.

43. Ans. a. Mediated by T cells *Ref: Hoffman 7/e p1651*

Engraftment syndrome is a clinical condition that is characterized by fever, skin rash, pulmonary edema, weight gain, liver, and renal dysfunction in addition to encephalopathy and it occurs at the time of neutrophil recovery after hematopoietic stem cell transplantation (HSCT). The clinical findings of engraftment syndrome reflect the manifestations of increased capillary permeability or capillary leak syndrome. While described most often following autologous stem cell transplantation, a similar clinical syndrome has been observed followed allogeneic stem cell transplantation. Engraftment syndromes are likely associated with an increased transplant-related mortality, mostly from pulmonary and associated multiorgan failure. Although this syndrome's pathophysiology is poorly understood, it is thought to be caused by a wave of cytokine production as the graft starts to recover. These symptoms are related to, but distinct from, the "cytokine storm" of acute GVHD because there is no concomitant T-cell-mediated attack. This syndrome responds immediately to steroids in most patients, and it typically presents earlier than acute GVHD.

44. Ans. c. Nonmyeloablative conditioning

Ref: Corbacioglu S. Risk factors for development of and progression of hepatic veno-occlusive disease/sinusoidal obstruction syndrome. Biol Blood Marrow Transp. 2019;25:1271-80.

The risk factors related to hepatic sinusoidal obstruction syndrome post-SCT may be patient related or treatment related. The patient-related factors include preexisting hepatic condition, previous abdominal radiation, impaired pulmonary function, and ferritin >1,000 ng/mL pre-HSCT. The treatment-related factors include the type of conditioning therapies used, e.g., high-intensity/MAC regimens and the GVHD prophylaxis used.

45. **Ans. e. All of the above**   *Ref: Hoffman 7/e p1676*

Risk factors associated with the development of sinusoidal obstruction syndrome (SOS) include history of pretransplant hepatitis or liver injury, intensive preparative regimens, increased TBI dose, and dose rate and increased busulfan dose. SOS may also be more frequent after mismatched related or matched unrelated donor transplantation. Prior therapy with gemtuzumab ozogamicin also increases the risk of post-transplant SOS. Sirolimus has also been shown to increase the risks of SOS after myeloablative allogeneic HCT, particularly using busulfan-based regimens.

46. **Ans. e. None of the above**   *Ref: Hoffman 7/e p1679*

Post-transplant lymphoproliferative disorders (PTLD) comprise a heterogeneous group of lymphoid proliferations, primarily involving B-lymphocytes that develop as a result of uncontrolled Epstein-Barr virus (EBV) infection. They occur almost exclusively in allogeneic HCT recipients, with an overall incidence of 1-2%. They typically manifest soon after transplantation with more than 80% of cases diagnosed within the first year. Since, T cells play an important role in preventing proliferation of EBV-infected lymphocytes, removal of T cells from the hematopoietic graft or anti-T-cell serotherapy with ATG or alemtuzumab are strong risk factors for PTLD. Withdrawal of immunosuppression is usually attempted first, but can be difficult in patients with active GVHD. Active surveillance for EBV reactivation in high-risk settings and initiation of preemptive therapy, often with rituximab, is important.

47. **Ans. a. 21 years old sister**
Ref: Kongtim P. Who is the best donor for haploidentical stem cell transplantation? Semin Hematol. 2019;56:194-200.

Several donor factors have been shown to influence outcomes of Haplo SCT. The association between donor-specific anti-HLA antibodies (DSAs) and the risk of primary graft failure (PGF) has been well-recognized in patients receiving transplantation with HLA mismatched donors. Using a donor without target HLA antigens is a desired option for a recipient with DSAs. Several studies in HLA-matched transplants have shown better outcomes in terms of acute and chronic GVHD as well as long-term survival when using HSC graft from a younger donor. It has been shown that minor HLAs encoded on Y chromosome (H-Y) can contribute to the alloreactive immunogenicity in a setting of female donor to male recipient, which leads to an increased risk of GVHD and NRM. Patients with ABO matched and minor mismatch grafts are preferred to major ABO mismatched grafts and, if this cannot be avoided, peripheral blood stem cells should be preferentially used in this setting. Mismatch between donor and recipient CMV serostatus has been shown to be associated with CMV disease and negatively influenced outcomes in HLA-matched transplantation. The presence of a greater number of HLA mismatches at either antigen or allele level did not worsen overall outcomes (GVHD, relapse rate, and NRM), while having three or more HLA-mismatches in the host versus graft (HVG) but not in graft versus host (GVH) direction was associated with improved event-free survival. Therefore, the degree of HLA mismatching should not be used as a criterion to select family haploidentical donors based on current available evidences.

48. **Ans. e. All of the above**
Ref: Thomas' Hematopoietic Cell Transplantation, 4/e, Chapter 3, p16.

The most common indications for autologous transplants are multiple myeloma (48%), non-Hodgkin's lymphoma (28%), Hodgkin's disease (12%), leukemia (5%), neuroblastoma (5%), and other cancers.

49. **Ans. a. The dose of palifermin is 60 μg/kg/day for 3 days prior to high-dose chemotherapy**
Ref: Thomas' Hematopoietic Cell Transplantation, 4/e, p653.

Keratinocyte growth factor (palifermin) is naturally produced in mesenchymal cells and acts on a wide variety of epithelial cells. A dose of 60 μg/kg/day for 3 days prior to high-dose BEAM chemotherapy was chosen based on safety and preliminary efficacy. Palifermin has been proved to significantly reduce the duration and severity of oral mucositis after high-dose TBI-containing therapy. Palifermin has been proved to significantly reduce the duration and severity of oral mucositis after high-dose TBI-containing therapy in a randomized trial. It is not effective in treating mucositis. Palifermin had no significant effect on engraftment, acute GVHD or survival.

50. **Ans. b. Valganciclovir, Ganciclovir, Foscarnet, Cidofovir, Maribavir, CMX001, Leflunomide**
Ref: Thomas' Hematopoietic Cell Transplantation, 4/e, Chapter 90, p1376.

Acyclovir is not a first-line agent for prevention of CMV infection, but because of its safety profile, it can have an important role in preventing CMV reactivation. Valganciclovir at an oral dose of 900 mg, due to its excellent bioavailability, can result in similar levels to IV Ganciclovir at a dose of 5 mg/kg. Cidofovir has been used for the preemptive management at 5 mg/kg per dose in two doses given 1 week apart, followed by maintenance therapy provided every other week. Foscarnet is a phosphonate that requires no metabolism for activity and, because of its excellent antiviral profile, has become an important agent in the treatment of CMV infection in the immunosuppressed population.

Side effects include nephrotoxicity, hypocalcemia, and hypophosphatemia. Immunoglobulins are not recommended for the prevention of CMV infection after HCT. Other drugs such as leflunomide, maribavir and newer agents, e.g., CMX001 also have a role.

51. Ans. e. All of the above

Ref: Thomas' Hematopoietic Cell Transplantation, 4/e, Chapter 86, p1288.

The incidence of acute GVHD is increased with HLA-nonidentical donors when compared with HLA-identical donors. HLA-C, HLA-DRB1, and HLA-DP allele disparity is independently associated with an increased risk of acute GVHD. Male recipients of female grafts having the highest rates of GVHD and previously parous donors may have experienced maternal alloimmunization from unshared minor antigens of the fetus. Increasing donor age is associated with an increased severe acute GVHD. Cord blood transplantation is associated with the lowest rates of acute and chronic GVHD. For CMV-seronegative recipients, matching with seronegative donors also appears to reduce the risk of both CMV infection and GVHD.

52. Ans. d. Isolated acute liver GVHD is commonly seen

Ref: Thomas' Hematopoietic Cell Transplantation, 4/e, Chapter 86, p1290,1293.

The skin is the most commonly affected organ in acute GVHD, with >75% of acute GVHD patients having some cutaneous involvement, and 44% of patients having skin involvement as their only manifestation. The gastrointestinal tract is the second most commonly involved organ in acute GVHD, with up to half of individuals being affected. The liver is the least commonly affected organ in acute GVHD, with less than 20% of acute GVHD patients having some degree of hepatic involvement.

53. Ans. e. Eculizumab is a very effective drug

Ref: Eleanor G. Thrombotic microangiopathy following hematopoietic stem cell transplant. Pediatr Nephrol. 2018;33:1489-500.

Eculizumab is a recombinant, fully humanized, monoclonal antibody that binds complement C5 and blocks production of proinflammatory C5a and the membrane attack complex C5b-9. Its use in atypical hemolytic uremic syndrome (aHUS) has proved to be life-saving. With considerable overlap between aHUS and transplant associated-thrombotic microangiopathy (TA-TMA), eculizumab has been used for both the prevention and treatment of TA-TMA. TA-TMA does not usually respond to plasma exchange, rituximab or IVIG and has poor prognosis with high risk of mortality.

54. Ans. a. HSCT is the only curative treatment for all patients with JMML

Ref: How I treat juvenile myelomonocytic leukemia, Franco Locatelli, Charlotte M. Niemeyer, Blood Feb. 2015. Thomas' Hematopoietic Cell Transplantation: Stem Cell Transplantation, 4/e, Chapter 352, p755

Indications for HSCT in JMML depends upon type of mutation

	PTPN 11	K-RAS	N-RAS	NF-1	CBL
Patients with Germline mutations	Noonan's syndrome—wait and watch (or mild chemotherapy)	Noonan's syndrome—wait and watch (or mild chemotherapy)	Noonan's syndrome—wait and watch (or mild chemotherapy)	Neuro fibromatosis—Type 1	Noonan's syndrome-wait and watch, HSCT if disease progresses
Patients with somatic mutations	HSCT	HSCT	HSCT for most	–	–

The current JMML study of the Children's Oncology Group includes cytoreductive therapy consisting of fludarabine and high-dose cytarabine concomitantly with 13-*cis*-retinoic acid prior to HSCT. Relapse is the major cause of treatment failure of HSCT in patients with JMML undergoing HCT. It generally occurs within the first year after transplantation. Splenectomy pre transplant does not help to improve engraftment, survival and reduces relapse.

55. Ans. e. All of the above

Ref: Thomas' Hematopoietic Cell Transplantation: Stem Cell Transplantation, 4/e, Chapter 70, p1031

Selected rare hematologic malignancies for which HSCT has been performed

Langerhans cell histiocytosis
Systemic mastocytosis
Hypereosinophilic syndrome
Acute megakaryoblastic leukemia
Acute erythroleukemia
Chronic myelomonocytic leukemia
Adult T-cell leukemia/lymphoma
Natural killer cell leukemia/lymphoma
Mycosis fungoides
Sézary syndrome
Angioimmunoblastic T-cell lymphoma
Primary central nervous system lymphoma
Hepatosplenic T-cell lymphoma (gamma/delta T-cell lymphoma)
T-cell prolymphocytic leukemia
Subcutaneous panniculitic T-cell lymphoma
Hematodermic neoplasm (blastic natural killer cell lymphoma)

56. Ans. e. All of the above
Ref: Thomas' Hematopoietic Cell Transplantation: Stem Cell Transplantation, 4/e, Chapter 44, p634-5

Glycerol and DMSO are colligative cryoprotectants that protect the cell from excessive dehydration as extracellular water is drawn into growing ice crystals. Plasma proteins exert cryoprotectant effects, possibly by modifying the viscosity or temperature of the cryoprotectant solution. HES is a polymeric substance containing chains of different molecular weights. Successful cryopreservation has been achieved using commercially available pharmacologic salt solutions.

57. Ans. e. None of the above
Ref: Thomas' Hematopoietic Cell Transplantation: Stem Cell Transplantation, 4/e, Chapter 79, p1187-8

Early experience with HSCT in FA had very poor outcomes. Poor outcome was primarily the result of excessive regimen related toxicity (RRT), including severe acute GVHD. Minimizing exposure to DNA crosslinking agents, such as high-dose CY or total body irradiation (TBI) ultimately led to markedly reduced risks of RRT, enhanced survival, and improved health quality of life. The optimum time for HCT is when the patient is young, has had few red cell and/or platelet transfusions, and is free of MDS or leukemia.

58. Ans. a. Serious VZV disease after transplantation is related to the compromise of B-lymphocyte function
Ref: Thomas' Hematopoietic Cell Transplantation: Stem Cell Transplantation, 4/e, Chapter 92, p1388-9

Serious VZV disease after transplantation is related to the compromise of T-lymphocyte function. Immunization with inactivated varicella vaccine has the potential to reduce the morbidity of VZV reactivation after HSCT. Prophylaxis with acyclovir in general delays but does not prevent VZV reactivation. VZV prophylaxis in HSCT recipients with risk factors, such as those with T-cell depletion, ATG therapy, anti-CD3 antibody therapy, or unrelated or HLA-mismatched transplantation. The rationale for avoiding routine use is that prolonged administration of antiviral prophylaxis enhances the emergence of VZV strains that are resistant to the drug.

59. Ans. b. There is no decrease in CMV infection/disease and improved survival in HSCT recipients after high doses of acyclovir prophylactically
Ref: Thomas' Hematopoietic Cell Transplantation: Stem Cell Transplantation, 4/e Chapter 91, p1385

The drug of choice for the treatment of HSV mucocutaneous infection in the HSCT recipient is acyclovir. The current standard of therapy: acyclovir 250 mg/m^2 (or 5 mg/kg) intravenously every 8 hours for at least 7 days. Oral Acyclovir can be given as 400 mg orally five times a day for 10 days. When acyclovir-resistant HSV is suspected or proven, the drug of choice is foscarnet at 40 mg/kg intravenously every 8 hours. For foscarnet/acyclovir-resistant cases cidofovir is recommended at 5 mg/kg intravenously once a week for 2 weeks, and then once every 2 weeks. A significant decrease in CMV infection and disease and significantly improved survival is seen in those HSCT recipients given high doses (500 mg/m^2 every 8 hours) of intravenous acyclovir prophylaxis until 30 days after HSCT.

60. Ans. b. HSV infection
Ref: Thomas' Hematopoietic Cell Transplantation: Stem Cell Transplantation, 4/e, Chapter 92, p1389

HSV-1 causes clinically apparent disease at about 2-3 weeks, and CMV disease usually occurs during the second to third months after transplantation. Epstein-Barr virus may also reactivate in the third month, whereas VZV recurrences present at a median of 5 months after HCT. In general, the risk of recurrent VZV infection is highest between 2 and 10 months after transplantation.

61. Ans. a. Use of TBI 200 cGy in conditioning
Ref: Thomas' Hematopoietic Cell Transplantation: Stem Cell Transplantation, 4/e, 96, p1459

Risk factors for IPS include TBI (>1200 cGy), increasing recipient age, myeloablative conditioning, HLA mismatch, transplantation for malignancies other than leukemia and use of methotrexate.

62. Ans. c. Higher doses are associated with lower risk of GVHD
Ref: Thomas HSCT Book

In matched sibling donor transplantation, higher cell doses were associated with faster engraftment, lower transplant related mortality and reduced risk of relapse. However, not all these studies demonstrated an improvement in overall survival because of increased risk of GVHD.

63. Ans. a. 2% viscous lidocaine + diphenhydramine + antacid

Topical anesthetics may be combined with an antacid suspension and/or diphenhydramine with or without nystatin in a cocktail referred to as "miracle or magic mouth wash". Formulations may vary but may also include steroids and antibiotics. One such cocktail consists of 2% lidocaine viscous, diphenhydramine and Maalox. Other cocktails add dexamethasone solutions as an anti-inflammatory or add antibiotics such as tetracycline. Care should be advised for patients using rinses containing lidocaine to avoid further trauma to the anesthetized mucosa. Another cocktail using diphenhydramine, lidocaine and an antacid demonstrated a statistically decrease in pain associated with oral mucositis compared to placebo.

CHAPTER 38

Graft versus Host Disease

1. The treatment of choice for grade III acute GVHD is:
   a. 1 mg/kg prednisolone
   b. 2 mg/kg prednisolone
   c. 1 mg/kg methylprednisolone
   d. 2 mg/kg methylprednisolone

2. The recommended dose of steroids for chronic GVHD is:
   a. 1 mg/kg prednisolone
   b. 2 mg/kg prednisolone
   c. 1 mg/kg methylprednisolone
   d. 2 mg/kg methylprednisolone

3. Severity of chronic skin GVHD is assessed by all, *except*:
   a. Clinical grading
   b. Skin biopsy
   c. Plasma levels of elafin
   d. All of the above

4. Biopsy in acute gut GVHD is most informative when done from:
   a. Rectosigmoid region
   b. Ascending colon
   c. Cecum
   d. Duodenum

5. Response to corticosteroids in patients with grade II–IV acute GVHD is:
   a. 30–35%
   b. 40–45%
   c. 50–55%
   d. 60–65%

6. Diagnostic features of chronic GVHD are all, *except*:
   a. Poikiloderma
   b. Lichen planus-like features
   c. Keratoconjunctivitis sicca
   d. All of the above

7. Poor prognosis in chronic GVHD includes:
   a. Extensive (>50%) skin involvement
   b. Platelet count of <100 × 10^9/L
   c. Progressive onset from acute GVHD
   d. All of the above

8. Cyclosporine acts by inhibiting:
   a. B cells
   b. T cells
   c. Both B and T cells
   d. NK cells

9. Second-line agents for acute GVHD are considered if patient does not respond to steroids for:
   a. 3 days
   b. 5 days
   c. 7 days
   d. 14 days

10. Second-line treatment of steroid-refractory acute GVHD includes all, *except*:
    a. Extracorporeal photopheresis
    b. Antitumor necrosis factor antibodies
    c. Mycophenolate mofetil
    d. Interleukin-2 receptor antibodies
    e. Rituximab

11. Which of the following is effective for the treatment of acute GVHD?
    a. Ruxolitinib
    b. Bortezomib
    c. Natalizumab
    d. Brentuximab vedotin
    e. All of the above

12. True about graft rejection and GVHD is:
    a. Graft rejection is mediated by donor cells and GVHD by recipient cells
    b. Graft rejection is mediated by recipient cells and GVHD by donor cells
    c. Both are mediated by donor cells
    d. Both are mediated by recipient cells
    e. Depends upon the type of donor

13. True regarding acute GVHD is:
    a. Mediated by donor antigen presenting cells
    b. Mediated by recipient antigen presenting cells
    c. Mediated by both recipient and donor antigen presenting cells
    d. Antigen presenting cells are not involved in GVHD

14. Which of the following in not produced by the hematopoietic cells?
    a. IL-6
    b. IL-21
    c. IL-23
    d. IL-33
    e. None of the above

15. Which of the following is required for the development of GVHD?
    a. The transplanted graft must contain immunologically competent cells
    b. The recipient must be incapable of rejecting or eliminating transplanted cells
    c. The recipient must express tissue antigens that are not present in the transplant donor
    d. All of the above

16. GVHD is due to:
   a. Major HLA mismatch
   b. Blood group mismatch
   c. Minor HLA mismatch
   d. All of the above

17. True about ABO mismatch transplant is:
   a. Plasma depletion is needed in minor ABO mismatched bone marrow transplant
   b. RBC depletion is needed in major ABO mismatched bone marrow transplant
   c. Both plasma and RBC depletion is needed in bidirectional mismatched bone marrow transplant
   d. Neither RBC nor plasma depletion is needed in peripheral blood stem cell transplant
   e. All of the above

18. The pathogenesis of chronic GVHD includes:
   a. Pre-existing inflammation
   b. Deregulation of adaptive immunity
   c. Excessive fibrosis
   d. All of the above
   e. None of the above

19. True about mesenchymal stem cells is:
   a. They can migrate to the site of inflammation
   b. They can differentiate into various cell types
   c. They are inhibitory to T cells
   d. They lack immunogenicity
   e. All of the above

20. The surface antigen expression of mesenchymal stem cells is:
   a. CD45, CD34, CD29, CD105
   b. CD3, CD14, CD19, CD90
   c. CD45, CD34, HLA-DR, CD73
   d. CD29, CD105, CD73, CD90

21. In GVHD, overlap syndrome refers to:
   a. Acute GVHD presenting after day 100
   b. Chronic GVHD presenting before day 100
   c. Features of both chronic GVHD and acute GVHD
   d. All of the above

22. Ribbon sign is seen in:
   a. Gut GVHD
   b. *Clostridium difficile* enterocolitis
   c. CMV enterocolitis
   d. Mycophenolate-induced diarrhea

23. Drug which inhibits de novo purine synthesis is:
   a. Sirolimus
   b. Mycophenolate mofetil
   c. Tacrolimus
   d. Cyclosporine A

24. True about sirolimus is:
   a. Obtained from Streptomyces
   b. Has antifungal activity
   c. Inhibits B and T cells
   d. Inactivates m-TOR
   e. All of the above

ANSWERS WITH EXPLANATIONS

1. Ans. d. 2 mg/kg methylprednisolone

Ref: Dignan FL. Diagnosis and management of acute graft-versus-host disease. BJH. 2012.

Acute GVHD occurs after allogeneic hematopoietic stem cell transplant and is a reaction of donor immune cells against host tissues. Activated donor T cells damage host epithelial cells after an inflammatory cascade that begins with the preparative regimen. Corticosteroids are the standard first-line treatment for acute GVHD. Their effect is likely to be due to lympholytic effects and anti-inflammatory properties. A dose of 2 mg/kg/day of methylprednisolone is recommended as the starting dose for patients with grades III-IV acute GVHD. There is no consensus on the optimal dose and duration of steroid therapy due to the lack of data. A prospective study comparing 2 mg/kg/day of methylprednisolone with 10 mg/kg/day of methylprednisolone showed no advantage of high-dose steroids over low-dose steroids. The use of methylprednisolone at doses higher than 2 mg/kg/day is not routinely recommended.

2. Ans. a. 1 mg/kg prednisolone

Ref: Dignan FL. BCSH/BSBMT Guideline: diagnosis and management of chronic graft- versus-host disease. BJH. 2012.

Alloreactivity forms the basis of the pathogenesis of chronic GVHD, but the phenotypes and origins of the alloreactive cells involved remain somewhat ambiguous. Attempts to study chronic GVHD experimentally have been somewhat hampered by the absence of a reliable animal model that exactly represents variable manifestations in humans. Chronic GVHD remains a major complication of allogeneic stem cell transplantation and is the leading cause of late nonrelapse death. The prevalence varies from 25 to 80% in long-term survivors. Chronic GVHD should be graded as mild, moderate, or severe according to NIH consensus criteria.

Corticosteroids are recommended in the first-line treatment of chronic GVHD. An initial starting dose of 1 mg/kg prednisolone is recommended by BCSH. The regimen involves using a daily dose of 1 mg/kg for 2 weeks and subsequently tapering to 1 mg/kg on alternate days over 4 weeks if chronic GVHD is stable or improving. In severe GVHD, this dose may be maintained for 2–3 months and then tapered by 10–20% per month for a total duration of 9 months. In patients who are receiving other immunosuppressive agents, it is recommended that steroids are tapered first. Calcineurin inhibitors may be helpful in the initial treatment of GVHD as a steroid sparing agent. Extracorporeal photopheresis (ECP) has been considered as a second-line treatment in skin, oral, or liver chronic GVHD.

3. Ans. b. Skin biopsy

Ref: Dignan FL. BCSH/BSBMT Guideline: diagnosis and management of chronic graft-versus-host disease. BJH. 2012.

Chronic GVHD should be graded as mild, moderate or severe according to NIH consensus criteria. The consensus conference also identified "diagnostic" and "distinctive" features of chronic GVHD. Diagnostic signs are clinical features that establish the diagnosis of chronic GVHD without the need for further investigations. Diagnostic manifestations include poikiloderma and lichen planus-like features of the skin, lichen planus in the mouth or genitals, fasciitis, and joint contractures. Distinctive findings include skin depigmentation, nail dystrophy, alopecia, xerostomia, mucoceles, ulceration of the mouth, keratoconjunctivitis sicca, and myositis. Cutaneous biopsy has not been found to be useful in predicting severity of disease, though it may be helpful in making the diagnosis. Elafin is overexpressed in GVHD skin biopsies. Plasma levels of elafin have been found to be significantly higher in skin GVHD and correlate with severity of GVHD, with a greater risk of death relative to other known risk factors and may have prognostic value as a biomarker of skin GVHD. Histological features on skin biopsy include apoptosis at base of epidermal rete pegs, dyskeratosis, exocytosis of lymphocytes, satellite lymphocytes adjacent to dyskeratotic epidermal keratinocytes, and perivascular lymphocytic infiltration in the dermis.

4. Ans. a. Rectosigmoid region

Ref: Dignan FL. Diagnosis and management of acute graft-versus-host disease. BJH. 2012.

Gastrointestinal acute GVHD typically causes secretory diarrhea. Patients can also have nausea, vomiting, anorexia, weight loss, and abdominal pain. Diarrhea can be copious and, in severe acute GVHD, patient may have bleeding due to mucosal ulceration. Biopsy of the rectosigmoid has been found to be the most informative in acute gut GVHD. Biopsies taken at endoscopy may show patchy ulceration, apoptotic bodies at crypt bases, crypt ulceration, and flattening of surface epithelium.

5. Ans. b. 40–45%

Ref: Dignan FL. Diagnosis and management of acute graft-versus-host disease. BJH. 2012.

Response to steroid as first-line therapy varies in patients with acute gut GVHD. Martin et al. reported overall complete or partial responses in about 44% of patients. Improvement rates were 43% for skin disease, 35% for evaluable liver disease, and 50% for evaluable gut disease. Weisdorf et al. reported a complete and continued resolution of acute GVHD in 41% of patients after a median of 21 days of corticosteroids. The 5-year survival was 51% for steroid responders compared to 32% for steroid nonresponders. An International Bone Marrow Transplant Registry (IBMTR) survey confirmed that most centers considered patients to be steroid refractory after 5 days of treatment.

6. Ans. c. Keratoconjunctivitis sicca

Ref: Dignan FL. BCSH/BSBMT Guideline: diagnosis and management of chronic graft-versus-host disease. BJH. 2012.

Diagnostic signs are clinical features that establish the diagnosis of chronic GVHD without the need for further investigations. Diagnostic manifestations include poikiloderma and lichen planus-like features of the skin, lichen planus in the mouth or genitals, fasciitis, and joint contractures. Distinctive signs are clinical features not associated with acute GVHD but which would be insufficient to make the diagnosis of chronic GVHD unless supported by positive biopsy or laboratory findings. Distinctive findings include skin depigmentation, nail dystrophy, alopecia, xerostomia, mucoceles, ulceration of the mouth, keratoconjunctivitis sicca, and myositis. Additional investigations are helpful in confirming the diagnosis of chronic GVHD in patients with distinctive features and excluding other conditions, e.g., infection or drug toxicities.

7. Ans. d. All of the above

Three conditions have been associated with poor prognosis in chronic GVHD—(1) extensive (>50% of body surface area) skin involvement, (2) a platelet count of $<100 \times 10^9/L$ (thrombocytopenia), and (3) progressive onset from acute GVHD.

8. Ans. b. T cells

Cyclosporin is used in the prophylaxis of GVHD. Cyclosporin binds to cyclophilin and prevents generation of NF-AT which is a nuclear factor for initiating gene transcription for lymphokines including interleukin-2 and interferon gamma. This action leads to suppression of cytokine production and subsequent inhibition of T-cell activation. A combination regimen of cyclosporin and prednisolone may have a steroid-sparing effect and reduce the incidence of steroid associated complications in the management of GVHD.

9. Ans. b. 5 days *Ref: See Q. No. 5.*

Second-line agents can be considered in patients who have failed to respond despite 2 mg/kg of IV methylprednisolone in conjunction with a calcineurin inhibitor for acute GVHD for 5 days or progressive disease for 3 days.

10. Ans. e. Rituximab

The following agents are used in the second line treatment of steroid-refractory acute GVHD: Extracorporeal photopheresis, antitumor necrosis factor alpha antibodies, mammalian target of rapamycin (mTOR) inhibitors, mycophenolate mofetil, and interleukin-2 receptor antibodies. Rituximab is an anti-CD20 monoclonal antibody that has been used in the treatment of chronic GVHD but its role in acute GVHD is limited to case reports.

11. Ans. e. All of the above

Ref: Hill LQ. New and emerging therapies for acute and chronic graft versus host disease. Ther Adv Hematol. 2018.

It has been shown that interferon gamma receptor (INFγR) signaling is mediated via JAK1/JAK2 and is upregulated in activated T cells. T cells deficient in INFγR cause significantly less GVHD compared with wild-type T cells, and pharmacologic inhibition of JAK1/2 by ruxolitinib leads to less GVHD, in addition to preserving antileukemic effects. Inhibition of JAK1/2 (nonspecific inhibition) significantly reduces T-cell function. Immune-modulating effects of bortezomib include deletion of alloreactive T cells, inhibition of APCs, inhibition of IL-6, increased survival of Tregs, and decrease in levels of B-cell activating factor (BAFF). Natalizumab is a humanized monoclonal antibody against α4-integrin containing adhesion molecules which are widely expressed on leukocytes, primarily lymphocytes. Natalizumab inhibits adhesion molecules, preventing leukocyte migration from the circulation into inflamed gut mucosa. CD30 is a tumor necrosis factor receptor family member and is highly expressed on activated lymphocytes with minimal expression on normal tissues. Patients with acute GVHD had a higher percentage of CD30 expressing CD8+ T cells, significantly higher plasma levels of soluble CD30, and increased CD30+ lymphocytes in affected intestinal tissue compared with patients without acute GVHD.

12. Ans. b. Graft rejection is mediated by recipient cells and GVHD by donor cells

Graft rejection involves immune reactivity of the recipient against transplanted allografts, while GVHD is triggered by the reactivity of donor-derived immune cells against allogeneic recipient tissues. Mature donor T cells contained within the infused graft mediate both GVHD and graft-versus-tumor with both being reduced when T cells are depleted.

13. Ans. c. Mediated by both recipient and donor antigen presenting cells

Ref: Perkey E. New insights into graft-versus-host disease and graft rejection. Ann Rev Pathol Mech Dis. 2018;13:219-45.

Donor T cells can recognize alloantigen either on host antigen presenting cells (APCs), known as direct antigen presentation, or on donor APCs, known as indirect presentation. Recipient-derived APCs are essential to initiate acute GVHD; however, donor APCs can amplify later disease states. For example, dendritic cells derived from the donor bone marrow restimulate alloreactive CD4+ T cells in target GVHD organs. After T cells are initially primed by recipient cells, donor CD103+ dendritic cells seed the gut, capturing alloantigens, and becoming activated by innate inflammatory signals before migrating to mesenteric lymph nodes, driving a potent positive feedback loop of T cell alloactivation through the provision of recipient alloantigen, IL-12, IL-6, and CD40 costimulatory signals.

14. Ans. d. IL-33

Ref: Piper C, Drobyski WR. Inflammatory cytokine networks in gastrointestinal tract graft vs. host disease. Front Immunol. 2019;10:163.

The STAT-dependent cytokines which have been most critically examined with respect to GVHD within the GI tract are IL-6, IL-21, and IL-23. IL-6 is a factor produced by monocytes and macrophages. IL-6 is a proinflammatory cytokine that is crucial in initiating a TH17 immune response. In the presence of IL-6 and TGF-β, naive T cells are able to differentiate into cells of the TH17 lineage, whereas in the absence of this cytokine, these same cells are directed to become Tregs. Blockade of IL-6 signaling by the administration of an antibody (tocilizumab) that binds to the IL-6 receptor significantly reduces GVHD-associated mortality and, specifically, pathologic damage within the colon. IL-23 is a member of the IL-12 family, signals through STAT3, and is secreted by dendritic cells, as well as other APCs such as macrophages and monocytes. IL-21 is produced by CD4+ T cells, CD8+ T cells, and NK-T cells, while the receptor for IL-21 is expressed on T cells, B cells, NK cells, dendritic cells, macrophages, and epithelial cells. Blockade of IL-21 signaling by either antibody-based strategies or genetic approaches is able to significantly reduce the severity of GVHD. IL-33 is produced primarily by a variety of nonhematopoietic cells which include endothelial cells, fibroblasts, and epithelial cells in the intestines and bronchi. Release of IL-33 leads to binding to its membrane receptor, ST2, which is expressed on a large number of immune cells (i.e., TH2 cells, regulatory T cells, type 2 innate lymphoid cells, macrophages, and granulocyte populations). The IL-33/ST2 axis is involved in acute GVHD. Exogenous IL-33 administration during the peak inflammatory response worsens the GVHD. Blockade of IL-33/ST2 interactions during allogeneic-hematopoietic cell transplantation by exogenous ST2-Fc infusions results in marked reduction in GVHD lethality. Transplant recipients that are deficient for IL-33 are protected from GVHD and administration of IL-33 in the early post-transplantation period (days 3–7 post-transplant) exacerbates this disease. Post-transplantation blockade of IL-33 with an sST2-Fc receptor fusion protein also attenuates GVHD.

15. Ans. d. All of the above

Ref: Billingham RE. The biology of graft-versus-host reactions. Harvey Lect. 1967;62:21-78.

The histocompatibility differences between the donor and the recipient, the presence of donor's immunocompetent cells, and the inability of the recipient to reject these cells were defined as the basic pathogenic prerequisites for GVHD development by Billingham in 1966. The immunocompetent cells are T lymphocytes that are present in the stem cell inoculum and are required to mount an effective immune response. A normal immune system is able to reject T cells from a foreign donor. However, when recipient's immune system is compromised through the use of various immune-ablative agents (chemotherapy and/or radiotherapy), the recipient is incapable of rejecting the transplanted cells.

16. Ans. d. All of the above

Ref: Worel N. ABO-mismatched allogeneic hematopoietic stem cell transplantation. Transfus Med Hemother. 2016;43:3-12.

The tissue antigens that differ in donor and recipient are major and minor human leukocyte antigens (HLA), and their expression on cell surfaces is crucial for the activation of allogenic T cells and initiation of GVHD. GVHD occurs when donor T cells activate and respond to HLA differences on recipient's tissue. Transplants carried out in the HLA-matched sibling or identical twin setting can still give rise to GVHD due to differences in minor HLA. Therefore, patients with major and minor incompatibility have higher risk of acute GVHD. Though some studies have found increased risk of GVHD with blood group mismatch, others have not found any significant association. Ludajic K et al. (BBMT 2009) have reported that patients with minor ABO incompatibility are at high-risk of massive immune hemolysis and acute GVHD after SCT. So, in this question, choice "d" seems to be the most reasonable answer as it includes minor HLA mismatch also.

17. Ans. e. All of the above

Ref: Worel N. ABO-mismatched allogeneic hematopoietic stem cell transplantation. Transfus Med Hemother. 2016;43:3-12.

Immediate hemolysis is commonly seen when bone marrow grafts are used as they contain more red blood cells (RBCs; approximately 200–450 mL) and plasma (up to 1,000 mL or more) compared to peripheral blood stem cell (PBSC) grafts. Therefore, in ABO-mismatched bone marrow transplant (BMT), it is clinical routine either to remove isohemagglutinins/antibodies (in case of minor ABO mismatch) or incompatible RBCs (in case of major ABO mismatch) from the graft or to reduce antidonor RBC antibodies or residual RBCs in the recipient by various techniques. Due to a lesser content of RBCs (approximately 8–15 mL) and plasma (approximately 200–500 mL) in PBSC grafts, it is usually not necessary to manipulate these products in case of ABO mismatch.

18. Ans. d. All of the above

Ref: Cooke KR, Luznik L, Sarantopoulos S, Hakim FT, Jagasia M, Fowler DH, et al. The biology of chronic graft-versus-host disease. NIH criteria. Biol Blood Marrow Transplant. 2017;23:211-34.

The three phase-based concepts of chronic GVHD pathogenesis include pre-existing inflammation, deregulation of adaptive immunity, and excessive fibrosis. Pre-existing inflammation is mediated by innate immunity mechanisms resulting in acute inflammation and nonspecific tissue damage caused by the administration of cytotoxic medications, infections, or previous Th1- and Th17-mediated acute GVHD activities. Thymus damage plays a key role in the second phase, manifesting as chronic inflammation and adaptive immunity deregulation. Thymus dysfunction results in decreased heterogeneity of tissue specific autoantigens mostly present in chronic GVHD target organs such as the skin, liver, salivary glands, lungs, eyes, and GI tract. The third phase of chronic GVHD pathogenesis is based on deregulated processes in response to chronic inflammation resulting in excessive fibrosis, disruption of the architecture of target tissues and organs, and their dysfunction. Exuberant or excessive repair lead to fibrosis, scaring, and end organ dysfunction.

19. Ans. e. All of the above

Ref: Amorin B, Alegretti AP, Valim V, Pezzi A, Laureano AM, da Silva MA, et al. Mesenchymal stem cell therapy and acute graft-versus-hostdisease: A review. Hum Cell. 2014;27(4):137-50.

Mesenchymal stem cells (MSCs) have the ability to migrate to sites of inflammation when injected intravenously. They can differentiate into various cell types, with distinct functions and can secrete multiple bioactive molecules capable of inhibiting inflammation and healing injured tissues. Another important characteristic of MSCs is their ability to perform immunomodulatory functions while lacking immunogenicity. MSCs have been shown to inhibit B- and T-cell activation, block the function of antigen presenting cells, inhibit NK cells, and increase Tregs. As they inhibit the proliferation and cytotoxic action of immune cells, MSCs have been employed in the treatment of several diseases, including GVHD, due to their inhibitory effects on the proliferation and cytotoxic activity of immune system cells.

20. Ans. d. CD29, CD105, CD73, CD90

Ref: Dominici M, Le Blanc K, Mueller I, Slaper-Cortenbach I, Marini F, Krause D, et al. Minimal criteria for defining multipotent mesenchymal stromal cells. The International Society for Cellular Therapy position statement. Cytotherapy. 2006;8(4):315-7.

Mesenchymal stem cells are ontogenetically and functionally different from hematopoietic stem cells. The antigens present on mesenchymal stem cells include CD29, CD105, CD73, and CD90 in >95% of cells, and there is lack of expression of hematopoietic antigens on MSCs. Therefore, MSCs are negative for CD45, CD34, CD3, CD14, CD19, or HLA-DR. CD45 is a pan-leukocyte marker and CD34 marks primitive hematopoietic progenitors and endothelial cells. CD14 and CD11b are prominently expressed on monocytes and macrophage, and CD79a and CD19 are markers of B cells. HLA-DR molecules are also not expressed on MSCs unless stimulated.

21. Ans. c. Features of both chronic GVHD and acute GVHD

GVHD has been classically divided into acute and chronic variants based on the time of onset using a cutoff of 100 days. However, this conventional division has been challenged by the recognition that signs of acute and chronic GVHD may occur outside of these designated periods. GVHD is now divided into four types: (1) Classic acute GVHD—cases present within 100 days of hematopoietic cell transplant (HCT) and display features of acute GVHD. Diagnostic and distinctive features of chronic GVHD are absent. (2) Persistent, recurrent, late onset acute GVHD—cases present greater than 100 days post-HCT with features of acute GVHD. Diagnostic and distinctive features of chronic GVHD are absent. (3) Classic chronic GVHD—cases may present at any time post-HCT. Diagnostic and distinctive features of chronic GVHD are present. There are no features of acute GVHD. (4) Overlap syndrome—cases may present at any time post-HCT with features of both chronic GVHD and acute GVHD. On occasion, this is colloquially referred to as "acute on chronic" GVHD.

22. Ans. a. Gut GVHD

Ref: Hoffman R, Benz EJ, Silberstein LE, Heslop H, Weitz J, Anastasi J. Hematology, 7th edition. Amsterdam: Elsevier; 2017. p1652.

Radiologic findings of the gastrointestinal tract in GVHD include luminal dilatation with thickening of the wall of the small bowel and air/fluid levels suggestive of an ileus on abdominal flat plates or small bowel series. Abdominal computed tomography may show the "ribbon" sign of diffuse thickening of the small bowel wall.

23. Ans. b. Mycophenolate mofetil

Sirolimus is an mTOR inhibitor. Mycophenolate mofetil is a prodrug of mycophenolic acid (MPA), an inhibitor of inosine monophosphate dehydrogenase (IMPDH). This is the rate-limiting enzyme in de novo synthesis of guanosine nucleotides. T- and B-lymphocytes are more dependent on this pathway than other cell types are. MPA depletes guanosine nucleotides preferentially in T and B lymphocytes and inhibits their proliferation, thereby suppressing cell-mediated immune responses and antibody formation. Tacrolimus, formerly known as FK506, is a macrolide antibiotic with immunosuppressive properties. Although structurally unrelated to cyclosporin A (CsA), its mode of action is similar. It exerts its effects principally through impairment of gene expression in target cells. Tacrolimus bonds to an immunophilin, FK506 binding protein (FKBP). This complex inhibits calcineurin phosphatase. The drug inhibits calcium-dependent events, such as interleukin-2 gene transcription, nitric oxide synthase activation, cell degranulation, and apoptosis.

24. Ans. e. All of the above

Ref: Sehgal SN. Sirolimus: Its discovery, biological properties, and mechanism of action. Transplant Proc. 2003;35(3 Suppl):7S-14S.

Sirolimus is produced by a strain of bacterium *Streptomyces hygroscopicus*, isolated from a soil sample collected from Rapa Nui commonly known as Easter Island. The compound was originally named rapamycin after the native name of the island, Rapa Nui. Although sirolimus was isolated as an antifungal agent with potent anticandida activity, subsequent studies revealed impressive antitumor and immunosuppressive activities. Sirolimus is a potent inhibitor of antigen-induced proliferation of T cells, B cells, and antibody production. The molecular mechanism underlying the antifungal, antiproliferative, and immunosuppressive activities of sirolimus is the same. Sirolimus forms an immunosuppressive complex with intracellular protein, FKBP12. This complex blocks the activation of the cell cycle-specific kinase, TOR. The downstream events that follow the inactivation of TOR result in the blockage of cell cycle progression at the juncture of G1 and S phase.

SECTION 5
Consultative Hematology

39. Consultative Hematology

CHAPTER 39

Consultative Hematology

1. A patient of rheumatic heart disease with mitral valve replacement on warfarin has developed severe headache. His CT scan shows small parieto-occipital bleed. His prothrombin time-international normalized ratio (PT-INR) is 13.5. The preferred management will be:
   a. Give vitamin K
   b. Give fresh frozen plasma and vitamin K
   c. Give prothrombin complex concentrate and vitamin K
   d. Give recombinant factor VIIa
   e. Urgent craniotomy

2. A patient with coronary artery disease has undergone coronary artery stenting 3 weeks back and is on Ecosprin. He presented with mild hematemesis. Platelet count is 1,20,000/µL. Next step is:
   a. Stop ecosprin along with evaluating cause of hematemesis
   b. Continue ecosprin along with evaluating cause of hematemesis
   c. Start clopidogrel
   d. Transfuse platelets and FFP
   e. Start another antiplatelet drug

3. A 40-year-old female patient with abdominal mass on evaluation was found to have prolonged activated partial thromboplastin time (patient's APTT—78 seconds, control 30 seconds). There is no past personal or family history of bleeding or thrombosis. Further evaluation shows presence of anticardiolipin antibodies. The best advice will be:
   a. The patient should be put on lifelong anti-coagulation
   b. The patient should be given anticoagulation during perioperative period
   c. The patient has high risk of bleeding
   d. All of the above

4. A pregnant female with 6 months of pregnancy on monthly follow-up found to have platelet count of 30,000/µL. The treatment is:
   a. Steroids
   b. Intravenous immunoglobulins
   c. Anti-Rh-D
   d. Platelet transfusion with steroids
   e. Wait and watch

5. A patient with carcinoma colon on evaluation found to have platelet count of 654,000/µL. He should undergo:
   a. Bone marrow biopsy for bone metastasis
   b. JAK-2 mutation analysis
   c. Treatment with hydroxyurea
   d. None of the above

6. A 35-year-old male patient with chronic obstructive lung disease on oral steroids found to have WBC 46,000/µL. Next step is:
   a. BCR-ABL to rule out CML
   b. Immunophenotyping to rule out CLL
   c. Bone marrow examination
   d. Hydroxyurea to maintain WBC less than 11,000/µL
   e. LAP score

7. A patient with hepatic hemangioma planned for surgery on routine evaluation found to have hemoglobin of 18.8 g/dL. The management of patient will be:
   a. JAK-2 mutation analysis
   b. BCR-ABL mutation analysis
   c. Surgery of hemangioma
   d. Regular phlebotomy

8. A patient with renal failure with Klebsiella sepsis and ecchymotic patches over limbs, found to have platelets 15,000/µL. Prothrombin and APTT were markedly prolonged. The treatment will be:
   a. Platelet transfusion   b. FFP transfusion
   c. Antibiotics   d. All of the above

9. A postrenal transplant patient on immuno-suppressive therapy presented with right axillary lymphadenopathy, weight loss, and fever. The treatment for the patient is:
   a. Wait and watch
   b. Trial of antitubercular therapy
   c. Decrease immunosuppressive therapy
   d. Increase immunosuppressive therapy

10. An 8-year-old child was admitted with high fever for 5 days, jaundice, and mild splenomegaly. The workup for hemolysis revealed mildly increased osmotic fragility and mildly positive Coombs test. The patient should be evaluated for:
    a. Hereditary spherocytosis
    b. Autoimmune hemolytic anemia

c. Parasitic infection
d. Serum iron and vitamin B_{12} levels
e. The hemolytic workup is fallacious

11. A 7-year-old child with cyanotic congenital heart disease is found to have hemoglobin level of 21 g/dL. True statement regarding this is:
a. There is increased erythropoietin production
b. Hematocrit level should be maintained around 60% through the use of exchange transfusions
c. Iron deficiency in polycythemia should be corrected
d. All of the above

12. Which of the following treatments should not be used in immune thrombocytopenia in HIV patients?
a. Intravenous immunoglobulin
b. Anti-RhD
c. Steroids
d. Splenectomy
e. All can be used

13. A 56-year-old patient with alcoholic liver disease, with Eastern Cooperative Oncology Group (ECOG) performance status of 1, developed fever with diffuse lymphadenopathy. His PT-INR was 1.4. He has been planned for cervical lymph node biopsy and bone marrow examination. True regarding the planned interventions is:
a. These procedures cannot be done in view of increased risk of bleeding
b. Patient should be given prophylactic FFP transfusions before the procedure even if there is no bleeding
c. Procedures should only be done after complete correction of coagulation abnormalities
d. The procedures can be performed without any prophylactic transfusions

14. True about antiphospholipid antibodies in pregnancy is:
a. Thrombotic events occur in approximately 5% of pregnant women with antiphospholipid antibodies
b. All pregnant women with SLE should undergo testing for antiphospholipid antibodies
c. Pregnant woman with antiphospholipid antibodies but no manifestations of the clinical syndrome should receive prophylactic anticoagulation
d. All of the above

15. A 5-year-old girl child presented with intracranial hemorrhage. She also had history of prolonged bleeding from umbilical cord at birth. His PT and APTT were normal. The next evaluation should include:
a. Mixing studies
b. Platelet function assays
c. von-Willebrand assay
d. Urea clot solubility test

16. Risk of which of the following complications increases with low hemoglobin in sickle cell anemia?
a. Painful crises
b. Avascular necrosis
c. Acute chest syndrome
d. Stroke

17. True about fertility preservation for lymphoma treatment are all, *except*:
a. The pretreatment semen quality is poor
b. Gonadal doses of 200–300 cGy cause prolonged and often irreversible azoospermia
c. Patients receiving CHOP therapy have very low risk of developing gonadal dysfunction
d. BEACOPP causes less infertility than ABVD therapy
e. All of the above

18. True regarding fertility status of patients treated with conventional chemotherapy for acute leukemia are all, *except*:
a. Male leukemia patients have lower pretreatment semen quality than healthy donors
b. The reproductive function of women treated with chemotherapy alone for acute lymphoblastic leukemia seems to be mostly preserved
c. Induction chemotherapy is as gonadotoxic as stem cell transplant
d. Standard chemotherapy regimens used to treat ALL and AML have low gonadotoxic potential
e. Cranial irradiation impairs fertility

19. A 5-year-old child was planned for surgery for tetralogy of Fallot, but on preoperative evaluation, was found to have hemoglobin of 21 g/dL and platelet count of 50×10^9/L. The most likely cause of thrombocytopenia in this case is:
a. Immune-mediated destruction
b. Destruction of platelets by cardiac defect
c. Right-to-left shunt
d. Pseudothrombocytopenia because of high hematocrit
e. Chronic disseminated intravascular dissemination

20. A 14-year-old girl presents to the outpatient clinic with easy bruising and fatigue. Complete blood count shows a white cell count of 2.5×10^9/L with 50% neutrophils, hemoglobin 7.4 g/dL, and platelet count of 7×10^9/L. Past medical history is significant for cardiac defect surgery at age of 10 years. Examination shows short stature, pallor, and ecchymoses. Which of the following investigations will be most pertinent in planning her treatment?
a. Whole body PET-CT
b. Immunoflowcytometry for acute lymphoblastic leukemia
c. Iron studies
d. Chromosomal breakage analysis

ANSWERS WITH EXPLANATIONS

1. Ans. c. Give prothrombin complex concentrate and vitamin K

Ref: Guidelines on oral anticoagulation with warfarin, 4th edition, Keeling D. BJH. 2011; Guidelines for management of anticoagulation with warfarin. NHS. 2012.

Warfarin acts by inhibiting the enzymes involved in the formation of a reduced form of vitamin K, which is essential for γ-carboxylation of glutamate residues at the amino terminus of coagulation factors II, VII, IX, and X and anticoagulant factors protein C and S.

Unlike older mechanical heart valves (MHV), the newer valve design with very low thrombogenicity has reduced markedly the rate of valve thrombosis and thromboembolism events (TEs), along with the required level of anticoagulation [<3.5 international normalized ratio (INR)], which has led to use of a lower dosage of warfarin as well as bleeding complications. The incidence of major bleeding complications in patients with MHV and taking oral anticoagulants has varied from 0.34 to 1.32% per patient-year.

British Committee for Standards in Haematology (BCSH) guidelines define major bleeding in terms of anticoagulation reversal as limb or life-threatening bleeding that requires complete reversal within 6-8 hours. Patients on warfarin have reduced levels of factors II, VII, IX, and X and rapid correction involves replacement of the preformed factors. Rapid correction is most effectively achieved by the administration of prothrombin complex concentrate (PCC, 4-factor PCCs).

International Society on Thrombosis and Hemostasis in 2005 defined major bleeding in nonsurgical patients as:
- Fatal bleeding
- Symptomatic bleeding in a critical area or organ, such as intracranial, intraspinal, intraocular, retroperitoneal, intra-articular or pericardial, or intramuscular (iliopsoas) with compartment syndrome
- Bleeding causing a fall in hemoglobin level of 2 g% or more, or leading to transfusion of two or more units of whole blood or red cells.

Among the factors, increasing warfarin-induced major bleeding, an INR level over the therapeutic range is the most important risk factor, independent of the indication for therapy, with the risk increasing dramatically with INR >4-5. Other risk factors which can increase major bleeding in patients on oral anticoagulation include age >75 years, hypertension, previous stroke, concomitant antiplatelet agents, and a previous history of bleeding. Management of warfarin-induced major bleeding in patients with MHV is challenging. There is vast controversy and confusion in the type of treatment required to reverse anticoagulation and stop bleeding as well as the ideal time to restart warfarin therapy safely without recurrence of bleeding and/or thromboembolism. Presently, the treatments available to reverse warfarin-induced bleeding are vitamin K, fresh frozen plasma (FFP), PCCs, and recombinant activated factor VIIa. Currently, vitamin K and FFP are the recommended treatments in patients with MHV and warfarin-induced major bleeding. Administration of vitamin K (10 mg intravenously at an infusion rate of 1 mg/min, diluted in dextrose 5% in water or dextrose 5% in normal saline) alone will require 12-24 hours (reversal begins within 6 hours) to reverse warfarin-induced coagulopathy. FFP contains vitamin K-dependent clotting factors. The suggested dose is 15 mL/kg infusion (range 10-30 mL/kg), about 3-4 units of plasma in the average-sized adult (one unit = 250 mL). Time to effect of FFP is 10 minutes, but it takes a few hours for partial reversal and at least 9-10 hours for complete reversal of INR (INR < 1.5). Other limitations in using FFP include fluid overload and transfusion-related acute lung injury. Although FFP is commonly used, as it is widely available and costs less, PCC has been noted to have significant benefits over FFP and according to a few authors it is the "gold standard" therapy. This is because of the concentration of clotting factors in PCCs being approximately 25 times higher than in FFP and because FFP contains an inadequate concentration of factor IX. Approximately 60 mL of PCC corresponds to 1,500 mL of FFP leading to a minimal risk of volume overload. The advantages of PCC are rapid preparation (time taken getting PCC 15 minutes vs. 1-2 hours for FFP), and complete reversal of warfarin effect within 10-30 minutes of administration. INR should be measured within 30 minutes of PCC administration. If it remains ≥1.5, a further PCC dose should be administered. If either FFP or PCCs are administered without vitamin K, initially there will be rapid normalization of the INR with a "rebound" increase 12-24 hours later; this phenomenon is commonly seen when vitamin K is not given simultaneously with FFP or PCC or an inadequate dose of vitamin K is administered. This is because the half-life of warfarin far exceeds the half-life of the administered coagulation factor complexes. FFP produces suboptimal anticoagulation reversal and should only be used if PCC is not available (BJH 2011).

For most patients, discontinuation of warfarin for 1-2 weeks should be sufficient to observe the evolution of a parenchymal hematoma to prevent its expansion, to clip or coil a ruptured aneurysm, or to evacuate an acute subdural hematoma.

Recombinant FVIIa (used in hemophilia patients) is also effective in reversing elevated INR at doses of 10-40 µg/kg bolus dose. Recombinant FVIIa gives a rapid and complete biochemical reversal of INR within 10 minutes, but has a short half-life of <1 hour. The disadvantage of rFVIIa is that it does not replace all clotting factors and even though INR is reduced immediately, clotting may not be restored in vivo. The most recent guidelines on management of these patients advise against use of rFVIIa in the treatment of warfarin-associated bleeding/ICH. So, in a patient with warfarin-associated bleeding, both vitamin K and FFP can be used depending upon the severity of bleeding.

2. Ans. b. Continue ecosprin along with evaluating cause of *hematemesis*

Ref: Oscarsson A, Gupta A, Fredrikson M, Järhult J, Nyström M, Pettersson E, et al. To continue or discontinue aspirin in the perioperative period: A randomized, controlled clinical trial. Br J Anaesth. 2010;104(3):305-12.

Veitch AM, Baglin TP, Gershlick AH, Harnden SM, Tighe R, Cairns S, et al. Guidelines for the management of anticoagulant and antiplatelet therapy in patients undergoing endoscopic procedures. Gut. 2008;57(9):1322-9.

Assia EI, Raskin T, Kaiserman I, Rotenstreich Y, Segev F. Effect of aspirin intake on bleeding during cataract surgery. J Cataract Refract Surg. 1998;24(9):1243-6.

Thrombosis of a drug-eluting stent (DES) is a catastrophic complication. The risk of stent thrombosis is increased in the perioperative setting and is strongly associated with the cessation of antiplatelet therapy. In a patient with DES on aspirin, the patient's inherent risk for bleeding, concomitant treatments that may increase this risk of bleeding, the type of surgery to cause bleeding, and the patient's risk for ischemic cardiac events if antiplatelet therapy is stopped, all must be taken into consideration before stopping antiplatelet drugs.

Studies have shown that discontinuation of aspirin therapy increases the risk of myocardial infarction (MI) and stroke. Patients at particularly high risk are those with recent or recurrent acute coronary syndrome (ACS) with dual oral antiplatelet therapy, recent percutaneous coronary intervention (PCI; less than 4 weeks), left ventricular ejection fraction ≤30%, triple-vessel disease, stent of length >25 mm or, a DES, history of thrombosis in a vessel of diameter ≤2.5 mm, incomplete revascularization, and ≥2 locations of symptomatic atherothrombosis.

Guidelines developed by the Oral Medicine and Oral Surgery Francophone Society found that interruption of aspirin or thienopyridine (clopidogrel) therapy before most of the dental procedures is unnecessary. Most such procedures carry a low risk of bleeding, and any bleeding that occurs can usually be controlled by local hemostasis. In general, discontinuation of antiplatelet therapy is considered unnecessary in procedures that are not highly invasive and therefore have a low bleeding risk. Oral, periodontal, and implant dental surgery are not associated with high rates of bleeding.

The French Society of Anesthesiology and Intensive Care (SFAR) considers discontinuation of aspirin unnecessary before eye surgery. Because aspirin and clopidogrel have additive effects on bleeding time, a suggestion has been made to continue aspirin but discontinue clopidogrel before eye surgery in patients on combination therapy. Similarly, cataract surgery can be done without the increased risk of bleeding in a patient on aspirin, so discontinuation of aspirin before cataract surgery is usually not indicated. In tonsillectomy, pre- or postoperative aspirin may contribute to perioperative bleeding and increase the number of revision procedures for hemostasis.

The Task Force on the Management of Acute Coronary Syndromes of the European Society of Cardiology Force recommended that in patients with a low risk of progressing to MI or death, oral antiplatelet agents should be discontinued 5 days before the procedure and reinstituted as soon as possible thereafter. Discontinuation of antiplatelet therapy is associated with increased rates of stent thrombosis. If possible, at least 2–4 weeks should elapse between placement of a stent and major noncardiac surgery. If the patient is not at high risk of bleeding and if the surgery is not associated with significant blood loss, aspirin therapy should be continued. Thienopyridine discontinuation 5 days before the procedure should be considered on a case-by-case basis. If there is a high risk of bleeding, withdrawal of both agents should be considered. If surgery is urgent or cannot be postponed for 5 days, discontinuation will not be possible or effective at the time of surgery and optimal surgical and pharmacological hemostasis must be employed. If bleeding occurs in a surgical patient whose antiplatelet therapy has not been discontinued, all antiplatelet drugs should be stopped immediately.

Because of the hypercoagulable state induced by surgery, early withdrawal of antiplatelet therapy for secondary prevention of cardiovascular disease increases the risk of postoperative myocardial infarction and death 5- to 10-fold in stented patients who are on continuous dual antiplatelet therapy. The shorter the time between revascularization and surgery, the higher the risk of adverse cardiac events. Elective surgery should be postponed beyond these periods, whereas vital, semiurgent, or urgent operations should be performed under continued dual antiplatelet therapy.

The risk of surgical hemorrhage is increased approximately 20% by aspirin or clopidogrel alone, and 50% by dual antiplatelet therapy. The risk of a cardiovascular event when stopping antiplatelet agents preoperatively is higher than the risk of surgical bleeding when continuing these drugs, except during surgery in a closed space (e.g., intracranial, posterior eye chamber) or surgeries associated with massive bleeding and difficult hemostasis. The mean delay between aspirin withdrawal and late thrombosis from DES is 7 days. Therefore, aspirin is a lifelong therapy that should not be interrupted. So, minor surgical procedures without significant bleeding and bone marrow aspiration and biopsy can be performed in patients taking aspirin, without withholding it.

3. Ans. b. The patient should be given anticoagulation during perioperative period

Ref: Metjian A, Lim W. ASH evidence-based guidelines: should asymptomatic patients with antiphospholipid antibodies receive primary prophylaxis to prevent thrombosis? Hematology Am Soc Hematol Educ Program. 2009:247-9.

The presence of antiphospholipid antibodies in the normal healthy population has been estimated to range from 1.0 to 5.6%. In patients with systemic lupus erythematosus, the prevalence ranges from 11 to 86%. In asymptomatic antiphospholipid antibodies positive patients, thromboprophylaxis with aspirin or low-molecular weight heparin (LMWH) during high-risk periods (i.e., surgery or prolonged immobilization) appears to be effective in reducing thrombotic complications.

Surgery can be done though mild risk of thrombosis may be there which can be managed by thromboprophylaxis. Antiphospholipid syndrome is diagnosed in a patient with thrombosis and/or defined pregnancy morbidity who has persistent antiphospholipid antibodies (aPL). The diagnosis should be suspected in someone with a prolonged activated partial thromboplastin time with other standard coagulation tests normal, along with the presence of an increased antiphospholipid or anticardiolipin anti-body titer and elevation of B2-glycoprotein-1. In the absence of an underlying connective tissue or other rheumatic disorder, antiphospholipid syndrome is considered as primary. Incidental detection of antiphospholipid antibodies is also common. BCSH recommends that primary thromboprophylaxis should not be used in those incidentally found to have antiphospholipid antibodies. Patients with an antiphospholipid syndrome and previous thrombosis usually are chronically anticoagulated. Oral treatment may be replaced with either unfractionated heparin or LMWH prior to surgery. Treatment should be tailored so that on the day of surgery, the INR is normal in range. Patients with APL titers <40 IU and with no past history of thrombosis also should receive LMWH in the perioperative period. In the case of patients who are discovered to have the antiphospholipid antibodies without any known thrombotic problems, the question of preventive treatment is unresolved. Long-term anticoagulation therapy is not currently recommended for asymptomatic patients. In the group of patients who have experienced venous thrombosis should be offered initial treatment with intravenous unfractionated heparin or LMWH. Long-term warfarin therapy should be commenced as soon as possible. For obstetric patients—subcutaneous heparin (unfractionated or LMWH) and low-dose aspirin are used. Therapy is held at the time of delivery; it is restarted after delivery and should be continued for as long as 6 weeks postpartum. Because of the controversial results of thromboprophylaxis (primary prevention) in patients positive for antiphospholipid antibodies without thrombosis, the continuous administration of aspirin and/or coumarins cannot be recommended to those patients, their use being reserved to situations with an elevated risk of thrombosis. Similarly, pregnant patients with antiphospholipid antibodies and no history of thrombotic events/abortions should not receive pharmacological treatment during pregnancy. The optimal perioperative treatment for these patients remains largely unclear. In most patients, these antibodies persist for a lifetime and therefore, put these patients at risk of major thrombotic events.

4. Ans. e. Wait and watch

Ref: Gernsheimer T, James AH, Stasi R. How I treat ITP in pregnancy. Blood. 2013;121:38-47.

ITP is the second most common cause of an isolated thrombocytopenia in pregnancy, accounting for about 3% of women with thrombocytopenia at delivery. Incidental thrombocytopenia of pregnancy, also called gestational thrombocytopenia, accounts for 70-80% of cases. It usually presents in the mid-second to third trimester. A diagnosis of gestational thrombocytopenia is unlikely if the platelet count is less than 50,000/µL. Developing a platelet count of less than 100,000/µL early in pregnancy, with declining platelet counts as gestation progresses, is most consistent with ITP. Bone marrow examination is rarely necessary to evaluate a thrombocytopenic pregnant patient and is not required to make the diagnosis of ITP. ITP is treated in the first and second trimesters when the patient has symptomatic bleeding, platelet counts are less than 30,000/µL or planned procedure requires a higher platelet count. Despite remaining relatively stable through most of the pregnancy, platelet counts may fall during the third trimester and monitoring should be more frequent. Women with no bleeding manifestations and platelet counts more than 30,000/µL do not require any treatment until delivery. Treatment is similar to that of nonpregnant women with newly diagnosed ITP with oral prednisone or prednisolone. If the platelet response to prednisone is suboptimal or when side effects of the drug are poorly tolerated, IVIG can be used (1 g/kg in a single or two divided doses), either alone or in combination with small doses of prednisone, to maintain safe platelet counts. Anti-RhD immunoglobulin is not recommended as a first-line agent because of concerns of acute hemolysis and anemia. Azathioprine has been safely administered during pregnancy. ITP is not an indication for cesarean delivery.

5. Ans. d. None of the above

Ref: Harrison CN, Bareford D, Butt N, Campbell P, Conneally E, Drummond M, et al. Guideline for investigation and management of adults and children presenting with a thrombocytosis. Br J Haematol. 2010;149(3):352-75.

The most common secondary (or reactive) causes of thrombocytosis are infection, inflammation, iron deficiency, tissue damage, hemolysis, severe exercise, malignancy, hyposplenism, and other causes of an acute phase response. The blood film may show other features to indicate an underlying cause, including acute infective, or inflammatory processes. A bone marrow aspirate or trephine is not usually required for reactive thrombocytosis. The diagnosis of essential thrombocythemia requires a sustained thrombocytosis of more than 450,000/μL and the exclusion of reactive causes. In this case, carcinoma colon along with iron deficiency might have caused reactive thrombocytosis and thrombocytosis per se does not require any treatment.

6. Ans. e. LAP score

Most changes in the white blood cell count are reactive and due to an increase or decrease of cells of the myeloid series. By definition, a leukocytosis is present if leukocytes are increased to more than 10,000/μL; in leukopenia, leukocytes are below 4,000/μL. In leukemoid reactions, leukocytes are increased to more than 30–50,000/μL. A left shift in the differential count means that the number of band forms (and other precursors such as metamyelocytes) is increased to more than 5%. In a pathological left shift, more immature precursors such as promyelocytes/myelocytes can be seen in the peripheral blood; this is almost always a sign of a hematological disorder. Serum leukocyte alkaline phosphatase is normal or elevated in leukemoid reaction, but is depressed in chronic myeloid leukemia (CML). The bone marrow in a leukemoid reaction, if examined, may be hypercellular but is otherwise typically unremarkable. Activated neutrophils (e.g., toxic granulation, Dohle bodies, and cytoplasmic vacuoles) are more characteristic of a reactive neutrophilia such as that seen in patients with bacterial infections or those receiving growth factor. Leukocytosis in a patient should prompt confirmation of the CBC and WBC differential. Examination of the blood smear should be performed to establish a manual differential. This will allow the distinction of myeloid from lymphoid disorders. Distinguishing myeloid leukemoid reactions from myeloid malignancies is difficult, with features such as dysplasia, basophilia, WBC count more than 50,000/μL, a pronounced left shift, and increased blasts favoring a myeloid malignancy with recommended BM examination and appropriate ancillary testing. With respect to lymphocytosis, pleomorphic lymphocytosis in the appropriate clinical context favors a reactive lymphocytosis, whereas a homogeneous population of lymphoid cells favors a lymphoproliferative disorder, particularly chronic lymphocytic leukemia (CLL). The major causes of leukemoid reactions are severe infections, intoxications, malignancies, severe hemorrhage, or acute hemolysis. This patient has leukemoid reaction which could be infection or steroid induced.

The leukocyte alkaline phosphatase (LAP) score is often used in patients with an elevated WBC to differentiate a reactive process from chronic myelogenous leukemia. Naphthyl AS-B1 phosphate is hydrolyzed to phosphate and an aryl maphthylthalamide by alkaline phosphatase in the cytoplasm of WBCs. In normal individuals, it is rare to find any neutrophils with a LAP score of 3, and a score of 4 should not be present. There is some physiological variation in LAP scores. Newborn babies, children, and pregnant women have high scores, and premenopausal women have, on an average, scores one-third higher than those of men. In pathological states, the most significant diagnostic use of the LAP score is in CML. In the chronic phase of the disease, the score is almost invariable low, usually zero. Transient increases may occur with intercurrent infection. In myeloid blast transformation or accelerated phase, the score rises. Low scores are also commonly found in paroxysmal nocturnal hemoglobinuria (PNH) and the very rare condition of hereditary hypophosphatasia. There are many causes of raised LAP score, notably in the neutrophilia of infection, polycythemia vera, leukemoid reactions, and Hodgkin's disease. In aplastic anemia, the LAP score is high, but it falls if PNH supervenes.

7. Ans. c. Surgery of hemangioma

Ref: McMullin MF, Bareford D, Campbell P, Green AR, Harrison C, Hunt B, et al. Guidelines for the diagnosis, investigation and management of polycythaemia/erythrocytosis. Br J Haematol. 2005;130(2):174-95.

Secondary polycythemia is an elevated absolute red blood cell mass caused by enhanced stimulation of red blood cell production by an otherwise normal erythroid lineage that may be congenital or acquired. Diagnosis is based on evidence of increased total red blood cells and normal to high-serum erythropoietin (EPO) levels. Differential diagnoses include polycythemia vera and primary familial polycythemia, which can be excluded on the basis of low EPO levels and the presence of a mutation in the *JAK2* gene for polycythemia vera. In acquired cases of secondary polycythemia, management is based on treating the underlying condition. Hemangiomas are known cause of secondary erythrocytosis and treatment of hemangioma results in normalization of hemoglobin.

8. Ans. d. All of the above

Ref: Levi M, Toh CH, Thachil J, Watson HG. Guidelines for the diagnosis and management of disseminated intravascular coagulation. Br J Haematol. 2009;145(1):24-33.

This patient has disseminated intravascular coagulation (DIC). DIC is a clinicopathological syndrome which complicates a range of illnesses. It is characterized by systemic activation of pathways leading to and regulating coagulation, which can result in the generation of fibrin clots that may cause organ failure with concomitant consumption of platelets and coagulation factors that may result in clinical bleeding. The diagnosis of DIC should include both clinical and laboratory information. The International Society for Thrombosis and Haemostasis (ISTH) DIC scoring system provides objective measurement of DIC. The scoring system for DIC includes four parameters of coagulation—prothrombin time, platelet count, fibrinogen, and fibrin degradation products. Platelet count (more than 100,000/µL = 0, less than 100,000/µL = 1, less than 50,000/µL = 2), elevated fibrin marker (e.g., D-dimer, fibrin degradation products; no increase = 0, moderate increase = 2, strong increase = 3), prolonged PT (<3 s = 0, >3 but <6 s = 1, >6 s = 2), fibrinogen level (>1 g/L = 0, <1 g/L = 1). The score is then calculated more than 5 compatible with overt DIC: Repeat score daily, less than 5 suggestive for nonovert DIC. A reduction in the platelet count or a clear downward trend at subsequent measurements is a sensitive (though not specific) sign of DIC. Thrombocytopenia is a feature in up to 90% of DIC cases. The PT or aPTT is prolonged in about 50-60% of cases of DIC at some point during the course of illness. This is mainly attributed to the consumption of coagulation factors but impaired synthesis, due to abnormal liver function, vitamin K deficiency or loss of the coagulation proteins, due to massive bleeding, may also play a role. In patients with DIC and bleeding or at high risk of bleeding (e.g., postoperative patients or patients undergoing an invasive procedure) and a platelet count of less than 50,000/µL transfusion of platelets should be considered. In nonbleeding patients with DIC, prophylactic platelet transfusion is not given unless there is a high risk of bleeding. In bleeding patients with DIC and prolonged prothrombin time and activated partial thromboplastin time, administration of FFP, cryoprecipitate or PCC may be useful. It should not be instituted based on laboratory tests alone but should be considered in those with active bleeding and in those requiring an invasive procedure. Patients with severe sepsis and DIC can be considered for recombinant human activated protein C. In cases of DIC where thrombosis predominates, such as arterial or venous thromboembolism, severe purpura fulminans associated with acral ischemia or vascular skin infarction, therapeutic doses of heparin should be considered. Treatment of the baseline infection and sepsis should be of prime concern.

9. Ans. c. Decrease immunosuppressive therapy

Ref: Parker A, Bowles K, Bradley JA, Emery V, Featherstone C, Gupte G, et al. Management of post-transplant lymphoproliferative disorder in adult solid organ transplant recipients – BCSH and BTS Guidelines. Br J Haematol. 2010;149(5):693-705.

Zimmermann H, Trappe RU. EBV and post-transplantation lymphoproliferative disease: What to do? Hematology Am Soc Hematol Educ Program. 2013;2013:95-102.

Post-transplant lymphoproliferative disorders (PTLDs) are serious, life-threatening complications of solid organ transplantation (SOT) and bone marrow transplantation leading to a high mortality (30-60%). PTLD is a group of lymphatic and plasmacytic proliferations arising in the setting of immunosuppression after transplantation. The highest incidence from 5 to 20% is reported following lung and intestinal transplantation; in contrast, renal transplant recipients (RTRs) have an incidence of 1-3%. In liver transplant recipients, the occurrence ranges from 2 to 10%. EBV infection is a risk factor and a cause of PTLD present in more than 80% of B-lymphocyte phenotypic disorders and, less commonly, in T-lymphocytic proliferations. The final diagnosis is always based on histopathology. The common types of monomorphic PTLDs are DLBCL, other may have Burkitt lymphoma, Hodgkin lymphoma etc. Once the diagnosis is suspected, immediate reduction in immunosuppression (RIS) should be considered under the direction of the transplant team. The evidence that immunosuppression of cytotoxic T lymphocytes enables proliferation of (EBV-transformed B) cells favors reduction of immunosuppression in patients with EBV-related PTLD. In some patients, this may be adequate to achieve complete remission, whilst facilitating further treatment in others. BCSH and American guidelines recommend steroid maintenance alone or reducing calcineurin inhibitors, e.g. ciclosporin by 50% and stopping all other agents, e.g. mycophenolate or azathioprine. A response to RIS is usually seen within 2-4 weeks. If the PTLD fully resolves with RIS, then no further treatment may be required. Resection or radiotherapy may be adequate treatment of localized PTLD. In patients with life-preserving grafts or those with nonlife preserving grafts in whom resection would mean loss of the transplanted organ, and who are deemed suitable, alternative treatments, such as rituximab and/or chemotherapy, are preferred. Rituximab monotherapy is recommended for clinical low-risk PTLD who fail to respond adequately to RIS. Rituximab plus anthracycline-based chemotherapy is recommended for patients who fail to achieve an adequate remission or progress despite previous RIS and rituximab monotherapy.

10. Ans. c. Parasitic infection
Ref: Hoffbrand AV, Moss PAH. Essential Haematology, 6th edition. Oxford, UK: Wiley-Blackwell; 2011. pp. 952.

The patient should be evaluated for malaria in view of high-grade fever. His peripheral blood film should be screened for malarial parasite. Anemia is the most prominent hematological manifestation of malarial infection. It is mostly seen with *Plasmodium falciparum*, because it invades erythrocytes of all ages whereas *P. vivax* and *P. ovale* invade only reticulocytes and *P. malariae* affects only mature cells. Cellular disruption and hemoglobin digestion lead to hemolysis characteristically seen in heavy parasitemia. Parasitized cells have an increased osmotic fragility and decreased deformability, causing their sequestration and destruction within the spleen, which often becomes massively enlarged. The malarial antigens may also attach to nonparasitized red cells to give rise to a positive direct Coombs test and hemolysis via a complement-mediated immune response. Acute intravascular hemolysis with hemoglobinuria, often leading to renal failure (called blackwater fever), occurs rarely in *P. falciparum* infection. So, multiple mechanisms including autoimmune mechanisms, splenic sequestration, DIC, and ADP release from damaged red cells leading to platelet activation and consumption, may occur in malaria, and may complicate the picture. This child has all these manifestations due to multiple factors generating from malarial infection.

11. Ans. d. All of the above *Ref: Hoffman 7/e p2222*

Because there is direct relationship between the hematocrit and blood viscosity, minor increases in the hematocrit above 70% cause marked increases in blood viscosity. This higher viscosity results in impaired perfusion within the microvasculature with ultimately less tissue oxygen delivery and resulting in complications. Therefore, the hematocrit level should be maintained at around 60% through the use of exchange transfusions. The blood should be removed slowly because vascular collapse, cyanosis, stroke, and seizures have been reported with rapid exchange. Children with polycythemia who have iron deficiency anemia are at increased risk for cerebral vein thrombosis because of the poor deformability of the iron-deficient RBCs, which further increases blood viscosity. To prevent this complication and to allow for maximal tissue oxygenation, all infants should be fed iron-rich infant formula and receive iron replacement therapy as needed to normalize RBC indices.

12. Ans. e. All can be used *Ref: Hoffman 7/e p2274*

HIV-associated ITP is generally responsive to the treatment used for classic ITP. Therapy with prednisone produces a major hematologic response (platelet count >100 × 10^9/L) in over half of all patients. No deleterious effects of short-term treatment with prednisone have been noted in HIV-infected patients. IVIG and anti-RhD are equally effective in increasing platelet counts acutely. Splenectomy has proven to be safe and effective in refractory patients with HIV-associated ITP.

13. Ans. d. The procedures can be performed without any prophylactic transfusions
Ref: Hoffman 7/e p2309

Studies have shown that in patients with liver disease, INR values in the range of 1.3–2.0 generally correspond to levels of factors II, V, and VII that are adequate for hemostasis. In patients with mild liver disease and mild-moderate INR prolongation (<2.0), serious surgical bleeding is unlikely in the absence of other hemostatic abnormalities, and prophylactic intervention is rarely required for low- or moderate-risk surgery. It should be noted that the PT of fresh frozen plasma is approximately 15 seconds, which corresponds to an INR of 1.5, so complete correction of the PT/INR is unlikely to be achieved.

14. Ans. d. All of the above *Ref: Hoffman 7/e p2213*

Antiphospholipid antibodies can be detected in 5% of healthy pregnant women and 37% of pregnant women with systemic lupus erythematosus (SLE). Thrombotic events occur in approximately 5% of pregnant women with antiphospholipid antibodies. All pregnant women with SLE should undergo testing for antiphospholipid antibodies. Women who sustain recurrent spontaneous abortions or a thromboembolic event during pregnancy should also undergo evaluation for the disorder. Women with antiphospholipid antibody syndrome who have sustained prior thrombotic events receive therapeutic anticoagulation during pregnancy. Those with antiphospholipid antibodies but no manifestations of the clinical syndrome should receive prophylactic anticoagulation.

15. Ans. d. Urea clot solubility test *Ref: Hoffman 7/e p2195*

This child probably has FXIII deficiency. FXIII deficiency is inherited in an autosomal recessive manner. Homozygotes usually have FXIII levels of less than 1% and have a severe bleeding diathesis. Patients with heterozygous FXIII deficiency are usually asymptomatic but have reduced levels of FXIII. Neonates with FXIII deficiency may present with umbilical bleeding a few days after birth, a frequent finding that occurs in 80% of cases. FXIII deficiency is not detected with screening PT, APTT, or thrombin time assays. Specific assays for FXIII or urea clot solubility testing are used for diagnosis. The clot solubility test is sensitive to very low levels of FXIII (<1%) but is normal if FXIII levels are in the 1–3% range. Consequently, FXIII immunoassays are preferable. More severe bleeding, including intracranial hemorrhage, occurs in 25–30% of patients and is the major cause of death. Treatment of FXIII deficiency includes FFP, cryoprecipitate, plasma-derived FXIII concentrate, or recombinant FXIII A-subunit.

16. Ans. d. Stroke
Ref: Hoffbrand 7/e p101

Patients with more severe anemia at baseline have a greater probability of developing stroke and renal dysfunction. On the other hand, a higher hemoglobin level is associated with a higher incidence of painful episodes, avascular necrosis, and acute chest syndrome. Blood transfusions are therefore considered the standard of care for both primary and secondary stroke prevention.

17. Ans. d. BEACOPP causes less infertility than ABVD therapy
Ref: Leader A, Lishner M, Michaeli J, Revel A. Fertility considerations and preservation in hemato-oncology patients undergoing treatment. Br J Haematol. 2011;153:291-308.

The pretreatment semen quality of patients with Hodgkin lymphoma (HL) and non-Hodgkin lymphoma (NHL) has been shown to be significantly inferior when compared to healthy controls. In contrast with male HL patients, there is no clear evidence of pretreatment fertility impairment in females. The ABVD regimen, which contains no alkylating agents, causes only temporary azoospermia that is typically reversible in all patients. BEACOPP (bleomycin, etoposide, doxorubicin, cyclophosphamide, vincristine, procarbazine, and prednisone) causes higher rates of azoospermia. Gonadal doses of 200–300 cGy cause prolonged and often irreversible azoospermia. Chemotherapy-induced gonadal failure is most often caused by alkylating agents, among which procarbazine and cyclophosphamide are considered the main culprits. Patients rendered azoospermic during HL and NHL treatment may potentially regain spermatogenic capacity at varying times after treatment, even over a period of several years. Females under the age of 40 years receiving CHOP (cyclophosphamide, doxorubicin, vincristine, prednisone) or CHOP-based chemotherapy for NHL have a very low risk of developing gonadal dysfunction. Male and female survivors of conventional chemotherapy-based treatment for childhood NHL are at low risk of infertility and impaired puberty. Regimens devoid of alkylating agents carry a far lower risk of gonadal dysfunction.

18. Ans. c. Induction chemotherapy is as gonadotoxic as stem cell transplant
Ref: Leader A, Lishner M, Michaeli J, Revel A. Fertility considerations and preservation in hemato-oncology patients undergoing treatment. Br J Haematol. 2011;153:291-308.

Male leukemia patients have lower pretreatment semen quality than healthy donors. Standard chemotherapy regimens used to treat ALL and AML have low gonadotoxic potential. Treatment with chemotherapy alone for ALL results in immediate impairment in spermatogenesis; however, the majority of men subsequently recover reproductive capacity. The reproductive function of women treated with chemotherapy alone for ALL seems to be mostly preserved. Furthermore, postpubertal AML patients treated with chemotherapy alone infrequently have impaired fertility, compared with significantly higher rates among those who received allogeneic or autologous hematopoietic stem cell transplantation (HSCT). High-dose cranial irradiation is associated with impaired fertility in boys who are treated for ALL before the age of 10 years. Myeloablative pretransplant conditioning regimes are based on alkylating agents and/or TBI, both of which have been implicated in causing marked germ cell damage and infertility. Azoospermia is found among more than 70% of allogeneic HSCT survivors who underwent myeloablative conditioning.

19. Ans. c. Right-to-left shunt
Ref: Lill MC, Perloff JK, Child JS. Pathogenesis of thrombocytopenia in cyanotic congenital heart disease. Am J Cardiol. 2006;98(2):254-8.

The pathogenesis of thrombocytopenia in cyanotic congenital heart disease is based on the right-to-left shunts that deliver large precursors of platelets from the systemic venous into the systemic arterial circulation, thus circumventing the lungs and reducing the number of platelets produced in the pulmonary bed. Shunted megakaryocytes release platelets at systemic impact sites, but the released platelets remain in situ, without contributing to platelet counts in the blood. Polycythemia, increased blood viscosity, and other rheological factors stimulate lysis and adenosine diphosphate (ADP) release, which may also cause platelet aggregation and result in thrombocytopenia. Therefore, right-to-left shunts deliver megakaryocytic cytoplasm into the system arterial circulation, bypassing the lungs where megakaryocytic cytoplasm is fragmented into platelets, thus reducing platelet production.

20. Ans. d. Chromosomal breakage analysis
Ref: Wilson DB, Link DC, Mason PJ, Bessler M. Inherited bone marrow failure syndromes in adolescents and young adults. Ann Med. 2014;46:353-63.

Fanconi anemia (FA) is a genetically and phenotypically heterogeneous disorder characterized by birth defects, progressive bone marrow failure, and a predisposition to cancer. FA is associated with a variety of phenotypic abnormalities such as short stature, micrognathia, clinodactyly, and other skeletal abnormalities. A diepoxybutane (DEB) chromosome fragility test is characteristically abnormal and as such helpful in establishing the diagnosis of FA. Identifying Fanconi is extremely important to treatment planning since these patients are exquisitely sensitive to alkylating agents such as cyclophosphamide and radiation, and conditioning and drug doses during stem cell transplant have to be modified accordingly.

SECTION 6: Hematopathology

40. Hematopathology

CHAPTER 40

Hematopathology

1. **All of these are associated with prolonged activated partial thromboplastin time (aPTT) without bleeding manifestations, *except*:**
   a. Factor XII deficiency
   b. Factor XI deficiency
   c. Prekallikrein deficiency
   d. High-molecular-weight kininogen (HMWK) deficiency

2. **Which of these bleeding disorders is associated with a normal screening coagulation profile?**
   a. Factor XIII deficiency
   b. Factor VII deficiency
   c. Factor XI deficiency
   d. Factor V deficiency

3. **Regarding T-cell large granular lymphocytic leukemia, all are true, *except*:**
   a. It is an aggressive disease
   b. It is characterized by proliferation of cytotoxic "T" cells or "natural killer (NK)" cells
   c. It is associated with rheumatoid arthritis
   d. It is associated with cytopenias

4. **Adult T-cell leukemia/lymphoma is characterized by all, *except*:**
   a. Causally linked to Epstein-Barr virus (EBV) infection
   b. Skin is the most common extralymphatic site
   c. Hypercalcemia is common
   d. Associated with T-cell immunodeficiency

5. **Early T-cell precursor (ETP) acute lymphoblastic leukemia (ALL) is characterized by all, *except*:**
   a. Negative for CD8 and CD1a
   b. Lacks expression of CD7
   c. CD5 is negative or dim
   d. Expresses one or more myeloid/stem cell markers

6. **Refractory cytopenia of childhood is characterized by all, *except*:**
   a. It is a provisional entity in the WHO classification of myelodysplastic syndrome (MDS)
   b. It is characterized by hypocellular bone marrow
   c. It is the most common subtype of MDS in childhood
   d. Ring sideroblasts are commonly seen

7. **Which of these is not a glycosylphosphatidylinositol (GPI) anchor protein used for paroxysmal nocturnal hemoglobinuria (PNH) testing by flow cytometry?**
   a. CD157
   b. CD24
   c. CD33
   d. CD14

8. **Myelodysplastic syndrome with ring sideroblasts mandates:**
   a. Ring sideroblasts ≥5% with SF3B1 mutation
   b. Ring sideroblasts ≥15% with SF3B1 mutation
   c. Ring sideroblasts ≥25% with SF3B1 mutation
   d. Ring sideroblasts not needed if SF3B1 mutation is present

9. **Which of these is not an MDS defining cytogenetic abnormality?**
   a. Del7q
   b. Del5q
   c. Loss of Y chromosome
   d. All of the above define MDS

10. **Eosin-5-maleimide (EMA) dye in flow cytometry for erythrocyte membrane abnormalities binds to which antigen?**
    a. Ankyrin
    b. Spectrin
    c. Band 3 protein
    d. GPI anchor

11. **True about fluorescein-labeled proaerolysin (FLAER) is:**
    a. Derived from bacteria
    b. Binds to phosphatidylinositol glycan gene
    c. Useful for identifying PNH clone on red blood cells
    d. All of the above

12. **Clonal hematopoiesis of indeterminate potential (CHIP) has been found to be associated with which systemic disorder?**
    a. Cataract
    b. Accelerated atherosclerosis
    c. Osteoporosis
    d. Pancreatitis

13. **All of the following are predictors for unfavorable prognosis in chronic lymphocytic leukemia, *except*:**
    a. Del17p
    b. Del11q
    c. Mutated immunoglobulin heavy chain variable gene (IGVH) status
    d. Mutation in *TP53* gene

14. Wnt signaling pathway is associated with:
   a. Bone homeostasis in multiple myeloma
   b. Fibrosis in idiopathic myelofibrosis
   c. Erythrocytosis in polycythemia vera
   d. Checkpoint pathway in Hodgkin lymphoma

15. Photodiode in flow cytometry is the optical detector for:
   a. Forward scatter signal
   b. Side scatter signal
   c. Light scatter emitted by fluorochromes
   d. All of the above

16. In flow cytometric assay, normal T-lymphocytes are best identified with the following marker profile:
   a. Dim CD45, low side scatter, CD3 positive cells
   b. Bright CD45, low side scatter, CD22 positive cells
   c. Bright CD45, high side scatter, CD3 positive cells
   d. Bright CD45, low side scatter, CD3 positive cells

17. Human leukocyte antigen (HLA) class II proteins are expressed almost exclusively on:
   a. All nucleated cells
   b. Antigen-presenting cells
   c. Red blood cells
   d. Vascular endothelium

18. Plasmacytoid dendritic cells (PDCs) are characterized by:
   a. CD123 + HLADR+
   b. CD123 + HLADR−
   c. CD123 − HLADR+
   d. CD 23 − HLADR−

19. Progenitor compartment in CD45 versus side scatter plot normally shows presence of all of the following, *except*:
   a. Blasts
   b. Plasmacytoid dendritic cells
   c. Basophils
   d. NK cells

20. ETP-ALL is characterized by all of the following, *except*:
   a. CD8−
   b. CD1a+
   c. CD5+ (<75% blasts)
   d. Presence of myeloid/stem cell markers

21. Germinal center reaction is characterized by all of the following, *except*:
   a. Class switching
   b. Somatic hypermutation
   c. BCL2 expression
   d. CD10 expression

22. Blue laser in flow cytometry excites the following fluorochromes, *except*:
   a. FITC (fluorescein isothiocyanate)
   b. PE (phycoerythrin)
   c. APC (allophycocyanin)
   d. PerCP-Cy5.5 (peridinin chlorophyll protein-conjugated to a cyanine dye Cy5.5)

23. Natural killer cells express the following markers, *except*:
   a. CD2
   b. CD7
   c. CD16/CD56
   d. TCR αβ

24. False about hematogones is:
   a. Characteristic waterfall pattern on CD10/CD20 dot plot in flow cytometry
   b. Physiological precursors of B-cells
   c. Proliferate during marrow regeneration
   d. Morphologically indistinguishable from blasts
   e. None of the above

25. The correct statement for erythropoietin (EPO) is:
   a. Predominantly produced in the bone marrow
   b. Stimulates RBC production by inducing proliferation of reticulocytes
   c. Decreased in erythroid hyperplasia
   d. Increased in aplastic anemia

26. In which of the following distribution regions of the body do neutrophils spend the least amount of time?
   a. Bone marrow storage pool
   b. Circulating pool
   c. Tissue pool
   d. Marginated pool

27. The order of Ig heavy- and light-chain rearrangement is:
   a. V-D-J, cytoplasmic mu, kappa, and lambda
   b. V-D-J, cytoplasmic alpha, kappa, and lambda
   c. Cytoplasmic delta, V-D-J, kappa, and lambda
   d. Cytoplasmic gamma, V-D-J, kappa, and lambda

28. Which description of T-cell gene rearrangement is correct?
   a. The order of rearrangement is gamma, delta, beta, and alpha
   b. The order of rearrangement is alpha, beta, gamma, and delta
   c. Gamma and delta receptors present on 95% of the circulating T-cells
   d. *TCR* genes do not undergo V(D)J rearrangement

29. Which of the following statements regarding Cabot rings is correct?
   a. They may be seen in megaloblastic anemia within reticulocytes
   b. They are a remnant of extra copy of RNA
   c. They are frequently seen after splenectomy
   d. None of the above

30. Which of the following has an abnormal response to ristocetin-induced platelet aggregation?
   a. Bernard–Soulier syndrome
   b. Glanzmann's thrombasthenia
   c. Chediak–Higashi syndrome
   d. None of the above

31. Which of the following diseases does not have an autosomal recessive inheritance pattern?
   a. Wiskott-Aldrich syndrome
   b. Chediak-Higashi syndrome
   c. Glanzmann's thrombasthenia
   d. Bernard-Soulier's syndrome

32. Which of the following statements regarding sample collection and transport in routine coagulation study is correct?
   a. The sample should be collected in citrate tubes containing 0.105M-0.109M (c2.3%) aqueous trisodium citrate dihydrate, maintaining the proportion of blood to citrate as 1:9
   b. Samples should be tested within 4 hours of collection
   c. The sample should be maintained at temperatures between 2 and 8°C to prevent loss of coagulation factor
   d. Plasma that has been hemolyzed during collection and processing can easily be analyzed by any automated analyzer

33. One-stage factor assays based on aPTT are the most commonly used techniques. Which of the following statements is incorrect?
   a. FVIII- and FIX-deficient plasma must completely lack FVIII and FIX respectively, i.e. contain <1 IU/dL, and have normal levels of other clotting factors
   b. The reference/calibration plasma, whether commercial or locally prepared, must be calibrated in international units
   c. At least three different dilutions of the reference plasma and the test sample under analysis are needed for a valid assay
   d. None of the above

34. The coagulation laboratory is receiving samples for aPTT tests from a multispecialty hospital. The laboratory should select aPTT reagent having which of the following properties?
   a. Sensitive to deficiencies of factors VIII, IX, and XI at a concentration of 0.35-0.4 IU/mL
   b. Responsive to unfractionated heparin over the therapeutic range of 0.3-0.7 IU/mL
   c. Low responsiveness to lupus anticoagulant
   d. All of the above

35. Platelet-poor plasma (PPP) is used in routine coagulation studies. The platelet counts in PPP should be less than:
   a. 10,000/cmm
   b. 20,000/cmm
   c. 30,000/cmm
   d. 50,000/cmm

36. Food and Drug Administration (FDA)-approved drugs for sickle cell anemia are all, *except*:
   a. Voxelotor
   b. Crizanlizumab
   c. L-glutamine
   d. Sevuparin

37. Which of the following is *not true* for lymphoplasmacytic lymphomas?
   a. It is a neoplasm of small B lymphocytes, plasmacytoid lymphocytes, and plasma cells lacking CD5, CD10, CD23, with strong expression of sIg and CD20
   b. t(9;14)(p13;q32) and rearrangement of *PAX-5* gene
   c. Thalidomide and bortezomib are not active in these lymphomas
   d. Monoclonal serum IgM paraproteinemia, with or without hyperviscosity, characterizes Waldenstrom's macroglobulinemia

38. The diagnostic criteria of hereditary hemorrhagic telangiectasia include:
   a. Epistaxis
   b. Telangiectasia
   c. Visceral lesions
   d. Family history
   e. All of the above

39. True about severe anaphylaxis is:
   a. Can be associated with mastocytosis
   b. Serum tryptase should be measured
   c. Bone marrow examination may be needed
   d. All of the above

40. True regarding bone marrow iron stain are all, *except*:
   a. A Prussian Blue stain should be performed on a BM smear for the evaluation of storage iron and sideroblasts
   b. A BM smear with increased iron stores should be included as a positive control
   c. If there is a 'dry tap', a core biopsy section and imprint can be stained for iron
   d. Core biopsy sections are more reliable than the aspirate for the assessment of storage iron

41. *RAG* genes are involved in the synthesis of:
   a. CD4
   b. CD8
   c. TCR
   d. HLA

42. Inverted CD4/CD8 ratio is seen in:
   a. Aging
   b. Post-stem cell transplant
   c. CMV infection
   d. HIV infection
   e. All of the above

43. Central tolerance is mediated by:
   a. *RAG* gene
   b. *NOTCH* gene
   c. *AIRE* gene
   d. *ARTEMIS* gene

44. In the bone marrow, RBC precursors are located:
   a. In the center of the hematopoietic cords
   b. Adjacent to megakaryocytes along the adventitial cell lining
   c. Surrounding fat cells in apoptotic islands
   d. Surrounding macrophages near the sinus membrane

45. In the Iron cycle, the transferrin receptor carries:
a. Iron out of duodenal cells from the intestinal lumen
b. Iron out of duodenal cells into the plasma
c. Transferrin-bound iron in the plasma
d. Transferrin-bound iron into erythrocytes

46. True about Howell-Jolly bodies is:
a. These are diffuse fine and coarse blue dots in red cells
b. Commonly seen in lead poisoning
c. Can be seen post-splenectomy
d. Represents residual RNA

47. Which of the following is a false statement regarding basophilic stippling?
a. Basophilic stippling is also known as Pappenheimer bodies
b. It occurs in lead poisoning and pyrimidine 5'-nucleotidase deficiency
c. They do not give a positive Perl's stain
d. Presence of basophilic stippling helps differentiate thalassemia trait from iron deficiency anemia

48. True about hepatitis associated aplastic anemia is:
a. Occurs 3-5 years after hepatitis
b. Results in 10-15% of all aplastic anemia cases
c. Immune destruction is not involved in pathogenesis
d. Treatment is similar for idiopathic aplastic anemia

49. Loss of Heterozygosity of chromosome 6p is characteristic feature of:
a. Myelodysplastic syndrome
b. Acquired aplastic anemia
c. Fanconi anemia
d. Myelofibrosis

50. True about acquired aplastic anemia are all, *except*:
a. About 1/3 of patients with AA have significantly short telomeres in their leukocytes
b. Shorten telomeres are associated with poor response to immunosuppressive therapy
c. Mutations in telomere genes TERC and TERT are common
d. None of the above

51. Disorders of ribosome biogenesis include all, *except*:
a. Diamond Blackfan anemia
b. Shwachman–Diamond syndrome
c. Kostmann syndrome
d. All of the above

52. A 17-year-old female with Hb of 4 gm/dL was evaluated for anemia requiring blood transfusions. She had maxillary and frontal prominence of facial bones.

Peripheral smear showed microcytic hypochromic with ansiocytosis, reticulocyte count of 5%, Iron studies- S.iron- 152 mcg/mL, TIBC- 105, S. ferritin- 2000 ng/mL. HPLC of parents and patient are normal. Bone marrow shows erythroid hyperplasia with dyserythropoiesis in the erythroid lineage. PNH by Flowcytometry is negative. The likely diagnosis in this case is:
a. Thalassemia intermedia
b. Myelodysplastic syndrome
c. Congenital dyserythropoietic anemia
d. Hemochromatosis

53. All are sensors of apoptosis, *except*:
a. BIM
b. Puma
c. Noxa
d. None of the above

54. Anti-apoptotic molecules includes:
a. BCL2
b. BCL-XL
c. MCL1
d. All of the above

55. All are structural proteins of RBC membrane, *except*:
a. Spectrin
b. Glycophorin C
c. Protein 4.2
d. Beta-glycoprotein

56. Which of the following is true regarding hepcidin?
a. Kidney is the primary source of hepcidin
b. Binds to ferroportin
c. Increases the absorption of iron
d. Increases in iron deficiency anemia

57. Which of the following is not correct?
a. "Serum folate" is a reliable indicator of body's folate stores
b. Human body stores 2-3 month's supply of Folic acid
c. Vit-B12 stores of body is sufficient for 5-10 years
d. Methylmalonic acid (MMA) and Homocysteine, both are elevated in Vit-B12 deficiency

58. Which of the following is not correct?
a "G6PD deficiency" is the most common RBC enzyme disorder associated with haemolysis
b. Females may be affected though X-linked
c. G6PD is the only source of NADPH in RBCs that protects against oxidative stress
d. G6PD assay immediately after acute haemolysis is a better indicator of it's deficiency.

59. Which of the following is false regarding pitted or pocked erythrocytes:
a. It is a test of splenic function
b. Endocytic vesicles containing hemoglobin, ferritin and remenants of mitochondria are found in patients with hyposplenism
c. Number of pitted RBCs is inversely proportional to splenic function
d. Normal persons have more than 2% pitted RBC'S

60. Which of the following helps in differentiating Vitamin K deficiency and liver disease?
a. Thrombin clotting time
b. Performing a factor II assay with and without Echis venom
c. Euglobulin lysis test
d. Clot lysis test

61. All of the following are true about Th17 cells, *except*:
   a. Subset of CD4+ T cells
   b. IL-23 plays a key role in their development
   c. Kills intracellular bacteria
   d. Role in the development of autoimmune diseases

62. Which of the following hemoglobin has the same electrophoretic mobility as HbS on cellulose acetate electrophoresis at pH 8.4:
   a. HbC
   b. HbA2
   c. HbD
   d. HbE

63. The size of nucleus of large cell lymphoma is the equal to that of:
   a. Macrophage
   b. Twice the size of lymphocyte
   c. Twice the size of RBC
   d. None of the above
   e. All of the above

64. B-lymphoblastic lymphoma (B-LBL) is distinguished from Burkitt lymphoma (BL) by:
   a. B-LBL has finer chromatin than that in BL
   b. B-LBL cases do not show the clear vacuoles typically seen in BL
   c. BL does not express CD34 or TdT
   d. All of the above

65. DLBCL is distinguished from mantle cell lymphoma by all, *except*:
   a. Cyclin D1
   b. SOX-11
   c. t(11;14)(q13;q32)
   d. CD5

66. True regarding CD30 expression in DLBCL are all, *except*:
   a. 10% to 20% of DLBCL cases are CD30 positive
   b. Epstein-Barr virus (EBV)–positive DLBCL cases can be CD30 positive
   c. DLBCL cases with CD30 expression have poor overall survival
   d. All of the above

67. Plasmablastic lymphoma is positive for:
   a. CD45   b. CD20
   c. PAX5
   d. IRF4/MUM1

68. What percentage of B cells should be EBV positive to call it EBV positive B cell DLBCL?
   a. More than 10%
   b. More than 20%
   c. More than 30%
   d. More than 50%

69. Hans algorithm is used for:
   a. DLBCL   b. Follicular lymphoma
   c. T cell lymphoma d. All of the above

70. True about double expresser and double hit lymphoma is:
   a. Both are same things
   b. Both are evaluated by immunohistochemistry
   c. Both are evaluated by FISH
   d. Both have equal prognostic significance
   e. None of the above

71. A 50 years old female with polycythemia vera has developed covid-19 pneumonia. True regarding anticoagulant prophylaxis is:
   a. Not recommended
   b. Only aspirin is suggested
   c. Prophylactic anticoagulant
   d. Therapeutic anticoagulant

72. Myeloperoxidase stains all, *except*:
   a. Granules of basophils
   b. Primary granules of neutrophils
   c. Secondary granules of neutrophils
   d. Granules of eosinophils
   e. Granules of monocytes

73. The myeloid:erythroid (M:E. ratio is calculated as the ratio of):
   a. Ratio of granulocytes to erythroblasts
   b. Ratio of all granulocytes and monocytes and their precursors to erythroblasts
   c. Ratio of white blood cells to red blood cells
   d. Ratio of myeloid progenitors to erythroid progenitors

74. Early erythroid precursors are identified by:
   a. Large nucleoli with vacoules
   b. Aggregates of ferritin
   c. Presence of sideroblasts
   d. MPO positive

75. Blasts of AML M0 are positive for:
   a. MPO   b. SBB
   c. Naphthol AS-D chloroacetate esterase
   d. NSE   e. None of the above

76. Auer rods are detected by:
   a. MPO stain   b. SBB stain
   c. Romanowsky stain
   d. All of the above

77. In a patient with acute promyelocytic leukemia, auer rods in bone marrow macrophages may suggest:
   a. Aggressive disease
   b. Associated monocytic leukemia
   c. Poor response to therapy
   d. None of the above

78. Acute promyelocytic variant leukemia should be differentiated from:
   a. AML-M0
   b. AML-M2
   c. AML-M5
   d. AML-M7

79. Megakaryoblasts are positive for:
   a. PAS
   b. SBB
   c. CAE
   d. MPO

80. Which of the following statement is false?
   a. Presence of RUNX1-RUNXT1 or CBFB-MYH11 fusion genes confirms the diagnosis of AML rather than MDS
   b. Presence of KMT2A rearrangement suggests therapy-related AML
   c. Detection of ETV6-RUNX1 associated with cryptic t(12;21)(p13.2;q22.1) is associated with ALL
   d. All of the above are true

81. RUNX1-RUNX1T1 fusion can be seen in:
   a. t(1;21;8)
   b. t(8;11;21)
   c. t(8;13;21)
   d. t(8;21)
   e. All of the above

82. True about c-KIT mutations is:
   a. Associated with a higher WBC
   b. More extramedullary disease
   c. Greater risk of relapse
   d. Worse survival
   e. All of the above

83. True regarding genetic analysis in acute promyelocytic leukemia are all, *except*:
   a. Translocation (15;17) can be detected directly without culture
   b. About 30–40% of cases show secondary karyotypic abnormalities
   c. The breakpoints in therapy relapsed APL differ from that in de-novo APL
   d. None of the above

84. FAB subtype of AML with inv(16) is seen in:
   a. AML M1
   b. AML M2
   c. AML M4Eo
   d. AML M5
   e. All of the above

85. Translocation (1;22) is commonly associated with:
   a. Acute monocytic leukemia
   b. Acute basophilic leukemia
   c. Acute erythroblastic leukemia
   d. Acute megakaryoblastic leukemia

86. False about acute myeloid leukaemia with NPM1 mutation is:
   a. NPM mutation is more common in females
   b. Blasts with cup shaped nuclei
   c. NPM can be detected by flow cytometry
   d. NPM can be used for MRD assessment
   e. All are true

87. True about plasmacytoid dendritic cell neoplasm are all, *except*:
   a. Cutaneous involvement is common
   b. Lack of alpha-naphthyl butyrate esterase activity
   c. CD123 is expressed
   d. MPO positive

88. High hyperdiploidy in ALL refers to:
   a. Chromosomes 47-50
   b. Chromosomes 50-66
   c. Chromosomes 66-80
   d. All of the above

89. The cytochemical stains used for the diagnosis of MDS include:
   a. Perls stain
   b. MPO
   c. SBB
   d. All of the above

90. True about chronic neutrophilic leukemia is:
   a. Toxic granulations can be seen
   b. Pelger–Huet anomaly is not seen
   c. Serum granulocyte colony-stimulating factor (G-CSF) is reduced
   d. Serum protein electrophoresis should be done
   e. All of the above

91. Indication of bone marrow examination in chronic lymphocytic leukemia include all, *except*:
   a. Anemia
   b. Thrombocytopenia
   c. Lymphocytosis
   d. None of the above

92. True about immunophenotype of CLL is:
   a. A worse prognosis in CLL has been linked to expression of both IgM and IgD rather than expression of IgD alone
   b. Aberrant expression of myeloid or T-lymphocyte markers is also associated with a worse prognosis
   c. ZAP70 expression correlates with lack of somatic hypermutation of IGHV
   d. All of the above

93. True about chronic lymphocytic leukemia is:
   a. Strong expression of SmIg
   b. Strong expression of FMC7
   c. Strong expression of CD79b
   d. Strong expression of CD19
   e. None of the above

94. True for AML with t(8;21) blasts immunophenotype are:
   a. High intensity expression of CD 34
   b. Weak expression of CD33
   c. Coexpression of CD 34 and CD 55
   d. All of the above

95. All are true for acute myeloid leukemia with t(8;21) (q22; q22.1), *except*:
   a. RUNX1 codes the alpha subunit of CBF
   b. KIT mutations occurs in < 10% of cases
   c. High rate of complete remission
   d. Presence of KIT mutation has adverse impact

96. AML that usually shows monocytic and granulocytic differentiation and characteristically an abnormal eosinophil component in the bone marrow is:
   a. RUNX1- RUNX1T1
   b. CBFB- MYH11
   c. PML-RARA
   d. All of these

97. Most common mutation in acute myeloid leukemia with inv (16) or t(16;16) is:
   a. KIT
   b. NRAS
   c. KRAS
   d. ASXL2

98. AML with basophilia is seen in association with:
   a. t(8;21)
   b. t(6;9)
   c. t(9;11)
   d. t(3;3)

99. AML with t(1;22) (p13.3;q13.1); RBM15-MKL1 is most likely to present in which of the following patients?
   a. A 5-year-old girl with Down's syndrome
   b. A 5-month-old girl without Down's syndrome
   c. A 5-month-old boy with Down's syndrome
   d. A 15-year-old girl with Down's syndrome

100. Which of the following findings is not expected in acute myeloid leukemia with inv(3) (q21q26.2) or t(3;3) (q21q26.2); GATA2, MECOM?
   a. Thrombocytosis
   b. Basophilia
   c. Multilineage dysplasia
   d. Increased megakaryocytes

101. Distinct morphological features of microgranular (hypogranular) APL are:
   a. Predominantly bilobed nuclei
   b. Submicroscopic size of the azurophilic granules
   c. Markedly elevated TLC
   d. All of the above

102. APL with PML-RARA (hypergranular variant) is characterised by low or absent expression of all, *except*:
   a. HLA-DR
   b. CD34
   c. CD11a
   d. CD33

103. All are true for acute myeloid leukemia with mutated NPM1, *except*?
   a. Involve exon 12 of NPM1
   b. Aberrant cytoplasmic expression of NPM1
   c. Myelomonocytic or monocytes features
   d. Mostly presents in childhood

104. True for acute myeloid leukemia with biallelic CEBPA is/are?
   a. More than 70% cases have a normal karyotype
   b. Favourable prognosis
   c. Patients with biallelic CEBPA mutations should be evaluated for a familial syndrome
   d. All of the above

105. Which of the following is true for acute myeloid leukemia with mutated RUNX1, *except*?
   a. Higher frequency in older patients
   b. Associated with radiation exposure
   c. Associated with better overall survival
   d. Germline studies should be performed

106. True about Erdheim-Chester disease is:
   a. Disease of mast cells
   b. Progresses to acute myeloid leukemia
   c. Osteosclerosis is common
   d. All of the above

107. False about BIRC3-MALT1 translocation is:
   a. Most common translocation in extranodal marginal zone lymphoma
   b. Strongly correlates with H. pylori-independent variants of gastric EMZL
   c. Can also be seen in 20-30% cases of splenic marginal zone lymphoma or nodal marginal zone lymphoma
   d. None of the above

108. Inversion 14 or t(14;14) is seen in:
   a. Early T precursor ALL
   b. T-cell prolymphocytic leukemia
   c. Heavy chain disease
   d. Hairy cell leukemia variant

109. Which of the following is the most appropriate test for detecting iAMP21 in B cell acute lymphoblastic leukemia (B- ALL) patient?
   a. Conventional karyotyping
   b. Fluorescent in situ hybridization
   c. Polymerase chain reaction
   d. Next generation sequencing

110. Which of the following statements is false about Langerhans cell histiocytosis (LCH)?
   a. Caused by mutations in MAPK pathway
   b. Cell of origin is myeloid dendritic cells originating in bone marrow

c. Originates from cutaneous dendritic cells known as Langerhans cells
d. BRAF mutation is one of the perfect bar code for identifying LCH cell of origin

111. Patient was diagnosed with AML with immunophenotype on blasts showed positivity for CD19 alongwith CD34, MPO, HLA DR and CD13, the likely associated cytogenetic abnormality would be:
a. t(8;21)
b. inv(16)
c. t(9;22)
d. t(6;9)

112. FLT3 mutations (ITD or TKD) occurs in what percentage of APML patients?
a. <10%
b. 10-20%
c. 30-40%
d. 60-70%

113. Which of the following statement is/are true about AML with biallelic mutation of CEBPA?
a. Favourable prognosis
b. More than 70% cases have normal karyotype
c. Patients with biallelic mutations should be screened for familial syndrome
d. They may have expression of CD 7
e. All of the above

114. MPO stain is negative in all of the below, *except*:
a. Acute basophilic leukemia
b. Acute erythroid leukemia
c. Acute megakaryoblastic leukemia
d. Acute promyelocytic leukemia

115. The B-cell Acute lymphoblastic leukemia (ALL) with iAMP21 is characterized by amplification of a portion of chromosome 21, detected by FISH with a probe for RUNX1 that reveals:
a. ≥5 copies of the gene
b. ≤5 copies of the gene
c. ≥3 copies of the gene
d. ≤3 copies of the gene

116. True about myelodysplastic syndrome/chronic myelomonocytic leukemia with systemic inflammatory and autoimmune disease (SIAD) is:
a. This condition which is found in 20% of MDS and CMML cases
b. TET2 and IDH mutations are present
c. These mutations are associated with T cell imbalance
d. All of the above

117. Which of the following conditions can have small hypolobated megakaryocytes in the marrow?
a. Chronic myeloid leukemia
b. Essential thrombocythemia
c. Polycythemia vera
d. Systemic mastocytosis
e. Chronic neutrophilic anemia

118. True about Neutrophil extracellular traps is:
a. Critical role in innate immunity
b. Produced by neutrophils in response to inflammatory mediators
c. During NET formation, the neutrophils lost nuclei, leading to death of the cells
d. All of the above

119. The following statements about Thiamine responsive megaloblastic anemia (TRMA) are true, *except*:
a. The TRMA is characterized by megaloblastic anemia, progressive sensorineural hearing loss and diabetes mellitus
b. TRMA patients have biallelic pathogenic mutations in SLC19A2
c. Bone marrow reveals megaloblastic changes with often associated with ringed sideroblasts
d. Hearing loss is usually late in these patients

120. The following statements are true regarding Myeloid neoplasms with germline DDX41 mutation, *except*:
a. DDX1 is an RNA helicase
b. Significant number of cases has biallelic mutation
c. Patients who develop MDS/AML usually present with leukocytosis
d. Erythroid dysplasia is prominent feature
e. It has an autosomal dominant inheritance with high penetrance

121. Following statements are true for HHV-8 associated lymphoproliferative disorders, *except*:
a. Germinotropic lymphoproliferative disorder (GLPD) is commonly seen in immunocompetent individuals
b. HHV8-positive multicentric Castleman disease present with constitutional symptoms
c. HHV-8 associated DLBCL arise from naïve IgM-producing B cells
d. HHV-8 DLBCL are mostly positive for EBER
e. Plasmablasts in multicentric Castleman disease are almost always positive for lambda light chain

122. A 65-year-old lady, who is a known case of Rheumatoid arthritis, presented to the hematology clinic with complains of persistent neutropenia and Lymphocytosis. She was later diagnosed as T-cell large granular lymphocytic leukemia (T-LGLL). Following statements regarding T-LGLL are true, *except*:
a. T-LGLL is indolent lymphoma and usually present with persistent severe neutropenia.
b. Approximately 1/3rd of patients carry mutation of *STAT5B* gene.
c. Ultrastructure of T-LGLL granules has characteristic appearance with parallel tubular arrays

d. T-LGLL is typically a disorder of mature CD2+, CD3+, CD8+, CD57+, and alpha-beta TCR- positive cytotoxic T cells. The cells usually have diminished or lost expression of CD5 and/or CD7
e. CD57 and CD16 are expressed in >80% of cases

123. Enteropathy associated T-cell lymphoma (EATL) affects mainly small intestine. The following statements regarding EATL are true, *except*:
a. Homozygosity for HLA-DQ2 allele is a risk factor for EATL
b. EATL is less prevalent in Asians
c. Large cells or anaplastic morphology is rarely seen in EATL
d. The lymphoma cells are usually CD3+, CD5-, CD7+, CD4-, CD8-, and CD103+, and they express cytotoxic granule—associated proteins
e. Many cases of EATL are preceded by type 2 refractory coeliac disease AND the intraepithelial lymphocytes in adjacent mucosa exhibit an aberrant phenotype similar to that of the EATL

124. The following statements are true about Langerhans cell histiocytosis, *except*:
a. Lung LCH of adult is strongly associated with smoking
b. Skin is most commonly affected organ in solitary form.
c. LCH infiltrates are associated with eosinophils and multi-nucleate giant cells
d. indeterminate cell histiocytosis (ICH) closely mimics LCH but lacks CD207 expression
e. BRAFV600E or MAP2K1 mutations are seen in over 75% of cases.

125. The RAS/MAPK pathway plays a vital role in cell development. The following statements are true regarding RAS/MAPK pathway, *except*:
a. *RAS* genes constitute a multi-gene family that includes HRAS, KRAS and NRAS
b. RAS proteins are small guanosine nucleotide bound GTPases.
c. Neurofibromatosis 1 is a type of RASOpathy.
d. Noonan Syndrome is a type of RASOpathy mostly caused by activating mutations of PTPN11.
e. None of the above

126. The Ras-associated autoimmune leukoproliferative disorder (RALD) is a nonmalignant clinical syndrome. The following statements are true for this entity, *except*:
a. Almost all patients present with persistent relative or absolute monocytosis, hypergammaglobulinemia, B-cell lymphocytosis and splenomegaly
b. Associated with mutations in NRAS or KRAS
c. A prominent subset of circulating monocytes with increased expression of CD16 is seen
d. T-cell lymphocytosis is a common feature
e. Increased proportion of CD10 positive B-cells

127. The following statements about Extranodal NK/T-cell lymphoma nasal type is true, *except*:
a. Characterized by angiocentricity and destruction with prominent necrosis
b. Cytoplasmic CD3- beta is positive in most of cases
c. NK-associated antigens like CD16 and CD57 are usually negative
d. EBER is the most reliable way to demonstrate presence of EBV

128. ALK positive large B-cell lymphoma, following statement are true:
a. It is commonly seen in patients with immune suppression
b. Exclusively seen in lymph nodes
c. Granular cytoplasmic ALK positivity is seen in cases with NPM1-ALK fusion protein.
d. Strongly express CD138 and CD20 is usually negative

129. The following statements are true about Chronic lymphoproliferative disorders of NK cells (CLPD-NK), *except*:
a. Abnormally uniform expression of CD8.
b. Dasatinib can result in sustained increase of monoclonal NK-cells
c. One third cases show activating mutations in STAT3 SH2 domain.
d. KIR receptor expression is usually normal
e. Uniform, bright CD94/NKG2A heterodimer expression

130. A 42-year-old male presented to medicine outpatient department with fever, constitutional symptoms and hepatosplenomegaly. The peripheral blood smear shows lymphocytosis. Serum LDH is markedly elevated. After immunophenotypic analysis, patient was diagnosed as case of aggressive NK-cell leukemia. The following statements are true about aggressive NK-cell leukemia, *except*:
a. Neoplastic cells express FASL
b. *TCR* genes are in germline configuration
c. EBV is absent in a clonal episomal form
d. Most cases have a fulminant clinical course
e. Patients can show hemophagocytosis

131. Mastocytosis is clonal proliferation of Mast cells. Following statements are true about cutaneous mastocytosis, *except*:
a. There is no evidence of systemic involvement including bone marrow
b. Patients may present with one or two of the minor diagnostic criteria of ISM
c. Urticaria pigmentosa is most common form of cutaneous mastocytosis
d. Cutaneous mastocytosis is mostly seen in children above the age of 6 months

132. CD117 (cKIT) expression on flowcytometry can be seen in:
   a. CD34⁺ hematopoietic stem and progenitor cells
   b. CD56^{bright} natural killer cells
   c. Proerythroblasts
   d. Neoplastic cells from patients with monoclonal gammopathies, acute leukemias, and myelodysplastic syndromes
   e. All of the above

133. Mast cell leukemia (MCL) is characterized by following features, *except*:
   a. Bone marrow aspirate smears contains equal to or more than 20% mast cells.
   b. MCL should have more than 10% mast cells in peripheral blood
   c. Skin lesions are uncommon in MCL
   d. *KIT* gene sequencing is preferred

134. Obstetric TTP is characterized by following features, *except*:
   a. Usually occur in second half of pregnancy
   b. Fetal extraction corrects TTP symptoms
   c. As much as 50% cases with TTP in first pregnancy have Upshaw Schulman syndrome
   d. There is no role of fetal extraction on mitigation of TTP symptoms

135. Correct statements with reference to transfusion associated GVHD (TA-GVHD) are all, *except*:
   a. TA-GVHD bone marrow is uniformly affected
   b. Skin, gastrointestinal, and liver signs and symptoms similar to stem cell transplant-related GVHD also occur in patients with TA-GVHD
   c. Signs and symptoms of TA-GVHD usually begin 2–30 days after transfusion
   d. Granulocyte transfusions are not associated with TA-GVHD

136. Which of the following is true regarding childhood ALL with t(12;21):
   a. It is the most common chromosome translocation in childhood ALL
   b. It results in ETV6-RUNX1 fusion
   c. It present after infancy
   d. ETV6 deletion on chromosome 12p is the most common additional genetic abnormality
   e. All of the above

137. Most common transcription factor gene mutated in MDS is:
   a. ETV6
   b. RUNX1
   c. GATA2
   d. TP53

138. Most common class of genes mutated in MDS pathogenesis is:
   a. RNA splicing factor genes
   b. Epigenetic modifier genes
   c. Transcription factor genes
   d. Cohesin complex genes

139. Revised IPSS scoring in MDS includes all parameters, *except*:
   a. Bone marrow blasts percentage b. Cytogenetics
   c. Leukopenia   d. Hemoglobin

140. Which of the following is not Blast equivalent:
   a. Promyelocyte   b. Promonocyte
   c. Atypical pronormoblast
   d. Micromegakaryocyte

141. MPO positivity in what percentage of blasts confirms the diagnosis of AML:
   a. 1%   b. 2%
   c. 3%   d. 5%

142. A 65-years-old female was admitted with the complaints of fever for 3 weeks and diffuse body-aches for 2 weeks. On evaluation there was no lymphadenopathy or hepatosplenomegaly. Complete hemogram revealed Hb 6.8g/dL, white cell count 65000/micl and platelet count of 33,000/micl. Peripheral blood smear showed 70% blasts. The immunophenotype showed positivity as shown below:

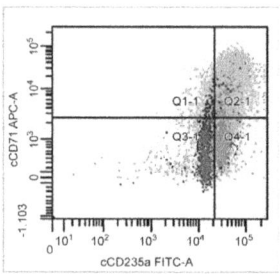

Courtesy: Dr Nishit Gupta, MD, DM

What is the most probable diagnosis?
   a. Acute myelomonocytic leukemia
   b. Acute erythroblastic leukemia
   c. Acute megakaryoblastic leukemia
   d. Acute undifferentiated leukemia

143. A 2-year-old girl was admitted with the complaints of fever, decreased oral intake and ecchymotic patches over body for 2 weeks. The peripheral blood showed 85% blasts. The bone marrow aspirate was dry. The peripheral blood blast immunophenotyping for acute leukemia analysis revealed the following:
   - The gated cells in the blast window expressed CD34, CD117, CD33, sCD61, sCD41a, cCD61 and CD56.
   - cMPO, CD13, CD14, CD15, CD64, CD4, CD11b, cCD41a, CD71, CD235a, CD19, CD10, CD20,

cCD79a, CD5, cCD3, CD7, CD38, CD123, TdT and HLA-DR are negative

The most probable diagnosis is:
a. Acute myelomonocytic leukemia
b. Acute monoblastic leukemia
c. Acute megakaryoblastic leukemia
d. Acute undifferentiated leukemia

144. A 5-year-old male child was admitted with the history of pain abdomen and intermittent vomiting for last 4 months. Abdominal examination revealed a distended abdomen with a diffuse mass palpable in right iliac fossa. Hemogram showed high white cell count with atypical cells. Bone marrow aspirate is shown below.

The immunophenotyping will show positivity for:
a. CD10, CD19, CD20, cCD79a, CD79b, CD22, sIgM, and HLA-DR
b. CD13, CD33, cMPO, CD34/CD117, TdT
c. CD2, cCD3, CD4, CD5, CD11b,
d. CD11c, CD14, CD15, CD64, TdT, CD38 and CD56
e. CD10, CD19, CD20, cCD79a, CD13, CD33, cMPO, CD34/CD117, TdT

145. In the above-mentioned case the treatment can involve any of the following, *except*:
a. R-CHOP
b. R-hyper-CVAD
c. CODOX-M/IVACA with rituximab
d. Dose-adjusted EPOCH with rituximab

ANSWERS WITH EXPLAXNATIONS

1. Ans. b. Factor XI deficiency

Factor XI (FXI) deficiency is also called hemophilia C, plasma thromboplastin antecedent deficiency, and Rosenthal syndrome. Severe FXI deficiency is inherited in an *autosomal recessive pattern*. In some cases, FXI deficiency can also be inherited in an *autosomal dominant pattern*. Men and women are affected by FXI deficiency equally. FXI deficiency is associated with bleeding manifestations of variable severity. Factor XII, prekallikrein, and HMWK are required for normal factor XI activation in the "contact phase" that initiates coagulation in the aPTT assay. Patients lacking one of these proteins have prolonged aPTTs, but do not have abnormal bleeding, even with surgery or injury. Therefore, either these proteins do not participate in hemostasis or redundant mechanisms compensate for their absence. No specific therapy is required to prepare deficient patients for surgery. Factor XII, prekallikrein, or HK deficiency must be distinguished from deficiencies of factors VIII, IX, or XI, which prolong the aPTT, but cause abnormal hemostasis. FXII/FXIIa deficiency influences thrombosis risk and inflammation.

2. Ans. a. Factor XIII deficiency

Ref: Hsieh L, Nugent D. Factor XIII deficiency. Haemophilia. 2008;14:1190-200

Factor XIII deficiency is associated with normal screening coagulogram. It is detected by abnormal clot solubility test. Inherited factor XIII (FXIII) deficiency is a rare bleeding disorder that can present with umbilical bleeding during the neonatal period, delayed soft-tissue bruising, mucosal bleeding, and life-threatening intracranial hemorrhage. FXIII deficiency has also been associated with poor wound healing and recurrent miscarriages. The results of standard laboratory clotting tests, such as prothrombin time, aPTT, fibrinogen level, platelet count, and bleeding time are all normal in FXIII-deficient patients. Using a solution of 1% monochloroacetic acid or 5M urea, clots will undergo lysis if a patient has FXIII levels of <1%. The clot solubility test is only sensitive at very low levels of FXIII (zero or very close to zero and will be normal if the FXIII activity level rises up to 1–3%).

3. Ans. a. It is an aggressive disease

Ref: Sokol L, Loughran TP Jr. Large granular lymphocyte leukemia. Oncologist. 2006;11:263-73.

T-cell large granular lymphocytes (LGL) is usually an indolent disease. Clonal disorders of LGLs represent a spectrum of biologically distinct lymphoproliferative diseases originating either from mature T cells ($CD3^+$) or from NK cells ($CD3^-$). The majority of patients with T-cell LGL leukemia have a clinically indolent course with a median survival time >10 years. Aggressive NK-cell LGL leukemia is usually a rapidly progressive disorder associated with Epstein-Barr virus (EBV), with a higher prevalence in Asia and South America.

4. Ans. a. Causally linked to Epstein-Barr virus (EBV) infection

Ref: Cook LB. Revised Adult T-Cell Leukemia-Lymphoma International Consensus Meeting Report. J Clin Oncol. 2019;8:677-87.

Adult T-cell leukemia-lymphoma (ATLL) is causally linked to human T-cell leukemia virus type 1 (HTLV1). ATLL is a distinct mature T-cell malignancy caused by chronic infection with human T-lymphotropic virus type 1 with diverse clinical features and prognosis. ATLL remains a challenging disease as a result of its diverse clinical features, multidrug resistance of malignant cells, frequent large tumor burden, hypercalcemia, and/or frequent opportunistic infection.

5. Ans. b. Lacks expression of CD7

Ref: Jain N, Lamb AV, O'Brien S, Ravandi F, Konopleva M, Jabbour E, et al. Early T-cell precursor acute lymphoblastic leukemia/lymphoma (ETP-ALL/LBL) in adolescents and adults: a high-risk subtype. Blood. 2016;127(15):1863-9.

Early T-cell precursors are recent immigrants from the bone marrow to the thymus, derived from hematopoietic stem cells, which retain a certain level of multilineage pluripotency. By gene expression profiling, ETP cells share similarities with hematopoietic stem cells and myeloid progenitor cells. The definition of ETP-ALL/LBL is based on the immunophenotype of the leukemic cells, which are typically CD1a−, CD8−, CD5− (dim), and positive for 1 or more stem cell or myeloid antigens. ETP-ALL is positive for CD7.

6. Ans. d. Ring sideroblasts are commonly seen

Ref: Hofmann I. Pediatric myelodysplastic syndromes. J Hematopathol. 2015;8:127-41.

Ring sideroblasts are typically absent in refractory cytopenia of childhood (RCC). RCC is the most common subtype of pediatric MDS accounting for about 50% of cases. There are major differences between pediatric and adult MDS. The majority of children present with hypocellular bone marrow resembling acquired or inherited bone marrow failure conditions. The implications of multilineage (compared to unilineage) dysplasia are uncertain in childhood, as opposed to adults where it has prognostic implications. Therefore, all pediatric MDS without excess blasts are grouped into the RCC category, regardless of the degree of dysplasia and cellularity. Pediatric patients commonly present with thrombocytopenia and neutropenia, as opposed to isolated anemia in adults. Therefore, the term refractory cytopenia is used in children rather than refractory anemia, which is used in adults. If ringed sideroblasts are observed in a pediatric bone marrow, other etiologies, particularly nutritional deficiencies, drug toxicity, and congenital sideroblastic anemias, including Pearson marrow-pancreas syndrome, should be considered.

7. Ans. c. CD33

The laboratory diagnosis of PNH, which is categorized by reduced synthesis of GPI anchor, is based on the detection of blood cells deficient in GPI-anchored proteins by flow cytometry. This involves different mutations, thus resulting in the deficient synthesis of GPI-anchored molecule and in partial or absolute deficiency, in all blood cell lineages, of the expression of GPI-anchored membrane proteins, such as CD55, CD59, CD14, CD16, CD24, and CD48, among others. CD33 is a gating antibody and is not GPI linked.

8. Ans. a. Ring sideroblasts ≥5% with SF3B1 mutation

Ref: Myelodysplastic syndromes. WHO 2017.

In the presence of SF3B1 mutation, ring sideroblasts ≥5% are enough to qualify as MDS-RS. The 2016 WHO classification categorizes patients with ≥5% ring sideroblasts and SF3B1 mutation as MDS-RS, in contrast to its prior MDS-RS classification (≥15% RS and no genotyping data).

9. Ans. c. Loss of Y chromosome

Loss of Y chromosome, del20q, and gain of chromosome 8 are not considered presumptive evidence of MDS in the absence of morphological dysplasia. Acquired loss of a sex-chromosome (−Y in males, −X in females) is an age-related phenomenon, but can also occur in association with hematological malignancies.

10. Ans. c. Band 3 protein

Ref: King MJ. Rapid flow cytometric test for the diagnosis of membrane cytoskeleton-associated haemolytic anaemia. Br J Haematol. 2000;111:924-33.

Eosin-5-maleimide (EMA) dye binds to band 3 protein. The RBC membrane is a lipid bilayer consisting of specific protein components such as α- and β-spectrin, ankyrin, band 3, protein 4.1, protein 4.2, and actin. These proteins maintain the structural integrity of the RBC membrane and defects in the genes encoding these proteins decrease cell membrane integrity. The basic principle of the EMA-RBC binding test involves the covalent binding of EMA to lysine-430 on the first extracellular loop of band 3 protein. Inadequate expression of band 3 protein will result in reduced binding of EMA. Flow cytometric analysis with EMA-labeled RBCs has shown a high sensitivity and specificity for diagnosing hereditary spherocytosis.

11. Ans. a. Derived from bacteria

Ref: Sutherland DR. Diagnosing PNH with FLAER and multiparameter flow cytometry. Cytometry B Clin Cytom. 2007;72:167-77.

Besides the specific monoclonal antibodies, FLAER, recently developed, has been used. It is a proaerolysin variant, secreted by the bacterium *Aeromonas hydrophila*, which selectively binds with high affinity to the glycan portion of GPI (not to phosphatidyl-inositol-glycan gene, PIG-A). Its usage allows direct assessment of the GPI expression in different cell lineages, except erythrocytes, and provides greater analytical sensitivity. The FLAER reagent presents excellent capacity in the detection of neutrophils and monocytes with a PNH phenotype. It also presents as advantages of the power of clear discrimination between normal and altered cells and the high accuracy in the analysis of samples presenting cells in different stages of maturation and/or dysplastic.

12. Ans. b. Accelerated atherosclerosis

Ref: Jaiswal S. Clonal hematopoiesis and risk of atherosclerotic cardiovascular disease. N Engl J Med. 2017;377(2):111-21.

Somatic mutations in leukemia-associated driver genes are commonly detected in apparently healthy older people with normal blood counts, and these clonally restricted mutations are associated with a risk for developing hematological neoplasms (especially myeloid) or cardiovascular events. An important mechanism of accelerated atherogenesis in the context of clonal hematopoiesis of indeterminate potential is endothelial inflammation driven by interaction between the vasculature and clonally derived circulating monocytes/macrophages.

13. Ans. c. Mutated immunoglobulins heavy chain variable gene (IGVH) status

Ref: Parikh SA. Prognostic factors and risk stratification in chronic lymphocytic leukemia. Semin Oncol. 2016;43(2):233-40.

Patients with higher degrees of somatic mutation in the IGHV of their chronic lymphocytic leukemia (CLL) clone experience longer overall survival (OS). Studies have shown that CLL patients with mutated IGHV (defined as a >2% difference from the germline nucleotide sequence) had a median OS > 20 years, whereas those with unmutated IGHV had median OS of ~8 years. 17p deletion and *TP53* mutation confer a poor prognosis. The unfavorable prognosis has been attributed to the critical role played by *TP53* on the apoptosis process control and by halting the cell cycle to allow time for the DNA-repair system to catch up. Such an effect is reinforced by the observation that more than 80% of patients with CLL carrying del(17p) in one allele have a *TP53* mutation on the remaining second allele, leading to complete loss of *TP53* protein function. Moreover, 4–5% of CLL cases carry a *TP53* mutation in the absence of del17p, shortening the progression-free survival (PFS) and OS, similar to those seen in cases with del 17p.

14. Ans. a. Bone homeostasis in multiple myeloma

Ref: Baron R. Wnt signaling in bone homeostasis and disease: from human mutations to treatments. Nat Med. 2013;19:179-92.

The relevance of Wnt signaling in myeloma was first acknowledged for its regulating role in bone homeostasis. Wnt signaling tightly controls the balance between bone-forming osteoblasts and bone-resorbing osteoclasts, by both direct and indirect mechanisms. Malignant plasma cells in myeloma severely disturb this system by secretion of Wnt antagonists in the bone marrow microenvironment. This skews the balance toward osteogenic bone resorption and results in development of the characteristic osteolytic bone lesions. In this process, a plethora of growth factors that were embedded in the bone matrix are released, which subsequently enhance myeloma cell growth and survival. Aberrant Wnt signaling plays a dual role in the pathogenesis of myeloma: (1) it mediates proliferation, migration, and drug resistance of myeloma cells and (2) myeloma cells secrete Wnt antagonists (Dickkopf, Dkk) that contribute to the development of osteolytic lesions by impairing osteoblast differentiation.

15. Ans. a. Forward scatter signal

Ref: Macey MG. Principles of flow cytometry. In: Flow Cytometry: Principles and Applications. New Jersey: Humana Press; 2007. p1-15.

Light scattered by particles as they pass through a laser or light source must be efficiently detected, and fluorescent light of a given wavelength requires specific identification. The amount of light scattered is generally higher in comparison with the amount of fluorescent light. Photodiodes are therefore used as forward angle light (FAL) sensors; they may be used with neutral density filters that proportionally reduce the amount of light received by the detector.

The sensors used for side light scatter and fluorochrome fluorescence are photomultiplier tubes (PMTs). These tubes serve as detectors and also as amplifiers of the weak fluorescent signals.

16. Ans. d. Bright CD45, low side scatter, CD3 positive cells

Ref: Lichtman MA. Williams Manual of Hematology. New York: McGraw Hill Professional; 2017. p1142-46.

Lymphocytes are a heterogeneous population of blood cells divided into several functional types and subtypes based on their organs of development and function. The major classes of lymphocytes include T cells, B cells, and NK cells. The T-lymphocytes have bright CD45 with CD3 expression and low side scatter and forward scatter. These cells are used as a reference cell for describing the cell size of different flow cytometric populations. Cells similar to T-cell size are small cells while those with higher forward scatter than T-lymphocytes are considered larger cells.

17. Ans. b. Antigen-presenting cells

Ref: Kumar V. Robbins Basic Pathology. Amsterdam: Elsevier Health Sciences; 2017. p126.

The genes encoding HLA are found on chromosome 6 and are inherited en-bloc such that half of each individual's HLA (an allele) will be from each parent. HLA is divided into class I and class II. Class I molecules are HLA A, B, and C while class II molecules are HLA DR, DP, and DQ. Class I molecules are expressed on all nucleated cells while class II molecule expression is restricted to cells such as antigen-presenting cells, e.g. dendritic cells, macrophages, and B cells.

18. Ans. a. CD123+ HLADR+

Ref: Swerdlow SH. WHO Classification of Tumours of Haematopoietic and Lymphoid Tissues, Revised 4th edition. Lyon: IARC; 2017. p174.

Plasmacytoid dendritic cells (also called professional type I interferon-producing cells or plasmacytoid monocytes) are characterized by expression of BDCA-2, CD123, and HLA-DR and are negative for CD14, CD11c, and CD1a. Blastic plasmacytoid dendritic cell neoplasm (BPOCN) is a clinically aggressive tumor derived from the precursors of PDCs.

19. Ans. d. NK cells

Ref: Gorczyca W. Flow Cytometry in Neoplastic Hematology: Morphologic-Immunophenotypic Correlation. Florida: CRC Press; 2017. p15-21.

Progenitor gate includes normal/abnormal myeloid blasts, hematogones, plasmacytoid dendritic cells, basophils, and normal plasma cells.

20. Ans. b. CD1a+

Ref: Swerdlow SH. WHO Classification of Tumours of Haematopoietic and Lymphoid Tissues, Revised 4th edition. Lyon: IARC; 2017. p212.

Early T-cell precursor acute lymphoblastic leukemia (ETP-ALL) is a neoplasm composed of cells committed to the T-cell lineage but with a unique immunophenotype indicating only limited early T-cell differentiation. ETP-ALL expresses CD7 but by definition lacks CD8 and CD1a and is positive for one or more of the myeloid/stem cell markers CD34, KIT (CD117), HLA-DR, CD13, CD33, CD11b, and CD65. Blasts also express cytoplasmic, or in rare cases surface CD3, and may express CD2 and/or CD4. CD5 is often negative; when positive, it is present on <75% of the blast population. It has been suggested that leukemias that express brighter or more uniform CD5 but otherwise meet the criteria for ETP-ALL be called near-ETP-ALL. By definition, myeloperoxidase (MPO) is negative, because a leukemia with an otherwise ETP immunophenotype that also expresses MPO would most likely meet the criteria for T/myeloid mixed-phenotype acute leukemia.

21. Ans. c. BCL2 expression

Ref: Swerdlow SH. WHO Classification of Tumours of Haematopoietic and Lymphoid Tissues, Revised 4th edition. Lyon: IARC; 2017. p190-91.

Germinal center centroblasts express low levels of surface immunoglobulins (sIg) and switch off expression of BCL2; therefore, they and their progeny are susceptible to apoptosis. Centroblasts express CD10 as well as BCL6, a nuclear transcription factor also expressed by centrocytes. In the germinal center, somatic hypermutation occurs in the *IGV* genes; these mutations can result in a nonfunctional gene or a gene that produces antibody with lower or higher affinity for antigen. Also, in the germinal center, some cells switch from IgM production to IgG or IgA production. Through these mechanisms, the germinal center reaction gives rise to the higher affinity IgG or IgA antibodies of the late primary or secondary immune response.

22. Ans. c. APC (allophycocyanin)

Ref: Macey MG. Principles of flow cytometry. In: Flow Cytometry. New Jersey: Humana Press; 2007. p78-79.

In a typical three-laser, eight-color configuration in flow cytometry, blue laser commonly excites FITC, PE, PerCP-Cy5.5, and PE-Cy7 (tandem conjugate of phycoerythrin and a cyanine dye, Cy7); red laser excites APC (allophycocyanin) and APC-H7 (modified tandem conjugate of allophycocyanin and Cy7); and violet laser excites pacific blue and pacific orange.

23. Ans. d. TCRαβ

Ref: Lichtman MA. Williams Manual of Hematology. New York: McGraw Hill Professional; 2017. p1142.

The NK cell is defined as an effector cell that is not MHC restricted and has the capacity for spontaneous cytotoxicity toward various target cells. Most NK cells have LGL morphology. Human NK cells characteristically express CD16 and CD56 but not TCRα/β or TCRγ/δ, CD3, or CD4. CD8 is found on approximately 30–50% of NK cells.

24. Ans. e. None of the above

Ref: Gorczyca W. Flow Cytometry in Neoplastic Hematology: Morphologic-Immunophenotypic Correlation. Florida: CRC Press; 2017. p84-90.

Hematogones are physiological precursors of B-cells, distinguished into three stages: Stage I, Stage II, and Stage III. Their numbers decrease with age but may be increased in regenerating marrows from patients after chemotherapy and stem cell transplant. Patients with MDS and myeloproliferative neoplasm (MPN) show lack/reduction in the number of hematogones. The identification of hematogones is important for distinguishing them from B-lymphoblasts. They are morphologically indistinguishable from B-lymphoblasts and can confound morphological counts for remission status assessment. Stage I hematogones express TdT, CD10, CD19, CD34, CD38, and CD58 and are negative for CD20. Stage II hematogones are positive for CD10, CD19, CD38 and cytoplasmic IgM and do not express CD34, CD58, TdT, and CD20, and Stage III hematogones start acquiring CD20 and surface immunoglobulin light chains.

25. Ans. d. Increased in aplastic anemia

Ref: Lichtman MA. Williams Manual of Hematology. New York: McGraw Hill Professional; 2017. p432-438.

Erythropoietin is predominantly produced in kidney and to a lesser part in the liver. Hypoxia increases production of EPO and induces committed progenitor cells [colony-forming unit-erythroid (CFU-E) and burst-forming unit-erythroid (BFU-E)] to proliferate in the marrow. These committed progenitor cells differentiate into pronormoblasts by shortening generation time and promoting early release of reticulocytes into blood, therefore stimulating proliferation. EPO gene is located on chromosome 7. The conditions associated with an increased EPO level include erythroid hyperplasia, aplastic anemia, cerebellar hemangioma, renal cell carcinoma, hepatocellular carcinoma, renal cysts, hydronephrosis, and ovarian carcinoma. The conditions associated with a decreased EPO level include polycythemia vera, after transfusion, chronic renal disease, and hypothyroidism.

26. Ans. b. Circulating pool

Ref: Lichtman MA. Williams Manual of Hematology. New York: McGraw Hill Professional; 2017.

The neutrophil count in the blood is maintained in a normal steady state by the balance of granulopoiesis in the marrow, distribution of neutrophils between the marginated pool (in the microvasculature) and the circulating pool (in the blood), and the rate of egress from blood to tissues. Neutrophils have a short life span in the blood, with a half disappearance time of approximately 7 hours. This process may be accelerated when inflammation is present and highlights the need for a sustained rate of production to maintain a normal blood neutrophil count. At least four compartments are involved: marrow storage pool, circulating pool, marginated pool, and tissue pool.

27. Ans. a. V-D-J, cytoplasmic mu, kappa, and lambda

Ref: Swerdlow SH. WHO Classification of Tumours of Haematopoietic and Lymphoid Tissues, Revised 4th edition. Lyon: IARC; 2017. p190-91.

The order of Ig heavy-chain and light-chain rearrangement is V-D-J, cytoplasmic mu, kappa, and lambda, which all takes place in the bone marrow. The earliest B-precursor cells in the bone marrow acquire cytoplasmic Ig heavy chain at the pre-B cell stage. The Ig heavy and light chains fuse on the cell surface to form the intact Ig molecule. IgH is located on chromosome 14q32 with 100 (V) variable regions and 15–20 (D) diversity regions and 6 (J) joining and the 9 (C) constant region genes that encode the particular Ig isotype: Cmu (IgM), Cdelta (IgD), Cgamma (IgG1-4), Calpha (IgA1-2), or Cepsilon (IgE). The heavy-chain rearrangement begins with D combining with J, followed by combination with V region gene. The exons are deleted. The DNA is transcribed and undergoes RNA splicing with removal of intron material with splicing of V, D, J, and Cmu (always Cmu first because it is the closest gene to the rearranged V-D-J segment) which now produces cytoplasmic IgH at the pre-B stage. This is followed by gamma 3,1 - alpha 1 - gamma 2,4 - epsilon - alpha 2 if nonproductive, due to termination or nonsense codon. The same process will begin on the other chromosome to make the same IgH. Next, the kappa light chain is made (no D regions and only one C region). If nonproductive, then the process will begin on lambda gene (no D region, 6 C region). The sequential kappa to lambda gene rearrangement process accounts for the 2:1 ratio of kappa to lambda.

28. Ans. a. The order of rearrangement is gamma, delta, beta, and alpha

Ref: Swerdlow SH. WHO Classification of Tumours of Haematopoietic and Lymphoid Tissues, revised 4th edition. Lyon: IARC; 2017. p192-193.

The order of rearrangement is gamma, delta, beta, and alpha. Alpha and beta receptors are present on 95% of the circulating T-cells. Like the rearrangement of the immunoglobulin gene in developing B-cells, the *TCR* genes also undergo V(D)J rearrangement.

Location of alpha, beta, gamma, and delta chains:
- Alpha: 14q11.2
- Beta: 7q34
- Delta: 14q11.2
- Gamma: 7p15.

29. Ans. a. They may be seen in megaloblastic anemia within reticulocytes

Ref: Lichtman MA. Williams Manual of Hematology. New York: McGraw Hill Professional; 2017. p467.

The ring-like or figure-of-eight structures sometimes seen in megaloblastic anemia within reticulocytes and in an occasional, heavily stippled, late-intermediate megaloblast are designated Cabot rings. Their composition is nuclear. Some investigators have suggested that Cabot rings originate from spindle material that was mishandled during abnormal mitosis. Others have found no indication of DNA or spindle filaments but have shown that the rings are associated with adherent granular material containing arginine-rich histone and nonhemoglobin iron.

30. Ans. a. Bernard–Soulier syndrome

Response to ristocetin is absent in Bernard-Soulier syndrome and von Willebrand disease (vWD) except vWD 2B which has a hyper-responsiveness to low dose of ristocetin.

31. Ans. a. Wiskott–Aldrich syndrome

Ref: Lichtman MA. Williams Manual of Hematology. New York: McGraw Hill Professional; 2017. p1224-6.

- *X-linked diseases*: VIII and IX, Wiskott-Aldrich syndrome
- *Autosomal dominant diseases*: vWD, platelet-type vWD, dysfibrinogenemia, antithrombin III, protein C, protein S, activated protein C resistance/factor V Leiden
- *Autosomal recessive diseases*: (All of the rest) II, V, VII, X, XI, XIII, alpha2-plasmin, Glanzmann's thrombasthenia, Bernard-Soulier's disease, dense granule deficiency (Hermansky-Pudlak, Chediak-Higashi, TAR syndrome).

32. Ans. b. Samples should be tested within 4 hours of collection

Ref: World Federation of Hemophilia. Guidelines for the Management of Hemophilia, 2nd edition. Quebec, Canada: World Federation of Hemophilia. p30.

The sample should be collected in citrate tubes containing 0.105M–0.109M (c3.2%) aqueous trisodium citrate dihydrate, maintaining the proportion of blood to citrate as 9:1. The sample should be maintained at temperatures between 20 and 25°C where possible, but for no more than 4 hours. Higher temperatures (>25°C) lead to loss of FVIII activity over time, whereas sample storage in the cold (2–8°C) leads to cold activation. If the sample cannot be processed within 4 hours of collection,

33. Ans. d. None of the above
Ref: World Federation of Hemophilia. Guidelines for the Management of Hemophilia, 2nd edition. Quebec, Canada: World Federation of Hemophilia. p31.

34. Ans. d. All of the above
Ref: Update of ISTH guidelines for LA detection. J Thromb Hemost. 2009;7:1737-40.

35. Ans. a. 10,000/cmm

Platelet-poor plasma shall be made (using a calibrated centrifuge) spun at 1,500–2,000 g for 15 minutes to achieve a platelet count of <10,000/cmm. The counts must be verified on randomly selected specimens once in 6 months or following a major repair on the centrifuge which requires recalibration.

36. Ans. d. Sevuparin *Ref: ASH updates 2018.*

Voxelotor is a small molecule that binds the alpha chain of HbS and increases its affinity for oxygen. FDA approved it on November 25, 2019. Crizanlizumab is a humanized monoclonal antibody against P-selectin, approved by FDA on November 15, 2019. L-glutamine was approved in July 2017. Sevuparin (antiadhesive and anti-inflammatory agent), a novel polysaccharide, interacts with multiple targets during a vaso-occlusive crisis. These interactions cause the release of blood components bound to each other and bound to the endothelial wall, preventing further occlusions from occurring. Sevuparin is under Phase 2 trial.

37. Ans. c. Thalidomide and bortezomib are not active in these lymphomas

Immunomodulatory drugs (IMiDs), such as thalidomide and lenalidomide, as well as proteasome inhibitors, such as bortezomib, have proven activity in LPLs. Like most CD20 positive B-cell lymphomas, the combined use of chemotherapy and immunotherapy with rituximab has improved the disease-free interval in such patients.

38. Ans. e. All of the above
Ref: Shovlin CL. Diagnostic criteria for hereditary hemorrhagic telangiectasia, Rendu-Osler-Weber syndrome. Am J Med Gene. 2000;91:66-7.

Hereditary hemorrhagic telangiectasia (HHT) is easily recognized in individuals displaying the classical triad of epistaxis, telangiectasia, and a suitable family history, but the disease is more difficult to diagnosis in many patients. Serious consequences may result if visceral arteriovenous malformations, particularly in the pulmonary circulation, are unrecognized and left untreated. In spite of the identification of two of the disease-causing genes (endoglin and ALK-1), only a clinical diagnosis of HHT can be provided for the majority of individuals. Diagnostic criteria suggested for hereditary haemorrhagic telangiectasia are that the patient should have at least three out of four of (a) epistaxis; (b) telangiectasia (typically affecting lips, mouth, fingers or nose); (c) visceral lesions (such as gastrointestinal telangiectasia or arteriovenous malformations in the lung, liver, brain or spinal cord) and (d) an appropriate family history.

39. Ans. d. All of the above *Ref: Muller UR and Haeberli G. (2009) The problem of anaphylaxis and mastocytosis. Curr Allergy Asthma Rep 2009;9:64–70.*

Mastocytosis is a rare disease characterized by an elevated whole body mast cell number. Anaphylaxis is a severe, generalized hypersensitivity reaction with rapid onset. The problem of anaphylaxis and mastocytosis is due to strongly increased mediator release from the elevated mast cell number during allergic reactions. This explains the much higher prevalence of anaphylaxis in mastocytosis than in the general population and its severe and sometimes fatal course. Because of the increased risk of anaphylaxis in mastocytosis, all patients with severe or recurrent anaphylaxis should be analyzed for underlying mastocytosis by estimation of baseline serum tryptase. So, recurrent anaphylaxis, often unprovoked, should raise the suspicion of systemic mastocytosis. A serum tryptase concentration above 20 ng/mL is an important diagnostic criterion, assay not being performed immediately after an attack. The patient should also undergo a bone marrow aspirate and trephine biopsy.

40. Ans. d. Core biopsy sections are more reliable than the aspirate for the assessment of storage iron
Ref: Lee SH. ICSH guidelines for the standardization of bone marrow specimens and reports. Int Jnl Lab Hem. 2008;30:349-64.

A Prussian Blue stain should be performed on a BM smear for the evaluation of storage iron and sideroblasts. A BM smear with increased iron stores should be included as a positive control. Squash preparations and particle clot sections can also be stained for iron. If there is a 'dry tap', a core biopsy section and imprint can be stained for iron. Core biopsy sections are less reliable than the aspirate for the assessment of storage iron, since decalcification removes storage iron.

41. Ans. c. TCR
Ref: Sharma SK. What a clinical hematologist should know about T cells? IBRR. 2020;11(4):20-32.

The TCR is formed by the product of variable (V), diversity (D) and joining (J) (VDJ) genes recombination and requires recombinase-activating genes (RAG 1 and 2). RAG genes break the DNA containing the VDJ genes at specific points to construct the TCR.

42. Ans. e. All of the above

Ref: Sharma SK. What a clinical hematologist should know about T cells? IBRR. 2020;11(4):20-32.

The normal CD4/CD8 ratio in healthy hosts is about 2 (range 1.5 and 2.5). Normal ratios can invert (<1) through isolated apoptotic or targeted cell death of circulating CD4 cells, expansion of CD8 cells, or a combination of both. The prevalence of an inverted CD4/CD8 ratio increases with age and after HSCT (when peripheral expansion of CD8 T cells and decreased thymic output of CD4 T cells results, which normalizes only after thymic recovery). Cytomegalovirus (CMV) infection has a significant impact on the CD4/CD8 ratio through the expansion of CMV specific CD8 cells, whereas human immunodeficiency virus (HIV) infection decreases CD4 T cells.

43. Ans. c. AIRE gene

Ref: Sharma SK. What a clinical hematologist should know about T cells? IBRR. 2020;11(4): 20-32.

Thymus has an extraordinary capacity to express and present proteins from all over the body, which is due to the expression of the AIRE gene by the epithelial cells that allow them to express, process and present proteins to the developing T cells in the thymus from the respective organs only. The characteristic feature of this gene is that it represents the tissue-specific-antigens of the whole of the host body which the T cells would encounter once they leave the thymus. Developing T cells that bind tightly to these organ-specific proteins in the context of MHC molecules undergo negative selection (i.e. they undergo apoptosis). These tissue-specific-antigens are the antigens of different organs, which the T cells have to recognize as self-antigens and are taught not to react against them. If these developing T cells fail to undergo this training of identification of self-antigens in the medulla, they will react against body's own tissue-antigens and will lead to autoimmunity, which will be self-destructive. This deletion of auto-reactive T cells (negative selection) results in development of central tolerance. This is one of the most remarkable features of thymic medullary epithelial cells, who have the provision of training the T cells about all the human body antigens at one place, rather than the T cells wandering from tissue to tissue to identify self-antigens, which is not practically possible for T cells.

44. Ans. d. Surrounding macrophages near the sinus membrane

Within the bone marrow, erythroid precursors are located along the macrophage lining. The reason for the same being macrophages are the ready source of iron for the growing erythroids.

45. Ans. d. Transferrin-bound iron into erythrocytes

Iron absorption occurs mainly from duodenum, via endocytosis of transferrin receptor 1 or via ferrous ron importer DMT1. Intracellular iron can be stored as ferritin. Export of this iron occurs through ferroportin, aided by hepaestin and ceruloplasmin.

46. Ans. c. Can be seen post-splenectomy

Ref: Interpretation of peripheral blood smears, Harrison, 20th edition, chapter 58, p379.

Howell-Jolly bodies are dense blue circular inclusions that represent nuclear remnants. They are seen in patients with asplenia. Basophilic stippling are red cell inclusion characterized by diffuse fine or coarse blue dots in the red cell representing RNA residue and are commonly seen in lead poisoning.

47. Ans. a. Basophilic stippling is also known as Pappenheimer bodies

Ref: Dacie 11th edition, p74-75, 85.

Basophilic stippling means the presence of many basophilic granules present throughout the cell. They do not stain with Perl's stain. These can be seen in thalassemia, megaloblastic anemia, lead poisoning, liver disease, and pyrimidine 5'- nucleotidase deficiency. The presence of basophilic stippling points towards thalassemia rather than iron deficiency anemia. Pappenheimer bodies are erythrocyte inclusions composed of hemosiderin and their presence is related to sideroblastic erythropoiesis and hyposplenia. These are not distributed throughout the cell as seen in basophilic stippling and stain positively for Perl's stain.

48. Ans. d. Treatment is similar for idiopathic aplastic anemia

Ref: Alshaibani A. Hepatitis-associated aplastic anemia. Hematol Oncol Stem Cell Ther. 2020.

Hepatitis-associated aplastic anemia (HAAA) is a rare illness, characterized by onset of pancytopenia with a hypoplastic bone marrow that traditionally occurs within 6 months of an increase in serum aminotransferases. HAAA is observed in 1% to 5% of all newly diagnosed cases of acquired aplastic anemia. Several hepatitis viruses have been linked to the disease, but in many cases no specific virus is detected. The exact pathophysiology is unknown; however, immune destruction of hematopoietic stem cells is believed to be the underlying mechanism. HAAA is a potentially lethal disease if left untreated. Management includes immunosuppression with antithymocyte globulin and cyclosporine and allogeneic hematopoietic stem cell transplantation.

49. Ans. b. Acquired aplastic anemia

Ref: Schoettler M. The Pathophysiology of Acquired Aplastic Anemia: Current Concepts Revisited. Hematol Oncol Clin North Am. 2018.

An acquired copy number neutral loss of heterozygosity (LOH) has been identified in approximately 11–13% of patients with acquired AA, usually involving the 6p locus and this finding is the second most common mutation detected in acquired AA. Acquired 6pLOH is characteristic and relatively specific to acquired AA, as it is exceedingly rare in the general population (prevalence ~0.09%). It is also not commonly identified in other bone marrow failure syndromes or MDS.

50. Ans. c. Mutations in telomere genes TERC and TERT are common

About 1/3 of patients with AA have significantly short telomeres in their leukocytes. Shorten telomeres are associated with poor response to immunosuppressive therapy (IST). Telomeres are structures that stabilize the ends of each chromosome to prevent excessive shortening with replication. Majority of patients with aplastic anemia and short telomeres do not have mutations in *TERC* and *TERT* genes which are found in dyskeratosis congenital.

51. Ans. c. Kostmann syndrome

Ref: Dokal I. Inherited bone marrow failure syndromes. Hematologica. 2010.

Heterozygous mutations in the neutrophil elastase gene (ELA2) have been demonstrated in the majority of patients with Kostman syndrome (Severe congenital neutropenia). Diamond Blackfan anemia, and Shwachman–Diamond syndrome are associated with mutation in ribosome biogenesis.

52. Ans. c. Congenital dyserythropoietic anemia

Ref: Hoffman's 6/e p 343-48.

Congenital dyserythropoietic anemia can present much later in life in certain cases. CDAs are classified into the 3 major types (I, II, III), plus the transcription factor-related CDAs, and the CDA variants, on the basis of the distinctive morphological, clinical, and genetic features. Next-generation sequencing has revolutionized the field of diagnosis of and research into CDAs, with reduced time to diagnosis, and ameliorated differential diagnosis in terms of identification of new causative/modifier genes and polygenic conditions.

53. Ans. d. None of the above *Ref: Robbins 9/e p 55.*

Members of this group, including BAD, BIM, BID, Puma, and Noxa, contain only one BH domain, the third of the four BH domains, and hence are sometimes called BH3-only proteins. BH3-only proteins act as sensors of cellular stress and damage, and regulate the balance between the other two groups, thus acting as arbiters of apoptosis.

54. Ans. d. All of the above *Ref: Robbins 9/e p55.*

BCL2, BCL-XL, and MCL1 are the principal members of this group; they possess four BH domains (called BH1-4). These proteins reside in the outer mitochondrial membranes as well as the cytosol and ER membranes. By keeping the mitochondrial outer membrane impermeable they prevent leakage of cytochrome c and other death-inducing proteins into the cytosol.

55. Ans. d. Beta glycoprotein *Ref: Hoffmann 6/e p627.*

In most patients with Hereditary elliptocytosis (HE) and the related disorder, the principal lesion involves defect in horizontal membrane-protein associations, primarily spectrin dimer-dimer interactions. In a subset of HE patients with a deficiency or a dysfunction of protein 4.1R or glycophorin C (GPC), the horizontal defect resides in the junctional complex, where the distal ends of spectrin tetramers connect to actin, in conjunction with protein 4.1R. In patients with severely dysfunctional spectrin mutations, the weakened spectrin dimer-dimer self-association disrupts the skeletal lattice, leading to a marked skeletal instability and cell fragments. In patients with mildly dysfunctional spectrins, RBC shape is that of biconcave elliptocytes.

56. Ans. b. Binds to Ferroportin

Ref: Robbins 9/e p649-50.

Iron absorption is regulated by hepcidin, a small circulating peptide that is synthesized and released from the liver in response to increases in intrahepatic iron levels. Hepcidin inhibits iron transfer from the enterocyte to plasma by binding to ferroportin and causing it to be endocytosed and degraded. As a result, as hepcidin levels rise, iron becomes trapped within duodenal cells in the form of mucosal ferritin and is lost as these cells are sloughed. Thus, when the body is replete with iron, high hepcidin levels inhibit its absorption into the blood. Conversely, with low body stores of iron, hepcidin synthesis falls and this in turn facilitates iron absorption. By inhibiting ferroportin, hepcidin not only reduces iron uptake from enterocytes but also suppresses iron release from macrophages, which are an important source of the iron that is used by erythroid precursors to make hemoglobin. This, as we shall see, is important in the pathogenesis of anemia of chronic diseases.

57. Ans. a. Serum folate" is a reliable indicator of body's folate stores *Ref: Hoffmann 6/e p512-15.*

The use of red-cell folates as a measure of long-term folate status is valid during clinical trials in which a single kit is used for a cohort of patients; however, it is not valuable for routine clinical diagnosis because of the significant variability of performance between different commercial kits and lack of clinical validation. For these reasons, the serum folate level, although labile, is a good initial choice. Of the total-body content of 2 to 5 mg in adults, about 1 mg is in the liver. There is an obligatory loss of 0.1% per day (1.3 µg) regardless of total-body cobalamin content. It takes about 3 to

4 years to deplete cobalamin stores when dietary cobalamin is abruptly malabsorbed, but it may take longer to develop nutritional cobalamin deficiency, because of an efficient enterohepatic circulation, which accounts for turnover of 5 to 10 µg/day of cobalamin. The body's reserves of folate are relatively modest, and a deficiency can arise within weeks to months if intake is inadequate. The combined use of homocysteine and methylmalonic acid (MMA) levels can differentiate cobalamin from folate deficiency, because most patients with folate deficiency have normal MMA levels, and the remainder have only mild elevations. These two tests are useful diagnostically. The abnormally high levels of metabolites return to normal only when the patient receives replacement with the appropriate (deficient) vitamin.

58. Ans. d. G6PD assay immediately after acute hemolysis is a better indicator of it's deficiency.

Ref: Hoffmann 6/e p616-18.

G6PD deficiency is the most prevalent human enzyme deficiency in the world, affecting an estimated 500 million people, although the vast majority of affected individuals are not symptomatic. Females heterozygous for G6PD are particularly difficult to diagnose because of their mosaicism for X chromosome enzymes and may have total RBC enzymatic activity ranging anywhere from hemizygote to normal; however, these females have a variable mixture of deficient and nondeficient RBCs and their deficient RBCs are subject to hemolytic crises. False-negative results are not unusual, however, especially if enzymatic analysis is performed shortly after resolution of acute hemolytic episodes or in heterozygous females. After acute hemolysis, reticulocytes and young RBCs, which have much higher enzymatic activity, predominate. These false-negative test results are more likely to occur when a screening test rather than a quantitative spectrophotometric analysis of the enzyme activity is used.

59. Ans. d. Normal persons have more than 2% pitted RBCs

To confirm suspected hyposplenism the simplest assay is a count of pitted or pocked erythrocytes. Fixation in 0.5% to 1% of glutaraldehyde and examination under interference optics should reveal endocytic vesicles containing hemoglobin, ferritin and remnants of mitochondria. These form in mature erythrocytes and are normally removed by functioning spleen. The number of pitted cells is inversely proportional to splenic function. Normal persons have less than 2% pitted RBCs. The absence of Howell-Jolly bodies on PBF cannot be used as evidence of adequate splenic function.

60. Ans. b. Performing a factor II assay with and without Echis venom. *Ref: Hoffman, 7th ed, p2242.*

Differentiating between Vitamin K deficiency and liver disease can be challenging with conventional lab tests. If available performing a factor II assay with and without Echis venom may be useful. Ecarin is derived from echis carinatus and can activate prothromin irrespective of gamma carboxylation. Factor II activity is reduced in both Vitamin K deficiency and liver disease, but factor II Echius is reduced in liver disease and is normal in Vitamin K deficiency.

61. Ans. c. Kills intracellular bacteria

Th17 cells kill extracellular bacteria and fungi by activating macrophages and neutrophils via IL-17 and IL-23 cytokines which kill extracellular microbes by phagocytosis.

62. Ans. c. HbD

Due to limited sensitivity and because some hemoglobins are electrophoretically similar though structurally different, an alternative procedure must be incorporated into the screening algorithm for differentiation of these hemoglobins. For example, HbS, HbD, HbG and Hb Lepore co-migrate, so they are indistinguishable on alkaline electrophoresis. The same is true for HbC, HbA2, HbO-Arab and HbE. Acid electrophoresis allows confirmation of variant hemoglobins observed in the Cellulose Acetate Electrophoresis procedure and allows good separation of HbC from HbE and HbO-Arab. It permits additional separation of HbS from HbD and HbG. So, several Hb variants, including HbD, HbG and Hb Lepore, have an electrophoretic mobility identical to that of HbS on cellulose acetate but may be distinguished by the negative sickle solubility test and citrate agar gel electrophoresis at acid pH (6.0). Similarly, hemoglobin C, E and O, which co-migrate on cellulose acetate at alkaline pH, can be differentiated by citrate agar electrophoresis. Cellulose acetate electrophoresis at a pH of 8.4 is a standard method of separating Hb S from other variants. However, **Hb S, G, and D** have the same electrophoretic mobility with this method.

63. Ans. e. All of the above
Ref: Joy King. A Practical Approach to Diagnosis of B-Cell Lymphomas With Diffuse Large Cell Morphology. Arch Pathol Lab Med. 2020;144:160–67.

Large lymphoma cells by definition have nuclei at least as large as normal macrophage nuclei or at least twice the size of a normal lymphocyte. Red blood cells are consistently seen even in small needle core lymphoma samples and serve as more reliable standards for lymphoma cell size estimation, because normal red blood cells should have a diameter essentially identical to those of lymphocytes. So, if 2 or more red blood cells can be estimated to fit in a lymphoma nucleus, that should be considered a large lymphoma cell.

64. Ans. d. All of the above
Ref: Joy F. King. A Practical Approach to Diagnosis of B-Cell Lymphomas With Diffuse Large Cell Morphology. Arch Pathol Lab Med. 2020;144:160–67.

B-LBL should be distinguished from BL as both are aggressive malignancies. B-LBL cell has finer chromatin than that in BL. B-LBL cases do not show the clear vacuoles typically seen in BL. BL expresses CD10 and surface immunoglobulin light chains and seldom expresses BCL2, but it does not express CD34 or TdT. Cases of B-LBL usually express CD10, CD34, TdT, or BCL2 but do not express surface light chains.

65. **Ans. d. CD5**

Ref: Vose JM. Mantle cell lymphoma: 2017 update on diagnosis, risk stratification, and clinical management. Am J Hematol. 2017; 92(8):806–13.

Cyclin D1 overexpression represents a sensitive marker for detection of MCL. In order to distinguish MCL from DLBCL, cyclin D1 expression should be assessed by IHC in every B-cell lymphoma case with medium or large cell size regardless of CD5 expression. The rearrangement of CCND1 with IGH, t(11;14)(q13;q32), causes overexpression of cyclin D1 and is present in nearly all MCL cases. Detection by FISH for this IGH/CCND1 translocation shows more than 95% sensitivity for MCL. Cyclin D1 also has been shown to be detected by IHC in 98% of MCL cases. In rare cases of cyclin D1–negative MCL, immunohistochemical staining for SOX11 is useful. SOX11, a SOX family transcription factor with a role in cell fate and differentiation, has been identified as a reliable diagnostic and prognostic marker of MCL in both cyclin D1–positive and cyclin D1–negative disease.

66. **Ans. c. DLBCL cases with CD30 expression have poor overall survival**

Ref: Hu S, et al. CD30 expression defines a novel subgroup of diffuse large B-cell lymphoma with favorable prognosis and distinct gene expression signature: a report from the International DLBCL Rituximab-CHOP Consortium Program Study. Blood. 2013;121(14):2715-24.

Testing for expression of CD30 should be considered in large B-cell lymphomas, especially those with anaplastic morphologic features, because 10% to 20% of DLBCL cases are CD30 positive. Also, most Epstein-Barr virus (EBV)–positive DLBCL cases are CD30 positive. The DLBCL cases with CD30 expression may have better overall survival.

67. **Ans. d. IRF4/MUM1**

Ref: Joy F. King. A Practical Approach to Diagnosis of B-Cell Lymphomas With Diffuse Large Cell Morphology. Arch Pathol Lab Med. 2020;144:160-67.

Positive expression of CD138 along with CD38 and IRF4/MUM1 is seen in plasmablastic lymphoma which often presents as oral cavity or extranodal masses in patients with HIV infection, immunodeficiency, or advanced age. These unusual B-cell lymphomas typically show plasmacytic, plasmablastic, or immunoblastic features and are notably negative or weakly positive for CD45, CD20, and PAX5.

68. **Ans. d. More than 50%**

All large B-cell lymphomas should be tested with in situ hybridization for EBV-encoded small RNA (EBER) for detection of EBV-positive DLBCL, NOS, a rare form of DLBCL mostly affecting patients older than 50 years. To receive a diagnosis of EBV positive DLBCL NOS, more than 50% of the lymphoma cells must be positive for EBV-encoded small RNA.

69. **Ans. a. DLBCL**

Ref: Hans CP, et al. Confirmation of the molecular classification of diffuse large B-cell lymphoma by immunohistochemistry using a tissue microarray. Blood. 2004;103(1):275–82.

The Hans algorithm provides prognostic information that favors either the germinal center or activated B-cell subtype of DLBCL. The Hans algorithm employs IHC for CD10, BCL6, and IRF4/MUM1 to predict either germinal center or activated B-cell phenotype. These markers are each considered positive if 30% or more of lymphoma cells are positive.

70. **Ans. e. None of the above**

Double expresser DLBCL is detected by immunohistochemistry (IHC) staining for BCL2 and MYC. DLBCLs, which are positive for both these markers have been shown to have a relatively poor prognosis, although not as unfavorable as the double hit lymphoma. Most double expresser DLBCL cases are not double hit lymphomas. Cytogenetic FISH testing must be performed to evaluate for the presence of double hit/triple hit lymphoma (high grade B cell lymphoma with MYC and BCL2 and/or BCL6. FISH is both sensitive and specific and is the gold standard in diagnosing double hit/triple hit lymphoma. A cost-effective approach is to analyze all cases for MYC rearrangements, and then do BCL2 and BCL6 FISH testing. A faster strategy is to test for all 3 markers simultaneously. So, double expression is seen by IHC and double hit is assessed by FISH.

71. **Ans. c. Prophylactic anticoagulation**

Ref: ASH Guidelines on Use of Anticoagulation in Patients with COVID-19.

The ASH guideline panel suggests using prophylactic-intensity over intermediate-intensity or therapeutic-intensity anticoagulation in patients with COVID-19 related acute illness who do not have suspected or confirmed VTE.

72. **Ans a. Granules of basophils**

MPO stains primary and secondary granules of cells of neutrophil lineage, eosinophil granules (granules appear solid., granules of monocytes and Auer rods, however granules of normal mature basophils do not stain.

73. **Ans. b. Ratio of all granulocytes and monocytes and their precursors to erythroblasts**

Ref: Lee SH. ICSH guidelines for the standardization of bone marrow specimens and reports. Int. Jnl. Lab. Hem. 2008;30:349–64.

The myeloid:erythroid (M:E. ratio should be calculated by expressing the ratio of all granulocytes and monocytes and their precursors (i.e. myeloblasts, promyelocytes, myelocytes, metamyelocytes, band forms, segmented neutrophils, eosinophils, basophils, promonocytes and monocytes) to erythroblasts (at all stages of differentiation).

74. Ans. b. Aggregates of ferritin

Ref: Leukaemia Diagnosis. Barbara Bain. 5/e, Hoboken, NJ : John Wiley & Sons, Inc., 2017.

Immature cells can be identified as erythroid when they contain aggregates of ferritin molecules or iron-laden mitochondria or when there is rhopheocytosis (invagination of the surface membrane in association with extracellular ferritin molecules).

75. Ans. e. None of the above

Ref: Leukaemia Diagnosis. Barbara Bain. 5/e, Hoboken, NJ : John Wiley & Sons, Inc., 2017.

By definition fewer than 3% of AML M0 blasts are positive for MPO, SBB and naphthol AS-D chloroacetate esterase (chloroacetate esterase, CAE. since a greater degree of positivity would lead to the case being classified as M1 AML. Similarly, blast cells do not show non-specific esterases (NSE) activity, since positivity would lead to the case being classified as M5 AML.

76. Ans. d. All of the above

Auer rods give positive MPO and SBB reactions and occasionally weak PAS reactions. The reaction for CAE is usually weak or negative. Although Auer rods are often detectable on a Romanowsky stain, they are more readily detectable on an MPO or SBB stain and larger numbers are apparent.

77. Ans. d. None of the above

Ref: Brown C and Opat S. An unusual case of indigestion: persistence of phagocytosed Auer rods in acute promyelocytic leukemia. Br J Hematol. 2006;133:112.

Bone marrow macrophages may contain giant granules or Auer rods derived from ingested leukemic cells. Auer rods can persist in macrophages after the patient has entered complete remission.

78. Ans. c. Acute monocytic leukemia (AML-M5)

Ref: Leukemia Diagnosis. Barbara Bain. Fifth edition. Hoboken, NJ : John Wiley & Sons, Inc., 2017.

AML M3 variant (APL M3V) may be confused with acute monocytic leukemia (M5b). if blood and bone marrow cells are not examined carefully and if the diagnosis is not considered. The use of an automated blood cell counter based on cytochemistry (MPO or SBB) is useful for the rapid distinction between M3V and M5 AML. When M3V appears likely from the cytological and cytochemical features, the diagnosis can be confirmed by cytogenetic, molecular genetic or immunophenotypic analysis.

79. Ans. a. PAS

Megakaryoblasts are negative for MPO, SBB and CAE. The more mature cells of this lineage are PAS positive and have partially fluoride-sensitive NSE activity, On PAS staining there are positive granules on a diffusely positive background. A PAS stain can highlight the presence of micromegakaryocytes and megakaryoblasts with cytoplasmic maturation.

80. Ans. d. All of the above are true

Ref: Leukaemia Diagnosis. Barbara Bain. Fifth edition. Hoboken, NJ: John Wiley & Sons, Inc., 2017.

Molecular studies help in the confirmation of AML in patients with a low blast percentage in patients with RUNX1- RUNXT1 or CBFB-MYH11 fusion genes. These studies can also recognize therapy-related AML by demonstration of KMT2A rearrangement following exposure to topoisomerase II-interactive drugs, and can recognize of subtypes of ALL associated with cryptic chromosomal rearrangements by detection of ETV6-RUNX1 associated with cryptic t(12;21)(p13.2;q22.1).

81. Ans. e. All of the above

Patients with variant translocations, such as t(1;21;8), t(8;11;21) and t(8;13;21)can be associated with RUNX1-RUNX1T1 fusion and have the same disease characteristics as t(8;21)(q22;q22.1) rearrangement.

82. Ans. e. All of the above

c-KIT mutations, or at least KIT-D816 mutations, are associated with a higher WBC, more extramedullary disease, a greater risk of relapse and a worse survival. KIT mutations occur in 20-25% of t(8;21) and 30% of inv(16) cases. The NCCN guidelines have included KIT mutations as a prognostic marker that can change CBF-AML from favorable to intermediate risk group.

83. Ans. a. Translocation (15;17) can be detected directly without culture

Ref: Leukaemia Diagnosis. Barbara Bain. 5/e. Hoboken, NJ : John Wiley & Sons, Inc., 2017.

The frequency with which the specific t(15;17)(q24.1;q21.2) translocation is detected is method dependent since direct examination without culture may result in only non-clonal erythroid cells entering mitosis. In addition to the primary abnormality, 30–40% of cases show secondary karyotypic abnormalities. Among these the commonest are trisomy 8, abnormal 7q, and del(9q), 8q+ and +21 PML-RARA fusion is very rare among cases of AML not recognized morphologically as APL. When APL occurs as a therapy-related leukaemia the precise breakpoints in the *PML* gene are clustered and differ from those in de novo disease.

84. Ans. e. All of the above

AML with inv(16) subtype of AML is associated with granulocytic and monocytic differentiation with cytologically abnormal eosinophils, which are often prominent, so that it is often referred to as 'M4Eo' AML. However, a significant proportion of cases of AML with inv(16) lack prominent eosinophilia, monocytic differentiation or both, and are classified as FAB types M1, M2, M2Eo, M4 or M5. A small number of cases of M7 AML associated with inv(16) or t(16;16) have also been recognized.

85. Ans. d. Acute megakaryoblastic leukemia

AML associated with t(1;22)(p13.3;q13.1) represents less than 1% of cases of AML. This translocation is associated with acute megakaryoblastic leukemia occurring predominantly in infants and young children and has intermediate prognosis. There is expression of platelet glycoproteins such as CD41 and CD61.

86. Ans. e. All are true

These mutations are more common in women than in men. An association with blast cells with invaginated nuclei (cup-shaped nuclei) has been observed. expression of NPM1, detectable by immunohistochemistry or flow cytometry, acts as a surrogate marker for an NPM1 mutation, MRD can be monitored by RQ-PCR. MRD detected by RQ-PCR after the second cycle of chemotherapy is associated with an adverse prognosis.

87. Ans. d. MPO positive

Presentation is often with cutaneous lesions (nodules or tumors). Lack of alpha-naphthyl butyrate esterase activity can help in making a distinction from acute monoblastic leukemia. There is almost always expression of CD56 in the absence of B-lineage and most myeloid antigens (myeloperoxidase and lysozyme negative). Expression of CD4, CD56, CD123 and CD45RA with lack of expression of CD45RO and CD116 has been found to be highly specific for this condition. CD43 and plasmacytoid dendritic cell-associated markers, CD68, CD303 (BDCA-2), CD304 (BDCA-4), TCL1A and CLA, as well as CD123, are expressed. Cytogenetic analysis shows complex clonal abnormalities, in two-thirds of patients. Prognosis is poor.

88. Ans. b. Chromosomes 50-66 *Ref: Hoffbrand's essential Haematology, 7th ed.*

The term 'high hyperdiploidy' indicates that leukemic cells have more than 50 (but usually fewer than 66) chromosomes. Cases of ALL with 'low hyperdiploidy' (47-50 chromosomes) have somewhat different characteristics, including a worse prognosis.

89. Ans. d. All of the above

The only cytochemical reactions essential in the diagnosis and classification of MDS are a Perls stain for iron, which is necessary for assessing the presence and number of ring sideroblasts, and a Sudan black B (SBB) or myeloperoxidase (MPO) stain to ensure that all cases with Auer rods are recognized.

90. Ans. e. All of the above
Ref: WHO book 2017, Hoffman 7th ed.

Chronic neutrophilic leukemia (CNL) is characterized by an increased neutrophil count with only small numbers of circulating granulocyte precursors and no dysplastic features. The neutrophil count is markedly increased but the peripheral blood shows few granulocyte precursors. Toxic granulation and Dohle bodies are often present, and ring shaped neutrophil nuclei have also been described. Typical myelodysplastic features such as hypogranular neutrophils, the acquired Pelger–Huet anomaly and micromegakaryocytes are not usually seen. Serum granulocyte colony-stimulating factor (G-CSF) is reduced. The presence of toxic granulation, Dohle bodies or an elevated LAP do not help in making a distinction. It is important to distinguish CNL from the neutrophilic leukemoid reaction that can occur in association with multiple myeloma and other plasma cell neoplasms. Serum protein electrophoresis is indicated in all patients who lack definitive evidence of a myeloid neoplasm.

91. Ans. c. Lymphocytosis

Bone marrow aspiration and trephine biopsy are not necessary for diagnosis of CLL but are recommended in the investigation of cytopenia and before initiation of therapy. In AIHA the bone marrow shows erythroid hyperplasia while in pure red cell aplasia there is a striking reduction in red cell precursors. In autoimmune thrombocytopenia, the bone marrow aspirate shows normal numbers of megakaryocytes. When a patient with CLL develops hemophagocytic lymphohistiocytosis, there is phagocytosis of lymphocytes as well as of myeloid cells.

92. Ans. d. All of the above
Ref: Leukaemia Diagnosis. Barbara Bain. 5/e, Hoboken, NJ : John Wiley & Sons, Inc., 2017.

A worse prognosis in CLL has been linked to expression of both IgM and IgD rather than expression of IgD alone. Aberrant expression of myeloid or T-lymphocyte markers is also associated with a worse prognosis. The most important immunophenotypic indicators of poor prognosis are ZAP70 expression and CD38 expression. Since CD38 and ZAP70 are expressed strongly by T cells and NK cells, it is important that measurements are made on CD5+CD19+ B cells. ZAP70 expression correlates with lack of somatic hypermutation of IGHV and also with CD38 expression.

93. Ans. e. None of the above
Ref: WHO Book 2017, Hoffman 7/e

The cells of CLL express SmIg weakly. The expression of CD19 and CD20 is also weaker in CLL, FMC7, CD22 and CD79b are usually absent or weak. CD200 is more strongly expressed than by normal B lymphocytes or the cells of other lymphoproliferative disorders (except hairy cell leukemia..

94. Ans. d. All of the above
Ref: WHO book 2017, p130.

Most cases of AML with t(8;21) display a characteristic immunophenotype, with a subpopulation of blast cells showing high- intensity expression of CD34, HLADR, MPO, and CD13, but relatively weak expression of CD33. There are signs of neutrophilic differentiation, with subpopulations of cells showing neutrophilic maturation demonstrated by CD15 and/or CD65 expression. Populations of blasts showing maturation asynchrony (e.g. coexpressing CD34 and CD15) are sometimes present.These leukemias frequently express the lymphoid markers CD19 and PAX5, and may express cytoplasmic CD79a.

95. Ans. b. KIT mutations occurs in < 10% of cases
Ref: WHO book 2017, p132.

The genes for both heterodimeric components of core-binding factor (CBF), RUNX1 and CBFB, are involved in rearrangements associated with acute leukemias. The t(8;21)(q22;q22.1) involves RUNX1, which encodes the alpha subunit of CBF. KIT mutations occur in 20-30% of cases. AML with t(8;21)(q22;q 22.1) is usually associated with a high rate of complete remission and long-term disease-free survival when treated with intensive consolidation therapy (e.g. high-dose cytarabine). Some factors appear to adversely affect prognosis, including the presence of KIT mutations in adults and CD56 expression.

96. Ans. b. CBFB- MYH11
Ref: WHO book 2017, p132

Acute myeloid leukaemia (AML) with inv(16)(p13.1 q22) or t(16; 16) (p13.1 ;q22) resulting in CBFB-MYH1 is an AML that usually shows monocytic and granulocytic differentiation and characteristically an abnormal eosinophil component in the bone marrow.

97. Ans. b. NRAS
Ref: WHO 2017, p133.

Secondary gene mutations are very common in this AML type; present in > 90% of cases. Mutations of KIT (most commonly in exons 8 and 17) occur in 30- 40% of cases. Mutations of NRAS (in 45% of cases), KRAS (in 13%), and FLT3 (in 14%) have also been reported. ASXL2 mutations, although common in AML with t(8;21), are uncommon in AML with inv(16) or t(16;16).

98. Ans. b. t(6;9)
Ref: WHO Book 2017, p137.

Marrow and peripheral blood basophilia, defined as 2% basophils, is generally uncommon in AML, but is seen in 44-62% of cases of AML with t(6;9)(p23;q34.1). Most cases Show evidence of granulocytic and erythroid dysplasia. Ring sideroblasts are present in some cases.

99. Ans. b. A 5 month old girl without Down's syndrome
Ref: WHO Book 2017, p139.

The t(1;22)(p13.3;q13.1) is an uncommon abnormality in AML, occurring in < 1% of all cases. It occurs most commonly in infants without trisomy 21 (Down syndrome), with a female predominance. Some cases are congenital.

100. Ans. b. Basophilia
Ref: WHO Book 2017, p138.

Acute myeloid leukemia (AML) with inv(3)(q21.3q26.2) or t(3;3)(q21.3;q26.2) resulting in deregulated MECOM (also called EV/1) and GATA2 expression is an AML with 20% peripheral blood or bone marrow blasts. It is often associated with normal or elevated platelet counts and has increased dysplastic megakaryocytes with unilobed or bilobed nuclei and multilineage dysplasia in the bone marrow.

101. Ans. d. All of the above
Ref: WHO Book 2017, p134.

Cases of microgranular (hypogranular) APL are characterized by distinct morphological features such as an apparent paucity or absence of granules, and predominantly bilobed nuclei. The hypogranular appearance of the cytoplasm is due to the submicroscopic size of the azurophilic granules.

102. Ans. d. CD33
Ref: WHO Book 2017, p134.

APL with PML-RARA (hypergranular variant) is characterized by low or absent expression of HLA-DR, CD34, and the leukocyte integrins CD11a, CD11b, and CD18. It shows homogeneous bright expression of CD33 and heterogeneous express ion of CD13. Most cases show expression of KIT (CD117), although this is sometimes weak.

103. Ans. d. Mostly presents in childhood
Ref: WHO Book 2017, p141.

Acute myeloid leukemia (AML) with mutated NPM1 carries mutations that usually involve exon 12 of NPM1. Aberrant cytoplasmic expression of NPM1 is a surrogate marker of such mutations. This AML type frequently has myelomonocytic or monocytic features and typically presents de nova in adults with a normal karyotype. it occurs in 2-8% of childhood cases and 27% - 35% of adult cases overall, as well as in 45-64% of adult cases with a normal karyotype.

104. Ans. d. All of the above
Ref: WHO Book 2017, p142.

The favourable prognosis associated with CEBPA mutation in AML is now known to be related to biallelic mutations only; therefore, biallelic mutation is now required for assignment to this category. The biallelic mutation is associated with a specific gene expression profile that is not associated with the single mutation. More than 70% of cases of AML with biallelic mutation of CEBPA have a normal karyotype. AM L with biallelic mutation of CEBPA is associated with a favorable prognosis, similar to that of AML with inv (16) (p13.1q22) or t(8;21)(q22;q22.1).

105. Ans. c. Associated with better overall survival

Ref: WHO Book 2017, p142.

Acute myeloid leukemia (AML) with mutated RUNX1 (a provisional entity in the current classification) is a de novo leukemia with 20% bone marrow or peripheral blood blasts that may have morphological features of most AML, NOS, categories and has a higher frequency among cases with minimal differentiation. Most studies find a higher frequency in older adults (aged > 60 years). One study reported a male predominance, but most have not identified a sex predilection. RUNX1 mutations in AML and myelodysplastic syndrome (MDS) are associated with radiation exposure and prior alkylating agent chemotherapy. In some studies, RUNX1 mutations in AML have been associated with worse overall survival in multivariate analysis. A subset of these patients have germline mutations of RUNX1; when RUNX1 mutation is detected, germline studies should be performed or careful family histories obtained. Affected family members may have autosomal dominant thrombocytopenia and dense granule platelet storage pool deficiency, as well as an increased risk of development of AML or MDS.

106. Ans. c. Osteosclerosis is common

Ref: Haroche J. Erdheim-Chester disease. Curr Rheumatol Rep. 2014 Apr;16(4):412.

Erdheim-Chester disease (ECD) is a rare, non-inherited, non-Langerhans form of histiocytosis of unknown origin. It is characterized by xanthomatous or xanthogranulomatous infiltration of tissues by foamy histiocytes, "lipid-laden" macrophages, or histiocytes, surrounded by fibrosis. Differential diagnosis includes Langerhans' cell histiocytosis, Rosai-Dorfman disease, Takayasu arteritis, Wegener's granulomatosis, primary hypophysitis, chronic recurrent multifocal osteomyelitis (see these terms), malignancies, neurosarcoidosis, mycobacterial infections and metabolic disorders. Diagnosis of ECD involves the analysis of histiocytes in tissue biopsies: these are typically foamy and CD68+ CD1a- in ECD, whereas in Langerhans cell histiocytosis (LCH) they are CD68+ CD1a+. The pathognomonic feature of ECD is osteosclerosis of the long bones manifesting as bone pain, mainly affecting the distal lowerlimbs (50% of cases). A «hairy kidney» appearance on abdominal CT scan is observed in approximately half of ECD cases. More than half of ECD patients carry the BRAF(V600E) mutation. Optimum initial therapy for ECD seems to be administration of interferon α and vemurafenib (in BRAF positive patients).

107. Ans. c. Can also be seen in 20-30% cases of splenic marginal zone lymphoma or nodal marginal zone lymphoma

Ref: Schreuder M. Novel developments in the pathogenesis and diagnosis of extranodal marginal zone lymphoma. Journal of Hematopathology. 2017:10:91-107.

BIRC3-MALT1 translocation represents t(11;18)(q21;q21) and is the most common translocation in extranodal marginal zone lymphoma (EMZL). It strongly correlates with H. pylori-independent variants of gastric EMZL. The BIRC3 MALT1 translocation is specific for EMZL and has not been detected in SMZL or NMZL.

108. Ans. b. T-cell prolymphocytic leukemia

Ref: Sun S. Current understandings on T-cell prolymphocytic leukemia and its association with TCL1 proto-oncogene. Biomedicine & Pharmacotherapy, 2020.

Inv14 or t(14;14)/TCL1A gene rearrangement is the hallmark of T-PLL and is found in 80% of T-PLL cases. T-cell leukemia/lymphoma 1 (TCL1) protein is detected by immunohistochemistry in most cases. Abnormal activation of proto-oncogene TCL1A at chromosome 14q32.1 is considered as the major recurrent genomic abnormality, which is associated with inversion [inv(14)(q11;q32)] and translocation [t(14;14)(q11;q32)]. TCL1A acts as a co-factor of protein kinase B/Akt and participates in the Akt signaling transduction pathway, leading to dysregulated cell metabolism, growth, proliferation and apoptosis.

109. Ans. b. Fluorescent in situ hybridization

Ref: Constitutional and somatic rearrangements of chromosome 21 in acute lymphoblastic leukemia. Nature. 2014

Intrachromosomal amplification of chromosome 21 (iAMP21) is a cytogenetic sub-group of B-ALL patients. FISH with probes specific for *RUNX1* gene help in detection of this genetic abnormality. Three or more extra copies of RUNX1 is suggestive of iAMP21. Break fusion bridge cycle is the initiating event followed by chromothripsis. It occurs This abnormality is seen in 2% of pediatric B cell ALL with a median age of around 9 years. It is associated with a poor event free survival.

110. Ans. c. Originates from cutaneous dendritic cells known as Langerhans cells

Ref: Histiocytic disorders: insights into novel biology and implications for therapy of Langerhans cell histiocytosis and Erdheim-Chester disease, ASH education book 2020, p395-99.

Langerhans cell histiocytosis (LCH) is a histiocytic disorder caused by mutations in the MAPK pathway most commonly BRAFV600E initiating in the myeloid dendritic cells of bone marrow. LCH occurs in both children and adults. BRAF mutation occurs in CD 34 + stem cells, CD11c + myeloid dendritic cells, CD 68+ macrophages. Patients with liver, spleen and bone marrow involvement are considered as high risk. Those patients with any other single organ involvement or multiple non -high risk organ system affected.

111. Ans. a. t(8;21)

Ref: WHO Book 2017, p 132.

AML with t(8;21) display a characteristic immunophenotype, with a subpopulation of blasts showing high intensity expression of CD34, HLA-DR, MPO and CD13, but relatively weak expression of CD33. Population of blasts showing maturation asynchrony (e.g. coexpressing CD34 and CD15). These leukemias frequently express the lymphoid markers CD19 and PAX5, and may express cCD79a. CD56 is expressed in a fraction of cases and may have adverse prognostic significance due to higher incidence of KIT mutation.

112. Ans. c. 30-40% *Ref: WHO Book 2017 p135.*

Mutations involving FLT3, including ITD and TKD, occur in 30-40% of APML cases and are associated with higher white cell count, microgranular morphology and involvement of bcr3 breakpoint of PML.

113. Ans. e. All of the above

Ref: WHO Book 2017 p 121, 143.

AML with biallelic mutation of CEBPA is associated with a favorable prognosis and is related to biallelic mutation only. More than 70% of cases have normal karyotype. Patients with biallelic CEBPA mutations should be evaluated for a familial syndrome (myeloid neoplasms with germline predisposition).

114. Ans. d. Acute promyelocytic leukemia

Ref: WHO Book 2017 p 69, 160-164.

Acute promyelocytic leukemia shows "burst positivity" on MPO staining. MPO negative leukemias are Acute erythroid leukemia, Megakaryoblastic leukemia, acute basophilic leukemia, acute mast cell leukemia, acute monoblastic leukemia.

115. Ans. a. ≥5 copies of the gene *Ref: WHO 4/e p308.*

The B-cell Acute lymphoblastic leukemia (ALL) with iAMP21 is characterized by amplification of a portion of chromosome 21, detected by FISH with a probe for RUNX1 that reveals ≥5 copies of the gene or gene (or ≥3 extra copies on a single abnormal chromosome 21)

116. Ans. d. All of the above *Ref: ASH 2020, Abstract 539.*

TET2 and IDH, but not SRSF2, mutations are enriched in patients with myelodysplastic syndrome/chronic myelomonocytic leukemia with systemic inflammatory and autoimmune disease (SIAD), a condition which is found in 20% of MDS and CMML cases. These mutations were associated with T cell imbalance in favor of effector memory T cells.

117. Ans. a. Chronic myeloid leukemia

Ref: WHO 2017 classification. p 31, 38, 52.

In Chronic phase CML, the megakaryocytes are smaller than normal and have hyposegmented nuclei (dwarf megakaryocytes), but are not true micromegakaryocytes such as those seen in MDS. Classical micromegakaryocytes are typically seen in MDS with del(5q). The other conditions, although they may also have dwarf forms, show a range of megakaryocyte abnormalities. In essential thrombocythemia, the megakaryocytes are often loosely clustered together and show stag-horn and cloud-like nuclei. In CNL the megakaryocytes may be cytologically normal or there may be increased smaller forms, but this is not typical micromegakaryocyte. In systemic mastocytosis and PV the megakaryocytes are normal in morphology.

118. Ans. d. All of the above

Ref: Robbins 9/e p36.

Neutrophil extracellular traps (NETs) are extracellular fibrillar networks that provide a high concentration of antimicrobial substances at sites of infection and prevent the spread of the microbes by trapping them in the fibrils. They are produced by neutrophils in response to infectious pathogens (mainly bacteria and fungi) and inflammatory mediators (e.g., chemokines, cytokines [mainly interferons], complement proteins, and ROS). The extracellular traps consist of a viscous meshwork of nuclear chromatin that binds and concentrates granule proteins such as antimicrobial peptides and enzymes. In the process of NET formation, the nuclei of the neutrophils are lost, leading to death of the cells. NETs have also been detected in the blood during sepsis, and it is believed that their formation in the circulation is dependent on platelet activation. The nuclear chromatin in the NETs, which includes histones and associated DNA, has been postulated to be a source of nuclear antigens in systemic autoimmune diseases, particularly lupus, in which individuals react against their own DNA and nucleoproteins.

119. Ans. d. Hearing loss is usually late in these patients

Ref: Oishi K et al. Thiamine-Responsive Megaloblastic Anemia Syndrome. 2003. Adam MP et al. editors. Gene Reviews® [Internet]. Seattle

TRMA (also called Rogers syndrome) is inherited in an autosomal recessive manner. At conception, each sib of an affected individual has a 25% chance of being affected, a 50% chance of being an asymptomatic carrier and a 25% chance of being unaffected. The diagnosis of TRMA is established in a proband with megaloblastic anemia with normal vitamin B12/folic acid levels, with or without diabetes or hearing loss in which there is a response to oral thiamine and/or identification of biallelic pathogenic variants in SLC19A2. The hearing defects usually develop in early age and in some even be present at birth. The hearing loss is sensorineural and irreversible. These patients develop Non-type I diabetes mellitus. The peripheral blood count shows macrocytic anemia and bone marrow shows megaloblastic erythropoiesis often with ringed sideroblasts.

120. Ans. c. Patients who develop MDS/AML usually present with leukocytosis *Ref: WHO 2017 Book, p125.*

Helicases are enzymes required for separation of double stranded nucleic acids in an energy dependent fashion. These enzymes also displace proteins from the nucleic acids. There are two types of helicases, RNA helicase and DNA helicase. RNA helicases are classified into multiple superfamilies. DEAD box RNA helicases belong to super family 2 and they are named DEAD box because members of this group have a conserved motif (Motif 2) with sequence D-E-A-D. Motif in biochemistry means - pattern of nucleotides in a DNA sequence or amino acids in a protein. Myeloid neoplasms with germline DDX41 mutation are recently defined autosomal dominant familial MDS/AML syndrome characterized by inherited mutations in the gene on chromosome 5 encoding the DEAD box RNA helicase-DDX41. In majority of cases the mutation is biallelic, with one mutation being germline. There is long latency (Mean age of 62 years for disease onset) and most patients either present with high grade MDS or AML. Patients usually present with leucopenia, hypocellular marrow with prominent erythroid dysplasia and a normal karyotype. The prognosis is generally poor.

121. Ans. d. HHV-8 DLBCL are mostly positive for EBER

Ref: WHO 2017 Book, p327.

Germinotropic lymphoproliferative disorder is HHV-8 associated lymphoproliferation, presenting as localized lymphadenopathy in asymptomatic immunocompetent individuals. The lymph node architecture is preserved and lymph node shows infiltration of germinal centre's by variable number of atypical Plasmablasts. The atypical cells show co-infection of HHV-8 and EBV. These cells are negative for B-cell markers and germinal center markers. CD138 and CD30 are also negative. Positive markers include CD38 and MUM1 and occasionally partial CD3. The atypical cells are polyclonal. Remember, crucial to diagnosis is plasmablasts like cells in germinal centre's negative for B/T/NK—associated markers, germinal center markers are negative. Dual positivity for EBV and HHV-8. IHC for EBV using LMP1 protein is usually negative and EBER is recommended. These cases have very good prognosis.

Multicentric Castleman disease (MCD) is clinical and pathological entity (Means you need both clinical and pathological findings to make a correct diagnosis). Multicentric in MCD means it's a systemic disease with generalized lymphoproliferation leading to generalized lymphadenopathy, constitutional symptoms and splenomegaly. The disease is characterized by proliferation of benign lymphocytes, plasma cells and vessels due to excessive production cytokines, in particular IL6. HIV positive patients with MCD, MCD are almost always related to HHV-8. In absence of HIV, MCD is associated with HHV8 in 50% cases in endemic areas. The diagnosis requires exclusion of infectious, neoplastic and autoimmune diseases that may have similar clinical presentations due to similar kind of cytokine profile.

Microscopy:

The B-cell follicles show varied degree of involution, hyalinization of germinal centres, prominent mantle zones, and prominent penetrating venules typical of Castleman disease.

The plasmablasts like cells are present in mantle zone cells or interfollicular areas, singly or in small clusters. Sometimes these plasmablasts like cells may undergo clonal transformation and there would be sheets of these cells (Transformation to HHV-8 positive DLBCL). These cells are positive for HHV-8 LANA1 and show strong cIgM expression and lambda light chain restriction. The plasmablastic cells immunophenotype: CD20+/-, CD79a-/+, CD138-, PAX5-, CD38-/+, CD27- and negative for EBER. The interfollicular areas are expanded by sheets of plasma cells. These plasma cells are cIgA positive and express polytypic light chains.

The HHV-8 positive DLBCL arises mostly in association with HHV-8 positive MCD. There is proliferation of HHV-8 positive plasmablastic cells expressing IgM lambda. These cells although appear like plasmablasts but don't show somatic hypermutation – indicating transformation of naïve IgM producing B-cells by HHV-8. The immunophenotype is similar to plasmablastic cells seen in HHV-8 positive MCD.

122. Ans. b. Approximately 1/3rd of patients carry mutation of *STAT5B* gene

Ref: WHO 2017 Book, p348-50.

T-LGLL is an indolent entity characterized by clonal expansion of T-LGLs. An LGL count of $>2 \times 10^9$/L is usually found but not mandatory. A lower number is compatible if the LGLs are clonal and patient displays other clinical or hematological features (Persistent neutropenia is common whereas thrombocytopenia is uncommon finding). Association with Rheumatoid arthritis and immune phenomenon are common in T-LGLL. The LGLs on peripheral blood smear can be identified by characteristic morphology with moderate to abundant cytoplasm containing typical azurophilic granules (Coarse, countable and patchy distribution), and reniform or round nucleus with mature chromatin. It is not possible to differentiate between reactive and clonal T-LGL expansion based just on morphology however clonal LGLs are usually more monotonous in morphology as compared to reactive T-LGL expansion which shows more heterogeneity in morphology with slightly deeper bluish shade of cytoplasm. Granules in the LGLs often exhibit ultrastructural appearance described as parallel tubular arrays. Bone marrow shows expansion of LGLs (>10% LGL). T-LGLL shows a constitutively activated mature post-thymic phenotype. Typically express CD2, CD3, CD8, CD57, TCR-αβ, CD45RA and CD16, in >80% of cases. Abnormally diminished or loss of expression of CD5 or/and CD7 is noted. Remember that loss would be such that there would be separate cluster formation on flowcytometry when compared to normal T-cells. CD56 expression is very infrequent and it indicates aggressive behavior and association with STAT5B mutation. STAT3 mutations (Not STAT5B. are found in almost one third of cases.

123. **Ans. c. Large cells or anaplastic morphology is rarely seen in EATL.** *Ref: WHO 2017 Book, p 372-75.*

EATL may be preceded by refractory coeliac disease (RCD). RCD is defined as persistent GI symptoms, with abnormal small intestinal mucosal architecture with increased intraepithelial lymphocytes (IELs) despite a strict gluten-free diet for ≥6–12 months. The intestinal changes seen are villous atrophy, crypt hyperplasia and increased IELs. Gut IELs are almost exclusively T cells. The significant proportion of these cells expresses TCR-γδ (around 60%). Normally, otherwise in most places TCR-αβ positive cells are more abundant. Also, gut IELs are antigen-experienced (Not naïve T-cells) and express activation associated markers, CD44 and CD69 and these cells don't recirculate. In addition, these T-cells have abundance of cytotoxic granule associated proteins and they characteristically express both activating and inhibitory types of innate natural killer (NK) cell receptors. So, gut IELs is ready to act cells. IELs constitutively express CD103 (also known as the αE integrin), which interacts with E-cadherin on intestinal epithelial cells. Also, especially in small intestine, the cells with TCR-αβ (around 40%) mostly express CD8αα, as compared to CD8αβ, are hallmark of activated T-cells. Some of these cells can co-express CD4 and CD8αβ. In contrast, T-cells in the Lamina propria are dominated by CD4 positive T-cells.

Coeliac disease, or gluten-sensitive enteropathy, predisposes to EATL. HLA-DQ2 homozygosity is considered a risk factor for development of EATL. The frequency of Coeliac disease and EATL is less in Asian countries due to the low frequency of coeliac HLA risk alleles. EATL is seen with greater frequency in areas with high prevalence of coeliac disease. The small intestine is involved in > 90% EATLs, most commonly the jejunum and ileum. The neoplastic cells exhibit a wide range of morphology. Most cases show medium to large pleomorphic cells with round to angulated nuclei, vesicular chromatin, visible nucleoli and abundant pale cytoplasm. Almost 40% cases show large cell or anaplastic cytomorphology. Admixture of inflammatory cells and angioinvasion, destruction and necrosis can also be present. The lymphoma cells are usually CD3+, CD5-, CD7+, CD4-, CD8-, and CD103+, and they express cytotoxic granule—associated proteins. All EATLs with large cell morphology express CD30. Almost 30-52% of patients with refractory coeliac disease develop EATL and the IELs exhibit aberrant immunophenotype in type 2 refractory coeliac disease whereas in type 1 refractory coeliac disease the lymphocytes show normal phenotype.

124. **Ans. b. Skin is most commonly affected organ in solitary form** *Ref: WHO 2017 Book, p472-74*

Normal histiocytes are distributed interstitially throughout the bone marrow, mainly in vicinity of erythroid islands. Histiocytes can be highlighted using CD68 immunostain (Dotted appearance because it stains lysosomes).

Histiocytosis term is usually used in context of neoplasms of Histiocytes, i.e., proliferation of macrophages, dendritic cells and monocyte derived cells. There are two types of histiocytosis, histiocytosis with clear cut malignant features and the other type which have overlapping cellular morphology with reactive increase in histiocytes. Histiocytosis with overlapping morphology with reactive increase in histiocytes is a true challenge for diagnosis. In this context, we need clinical presentation and radiological data to guide us for correct diagnosis. In addition, presence of mutations like BRAFV600E, definitely help in differentiating clonal histiocytosis from reactive histiocytosis. In context of biology of clonal histiocytosis, please remember RAS/RAF/MEK/ERK pathway. LCH is clonal proliferation of Langerhans-type cells that express CD1a, langerin (CD207), and S100 protein and show Birbeck granules by ultrastructural examination. The disease is more common in white population of northern Europe. Primary LCH of lung is almost always disease of smokers. The disease can involve single site, multiple sites in same organ or can involve multiple systems. The dominant site of involvement in solitary form is bone. The lesions are characterized by expansion of LCH cells. LCH cells have folded, indented, grooved nuclei, with fine chromatin, invisible nucleoli, slightly more eosinophilic cytoplasm and more well defined borders (compared to normal cells). Variable number of eosinophils and multi-nucleate giant cells are also noted. Lymph node involvement usually occurs in sinusoidal pattern and Liver involvement has strong preference for intrahepatic biliary involvement.

Indeterminate dendritic cell tumor or indeterminate cell histiocytosis, is proliferation of indeterminate cells (Alleged precursor of Langerhans cells). Mostly involve skin and show diffuse infiltration of dermis by cells resembling Langerhans cells. Eosinophilic infiltrate is usually not seen. So, just based on morphology it's difficult to differentiate between ICH and LCH. ICH cells also express CD1a, S-100 but are negative for langerin. ICH cells are also negative for Birbeck granules and lacks histiocytic marker CD163 and FDCs markers CD21, CD23, and CD35.

BRAF mutations are noted in almost 50% cases and about 25% cases show somatic mutations in MAP2K1. Both BRAF and MAP2K1 mutations are mutually exclusive.

125. **Ans. e. None of the above**

Ref: Rauen et al. Annu Rev Genomics Hum Genet. 2013;14:355-69

The RASopathies are a clinically defined group of medical genetic syndromes caused by germline mutations in genes that encode components or regulators of the Ras/

mitogen-activated protein kinase (MAPK) pathway. These disorders include neurofibromatosis type 1, Noonan syndrome, Noonan syndrome with multiple lentigines, capillary malformation–arteriovenous malformation syndrome, Costello syndrome, cardio-facio-cutaneous syndrome, and Legius syndrome. Because of the common underlying Ras/MAPK pathway dysregulation, the RASopathies exhibit numerous overlapping phenotypic features. *RAS* genes constitute a multigene family that includes *HRAS*, *NRAS*, and *KRAS*. as proteins are small guanosine nucleotide-bound GTPases that function as a critical signaling hub within the cell. Neurofibromatosis type 1 (*NF1*) was the first syndrome identified as being caused by mutation of a gene in the Ras/MAPK pathway (*NF1*). Noonan syndrome (NS) is also a type of RASopathy, caused by mostly activating mutations in *PTPN11*. The Ras/MAPK pathway has been studied extensively in the context of oncogenesis because its somatic dysregulation is one of the primary causes of cancer. Ras is somatically mutated in approximately 20% of malignancies, and BRAF is somatically mutated in approximately 7% of malignancies.

126. Ans. e. Increased proportion of CD10 positive B-cells

Ref: Calvo et al. Blood 2015;125(18):2753-8.

Ras-associated autoimmune leukoproliferative disorder (RALD) is a nonmalignant clinical syndrome initially identified in a subset of putative autoimmune lymphoproliferative syndrome (ALPS) patients. Similar to patients with ALPS, RALD patients present with lymphadenopathy, massive splenomegaly, increased circulating B cells, hypergammaglobulinemia, and autoimmunity. In contrast to ALPS, biomarkers such as CD4−/CD8− double negative T-cell receptor αβ (TCRαβ+) T cells and serum vitamin B_{12} levels are not always increased, and germline or somatic mutations in *FAS*, *FASL*, or *CASP10* are absent in RALD. Persistent absolute or relative monocytosis is a cardinal feature of RALD. Bone marrow and peripheral blood smear findings overlap with those of juvenile myelomonocytic leukemia (JMML) in children or chronic myelomonocytic leukemia (CMML) in older patients. Activating somatic mutations that cause amino acid substitutions that affect codons 12 or 13 in *KRAS* or *NRAS* were identified in myeloid and lymphoid lineages. Although both RALD and JMML share common *RAS* mutations, JMML cells apparently accumulate additional genetic abnormalities that contribute to the malignant phenotype. These include cytogenetic abnormalities and activating somatic mutations in *PTPN11*, c-CBL, ASXL1, and FLT-3. Atypical immunophenotypic changes in peripheral blood monocytes and granulocytes are detected in RALD. Increased CD16 expression on monocytes suggests that the monocytic population comprises increased nonclassical or activated monocytes that have features of tissue macrophages, cells that are also increased in sepsis and inflammation. Polyclonal B-cell lymphocytosis with circulating CD10+ B cells and increased CD14 expression on granulocytes are also common in RALD.

127. Ans b. Cytoplasmic CD3- beta is positive in most of cases

Ref: Tse E, Kwong YL. How I treat NK/T-cell lymphomas. Blood. 2013;121(25):4997-5005

NK-cells kill tumor cells and bacteria/virus infected cells. NK cells express T-lineage–associated antigens, including CD2 and CD7. Different from T cells, they are negative for surface CD3 but express cytoplasmic CD3. NK cells also express "NK-associated" antigens, including CD16, CD56, CD94, KIRs and CD57, with CD56 being the most consistently expressed. Molecularly, the T-cell receptor (*TCR*) genes are in germline configuration.

Majority of ENNTL are of NK-cell origin however a very small fraction is of true T-cell origin and show TCR gene rearrangement hence the name NK/T-cell lymphoma.

NK/T-cell lymphomas are almost exclusively extranodal. Initial sites involved are often the nose and nasopharynx and occasionally the paranasal sinuses, tonsil, Waldeyer ring, and oropharynx. Non-nasal NK/T-cell lymphomas are rare and a strict definition of non nasal NK/T-cell lymphoma requires absence of nasal involvement, shown by random nasopharyngeal biopsies and PET/CT. The involvement of peripheral blood and bone marrow is very rare.

Cytologically, neoplastic cells are small to medium-sized lymphoid cells possessing pale cytoplasm with azurophilic granules. Histopathologically, lymphoma cells may be admixed with a polymorphic population of small lymphocytes, plasma cells, eosinophils, and histiocytes, hence the old terminology "polymorphic reticulosis." Lymphomatous infiltrate may show angiocentricity and angiodestruction, leading to coagulative necrosis. Marrow hemophagocytosis may occur.

Immunophenotypically, lymphoma cells are typically CD2+, cytoplasmic CD3ε+, CD56+, and express perforin, granzyme B, and TIA-1. Neoplastic cells are invariably infected by Epstein-Barr virus (EBV) in a clonal episomal form (Not integrated with host genome), which is detected most reliably by in situ hybridization (ISH) for EBV-encoded RNA (EBER), constituting a diagnostic requisite.

128. Ans. d. Strongly express CD138 and CD20 is usually negative

Ref: Takeuchi K et al. Haematologica. 2011;96(3):464-67.

ALK positive large B-cell lymphoma (ALK+LBCL) is aggressive neoplasm of large monomorphic immunoblast like cells (Amphophilic look on H&E) involving mainly lymph nodes frequently with sinusoidal pattern and usually have plasma cell phenotype rather than B-cell phenotype. It is more frequent in young men and 1/3rd of cases occurs in pediatric age group. Most patients present with generalized lymphadenopathy or advanced stage. Bone marrow involvement is seen in almost 1/4th of cases.

Lymphoma cells are strongly positive for ALK protein with restricted granular cytoplasmic staining pattern highly indicative of CLTC-ALK fusion protein. Lymphoma cells also express EMA, CD138, other plasma cell markers, and negative for B-lineage associated antigens (CD20, CD79a, PAX5) or positive in only small fraction of cells. CD45 is weak or negative and CD30 is negative. Most tumors express cytoplasmic IgA. Like ALK positive ALCL, all cases are negative for EBV and HHV-8. T-cell markers are negative however rare cases can show CD4, CD57. Some cases may show CK positivity which can lead do misdiagnosis of Carcinoma.

Most common genetic abnormality is t(2;17) leading to CLTC-ALK fusion protein. CLTC is gene for Clathrin. Less commonly t(2;5) resulting in NPM-ALK fusion and rarely SQSTM1-ALK fusion protein is noted. The characteristic ALK staining is usually cytoplasmic and coarsely granular (attributed to the presence of the Clathrin-ALK fusion) and in cases with NPM-ALK fusion, ALK staining shows nuclear and cytoplasmic pattern. In cases with SQSTM1-ALK, a diffuse cytoplasmic staining pattern with ill-demarcated spots has been reported.

129. Ans. d. KIR receptor expression is usually normal

Ref: WHO 2017 Book, p 351.

CLPD-NK is characterized by persistent (>6 months) increase (>2 × 10^9/L) in NK-cells without a clearly identifiable cause. A transient increase in NK-cells can be encountered in many situations like autoimmune disorders and viral infections. The TKI dasatinib produces a sustained increase in NK cells that can be monoclonal. One third of cases have activating mutations in STAT3 SH2 domain.

The immunophenotyping shows NK-cell phenotype (Surface CD3 negative, cCD3- epsilon positive, CD16 positive and dim CD56). Cytotoxic markers are positive. There may be diminished or lost expression of CD2, CD7 and CD57, AND abnormal uniform expression of CD8 (A fraction of normal NK-cells show heterogenous CD8 expression). KIR family of receptors is usually abnormal. CD94/NKG2A expression is usually uniformly bright.

130. Ans. c. EBV is absent in a clonal episomal form

Ref: WHO 2017 Book, p 353-55.

Aggressive NK-cell leukemia is a systemic neoplastic proliferation of NK-cells frequently associated with EBV and an aggressive clinical course. This entity is more prevalent in Asians. The most commonly involve blood, bone marrow, liver and spleen. Patients present with leukemic blood picture with cytopenias. LDH levels are markedly elevated and Hepatosplenomegaly is common. The disease can be complicated by HLH, coagulopathy or multi-organ failure. Atypical cells show variable morphology and NK-cell related immunophenotype. Neoplastic cells express FASL. As it is NK-cell neoplasm, TCR-genes are in germline configuration. EBV can be detected in 85%-100% cases and EBV present in clonal episomal form.

131. Ans. d. Cutaneous mastocytosis is mostly seen in children above the age of 6 months

Ref: WHO 2017 Book, p65-66.

Diagnosis of Cutaneous mastocytosis (CM) requires two findings:
1. Classical clinical findings.
2. Histological proof of abnormal mast cell proliferation in dermis.

Plus, there is no systemic involvement (Bone marrow or any other organ), but patients might have elevated tryptase levels or abnormal morphology of mast cells in bone marrow. There are three major variants of CM: Urticaria pigmentosa (UP)/Maculopapular CM, Diffuse CM, Mastocytoma of skin. Among these, UP is most common variant of CM. The skin lesions in UP tends to be large and a few in most of cases. Indolent systemic mastocytosis also involve skin and lesions tends to be small and numerous. CM is mostly disease of young children and 50% children develop typical lesions before the age of 6 months. In adults, pure CM is rare and bone marrow must be done in adults to rule out systemic mastocytosis. Various KIT mutations, including D816V have been detected in childhood CM.

132. Ans. e. All of the above

Ref: Escribano L et al. Leuk Lymphoma. 1998;30(5-6):459-66.

CD117 can be found in CD34+ hematopoietic stem and progenitor cells, myeloid precursors, small fraction of erythroid precursors, CD56 bright natural killer cells, and neoplastic cells from patients with monoclonal gammopathies, acute leukemias, and myelodysplastic syndromes, among other hematologic malignancies. CD117 is also expressed by a small but important fraction of CD3–/CD4–/CD8– prothymocytes, so a small fraction of T-ALL can show CD117 expression. Rarely CD117 expression has been reported in atypical basophils.

133. Ans. b. MCL should have more than 10% mast cells in peripheral blood *Ref: WHO 2017 classification. p69-70.*

Mast cell leukemia is characterized by ≥ 20% mast cells. Mast cells in MCL are usually immature and atypical, and often with round nuclei. In most cases with MCL, no skin lesions are detected. The % mast cells in classical MCL cases ≥10% but percentages below 10% doesn't exclude diagnosis of MCL (aleukemic variants). KIT mutations in MCL may be atypical (non-D816V codon 816 mutation) or non-codon 816 mutations. So KIT gene sequencing is preferred method to detect atypical KIT mutations, which are more common in MCL.

134. Ans. b. Fetal extraction corrects TTP symptoms

Ref: Blood. 2017;129(21):2836-46.

TTP is characterized by acquired or congenital severe deficiency of ADAMTS13 enzyme. Overall, in ~2% cases the deficiency is congenital, inherited as recessive biallelic mutations, so called congenital TTP or Upshaw-Schulman syndrome (USS). Pregnancy-associated TTP mostly occurs during the second half of pregnancy. In the case of USS, TTP occurs as soon as the first pregnancy. In the acquired form of TTP, the first episode may occur during any pregnancy. In contrast to other obstetrical TMA (preeclampsia or hemolysis elevated liver enzymes low platelet count syndrome), the fetus extraction does not correct TTP symptoms; as a consequence, provided there are no fetal abnormalities, the pregnancy should not be interrupted, and the patient should be treated using the usual recommendations. Among adulthood-onset TTP, obstetric TTP is characterized by a very high frequency of USS (~33%), with this rate reaching almost 50% when considering only first pregnancies.

135. Ans. d. Granulocyte transfusions are not associated with TA-GVHD   *Ref: Vox Sanguinis 2008;95:85-93.*

Transfusion-associated graft-versus-host disease (TA-GVHD) is a rare complication of transfusion of blood components containing lymphocytes. Clinically, TA-GVHD presents like bone marrow transplant (BMT) or stem cell transplant-associated GVHD but, additionally, with findings due to marked bone marrow aplasia. Graft-versus-host is caused by donor T lymphocytes mounting a response to recipient tissues. In TA-GVHD, donor T lymphocytes are derived from blood components containing viable lymphocytes. Typically, in immunocompetent hosts, viable T lymphocytes are destroyed by the recipient's immune system. In susceptible patients, whether immunocompetent or with congenital or acquired cellular immune deficiency, transfused T cells are not destroyed; they proliferate and can induce an immune response 'rejecting' the host tissues. GVHD following stem cell transplants (e.g., bone marrow or peripheral blood progenitor cells) primarily affects the skin, the gastrointestinal tract and the liver. As the bone marrow and immune system cells are of donor origin in bone marrow or stem cell transplant-related GVHD, the bone marrow is not affected. However, with TA-GVHD, the bone marrow is of recipient origin, so in TA-GVHD, the marrow is uniformly affected and is the source of greatest morbidity and mortality. TA-GVHD is a more fulminant and lethal condition. Signs and symptoms of TA-GVHD usually begin 2–30 days after transfusion. TA-GVHD follows 0·1–1·0% of transfusions in susceptible recipients. As bone marrow failure is almost uniform in patients with TA-GVHD, the mortality rate of TA-GVHD is 87–100%. Any non-frozen blood component containing viable lymphocytes can potentially cause TA-GVHD, even fresh plasma. Frozen components, although shown to contain some viable lymphocytes after thawing, have not been definitively proven to have caused TA-GVHD. No documented cases of TA-GVHD have been attributed to fresh-frozen plasma (FFP). Granulocyte transfusions (which contain many lymphocytes) given fresh to immunocompromised patients have an increased propensity for causing TA-GVHD. Any blood component from relatives is considered to be at higher risk for causing TA-GVHD due to shared HLAs between donor and recipient. The patients most vulnerable to TA-GVHD are those with congenital or acquired cellular immunodeficiencies that leave the patient unable to recognize and destroy foreign cells. Patients with identified congenital cellular immunodeficiency defects, such as severe combined immunodeficiency disorder and DiGeorge syndrome, should always be given irradiated blood components when transfusion is needed. It is generally accepted that premature infants are in an immunocompromised state and should receive irradiated blood components, even up to 7 months of age. Similarly, intrauterine transfusions also require irradiated components. It has been suggested that all newborns, who have not had an opportunity to demonstrate immune competence, should receive irradiated components.

136. Ans. e. All of the above   *Ref: Hoffman 7/e*

t(12;21) resulting into ETV6-RUNX1 is detectable by molecular techniques in approximately 25% of childhood B-lineage ALL which makes it as the most common translocation in pediatric ALL. In contrast to MLL rearranged ALL, ETV6-RUNX1 leukemias present after infancy with concordance rate of only 10% in identical twins. This fusion can be found in 1% of cord blood samples of normal newborns, a frequency 100 times higher than the prevalence of this subtype of leukemia suggesting ETV6-RUNX1 initiates leukemogenesis and further genetic alterations are required for overt disease. ETV6 deletion on chromosome 12p is the most frequent additional genetic abnormality described in cases of B-ALL with ETV6-RUNX1. Absence of exposure to common infections in the first year of life is associated with higher risk of developing ETV6-RUNX1 positive and hyperdiploid ALL (>50 chromosomes) in older children. ETV6-RUNX1 fusion and hyperdiploidy both are favorable genetic features in B-ALL. Myeloid antigens CD15, CD33 are aberrantly expressed in cases with ETV6-RUNX1.

137. Ans. b. RUNX1   *Ref: Hoffman 7/e*

RUNX1 formerly known as AML1 is the most common transcription factor gene mutated in MDS. Germline point mutations in RUNX1 were seen in autosomal dominant familial platelet disorder with predisposition for AML and somatic mutations in sporadic AML and MDS. RUNX1 mutations confer poor prognosis in MDS patients irrespective of other prognostic factors. RUNX1 mutations confer poor prognosis. TP53 mutations seen in 10% cases of MDS while ETV6 and GATA2 mutations are rare.

138. Ans. a. RNA splicing factor genes

Ref: Hoffman 7/e

RNA splicing factor genes are the most commonly mutated class of genes in MDS. These are rare in other cancers than MDS and are associated with specific morphological phenotypes. SF3B1 is the most frequently mutated splicing factor gene seen in 20-30% cases and is associated with ring sideroblasts morphology. There is lower risk of progression to AML. SRSF2 is the second most commonly mutated splicing factor gene and patients with SRSF2 mutation tends to have more dysplasia in granulocytic lineage than in erythroid lineage. . It is seen in 10-15% of MDS cases and 40% of cases of CMML and is associated with poor prognosis in MDS. U2AF1 mutation occurs in 12% of cases of MDS with tendency to evolve into secondary AML. Epigenetic modifier mutations in MDS are the next most commonly mutated genes and includes TET2, DNMT3A, ASXL1,EZH2. Mutations in transcription factor, tyrosine kinase factors and cohesion factor genes are rare in MDS.

139. Ans. c. Leukopenia

Ref: Greenberg PL, et al. Revised international prognostic scoring system for myelodysplastic syndromes. Blood. 2012;120(12):2454-65.

Revised International Prognostic Scoring System (IPSS-R) includes five parameters- cytogenetics, BM blast percentage, hemoglobin, platelet counts and absolute neutrophil count (ANC).

140. Ans. d. Micromegakaryocyte

Ref: Hoffman 7/e

Promyelocytes in APL, promonocytes in acute monoblastic leukemia and abnormal pronormoblasts in acute erythroleukemia, pure erythroid type are considered as blast equivalents. Pronormoblasts and micromegakaryocytes are not blast equivalents.

141. Ans. c. 3%

Ref: Hoffman 7/e

Cytochemistry highlights the morphologic characteristics in AML. Myeloperoxidase (MPO) is the Most specific granulocytic marker and MPO positivity in at least 3% of the blasts is consistent with diagnosis of AML. However, lack of MPO staining does not rule out AML. MPO staining is absent in AML with minimal differentiation, acute monoblastic leukemia and acute megakaryocytic leukemia. Monoblastic leukemias are stained by nonspecific estarases.

142. Ans. b. Acute erythroblastic leukemia

Ref: Bain BJ. Morphological and Immunophenotypic Clues to the WHO Categories of Acute Myeloid Leukaemia. Acta Haematol. 2019;141:232-44.

Pure erythroid leukaemia can often be suspected morphologically since the primitive erythroblasts have round nuclei, very basophilic cytoplasm, and frequently vacuoles, which represent glycogen and thus can be elongated rather than round. Confirmation is by demonstration of the expression of CD235a (glycophorin A) and often also CD36 and strong CD71. Investigating for CD105 expression can also be useful in some cases, allowing for the fact that this marker is only transiently present during normal erythroid maturation. On immunohistochemistry, E-cadherin is useful since it is expressed earlier than CD235a.

143. Ans. c. Acute megakaryoblastic leukemia

Ref: Gruber TA. The biology of pediatric acute megakaryoblastic leukemia. Blood. 2015;126(8): 943-49.

Acute megakaryoblastic leukemia (AMKL) can sometimes but not always be suspected from cytological features (moderately basophilic, agranular cytoplasm with cytoplasmic blebs), with confirmation being by demonstration of expression of CD41, CD42, and/or CD61. However, the diagnosis of AML, not otherwise specified cannot be made until t(1; 22) has been excluded. Bone marrow biopsy frequently demonstrates extensive myelofibrosis, often making aspiration in these patients difficult. AMKL is extremely rare in adults, occurring in only 1% of AML patients. This is in contrast to children, where it comprises between 4% and 15% of AML patients. AMKL in children with Down syndrome (DS) is characterized by a founding *GATA1* mutation that cooperates with trisomy 21, followed by the acquisition of additional somatic mutations.

AMKL is the most frequent type of AML in children with DS, and the incidence in these patients is 500-fold higher than in the general population. Patients with trisomy 21 have, in essence, an extra copy of many genes on chromosome 21, and overexpression of one or more has been hypothesized to provide the cellular setting that is permissible for persistence and eventual transformation of *GATA1* mutant cells.

144. Ans. a. CD10, CD19, CD20, cCD79a, CD79b, CD22, CD38, FMC7, sIgM, and HLA-DR

Burkitt lymphoma (BL) is an aggressive non-Hodgkin B-cell lymphoma. The morphology is typical of FAB ALL-L3. Bone marrow aspirate smears show predominantly atypical cells having high N:C ratio, clumped chromatin, prominent nucleoli and scant basophilic cytoplasm, some of which show nuclear and cytoplasmic vacuolation, consistent with lymphoproliferative disorder favoring acute lymphoblastic leukemia (FAB ALL-L3). Immunohistochemistry and cytogenetics play a significant role in the diagnosis and management of Burkitt lymphoma. The malignant B-cells express surface IgM. The cells are positive for B-cell markers including CD19, CD20, CD79a, and PAX5. They are positive for germinal center markers CD10 and bcl-6. The neoplastic cells do not express T-cell markers and do not express immature markers TdT or CD34. Rapid cell turnover is reflected by high Ki67 positivity nearing 100%, which is a very helpful diagnostic clue. In sporadic (non-African) Burkitt lymphoma, abdominal disease predominates, often arising in the region of the ileocecal valve or the mesentery.

145. **Ans. a. R-CHOP**

Ref: Jacobson C. How I treat Burkitt lymphoma in adults. Blood. 2014.

Treatment must be initiated rapidly because these tumors grow rapidly. Standard chemotherapy regimens, such as cyclophosphamide, doxorubicin, vincristine, and prednisone (CHOP) are inadequate in treating Burkitt lymphoma both in children and adults. Current recommendations are offered by the National Comprehensive Cancer Network and include multiagent regimens with CNS prophylaxis. An intensive alternating regimen of cyclophosphamide, vincristine, doxorubicin, methotrexate, ifosfamide, etoposide, and cytarabine (CODOX-M/IVAC). plus rituximab results in a cure rate of > 80% for children and adults. For patients > 60 years, regimens such as rituximab plus etoposide, prednisone, vincristine, and doxorubicin (dose-adjusted R-EPOCH) are also commonly used with success. R-hyper-CVAD is also effective and is used in adults. For patients without CNS metastases, CNS prophylaxis is essential. Upfront transplant is not indicated.

SECTION 7
Transfusion Medicine

41. Blood Banking and Transfusion

Chapter 41: Blood Banking and Transfusion

1. **What is stored at 20–24°C?**
   a. Packed red blood cells (PRBCs)
   b. Platelets
   c. Fresh frozen plasma (FFP)
   d. Cryoprecipitate

2. **Transfusion-associated graft versus host disease (TA-GVHD) differs from GVHD by the presence of:**
   a. Skin rash
   b. Diarrhea
   c. Jaundice
   d. Pancytopenia

3. **Which of the following is not true about post-transfusion purpura?**
   a. Usually develops 1 week after transfusion
   b. Most patients have anti-human platelet antigen (HPA)-1a antibodies
   c. Treatment of choice is intravenous immunoglobulin (IVIg)
   d. Severe thrombocytopenia is rare

4. **Use of filter can prevent all of the following, except:**
   a. Cytomegalovirus (CMV) infection
   b. Hepatitis C virus (HCV) transmission
   c. Febrile nonhemolytic transfusion reaction
   d. Reduce the risk of alloimmunization

5. **Cryoprecipitate contains all of the following, except:**
   a. von Willebrand factor (VWF)
   b. Factor VIII
   c. Fibrinogen
   d. Factor IX

6. **All of the following should be irradiated, except:**
   a. FFP
   b. Granulocytes
   c. Red blood cells (RBCs)
   d. Platelets

7. **Which statement is not true about direct Coombs test (DCT)?**
   a. It detects agglutination of antibody-coated RBCs
   b. It may detect complements attached to RBC surface
   c. It is used for cross-matching
   d. It is positive in hemolytic disease of newborn because of Rh incompatibility

8. **Which is not a mandatory test in screening of blood donation?**
   a. Hepatitis C antibody
   b. Hepatitis B
   c. Malaria
   d. Venereal disease research laboratory
   e. Typhoid

9. **Which of the following situations will lead to intravascular hemolysis?**
   a. Group O RBC to group A recipient
   b. Group O RBC to group AB recipient
   c. Rh+ve RBC to Rh-ve recipient
   d. Group A RBC to group O recipient

10. **The Duffy blood group system is functionally associated with:**
    a. Invasion by *Plasmodium falciparum*
    b. Red blood cell urea transporter
    c. Maintenance of membrane integrity
    d. Invasion by *Plasmodium vivax*

11. **Antibody screening showed that all panel cells gave positive reaction and subsequent extended panels used to identify the antibody gave positive reactions with all cells. The possible cause(s) of this is(are):**
    a. Presence of autoantibody
    b. Alloantibody against a high-frequency antigen
    c. Presence of multiple alloantibodies
    d. All of the above

12. **A patient with acute promyelocytic leukemia who is on chemotherapy with disseminated intravascular coagulation with hemoglobin (Hb) of 7.0 g/dL requires blood transfusion. An RBC unit is removed from storage and should be transfused:**
    a. Within 30 minutes of removal from cold storage
    b. Within 2 hours or when the unit has come to room temperature
    c. After warming to 37°C
    d. Within 1 hour of removal from cold storage

13. **The one unit of PRBC must be completely transfused within:**
    a. 30 minutes
    b. 4 hours
    c. 6 hours
    d. 8 hours

14. **TRALI (transfusion-related acute lung injury) can be caused by the transfusion of:**
    a. RBCs
    b. Plasma
    c. Platelets
    d. All of the above

15. An 8-year-old female patient presented with marked anemia, Hb 6.1 g/dL, and dark urine following recent transfusion. She has undergone an allogeneic peripheral blood stem cell transplant 6 months prior for acute myeloid leukemia and has received RBC and platelet transfusions post-transplant. The transplant was a major ABO mismatch with the donor A and recipient O. The direct antiglobulin test (DAT) was weekly positive and eluate was positive against A1 cells at 37°C by the indirect antiglobulin test (IAT). Microspherocytes were present in the blood film. There were no mixed field reactions in the patient's blood group. What is the most likely cause of her dark urine?
    a. Hemolysis due to anti-A in donor RBCs
    b. Hemolysis due to anti-A in donor platelets
    c. Hemolysis due to autoimmune hemolytic anemia (AIHA)
    d. Hemolysis due to associated GVHD

16. Coomb's cross-match should be done in all of the following, except:
    a. Recipient having Rh–ve negative blood group
    b. Neonatal transfusion
    c. Postallogeneic transplant recipient
    d. Autoimmune hemolytic anemia

17. A young teenager with diagnosis of sickle cell disease (SCD) admitted with acute chest syndrome and his Hb fell from 8 to 5.5 g/dL for which he was given 3 units of PRBCs urgently. His Hb improved to 9.0 g/dL, but after 1 week he was found to have blackish urine, pain in back, and jaundice. His lactate dehydrogenase (LDH) was 1,000 U/L. Reticulocyte was 1% with DCT being negative, and no atypical antibody was found. All of the following can be done, except:
    a. IVIg
    b. Erythropoietin (EPO)
    c. Corticosteroids
    d. All of the above
    e. Transfusion of compatible blood

18. The result of a pregnant lady with RhD typing done using an anti-D reagent potentiating agent polyethylene glycol (PEG) showed that the patient was strong but had weak control. The next course of action will be:
    a. Report as D-positive
    b. Report as D-negative
    c. Perform a DCT and repeat D-typing using a different technique
    d. Perform a DCT and if it is positive report as D-negative

19. Administration of 500 IU of anti-D is sufficient prophylaxis for future hemolytic disease of the newborn which will cover a bleed of:
    a. 2 mL
    b. 4 mL
    c. 6 mL
    d. 8 mL

20. Irradiation of blood will:
    a. Decrease potassium leakage from RBCs
    b. Not be required for transfusions from close relatives
    c. Not be required for leukodepleted RBCs
    d. Reduce the shelf life of RBCs

21. An elderly gentleman is a known case of chronic lymphocytic leukemia (CLL; Binet stage A) for which he has never received any treatment. He was brought to casualty with Hb of 5.0 g/dL. Cross-matching was difficult because of DCT and indirect Coombs test (ICT) being positive against all panel cells. RBC morphology was normal with normal bilirubin and LDH. What is the most appropriate transfusion product?
    a. Irradiated PRBC
    b. ABO/Rh/matched "least incompatible" PRBCs
    c. Washed PRBCs
    d. Human leukocyte antigen (HLA)-matched RBCs

22. After centrifuging, human bone marrow is arranged in these layers from top to bottom:
    a. Plasma, platelet, white blood cells (WBCs), and RBCs
    b. Platelets, WBCs, RBCs, and plasma
    c. RBCs, WBCs, plasma, and platelet
    d. Plasma, RBCs, platelet, and WBCs

23. Buffy coat contains:
    a. Fat and WBCs
    b. WBCs and plasma
    c. WBCs and platelets
    d. WBCs and RBCs

24. A young man met with an accident and is brought to the ER with shock. The blood group of the patient is not known. This patient needs immediate blood transfusion, so which will be the most appropriate blood group to be given?
    a. O positive
    b. AB positive
    c. O negative
    d. AB negative

25. A 50-year-old man was given three units of blood transfusion and around 5 hours later he developed acute shortness of breath, fever, and dry cough. On evaluation he was having a blood pressure of 100/60 mm Hg, temperature of 101°F, and SpO$_2$ of 92%. The most likely diagnosis in this case is:
    a. Hemolytic transfusion reaction
    b. Delayed hemolytic transfusion reaction
    c. Febrile nonhemolytic transfusion reaction
    d. IgA deficiency
    e. Transfusion-associated lung injury

26. Packed RBCs are prepared by:
    a. Filtration
    b. Centrifugation
    c. Precipitation
    d. Sedimentation

27. Truth regarding leukodepletion of blood components is:
    a. Reduction in frequency of febrile nonhemolytic transfusion reactions (FNHTRs)
    b. Prevention of alloimmunization to human leukocyte antigens

c. Prevention of platelet refractoriness due to alloimmunization
   d. Reduction in the risk of cytomegalovirus transmission
   e. All of the above

28. Truth regarding red blood transfusion is:
   a. Transfusion should start within 1 hour of removal of blood unit from the refrigerator
   b. Transfusion of RBCs should be completed within 2 hours
   c. If transfusion is getting delayed, then it should be stored in a ward refrigerator
   d. If a unit of RBCs is out of a blood bank refrigerator for more than 1 hour, then it should be stored in the blood bank refrigerator for future use
   e. None of the above

29. Truth regarding platelet transfusion is:
   a. Transfusion should begin as soon as the platelets are received from the blood bank
   b. Stored at 20–24°C
   c. Kept on agitator
   d. All of the above

30. Truth regarding fresh frozen plasma is:
   a. If not used after thaw, it has to be discarded
   b. After thaw, it can be stored at 2–6°C for 24 hours
   c. It can be refrozen if not used
   d. All of the above

31. Indications for the use of blood warmers:
   a. Large volumes transfused rapidly
   b. Neonatal exchange transfusions
   c. Patient rewarming phase during cardiopulmonary bypass surgical procedures
   d. Transfusions for patients with clinically significant cold reactive antibodies
   e. All of the above

32. Transfusion of platelets is contraindicated in:
   a. Thrombotic thrombocytopenic purpura (TTP)
   b. Hemolytic uremic syndrome (HUS)
   c. Heparin-induced thrombocytopenia (HIT)
   d. Post-transfusion purpura (PTP)
   e. All of the above

33. Plasma should be frozen within:
   a. 8 hours   b. 12 hours
   c. 18 hours   d. 24 hours

34. Cryoprecipitate is indicated for:
   a. Fibrinogen deficiency   b. Factor XIII deficiency
   c. Hemophilia A   d. von Willebrand disease

35. False about leukodepletion is:
   a. Prestorage leukodepletion is preferable to poststorage
   b. A final white blood cell count should be $<5 \times 10^6$
   c. Reduces febrile hemolytic reactions
   d. Reduces platelet refractoriness
   e. All of the above

36. The following statements are true, *except*:
   a. Anti-A and anti-B antibodies are mainly of the IgM immunoglobulin class
   b. Antibodies against the Rh antigens are of the IgG type
   c. Blood group antibodies in plasma are demonstrated by the indirect antiglobulin test (IAT)
   d. Nearly all clinically significant RBC antibodies can be detected by an indirect antiglobulin antibody screen carried out at 37°C
   e. All are true

37. Which of the following is an Rh antigen?
   a. C   b. c
   c. D   d. E
   e. All of the above

38. Truth about transfusion-related acute lung injury (TRALI) is:
   a. Caused by antibodies to RBC antigens
   b. Present between 7 and 14 days of transfusion
   c. Diuretics are used for treatment
   d. Rarely associated with plasma or platelet transfusions
   e. None of the above

39. Truth about post-transfusion purpura is:
   a. Due to coagulopathy after massive blood transfusion
   b. Anti-PF4 antibodies are most commonly implicated
   c. Platelet transfusions improve the condition
   d. All of the above

40. Vasovagal reaction associated with blood donation is the result of the following attribute:
   a. Peripheral baroreceptor activity
   b. Orthostatic changes
   c. Anxiety and psychological stress
   d. Increased vagal tone
   e. All of the above

41. The following is the disadvantage of "Off-Line" method over the "In-Line" method for photophoresis:
   a. More economical
   b. Applicability for pediatric patients
   c. Better efficiency of buffy coat collection
   d. Separate equipment used for a single procedure

42. The following blood group system is not intrinsic to red cell surface protein:
   a. ABO
   b. Rh
   c. MNS
   d. Duffy

43. Which of the following is not true for "A2" blood group?
   a. This is the most common subgroup of blood group "A"
   b. Reagent called "lectin," prepared from *Dolichos biflorus,* is used to confirm "A2" blood group

c. Any "A2" individual will require "A2" RBCs for transfusion if there is the presence of anti-A1 antibody
d. RBCs prepared from "A2" blood donors should not be issued to "A1" patients

44. What is not true about the Bombay blood group?
a. It is a very rare genotype "hh" (phenotype O_h)
b. The RBCs of these individuals do not possess H antigen; hence, no "A" or "B" antigen can be made
c. The serum of these individuals contains anti-H with or without anti-A and anti-B
d. "Bombay phenotype" patients can safely be transfused "O" Rh "D" negative PRBCs

45. Maternal samples are mandatory for providing PRBCs for neonatal transfusions because:
a. It is difficult to collect enough sample from a newborn for compatibility testing
b. Mother and newborn blood groups are usually similar
c. Neonates do not produce any naturally occurring antibody at birth and may possess IgG type of antibodies from the mother, which might interfere with the compatibility testing
d. Neonates should always be transfused maternal blood group

46. Which is of the following is not true about whole blood transfusion?
a. Presently, the indication for whole blood transfusions is only in acute blood loss and neonatal exchange transfusions
b. Whole blood transfusion practices waste the other blood components (platelets and plasma) which can be given to other patients
c. Whole blood units can be safely transfused across ABO blood groups
d. The incidence of transfusion reactions such as FNHTRs and transfusion-associated circulatory overload (TACO) are more with whole blood transfusions

47. How many ABO phenotypes and genotypes exist?
a. 6,4   b. 4,6
c. 6,6   d. 4,4

48. All of the following are a potential cause of a false-positive direct Coombs test, *except*:
a. Use of EDTA anticoagulated blood
b. Use of refrigerated clotted whole blood
c. Bacterial contamination
d. Dirty glassware
e. Overcentrifugation of erythrocytes

49. The most frequent cause of ABO hemolytic disease of the newborn is:
a. Mother group O, baby group A
b. Mother group O, baby group B
c. Mother group A, baby group O
d. Mother group A, baby group B
e. Mother group B, baby group A

50. The acceptable interval between homologous whole blood (single unit) donation for males is:
a. 4 weeks   b. 6 weeks
c. 8 weeks   d. 10 weeks
e. 12 weeks

51. Which of the following is a characteristic of anti-I?
a. Often associated with hemolytic disease of the newborn
b. Frequently a cold agglutinin
c. Reacts best at 37°C   d. Is usually IgG

52. Red blood cell priming of the extracorporeal apheresis circuit is indicated in pediatric patients with the following conditions, *except*:
a. Weight less than 25 kg for hematopoietic progenitor cell collection
b. Weight less than 15 kg in plasma exchange
c. It is mandatory to rinse-back all the RBCs in the circuit at the end of such procedures
d. Priming is done using compatible donor RBCs

53. Screening for alloantibody and phenotyping of the patient are essential before initiating which monoclonal antibody?
a. Daratumumab (anti-CD38)
b. Rituximab (anti-CD20)
c. Infliximab (inhibits TNF-alpha)
d. Daclizumab (inhibits IL-2)

54. Truth about the development of anti-A and anti-B antibodies after birth is:
a. Develop in response to the development of corresponding B or A antigens on RBCs
b. Are inherited from the mother
c. Develop in response to exposure to blood products
d. Produced in response to antigens of bacteria, viruses, and other substances that are inhaled or ingested

55. Truth about red cell antibodies is:
a. Most naturally occurring antibodies are cold reacting
b. Cold antibodies that fail to react above 30°C are of no clinical significance and can be ignored for blood transfusion purposes
c. Any red cell antibody reacting above 30°C should be considered potentially capable of destroying RBCs in vivo
d. All of the above

56. Not true about cryoprecipitate is:
a. Prepared from blood while separating the fresh plasma
b. Contains equal amounts of factors VIII and IX
c. Is a poor source of fibrinogen
d. Contains 30 IU of factor VIII
e. All of the above

ANSWERS WITH EXPLANATIONS

1. Ans. b. Platelets *Ref: William's 8/e p2296, 2303*

Both whole blood-derived random platelets and apheresis platelet concentrates can be stored for 5 days at 20-24°C. The storage container should be made of plastic material that allows adequate diffusion of oxygen to meet the cells' metabolic needs, and the platelet concentrates must be agitated during storage. RBCs are preserved by either liquid storage at 4°C or frozen storage with various cryoprotective agents at –80°C. FFP and cryoprecipitates are stored at –80°C.

2. Ans. d. Pancytopenia *Ref: William's 8/e p2296*

A rare complication of transfusion is TA-GVHD, which develops after the engraftment of allogeneic lymphocytes that attack the recipient's tissue. It begins within 3–30 days after transfusion. It occurs because transfusions from close relatives or other genetically matched donors are administered to severely immune-compromised recipients (may occur in immune-competent hosts also). It presents as maculopapular rash, fever, watery diarrhea, liver dysfunction, and marrow failure. There is approximately 90% mortality rate.

3. Ans. d. Severe thrombocytopenia is rare
Ref: Hoffman's 5/e p2095-96

Post-transfusion purpura is an uncommon (1/7,000 transfusions), acquired thrombocytopenia that develops approximately 1 week after blood transfusion.

It typically affects multiparous, middle-aged, or elderly females who present with acute onset of bleeding due to severe thrombocytopenia.

The mean days of onset of symptoms after transfusion is 6–8 days (range 1–14 days).

It usually occurs after a blood product containing platelet material is transfused.

Subclinical cases have been reported, but the incidence of an asymptomatic, milder form is unknown:
- Sera from >90% of patients contain antibodies to HPA-1a
- Suspected if the patient's plasma lyses platelets from random normal donors
- Other causes such as drug-induced thrombocytopenia and heparin-induced thrombocytopenia to be ruled out
- Bleeding symptoms usually last for a mean of 10 days and fatality rates approach 10%
- Treatment of choice is IVIg with >90% response rates.

4. Ans. b. Hepatitis C virus (HCV) transmission
Ref: Hoffman 5/e p2213

There are three methods of leukoreduction:
1. Prestorage filtration (preferred method)
2. Prerelease (from blood bank) filtration
3. Bedside filtration.

Leukodepleted RBCs will lower the risk of febrile nonhemolytic transfusion reaction, lower the risk of cell-associated viral infection (e.g., CMV), and reduce the risk of alloimmunization.

5. Ans. d. Factor IX *Ref: Hoffman 5/e p2233*

Cryoprecipitate contains factor VIII, fibrinogen, fibronectin, VWF, and factor XIII, but not factor IX.

6. Ans. a. FFP
Ref: Treleaven J, Gennery A, Marsh J, Norfolk D, Page L, Parker A, et al. Guidelines on the use of irradiated blood components prepared by the British Committee for Standards in Haematology blood transfusion task force. Br J Hematol. 2010;152(1):35-51.

Components to be irradiated	Components not to be irradiated
• All red blood cells	• Stem cells (absolutely not)
• Platelets	• FFP
• Granulocytes	• Cryoprecipitate
	• Fractioned plasma

7. Ans. c. It is used for cross-matching
Ref: Dacie and Lewis 10/e p241, 247-248, 501-502, 537-8

Direct Coombs test or DAT is the test used for detecting antibody-coated RBCs. A patient's RBCs are taken and mixed with Coomb's polyspecific (anti-IgG, anti-IgM, anti-C3c, and anti-C3d) sera. ICT or IAT is the test for detecting soluble (auto or allo) in the plasma. Here, the patient's plasma is mixed with Coomb's sera (polyspecific or monospecific) with washed normal RBCs.

Majority of anti-RBC antibodies are noncomplement-binding IgG, so anti-IgG is a major component of polyspecific sera.

Anti-IgA is not required because IgG of the same specificity always coexists.

Anti-IgM is also not required because these can easily be identified with complement which can cause significant agglutination.

Ethylenediaminetetraacetic acid prevents complement activation, so if plasma is used only anti-IgG is necessary.

Laboratories using other than normal ionic strength saline, such as low ionic strength saline, PEG, or polybrene, may use only anti-IgG.

But anti-C3 is certainly required for DAT for diagnosis of AIHA.

Monospecific reagents are prepared against the heavy chain of IgG, IgM, IgA, C5, and C3.

For cross-matching, IAT is used to detect the low-frequency antigens in the screening for antibody. The advantages are:
- Acts as double check that the donation is negative for corresponding antigen(s)
- Ensures serological compatibility
- Allows detection of antibodies to low-frequency antigens not present in the screening cells.

IAT cross-match is recommended for:
- Patient who has had ABO-incompatible solid organ or bone marrow transplant
- Patient who has alloantibody of low clinical significance
- Patient whose DAT/DCT is positive.

8. Ans. e. Typhoid

The transmissible infections for which universal screening of all donations in all countries is recommended are:
- HIV
- HBsAg
- HCV
- Syphilis.

The transmissible infections for which universal screening is recommended in some countries are (based on endemicity of disease):
- Malaria
- Chagas disease
- HTLV (human T-lymphotropic virus)-I/II
- CMV.

9. Ans. d. Group A RBC to group O recipient
Ref: William's 8/e p2267

10. Ans. d. Invasion by *Plasmodium vivax*
Ref: William's 8/e p619-622, 2249

Duffy antigen is a receptor for *P. vivax*.

The receptor for *P. falciparum* on RBCs is glycophorins.

Red blood cell urea transporter is the Kidd antigen. Its absence can be associated with impaired urea transport and urine-concentrating defect.

Integral membrane proteins are band 3, glycophorins, Rh, Kell, Kidd, Duffy, and Lutheran glycoproteins. Duffy is not the major protein involved in the overall integrity of RBC membrane.

The peripheral membrane proteins are spectrin, ankyrin, actin, protein 4.1, 4.2, and 4.9, p55, and the adducins.

11. Ans. d. All of the above
Ref: Dacie and Lewis 10/e p532-40

Antibody screening is used for suspected presence of alloantibodies in recipient's sera. It is done by mixing the recipient's sera with RBCs of known low-frequency antigens. Antibody screening should always be carried out by IAT as the primary method.

In UK, the following antigens should be expressed as minimum: Cc, D, E, K, k, Fya, Fyb, Jka, Jkb, S, s, M, N, and Lea.

In AIHA, the antibody screen will show positive reaction with all the panels (pan-reactive).

If the alloantibody is directed against a high-frequency antigen or multiple low-frequency antigens, then also it will be positive with all panels. That is why it is recommended to do DCT and extended O group panel use (minimum 11-cell panel). In case of autoantibody, DCT will be positive.

12. Ans. a. Within 30 minutes of removal from cold storage

The universal rule is to start transfusion within 30 minutes from the release from cold storage. It should not be put back in cold storage if it is out for >30 minutes. Within 4 hours, the transfusion should be over. However, it can safely be given within 2 hours in adults without any comorbidities.

For pediatric patients, the rate is 5 mL/kg/h (max. 150 mL/h).

The volume required is calculated by the formula:

Vol (mL) = Desired Hb rise (g/dL) × weight (kg) × 3.

13. Ans. b. 4 hours *Ref: BCSH guidelines p47-49*

14. Ans. d. All of the above *Ref: William's 8/e p2294-5*

Transfusion-related acute lung injury is acute hypoxia due to noncardiogenic pulmonary edema that follows transfusion. All blood components have been implicated in TRALI, but most frequent products associated are those containing plasma (50-63% of TRALI fatalities).

The clinical features are sudden dyspnea, severe hypoxemia, hypotension, and fever that develop within 6 hours after transfusion and usually resolve with supportive care within 48-96 hours.

15. Ans. a. Hemolysis due to anti-A in donor RBCs
Ref: Blood 2008;112:3036-47

The differential diagnosis of hemolysis after hematopoietic stem cell (HSC) transplant is:

In this case, first we have to find the blood group of the patient. Since he is not showing any mixed field reaction, his blood group should be:
- Forward typing → group A
- Reverse typing → anti-B/only anti-A production.

This means that his blood group has changed to group A and he may or may not have stopped anti-A antibody production. Eluate from agglutinated RBC shows anti-A1 antibody which means that it is the A group RBCs which are getting hemolyzed. Donor RBCs are usually packed and contain very less plasma so it is the anti-A antibodies present in donor platelets that are destroying the recipient's group A RBCs. Moreover, it is assumed that he must be getting O group RBCs, so there is no point of donor RBCs getting hemolyzed.

16. Ans. d. Autoimmune hemolytic anemia
Ref: Dacie and Lewis 10/e p538; William's 8/e p2254

Nowadays, it is no longer needed to do full indirect antiglobulin test (IAT) cross-match if antibody screening has been done; thus a simple, less time-consuming immediate spin cross-match can be done. Doing IAT cross-match is still recommended in cases of neonates, postallogeneic bone marrow transplant, or solid organ transplant. Because RhD sometimes can have weak expression and can sometimes lead to in vivo hemolysis, it is always recommended to do IAT cross-match for all negative units.

17. Ans. d. All of the above
Ref. Transfusion Journal 48;1231-8

This patient has hyperhemolysis syndrome which is a rare complication of blood transfusion in patients with SCD, myelofibrosis, thalassemia, and anemia of chronic disorder. Presenting features include fever, joint pain, severe anemia after transfusion (posttransfusion Hb less than pretransfusion), hemoglobinuria, hyperbilirubinemia, high LDH, and marked reticulocytopenia. It can be acute and delayed.

Acute	Delayed
Occurs <7 days	Occurs >7 days
DAT is usually negative	DAT is usually positive
No RBC alloantibodies are identified	New alloantibodies are often identified

The possible mechanisms are:
- Bystander hemolysis
- Suppression of erythropoiesis
- RBC destruction due to contact lysis via activated macrophages
- Other antibodies may react with transfused foreign antigens (e.g., HLA and plasma proteins) which may cause complement activation.

Macrophages are usually activated in sickle cell disease patients. HbS RBCs adhere to macrophages via integrin $\alpha 4\beta 1$ to VCAM-1 on macrophages. HLA antibody formation is also common among SCD patients. RBC may get hemolyzed through bystander hemolysis:
- Transfused RBC → ICAM-4 → CD11c/CD18
- Sickle reticulocyte → ICAM-4 → CD11c/CD18
- Sickle reticulocyte $\alpha 4\beta 1$ → VCAM-1.

The various treatment options are steroids, IVIg, and EPO. Repeat transfusion should be avoided and is only indicated if there is severe anemia and should always be given along with IVIg and steroids. The dose of Inj. Methylprednisolone is 0.5–1 g (adult) and 4 mg/kg (pediatric) for 2–3 days. The dose of IVIg is 0.4 g/kg/day × 5 days.

18. Ans. c. Perform a DCT and repeat D-typing using different technique
Ref: Dacie and Lewis 10/e p532; William's 8/e p2254

Some individuals can have weak expression of D antigen (partial D) that can only be detected by the antiglobulin test (AT). That is why D-negative individuals should always be confirmed by repeat testing with different anti-D before assigning as D-positive. The AT can be potentiated by agents such as PEG-AT and albumin (Alb-AT). PEG-AT is generally regarded as superior to Alb-AT for the detection of clinically significant RBC antibodies.

19. Ans. b. 4 mL
Ref: Dacie and Lewis 10/e p544

125 IU anti-D immunoglobulin is sufficient for a fetomaternal hemorrhage of 1 mL cells.

20. Ans. d. Reduce the shelf life of RBCs

Irradiation increases membrane permeability, and thus the K^+ is lost and Na^- is gained inside the RBC.

Definitely required if transfusion is from closed relatives, although it is highly recommended not to use blood of close relatives.

Even leukodepleted RBC needs to be irradiated to prevent TA-GVHD and acute GVHD postallogeneic HSC transplantation.

The shelf life of RBC definitely decreases, and it is recommended to transfuse irradiated RBCs immediately and should not be restored.

Platelets can be stored after irradiation, and it does not decrease the shelf life of platelets.

21. Ans. b. ABO/Rh matched "least incompatible" PRBCs
Ref: Hoffman 5/e p1346

Autoimmune hemolytic anemia occurs in up to 37% of CLL patients at some point during the course of their illness. The DAT is positive in 74% of CLL patients, but not all patients develop hemolysis. Most of the antibodies produced are warm reactive, but patients can occasionally present with cold agglutination syndrome. The antibodies which are mostly polyclonal are produced by normal B cells rather than the leukemia clone.

This patient presented with anemia which seems not due to AIHA because there is no evidence of hemolysis. But he is having positive DCT and ICT, and the RBCs are coated with antibodies. Moreover, cross-matching was also difficult in this patient. Giving least incompatible blood is therefore advisable.

22. Ans. b. Platelets, WBCs, RBCs, and plasma
Ref: Hoffman's 6/e p1720

Blood components are prepared by the principle of density gradient centrifugation. After centrifugation at high spin (3,000 rpm), the blood is arranged in this order from top to bottom: plasma, platelet, buffy coat, and RBCs.

23. Ans. b. WBCs and plasma

Ref: Dacie and Lewis 10/e p68-9

Buffy coat is prepared by centrifuging the EDTA blood sample at 1,200–1,500 g. In healthy individuals, buffy coat contains WBCs and plasma; however, in a diseased state it can contain parasites, megakaryocytes, lupus erythematosus cells in SLE, and immature cells as well.

24. Ans. c. O-negative   *Ref: William's 7/e p2165*

If the urgency of the patient's need justifies the administration of uncross-matched blood, type O, Rh-negative blood with low plasma anti-A and anti-B titers can be used. Unfortunately, tests for donor anti-A and anti-B titers are not routinely done.

25. Ans. e. Transfusion-associated lung injury

Ref: William's 7/e p2166-8

The various transfusion-related complications and their clinical manifestations are:

- *Acute hemolytic transfusion reaction*: The signs and symptoms are fever, low backache, sensation of chest compression, hypotension, and nausea and vomiting and in severe cases hemoglobinuria and acute kidney injury, sometimes requiring dialysis. This is most likely caused by blood group incompatibility leading to both intravascular and extravascular hemolysis.
- *Febrile nonhemolytic transfusion reactions*: It is due to the sensitivity of leukocytes or platelets, bacterial pyrogens, and unidentifiable causes. Most of the times, it can be prevented by use of leukodepleted products, and if it happens paracetamol or antihistaminics are enough.
- *Transfusion-associated lung injury*: Incompatibility to leukocyte antigens may also produce pulmonary edema of noncardiac origin, with acute respiratory distress, chills, fever, and tachycardia, usually occurring within 4 hours of transfusion. Once considered to be a rare complication, it is now seen with increased frequency. Chest X-ray shows bilateral diffuse, patchy infiltrates without cardiac enlargement. Therapy is supportive only and the symptoms usually subside in less than 24 hours, with pulmonary infiltrates clearing in 4 days.
- *Allergic reactions*: Transfusion of blood products in some patients may result in generalized pruritus and urticarial. Occasionally, there may be bronchospasm, angioneurotic edema, or anaphylaxis. It usually responds to antihistaminics.
- *Anti-IgA in IgA-deficient recipients*: Severe anaphylactoid reactions can occur in IgA-deficient patients who have formed anti-IgA. The reaction is usually not associated with fever, but may produce dyspnea, nausea, chills, abdominal cramps, emesis, diarrhea, and profound hypotension. Diagnosis requires laboratory demonstration of IgA deficiency and the presence of circulating anti-IgA. If it is known, then the patient should be given IgA-deficient blood products.
- *Bacterial contamination*: Blood may be contaminated by cold growing organisms (Pseudomonas or colon-aerogenes group). These microorganisms can utilize citrate as the primary source of carbon, and contamination of blood by these organisms may deplete its citrate content and can lead to clotting. The infusion of large numbers of gram-negative microorganisms results in a serious reaction, entoxic shock, characterized by fever, marked hypotension, abdominal pain, vomiting, and diarrhea, and then further profound shock. The reaction may start with shaking chills following a latent period of 30 minutes or more. It is managed like septic shock with broad-spectrum antibiotics and other supportive care.
- *Circulatory overload*: Hypervolemia produced by administration of excess blood in patients with a compromised cardiovascular system may provoke the development of congestive heart failure and pulmonary edema, and it is usually managed with fluid restriction and diuretic therapy.
- *Delayed hemolytic reaction*: In the delayed hemolytic reaction, development of previously undetected alloantibodies occurs approximately 4–14 days after transfusion of apparently compatible blood. The principal clinical signs are onset of jaundice and absence of expected increment in RBC mass. These reactions are associated with positive DAT.

26. Ans. b. Centrifugation

Ref: AABB technical manual, 19/e, 2017

The PRBCs are prepared from whole blood by centrifuging at low spin at 1,200 rpm and then platelet-rich plasma (PRP) is expressed into the satellite bag. The additive is added in the RBC primary bag and preserved. The PRP bag is then centrifuged at high spin at 3,000 rpm to separate plasma in the satellite bag and the remaining bag with platelets is preserved.

27. Ans. e. All of the above

Leukodepletion is a process of removing white cells from blood components. This is achieved by means of differential centrifugation. Leukodepleted blood components should contain <5 × 10^6 white cells per unit. There is good evidence to support the value of leukodepletion in preventing transfusion-associated transmission of some infectious agents and in reducing the adverse immunomodulatory effects of allogeneic transfusion, mentioned above. It also reduces the risk of other leukocyte-associated blood-borne infections, such as transmission of human T-lymphotropic virus types I and II, and inadvertent bacterial contamination of blood components.

28. Ans. e. None of the above

Ref: Carson JL. Clinical Practice Guidelines from the AABB. JAMA. 2016;316:2025-35.

Transfusion should begin as soon as possible following removal of the unit from a monitored blood refrigerator. Transfusion of RBCs should be completed within 3–4 hours of removal from a monitored blood refrigerator. They must not be stored in a ward refrigerator, domestic refrigerator, or refrigerator intended for vaccine storage. If a unit of RBCs has been out of controlled storage for more than 30 minutes and there is no prospect of imminent transfusion, it should be returned to the blood bank for disposal. The unit cannot be accepted back into blood bank stock.

29. Ans. d. All of the above

Ref: Carson JL. Clinical Practice Guidelines from the AABB. JAMA. 2016;316:2025-35.

Transfusion should begin as soon as the platelets are received from the blood bank. Platelets are stored (usually in the blood bank) at room temperature 20–24°C with constant agitation. Platelets must not be transported or stored in a refrigerator or chilled transport container.

30. Ans. b. After thaw, it can be stored at 2–6°C for 24 hours

Ref: Carson JL. Clinical Practice Guidelines from the AABB. JAMA. 2016;316:2025-35.

If the plasma is not going to be used or transfusion cannot be started within 30 minutes, it must be returned to the blood bank immediately. If returned within 30 minutes of being issued, then it can be stored for up to 24 hours at 2–6°C during which time it may be reissued to the same or a different patient. If not used within 24 hours, the returned plasma expires. Once thawed, the plasma must not be refrozen.

31. Ans. e. All of the above

Clinical indications for the use of blood warmers are when large volumes of blood are transfused rapidly, e.g. >50 mL/kg/h in adults and >15 mL/kg/h in children, in neonatal exchange transfusions, in polytrauma situations in which core-rewarming measures are indicated, in patient rewarming phase during cardiopulmonary bypass surgical procedures, and in transfusions for patients with clinically significant cold reactive antibodies ("cold agglutinins"), i.e., symptomatic cold hemagglutinin disease. Blood warmers are not indicated for routine transfusion of blood. Blood warming is seldom necessary or desirable for elective transfusion at conventional rates, even for patients with asymptomatic cold agglutinins.

32. Ans. e. All of the above

Severe adverse reactions have been reported in patients with TTP and HIT following platelet transfusion. Platelet transfusion to these patients may also precipitate thrombotic events and can aggravate their clinical condition.

33. Ans. a. 8 hours

Fresh frozen plasma is collected using an apheresis procedure and rapidly frozen within 8 hours of collection to maintain labile coagulation factors.

34. Ans. a. Fibrinogen deficiency

Cryoprecipitate is indicated for bleeding associated with fibrinogen deficiencies. Routine use of cryoprecipitate as an alternative treatment for congenital fibrinogen deficiency, dysfibrinogenemia, factor XIII deficiency, hemophilia A, or von Willebrand disease is not recommended and should be considered only when the specific factor concentrate is not available.

35. Ans. c. Reduces febrile hemolytic reactions

Ref: Carson JL. Clinical Practice Guidelines from the AABB. JAMA. 2016;316:2025-35.

Leukodepletion can be done in-process during apheresis collection or by filtration of the blood product either in the blood bank (prestorage) or at the patient's bedside (poststorage). Prestorage leukocyte reduction is preferable to poststorage as it facilitates appropriate quality control and removes leukocytes prior to the release of cytokines, cellular debris, and intracellular microorganisms. Leukodepletion may also reduce erythrocyte storage-induced damage and transfusion reactions and decrease the risk of infections. Blood products that are customarily leukodepleted include RBCs, apheresis platelets, and whole blood-derived platelets. The average whole blood unit contains $\geq 1 \times 10^9$ leukocytes at collection. To meet quality standards, a leukodepleted component, whether a unit of RBCs, apheresis platelets, or prestorage-pooled whole blood-derived platelets, must have a final white blood cell count of $<5 \times 10^6$. It reduces the incidence of recurrent FNHTRs and HLA-mediated platelet refractoriness.

36. Ans. e. All are true

The ABO blood group system was the first to be discovered because anti-A and anti-B are mainly of the IgM immunoglobulin class and cause visible agglutination of group A or B RBCs in laboratory mixing tests. Many other blood group antibodies, such as those against the Rh antigens, are smaller IgG molecules and do not directly cause agglutination of RBCs. Blood group antibodies in plasma are demonstrated by the IAT. Nearly all clinically significant red cell antibodies can be detected by an IAT antibody screen carried out at 37°C. Anti-A and/or anti-B in the recipient's plasma binds to the transfused cells and activates the complement pathway, leading to destruction of the transfused RBCs (intravascular hemolysis) and the release of inflammatory cytokines that can cause shock, renal failure, and disseminated intravascular coagulation (DIC).

37. Ans. e. All of the above

There are five main Rh antigens on RBCs for which individuals can be positive or negative: C/c, D, and E/e. RhD is the most important in clinical practice. Antibodies to RhD (anti-D) are only present in RhD-negative individuals who have been transfused with RhD-positive RBCs or in RhD-negative women who have been pregnant with an RhD-positive baby.

38. Ans. e. None of the above

Ref: Carson JL. Clinical Practice Guidelines from the AABB. JAMA. 2016;316:2025-35.

Classical TRALI is caused by antibodies in the donor blood reacting with the patient's neutrophils, monocytes, or pulmonary endothelium. Inflammatory cells are sequestered in the lungs, causing leakage of plasma into the alveolar spaces (noncardiogenic pulmonary edema). Most cases present within 2 hours of transfusion (maximum 6 hours) with severe breathlessness and cough productive of frothy pink sputum. It is often associated with hypotension (due to loss of plasma volume), fever and rigors, and transient peripheral blood neutropenia or monocytopenia. It is usually associated with plasma or platelets transfusion. Chest X-ray shows bilateral nodular shadowing in the lung fields with a normal heart size. TRALI is often confused with acute heart failure due to circulatory overload, and treatment with powerful diuretics may increase mortality. Treatment is supportive, with high-concentration oxygen therapy and ventilatory support if required. Steroid therapy is not effective.

39. Ans. d. All of the above

Affected individuals develop a very low platelet count and bleeding 5-12 days after transfusion of RBCs. The typical patient is a parous female who is negative for a common platelet antigen, most commonly HPA-1a, and may have been initially sensitized by carrying an HPA-1a-positive fetus in pregnancy. Post-transfusion purpura is caused by restimulation of platelet-specific alloantibodies in the patient that also damage their own (antigen-negative) platelets by an "innocent bystander" reaction. This severe, and potentially fatal, complication has become rare since the introduction of leukodepleted blood components. Platelet transfusions are usually ineffective (but may be given in high doses in patients with life-threatening bleeding), but most patients show a prompt and sustained response to high-dose intravenous immunoglobulin (IVIg).

40. Ans. e. All of the above

The vasovagal attack appears to be a hypothalamic response mediated by either a central neural pathway or a peripheral pathway associated with the baroreceptors. Vasovagal reactions are typically biphasic, originating with a stress-induced elevation in pulse and blood pressure, and rapidly followed by the commonly recognized signs and symptoms of fainting. These effects result primarily from the action of the autonomic system, causing slowing of the heart, vomiting and sweating, and, perhaps most important, dilatation of the arterioles, leading to a sudden fall in blood pressure. The slow pulse rate (30-60 per minute) in the vasovagal attack is the most useful single sign in differential diagnosis.

41. Ans. d. Separate equipment used for a single procedure

Ref: Perotti C. A concise review on extracorporeal photochemotherapy: where we began and where we are now and where we are going! Transfus Apher Sci. 2015;4:11.

The "Off-Line" method may offer some advantages over the "In-Line" method, such as applicability to pediatric patients, as equipment for the "In-Line" method has a higher extracorporeal volume, hence limiting its applications. In "Off-Line" methods, new apheresis devices used offer higher collection efficiency of lymphocytes resulting in greater cellular harvest, which can be extracted in less time and with low concentration of anticoagulant exposure. Use of multiple equipment for "Off-Line" extracorporeal photopheresis exposes the patients to potential risks for infections induced from handling the product and processing.

42. Ans. a. ABO

The ABO blood group system along with H, LE, P, GLOBO, I, and FORS are carbohydrate structures which are synthesized by sequential addition of sugar residue to a common precursor substance. Others such as Rh, MNS, Duffy, Kid, and Lutheran blood group systems are transmembrane proteins in origin.

43. Ans. d. RBCs prepared from "A2" blood donors should not be issued to "A1" patients

The "A2" blood group is one of the most common subgroups of the "A" blood group system. The "A2" blood group is confirmed when the RBCs are tested with a reagent called lectin (prepared from *Dolichos biflorus*) which shows no agglutination if the individual is "A2" and confirms the blood group. Some "A2" patients also possess anti-A1 antibodies (IgG and/or IgM type); in that case, the "A2" patient should be transfused with either "A2" or group "O" RBCs. Components prepared from "A2" donors such as RBC may be used for both "A1" and "A2" patients.

44. Ans. d. "Bombay phenotype" patients can safely be transfused "O" Rh "D" negative PRBCs

The "Bombay phenotype" patients can only be transfused "Bombay phenotype" PRBCs due to the presence of naturally occurring anti-H antibody which may react with all blood group individuals except O_h blood group donors. The Bombay phenotype was first discovered in Bombay, India, in 1952. In this blood group, no "A" or "B" antigens are identified on RBCs or in secretions. By definition, this would fit the

"O" blood type. It is presumed that the H antigen is a precursor carbohydrate from which A and B blood groups are formed. All blood cells, except for Bombay, express the H antigen. There is no ill effect with being H deficient, but if a blood transfusion is ever needed, people with this blood type can receive blood only from other donors who are also H deficient (A transfusion of "normal" group O blood can trigger a severe transfusion reaction).

45. **Ans. c. Neonates do not produce any naturally occurring antibody at birth and may possess IgG type of antibodies from the mother, which might interfere with the compatibility testing**

The ABO blood group antigens are not completely developed in neonates as well as the corresponding anti-A and/or anti-B antibody also starts appearing after 4 months of age. At birth, the neonates only possess the IgG fraction of maternal antibodies, which cross the placenta. Hence, for any compatibility of PRBC for these neonates, the blood banks need the maternal samples for compatibility testing or cross-matching.

46. **Ans. c. Whole blood units can be safely transfused across ABO blood groups**

In present clinical practice, the indication of whole blood transfusions is only in acute blood loss and neonatal exchange transfusions. The whole blood is routinely separated into blood components such as PRBCs, platelets, and plasma that can be issued to three different patients, hence optimizing the blood component utilization. The across-ABO blood group barrier transfusion is limited to blood component therapy and not to whole blood transfusions as whole blood transfusions consist of both ABO antigen and ABO corresponding antibodies which might cause a transfusion reaction. The incidence of transfusion reactions such as FNHTRs and TACO are more common with whole blood transfusions as whole blood is not leukoreduced and the volume of transfusions is more as compared to component transfusions.

47. **Ans. b. 4,6**

The inheritance of ABO genes follows the simple laws of Mendelian genetics and the ABO genes are codominant in expression. One position, or locus, on each chromosome 9 is occupied by A, B, or O gene. The O gene is considered an amorphic as no detectable antigen is produced in response to the inheritance of this gene. Hence, there are four phenotypes O, A, B, and AB, which can result in six genotypes AO, AA, BO, BB, OO, and AB.

48. **Ans. a. Use of EDTA anticoagulated blood**
Ref: Zantek ND. The direct antiglobulin test: a critical step in the evaluation of hemolysis. Am J Hematol. 2012;87:707-9.

The direct Coombs test is done on a sample collected in EDTA anticoagulated samples. False-positive results tend to arise when (1) specimens degrade sufficiently to cause nonspecific binding of the DCT reagents, (2) overcentrifugation causes the RBC to be packed too tightly, (3) there is underagitation at the time of result interpretation, (4) there is a prolonged delay in testing, (5) there is a clotted specimen, and (6) there are patient factors such as spontaneous agglutination.

Causes of false-negative DCT include (1) improper cell washing, (2) delay in adding antiglobulin reagent after the washing step, (3) inactive, or forgotten, antiglobulin reagent, and (4) improper specimen agitation at the time of result interpretation.

49. **Ans. a. Mother group O, baby group A**

ABO hemolytic disease of newborn is reported most commonly when the mother is O and the baby is A due to the fact that O mothers have more fraction of anti-A antibody of IgG in nature which crosses the placenta and causes hemolysis in newborn if the blood group of newborn is A.

50. **Ans. e. 12 weeks**

The interval between two whole blood donations for males is 12 weeks (3 months) and for females is 16 weeks (4 months). These recommendations were issued by the National Blood Transfusion Council (NBTC) keeping in mind the estimated time which will be required for the donor to recover the total iron lost with each donation.

51. **Ans. b. Frequently a cold agglutinin**
Ref: Roelcke D. Cold agglutination. Transfus Med Rev. 1989:3;140-66.

Anti-I antibody is often encountered (IgM type) autoantibody which is associated with cold agglutinin. As it is of the IgM type, it does not cross the placenta and cause hemolytic disease of the newborn. Cold autoantibodies commonly show specificity against the "Ii" blood group system, with approximately 90% directed against the "I" antigen and most of the remaining ones directed against the "i" antigen.

52. **Ans. c. It is mandatory to rinse-back all the RBCs in the circuit at the end of such procedures**

Packed red blood cell priming of apheresis circuit is indicated when the total extracorporeal RBC volume is large enough to disturb the hemodynamic stability of a patient, which is usually the case in pediatric procedures. Priming is done using a compatible donor PRBC, so that there is no reduction in hematocrit levels of the patient during the procedure. Rinse-back is not mandatory in cases where PRBC priming is done as it may cause a volume overload.

53. **Ans. a. Daratumumab (anti-CD38)**
Ref: van de Donk NW. Clinical efficacy and management of monoclonal antibodies targeting CD38 and SLAMF7 in multiple myeloma. Blood. 2016;127:681-95.

Daratumumab is a human monoclonal IgG1κ antibody used for the treatment of multiple myeloma.

The antibody binds to CD38, which is expressed on lymphoid and myeloid cells. Therapeutic monoclonal antibodies may disturb laboratory diagnostics. Daratumumab interferes with myeloma cell detection by flow cytometry and disturbs the detection and quantitation of monoclonal proteins by immunofixation electrophoresis. Since CD38 is also expressed at low levels on RBCs, daratumumab causes positive reactions in IATs, e.g. antibody detection (screening) tests, antibody identification panels, and antihuman immunoglobulin cross-matches. Hence, these patients should undergo an allo-antibody screening and Rh and Kell phenotyping before starting daratumumab.

54. Ans. d. Produced in response to antigens of bacteria, viruses, and other substances that are inhaled or ingested   *Ref: Hoffbrand 7/e p197*

ABO antibodies are probably produced in response to antigens of bacteria, viruses, and other substances that are inhaled or ingested. Despite this probable antigenic stimulus, the term "naturally occurring" is retained for these "non-red-cell-induced" antibodies. "Immune" RBCs or alloantibodies are only produced after pregnancy or following transfusion or injection of blood or blood group substances.

55. Ans. d. All of the above   *Ref: Hoffbrand 7/e p197*

Cold antibodies give higher agglutination titers at low temperatures (0–4°C), and many of them will not agglutinate RBCs at 37°C. The most naturally occurring antibodies are cold reacting. Cold antibodies that fail to react above 30°C are of no clinical significance and can be ignored for blood transfusion purposes. Immune antibodies have a thermal optimum of 37°C. Any red cell antibody reacting above 30°C should be considered potentially capable of destroying RBCs in vivo.

56. Ans. e. All of the above   *Ref: Hoffbrand 7/e p224*

Cryoprecipitate is prepared from FFP that is allowed to thaw slowly (classically at 4°C overnight). After removal of the supernatant, factor VIII: C, von Willebrand factor (VWF), fibrinogen, fibronectin, and factor XIII are left as a precipitate, which is then refrozen in approximately 30 mL of plasma and stored at –30°C or below for up to 24 months. Each unit should contain a minimum of 70 IU of factor VIII: C and 140 mg of fibrinogen. Cryoprecipitate is now used mainly as a source of fibrinogen in cases of DIC, hepatic failure, and hypofibrinogenemia.

SECTION 8: Immunohematology

42. Immunohematology

CHAPTER 42

Immunohematology

1. **Which of the following statement is not correct?**
   a. The immunoglobulin heavy chain locus is present on chromosome 14
   b. The immunoglobulin kappa chain locus is present on chromosome 2
   c. The immunoglobulin lambda chain locus is present on chromosome 16
   d. All of the above are correct

2. **True about antibody response following an infection is:**
   a. The first response is IgM only, irrespective of the type of infection
   b. The first response is IgG only, irrespective of the type of infection
   c. The first response is IgA only, irrespective of the type of infection
   d. The first response can be either IgM, IgG, IgA, or IgE depending upon the type of infection

3. **The characteristic features of IgM include all, *except*:**
   a. Secreted from B cells as a pentamer
   b. Develops after class switch recombination and somatic hypermutation
   c. IgM is more effective than IgG in mediating agglutination
   d. It is mostly intravascular
   e. All are true

4. **The following are true about B cells, *except*:**
   a. B-cells act as antigen-presenting cells
   b. B-cells produce inflammatory cytokines
   c. Breg cells secrete IL-10
   d. All are true

5. **True about immunoglobulin class switching is:**
   a. IgM-producing cells multiply and start producing IgG
   b. Constant region portion of antibody heavy chain is changed but the variable region remains same
   c. It does not affect antigen specificity
   d. All of the above

6. **True about function of the various immunoglobulins are, *except*:**
   a. IgM enhances ingestion of cells by phagocytosis
   b. IgA aggregates the antigens and keeps them in the secretions
   c. IgE bind to mast cells and basophils
   d. IgG is involved in the ABO blood group antigens on the surface of RBCs

7. **True about hyper-IgM syndrome is:**
   a. Defect in CD40 ligand
   b. Disorder of immunoglobulin class switching
   c. Patient dies at young age
   d. All of the above

8. **Identification of B-cell reconstitution post stem cell transplant can be done by all, *except*:**
   a. Serum immunoglobulin levels
   b. B-cell quantification
   c. Antimicrobial antibody development in relation to vaccination
   d. Assessment of bone marrow plasma cells

9. **All are true about regulatory T-cells, *except*:**
   a. Tregs are CD4 negative and CD8 negative
   b. Foxp3 is critical for their function
   c. Helps in preventing allograft rejection
   d. Helpful in reducing graft versus host disease (GVHD)

10. **All have been used for treatment of CAR T-cell (chimeric antigen T-cell receptor) mediated cytokine release syndrome, *except*:**
    a. Tocilizumab
    b. Siltuximab
    c. Fontolizumab
    d. Steroids

11. **All are shown to be mechanisms of relapse after anti-CD19 CAR-T therapy for acute lymphoblastic leukemia, *except*:**
    a. Antigen escape
    b. Nonpersistence of infused CAR T-cells
    c. Leukemic lineage switch from lymphoid to myeloid
    d. All of the above

12. **Antithymocyte globulin (ATG) for clinical use can be derived from all sources, *except*:**
    a. Horse
    b. Rabbit
    c. Pig
    d. Rat

ANSWERS WITH EXPLANATIONS

1. Ans. c. The immunoglobulin lambda chain locus is present on chromosome 16

Human antibody molecules and B-cell receptors are composed of heavy and light chains [each of which contains both constant (C) and variable (V) regions], which are encoded by genes on three loci: (1) the immunoglobulin heavy locus is present on chromosome 14, containing the gene segments for the immunoglobulin heavy chain; (2) the immunoglobulin kappa (κ) locus is present on chromosome 2, containing the gene segments for part of the immunoglobulin light chain; and (3) the immunoglobulin lambda (λ) locus is present on chromosome 22, containing the gene segments for the remainder of the immunoglobulin light chain.

2. Ans. a. The first response is IgM only, irrespective of the type of infection

Ref: Racine R, Winslow GM. IgM in microbial infections: taken for granted? Immunol Lett. 2009;125:79-85.

The first response is IgM only irrespective of the type of infection. When the B-cell is not producing any specific antibody, the M region which is most adjacent to variable (VDJ) region is transcribed as default and so IgM is the initial antibody response. If the specific antibody has to be produced (after the B-cell has been activated by helper T-cell), the initial portion of constant region containing M (mu region) will be deleted and specific antibody to the pathogen, e.g., the G (gamma region) will be transcribed and hence IgG antibody will be produced, if the pathogen is a parasite then E (epsilon region) will be transcribed and IgE will be produced.

3. Ans. b. Develops after class switch recombination and somatic hypermutation

Ref: Racine R, Winslow GM. IgM in microbial infections: taken for granted? Immunol Lett. 2009;125:79-85.

IgM provides a first line of defense during microbial infections, prior to the generation of adaptive, high-affinity IgG responses that are important for long-lived immunity and immunological memory. Monomeric IgM (180,000 kDa) is expressed as membrane-bound antibody on all naive B-cells, but it is secreted from B-cells as a pentamer (five monomeric units held together by disulfide bonds that link the carboxy-terminal heavy chains and the J chain). The pentameric structure generates 10 linked antigen-binding sites, affording IgM a higher valency than other immunoglobulins. IgM is generated from germline configured transcripts in B-cells, prior to the onset of class switch recombination (CSR) and somatic hypermutation (SHM) and is typically of low affinity. IgM is 100–10,000 times more effective than IgG in mediating agglutination. Agglutination is considered to be a key component of the process of IgM-mediated virus neutralization, given that a single bound IgM can activate complement and lyse an erythrocyte, while a thousand or more IgG molecules are required.

4. Ans. d. All are true

Ref: Chen X, Jensen PE. The role of B lymphocytes as antigen-presenting cells. Arch Immunol Ther Exp. 2008;56(2):77-83.

In addition to their obvious role in humoral immunity, B-lymphocytes contribute directly to cellular immunity via three other mechanisms: (1) they serve as antigen-presenting cells that enhance T-lymphocyte-mediated immunity; (2) they function as cellular effectors that produce inflammatory cytokines; and (3) a subgroup of them, known as Bregs and characterized by IL-10 secretion, modulate immune response. B-cells are by far the largest population of antigen-presenting cells found in vivo. B-cell depletion therapy impairs T-cell responses by eliminating B-cell-mediated antigen presentation.

5. Ans. d. All of the above

Immunoglobulin class switching is a biological mechanism that changes a B-cell's production of immunoglobulin from one type to another, such as from the isotype IgM to the isotype IgG or IgA. During this process, the constant-region portion of the antibody heavy chain is changed, but the variable region of the heavy chain remains the same. Since the variable region does not change, class switching does not affect antigen specificity. Immunoglobulin class switching is important for the B-cells to respond to various pathogens by producing different types of antibodies.

6. Ans. d. IgG is involved in the ABO blood group antigens on the surface of RBCs

IgG provides long-term protection because it persists for months and years after the disappearance of the antigen that has triggered their production. IgG protect against bacteria, viruses, neutralize bacterial toxins, trigger compliment protein systems, and bind antigens to enhance the effectiveness of phagocytosis. Main function of IgA is to bind antigens on microbes before they invade tissues. It aggregates the antigens and keeps them in the secretions so when the secretion is expelled, so is the antigen. IgM is involved in the ABO blood group antigens on the surface of RBCs. IgM enhance ingestions of cells by phagocytosis. IgE bind to mast cells and basophils which participate in the immune response.

7. Ans. d. All of the above

Patients with hyper-IgM syndrome have an inability to switch from the production of antibodies of the IgM type to antibodies of the IgG, IgA, or IgE types. As a result, patients with this disease have decreased levels of IgG and IgA but normal or elevated levels of IgM in their blood. Normally, B-lymphocytes can produce IgM antibodies on their own, but they require interactive help from T-lymphocytes in order to switch from IgM to IgG, IgA, or IgE. Hyper-IgM syndrome results from a variety of genetic defects that affect this interaction between T-lymphocytes and B-lymphocytes. The most common form of hyper-IgM syndrome results from a defect or deficiency of a protein that is found on the surface of activated T-lymphocytes. The affected protein is called CD40 ligand because it binds, or ligates, to a protein on B-lymphocytes called CD40. Although low-affinity IgM antibodies circulate in the blood prior to encountering pathogens, high-affinity IgG and IgA antibodies are required to inactivate toxins, neutralize viruses, and promote the clearance of microorganisms. Individuals with hyper-IgM syndrome lack the ability to make high-affinity IgG and IgA antibodies and are unable to combat bacterial and viral infections and usually die at a young age.

8. **Ans. d. Assessment of bone marrow plasma cells**
Ref: Small TN. B cells and transplantation: an educational resource. Biol Blood Marrow Transplant. 2009;15:104-13.

B-cell reconstitution after stem cell transplant can be done by examining immunoglobulin levels, B-cell quantification, and antimicrobial antibody development in relation to donor/recipient serologic status or vaccination.

9. **Ans. a. T regs are CD4 negative and CD8 negative**
Ref: Fontenot JD. Foxp3 programs the development and function of CD4+CD25+ regulatory T cells. Nat Immunol. 2003;4:330-6.

Regulatory T (Treg) cells play a critical role in maintaining self-tolerance as well as in regulating immune responses. Increasing Treg numbers and/or enhancing their suppressive function may be beneficial for treating autoimmune diseases and for preventing allograft rejection and GVHD. Overexpression of Foxp3 in conventional T-cells converts them to a Treg phenotype and endows them with anergy and suppressive activity. Continuous expression of Foxp3 is critical for maintaining the suppressive activity of Treg cells. Diminishing the degree of Foxp3 expression may convert Treg cells to Th2 like cells, implying a close relationship of the Th2 and Treg lineages. Induced Treg cells are Foxp3+ CD4+ CD25+ cells.

10. **Ans. c. Fontolizumab**
Ref: Riegler LL. Current approaches in the grading and management of cytokine release syndrome after chimeric antigen receptor T-cell therapy. Ther Clin Risk Manag. 2019;15:323-35.

Chimeric antigen T-cell receptor cell therapy is US Food and Drug Administration approved for pediatric acute lymphoblastic leukemia and adult relapsed/refractory non-Hodgkin lymphoma. Cytokine release syndrome (CRS) is a major toxicity associated with CAR-T cell therapy (other being neurotoxicity, B-cell aplasia). Although grade I-II CRS may be managed symptomatically, grade 3-4 CRS may need treatment with tocilizumab (anti-IL-6 monoclonal antibody) with or without steroids. Siltuximab is also an IL6 antibody, and has been used at some centers. Fontolizumab is anti-INF-alpha monoclonal antibody that is not recommended as it impairs T-cell proliferation.

11. **Ans. d. All of the above**
Ref: Riegler LL. Current approaches in the grading and management of cytokine release syndrome after chimeric antigen receptor T-cell therapy. Ther Clin Risk Manag. 2019;15:323-35.

Main mechanism of CAR T-cell therapy failure is because of disappearance of circulating CAR T-cells, due to short life of viral vector used. Other mechanisms described include CD19 antigen escape from surface of tumor cells, and rarely switch from lymphoid to myeloid lineages.

12. **Ans. d. Rat**
Ref: X Ma. Comparison of porcine anti-human lymphocyte globulin and rabbit anti-human thymocyte globulin in the treatment of severe aplastic anemia: a retrospective single-center study. Eur J Haematol. 2016;96;260-8.

Antithymocyte globulin is used as an immuno-suppressive drug in aplastic anemia and in stem cell transplantation for various hematological conditions. It is a polyclonal antibody complex derived from sera of various animals like horse, rabbit, and pig after injecting human thymocytes into these animals. It is generally believed that smaller the organism more the potency of the ATG.

SECTION 9

Case-based Questions

43. Case-based Questions

CHAPTER 43

Case-based Questions

1. A 52-year-old man had dull and constant back pain for 3 months. He recently developed a cough productive of yellowish sputum. On physical examination, there were crackles at the right lung base. A plain film radiograph of the spine revealed several 1–2 cm lytic lesions of the vertebral bodies. Laboratory studies showed glucose 78 mg/dL, urea nitrogen 49 mg/dL, creatinine 5 mg/dL, total protein 8.3 g/dL, albumin 3.2 g/dL, alkaline phosphatase 176 U/L, AST (aspartate aminotransferase) 55 U/L, ALT (alanine aminotransferase) 33 U/L, and total bilirubin 1.3 mg/dL. A sputum culture grew *Streptococcus pneumoniae*. Which of the following pathologic findings is most likely to be seen in a bone marrow biopsy from this man?

a. Scattered small granulomas
b. Nodules of small mature lymphocytes
c. Occasional Reed-Sternberg cells
d. Numerous plasma cells
e. Hypercellularity with many blasts

2. A 43-year-old woman has experienced low-grade fevers, night sweats, and generalized malaise for the past 3 months. On physical examination, she has nontender cervical and supraclavicular lymphadenopathy. A cervical lymph node biopsy is performed. On microscopic examination at high magnification, there are occasional CD15+ and CD30+ Reed-Sternberg cells along with large and small lymphocytes and bands of fibrosis. Which of the following is the most likely diagnosis?

a. Burkitt lymphoma
b. Hodgkin lymphoma
c. Cat scratch disease (CSD)
d. Mycosis fungoides
e. Multiple myeloma

3. An 18-year-old adolescent has malaise for the past 4 weeks. He has mild pharyngitis on physical examination as well as tender axillary and inguinal lymphadenopathy. The spleen is palpable. A hemogram shows Hb 14.0 g/dL, mean corpuscular volume (MCV) 96 fL, platelet count 201,300/µL, and white blood cell (WBC) count 7,000/µL with "atypical lymphocytes" on the peripheral blood smear. His illness is most likely to be acquired via which of the following mechanisms?

a. Congenital genetic abnormality
b. From a close contact on a date
c. As a result of an insect bite
d. Through an environmental exposure at work
e. Without any known etiology

4. A 46-year-old man has had fevers for the past 4 weeks. On physical examination, his temperature is 37.8°C. Laboratory studies show Hb 12.8 g/dL, MCV 94 fL, platelet count 220,000/µL, and WBC count 70,000/µL. The WBC differential count shows 82 neutrophils, 6 bands, 6 metamyelocytes, 1 myelocyte, 4 lymphocytes, and 1 monocyte. The leukocyte alkaline phosphatase (LAP) score is high at 150. Which of the following laboratory test findings is most likely to be present in this man?

a. Bone marrow karyotype of 46, XY, t(9;22)
b. Serologic titer of 1:1024 for anti-double-stranded DNA
c. Serum vitamin B_{12} level of 100 pg/mL
d. 4+ ketonuria and 4+ proteinuria
e. Oral swab culture positive for *Streptococcus*, viridans group

5. A clinical study is conducted involving adults from 20 to 70 years of age who underwent splenectomy for blunt force abdominal trauma. An age-matched control group of patients consists of patients who have congestive splenomegaly. The laboratory findings from these subjects are analyzed. Which of the following laboratory test findings is most likely to be observed only in the study group following splenectomy?

a. Thrombocytopenia
b. Red blood cell (RBC) Howell-Jolly bodies
c. Decreased RBC distribution width (RDW)
d. Leukopenia
e. Nucleated RBCs

6. A 36-year-old man has had a sore throat with fever for 5 days. On physical examination, he has mildly tender generalized cervical lymphadenopathy. Laboratory findings include Hb 14 g/dL, platelet count 200,000/µL, and WBC count 12,000/µL with a

differential count of 75 neutrophils, 10 bands, and 15 lymphocytes. Which of the following is the most likely diagnosis?
a. Lymphocytic lymphoma
b. Hodgkin lymphoma
c. Group A *Streptococcus* infection
d. Human immunodeficiency virus (HIV) infection
e. Brucellosis

7. A 35-year-old man has had a progressively worsening productive cough for 1 month. On physical examination, a few small nontender lymph nodes are palpable in the axillae. Laboratory studies show Hb 10.2 g/dL, MCV 90 fL, WBC count 72,000/μL, and platelet count 46,000/μL. Microscopic examination of his peripheral blood smear shows many blasts with Auer rods. Which of the following is the most likely diagnosis?
a. Leukemoid reaction
b. Acute myelogenous leukemia (AML)
c. Chronic lymphocytic leukemia (CLL)
d. Lymphoblastic leukemia
e. Leukoerythroblastosis

8. A 60-year-old woman has had malaise for the past 1 year. On physical examination, there are no abnormal findings. Her Hb is 9.5 g/dL, MCV 88 fL, platelet count 200,000/μL, and WBC count 8,200/μL. Her total serum iron is 20 μg/dL, total iron binding capacity (TIBC) 240 μg/dL, and soluble serum transferrin receptor is normal. A bone marrow biopsy is performed, and microscopic examination shows that maturation is occurring in all cell lines and there are no abnormal cells seen. Stainable iron in the bone marrow has increased. Which of the following underlying diseases is she most likely to have?
a. Diverticulosis
b. Hepatitis C infection
c. Systemic lupus erythematosus (SLE)
d. Atrophic gastritis
e. Fanconi anemia

9. A 56-year-old man has noted the presence of several lumps on the right side of his neck for the past 5 months. On physical examination, he has firm, nontender, movable lymph nodes palpable in the right posterior cervical region. He does not have splenomegaly or hepatomegaly. Laboratory studies show Hb 11.8 g/dL, MCV 87 fL, platelet count 280,000/μL, and WBC count 8,000/μL. A cervical lymph node biopsy is performed and on microscopic examination shows numerous nodules of small, monomorphic lymphocytes. Which of the following is the most likely diagnosis?
a. Chronic lymphocytic leukemia
b. Follicular lymphoma
c. Infectious mononucleosis
d. Hodgkin lymphoma, lymphocyte predominance type
e. Reactive hyperplasia

10. A 49-year-old man has had increasing abdominal discomfort with abdominal enlargement for the past 2 years. An abdominal CT scan reveals massive (estimated 3,000 g size) splenomegaly. Laboratory data include Hb 9 g/dL, WBC count 6,000/μL, and platelet count 60,000/μL. Which of the following underlying conditions is he most likely to have?
a. Myelofibrosis
b. Sickle cell anemia
c. Portal hypertension
d. Infectious mononucleosis
e. Hemochromatosis

11. A 45-year-old woman has had fever and mental confusion for 1 week. Physical examination shows temperature 38.2°C, pulse rate (PR) 100/min, respiratory rate (RR) 22/min, and BP 110/60 mm Hg. She has widespread petechiae on skin and mucosal surfaces. Laboratory studies show her creatinine 6.3 mg/dL. She has a hemoglobin of 12.2 g/dL, MCV 93 fL, platelet count 19,000/μL, and WBC count 8,000/μL. Schistocytes are seen on her peripheral blood smear. Her prothrombin time, partial thromboplastin time, and D-dimer are not elevated. Which of the following is the most likely diagnosis?
a. Disseminated intravascular coagulopathy
b. Idiopathic thrombocytopenic purpura (ITP)
c. Thrombotic thrombocytopenic purpura (TTP)
d. Trousseau syndrome
e. Warm autoimmune hemolytic anemia (AIHA)

12. A 62-year-old previously healthy man has noted increasing fatigue and shortness of breath with minimal exercise for the last 4 months. He has felt some abdominal discomfort over the past month. On physical examination, he has nontender cervical lymphadenopathy. The liver span is 17 cm in the right mid-clavicular line; the edge is smooth and palpable just below the right costal margin. The spleen is palpated 3 cm below the left costal margin on inspiration. A complete blood count (CBC) shows WBC count 23,600/μL with 16 neutrophils, 2 bands, 78 lymphocytes, and 4 monocytes; Hb 11.9 g/dL; MCV 90; and platelet count 277,300/μL. The direct Coombs test (DCT) is positive. Which of the following is the most likely diagnosis?
a. Leukemoid reaction
b. Chronic myelogenous leukemia
c. Acute myelogenous leukemia
d. Acute lymphocytic leukemia
e. Chronic lymphocytic leukemia

13. A 17-year-old boy has had weakness for 3 months. On physical examination, he has a palpable spleen tip. A CBC shows Hb 8.8 g/dL, MCV 65 fL, platelet count 187,000/μL, and WBC count 7400/μL. His serum ferritin is 4,000 ng/mL. A bone marrow biopsy is performed and on microscopic examination reveals a myeloid:erythroid (ME) ratio of 1:4, and there is 4+ stainable iron. Which of the following is the most likely diagnosis?

a. Glucose-6-phosphate dehydrogenase (G6PD) deficiency
b. Beta-thalassemia
c. Sickle cell anemia
d. Hereditary spherocytosis
e. Malaria

14. A 43-year-old man has experienced increasing malaise and difficulty concentrating at work for the past 6 months. On physical examination, he has splenomegaly but no lymphadenopathy. He is afebrile. Laboratory studies show Hb 12.0 g/dL, MCV 92 fL, platelet count 400,000/μL, and WBC count 200,000/μL with differential count 73 neutrophils, 12 bands, 6 metamyelocytes, 2 myelocytes, 2 myeloblasts, and 5 lymphocytes. The LAP score is very low. A bone marrow biopsy is performed. Which of the following microscopic findings is most likely to be found in this biopsy?

a. Sheets of plasma cells
b. Atypical cytokeratin-positive glands
c. Numerous mature and immature myeloid cells
d. Predominance of adipocytes
e. Granulomas that have many acid-fast bacilli

15. A 39-year-old woman has the sudden onset of fever, abdominal pain, tachycardia, and nausea. On physical examination, her vital signs included temperature 38.6°C, PR 120/min, RR 28/min, and BP 100/60 mm Hg. She is icteric. Laboratory studies show Hb 8.0 g/dL, MCV 99 fL, platelet count 209,500/μL, and WBC count 6,840/μL. Her reticulocyte count is 0.15%. On microscopic examination of her peripheral blood smear, RBCs are small and lack central pallor. Which of the following most likely initiated this woman's acute illness?

a. Quinacrine use
b. Parvovirus infection
c. Decreased oxygen tension
d. Exposure to cold
e. Transfusion therapy

16. A 66-year-old man has had fatigue, fever, and episodes of epistaxis for the past 4 months. On physical examination, his temperature was found to be 37.4°C. Laboratory studies show Hb 12.5 g/dL, MCV 89 fL, platelet count 170,000/μL, and WBC count 62,000/μL. Examination of his peripheral blood smear shows large blasts with Auer rods. Which of the following risk factors most likely preceded the development of his current illness?

a. Malaria
b. Infectious mononucleosis
c. Diabetes mellitus
d. Beta-thalassemia
e. Myelodysplasia

17. A 42-year-old woman has noticed during the past month that even minor trauma produces major bruises over her body. On physical examination, she has areas of purpura on the skin of her arms and legs. Laboratory studies show that her prothrombin time is 12.9 seconds (control 13 seconds) and partial thromboplastin time 26.2 seconds (control 25 seconds). Her CBC shows Hb 11.1 g/dL, MCV 84 fL, platelet count 880,000/μL, and WBC count 55,400/μL. A bone marrow biopsy is performed and on microscopic examination shows hypercellularity with myeloid and megakaryocytic hyperplasia. Which of the following is the most likely diagnosis?

a. Epstein-Barr virus (EBV) infection
b. Myeloproliferative disorder
c. Drug reaction to recent antibiotic therapy
d. Wiskott-Aldrich syndrome
e. Megaloblastic anemia

18. A clinical study is performed with subjects who are adults and found to have anemia. Their clinical histories and laboratory findings are reviewed. It is observed that ingestion of a drug preceded development of the anemia in some of the subjects, but not in others. Which of the following conditions is most likely to be found in persons without a history of drug ingestion?

a. G6PD deficiency
b. Autoimmune hemolytic anemia
c. Macrocytic anemia
d. Aplastic anemia
e. Microcytic anemia

19. A 35-year-old man is given antimalarial prophylaxis for a trip to West Africa. Over the next week, he develops increasing fatigue. On physical examination, there are no abnormal findings. Laboratory studies show a hematocrit of 30%. Examination of his peripheral blood smear shows RBCs with numerous Heinz bodies. There is a family history of this disorder, with males, but not females, affected. Which of the following is the most likely diagnosis?

a. Beta-thalassemia
b. Sickle cell anemia
c. Alpha-thalassemia
d. Hereditary spherocytosis
e. G6PD deficiency

20. A study is conducted to determine what changes in the size of the spleen take place with hematologic disorders. The spleen sizes are estimated from CT scans for adult patients who developed complications of their hematologic disease. For which of the following diseases is the spleen most likely to remain normal in size?

a. Autoimmune hemolytic anemia
b. Chronic alcohol abuse
c. Myeloproliferative disorder
d. Idiopathic thrombocytopenic purpura
e. Sickle cell anemia

21. A 61-year-old man has become increasingly fatigued for the past 10 months. On physical examination, there are no abnormal findings. Laboratory studies show that his Hb is 9.2 g/dL, MCV 132 fL, platelet count 300,000/µL, and WBC count 7,590/µL. Which of the following morphologic findings is most likely to be present on examination of his peripheral blood smear?

a. Hypersegmented neutrophils
b. Nucleated RBCs
c. Blasts with Auer rods
d. Hypochromic, microcytic RBCs
e. Schistocytes

22. An 80-year-old man has been feeling tired for the past 8 months. On physical examination, there are no abnormal findings. Laboratory studies show Hb 9.4 g/dL, MCV 72 fL, platelet count 330,000/µL, and WBC count 8,200/µL with automated differential count of 70.1% neutrophils, 18.8% lymphocytes, and 11.1% monocytes. Which of the following morphologic findings is most likely to be seen on his peripheral blood smear?

a. Fragmentation
b. Many nucleated forms
c. Hypochromasia
d. Spherocytosis
e. Howell-Jolly bodies

23. A 24-year-old primigravida gives birth to a boy at 35 weeks' gestation. On physical examination, the infant is markedly hydropic. Laboratory studies show that his hematocrit is 17% and the peripheral blood smear reveals numerous nucleated RBCs and even a few erythroblasts. The RBCs display marked anisocytosis and poikilocytosis. Which of the following diseases is most likely to be present in this infant?

a. Sickle cell anemia
b. Alpha-thalassemia
c. Hemoglobin E disease
d. G6PD deficiency
e. Hereditary elliptocytosis

24. A 52-year-old man has had worsening arthritis and swelling of his feet for the past year. A chest radiograph shows cardiomegaly and pulmonary edema. Laboratory studies show Hb 13.0 g/dL, MCV 86 fL, platelet count 355,500/µL, and WBC count 6,720/µL. His serum iron is 564 µg/mL with iron-binding capacity 440 µg/mL and ferritin 930 ng/mL. Which of the following is the most likely diagnosis?

a. Beta-thalassemia
b. Autoimmune hemolytic anemia
c. Anemia of chronic disease (ACD)
d. Polycythemia vera
e. Pernicious anemia
f. Hereditary hemochromatosis

25. A 66-year-old man has had a fever with cough for a month. On physical examination, his temperature was found to be 37.5°C. There are crackles auscultated in upper lung fields. A chest radiograph shows a reticulonodular pattern with upper lobe cavitary lesions. His sputum is positive for acid-fast bacilli. A CBC shows Hb 14.2 g/dL, MCV 92 fL, platelet count 335,000/µL, and WBC count 50,500/µL with differential count of 59 neutrophils, 20 bands, 8 metamyelocytes, 4 myelocytes, 2 promyelocytes, 5 lymphocytes, and 2 monocytes. Which of the following laboratory test findings is most likely to be present in this man?

a. High LAP
b. Karyotype with 46, XY, t(9;22)
c. Monoclonal gammopathy
d. Elevated D-dimer
e. Positive terminal deoxynucleotidyl transferase (TdT) assay

26. A 6-year-old boy has become increasingly lethargic for the past 2 months. There are ecchymoses noted on the skin of his lower legs. Laboratory studies show Hb 9.2 g/dL, MCV 91 fL, platelet count 201,000/µL, and WBC count 14,128/µL. A bone marrow biopsy is performed and on microscopic examination shows nearly 100% cellularity with replacement by primitive cells that have large nuclei with delicate chromatin and indistinct nucleoli with scanty cytoplasm. These cells mark for CD10 (CALLA) antigen. Which of the following is the most likely diagnosis?

a. Acute myeloid leukemia
b. Hodgkin lymphoma
c. Acute lymphoblastic leukemia (ALL)
d. Epstein-Barr virus infection
e. Chronic myelogenous leukemia

27. A 72-year-old woman has developed increasing dyspne.a for the past 2 weeks. Scleral icterus is noted. A CBC shows Hb 7.1 g/dL, MCV 93 fL, platelet count 325,000/µL, and WBC count 7,500/µL with differential count of 60 neutrophils, 4 bands, 25 lymphocytes, 9 monocytes, and 2 eosinophils with 10 nucleated RBCs/100 WBCs. Which of the following is the most likely diagnosis?

a. Iron deficiency anemia (IDA)
b. Pernicious anemia
c. Anemia of chronic disease
d. Sickle cell anemia
e. Hemolytic anemia

28. A 62-year-old man has had constant dull pain in his lower right back for the past 4 months. On physical examination, there is tenderness on percussion of his right costovertebral angle. An abdominal CT scan reveals a 6 cm mass in the upper pole of the right kidney. A CBC shows Hb 21.3 g/dL, MCV 96 fL, platelet count 234,000/μL, and WBC count 9,230/μL. Serum chemistries include glucose 87 mg/dL and creatinine 1.3 mg/dL. Which of the following is the most likely cause for his findings?

a. Polycythemia rubra vera
b. Erythroleukemia
c. Hemophilia A
d. Diabetes insipidus
e. Increased serum erythropoietin

29. A 42-year-old woman has become increasingly fatigued for the past 3 months. During the past week, she has noted purpuric spots on her skin. She has no hepatosplenomegaly and no lymphadenopathy. Laboratory studies show Hb 6.8 g/dL, MCV 91 fL, platelet count 34,000/μL, and WBC count 2,140/μL. Which of the following is the most likely diagnosis?

a. Aplastic anemia
b. Myeloproliferative disorder
c. Immune thrombocytopenic purpura
d. Large B cell lymphoma
e. Hereditary spherocytosis

30. A 55-year-old man has noted a change in the appearance of his face over the past 7 months. On physical examination, his facial skin is thickened and reddened. A punch biopsy of skin is performed and on microscopic examination shows infiltration by neoplastic T lymphocytes that are CD4 positive. Which of the following is the most likely diagnosis?

a. Hodgkin lymphoma
b. Mycosis fungoides
c. Burkitt lymphoma
d. Acute lymphocytic leukemia
e. Hairy cell leukemia (HCL)

31. A 53-year-old man has had increasing fatigue for the past 4 months. On physical examination, he was found to have massive splenomegaly but no lymphadenopathy. Laboratory studies show Hb 10.1 g/dL, MCV 90 fL, WBC count 1,900/μL, and platelet count 52,000/μL. Examination of his peripheral blood smear shows increased numbers of peripheral blood lymphocytes containing tartrate-resistant acid phosphatase. Which of the following is the most likely diagnosis?

a. Chronic lymphocytic leukemia
b. Human T-lymphotropic virus type 1 (HTLV-1) infection with leukemia
c. Hairy cell leukemia
d. Gaucher disease
e. Myelodysplasia

32. A 12-year-old girl has exhibited increasing sluggishness with poorer performance in school over the past year. She has not had increased numbers of infections. The child now complains of headaches. A physical examination shows no hepatosplenomegaly or lymphadenopathy. A CBC shows Hb 11.8 g/dL, MCV 71 fL, platelet count 311,000/μL, and WBC count 8,160/μL. Examination of her peripheral blood smear shows basophilic stippling of erythrocytes. The serum haptoglobin is 5 mg/dL. Which of the following laboratory test findings is most likely to be present in this girl?

a. Hemoglobin S on electrophoresis
b. Increased osmotic fragility
c. Positive DCT
d. Decreased serum iron
e. Elevated free erythrocyte protoporphyrin

33. A 3-year-old boy has had a seborrheic eruption over the scalp and trunk over the past month. He then develops a right earache. On physical examination, the right tympanic membrane is erythematous and bulging. He has hepatosplenomegaly and generalized lymphadenopathy. Laboratory studies show Hb 9.5 g/dL, Hct 28.7%, MCV 90 fL, platelet count 58,000/μL, and WBC count 3,140/μL. A bone marrow biopsy is performed and on microscopic examination shows 98% cellularity with extensive infiltration by cells resembling macrophages that express CD1a antigen and, by electron microscopy, have prominent HX bodies (Birbeck granules). Which of the following conditions is most likely to produce this boy's findings?

a. Myeloproliferative disorder
b. *Plasmodium vivax* infection
c. Hodgkin lymphoma, lymphocyte depletion type
d. Langerhans cell histiocytosis (LCH)
e. AIDS

34. A 69-year-old woman has had increasing fatigue with 5 kg weight loss over the past 5 months. Her hands become purple and painful upon exposure to cold. On physical examination, she was found to have a palpable spleen tip. Laboratory studies show Hb

5 g/dL, MCV 99 fL, platelet count 193,600/μL, and WBC count 5,390/μL. The DCT is positive at 4°C and negative at 37°C. Which of the following underlying diseases is this woman most likely to have?

a. Non-Hodgkin lymphoma (NHL)
b. Systemic lupus erythematosus
c. Pernicious anemia
d. Scleroderma
e. Thalassemia minor

35. A 13-year-old girl has the sudden onset of severe abdominal pain and back pain. On physical examination her abdomen was found to be diffusely tender, but there are no masses. A CBC shows Hb 6.5 g/dL, MCV 99 fL, platelet count 211,000/μL, and WBC count 11,200/μL. Examination of her peripheral blood smear shows nucleated RBCs and sickled RBCs. Which of the following types of gene mutation is she most likely to have?

a. Deletion
b. Duplication
c. Insertion
d. Missense
e. Nonsense

36. A 41-year-old man has had worsening headaches for the past 3 months. He has no lymphadenopathy or hepatosplenomegaly. Laboratory studies show Hb 12 g/dL, platelet count 250,000/μL, and WBC count 8,200/μL with differential count of 80% granulocytes, 10% lymphocytes, and 10% monocytes. A head CT scan reveals a 3 cm mass lesion to the right of midline next to the lateral ventricle. A stereotactic brain biopsy is performed, and microscopic examination shows diffuse large B-cell lymphoma. Which of the following laboratory test findings is this patient most likely to have?

a. Elevated TdT transferase
b. Bence-Jones proteinuria
c. Elevated serum IgM
d. HIV-1 RNA of 80,000 copies/mL
e. Lymphoma positive for tartrate-resistant acid phosphatase

37. A 32-year-old woman has had worsening fatigue for the past 2 months. On physical examination, she was found to have an erythematous macular rash on her upper chest, forearms, and face. Laboratory studies show Hb 9.2 g/dL, MCV 101 fL, platelet count 219,000/μL, and WBC count 5,850/μL. The RDW is markedly increased. Her peripheral blood smear shows polychromasia. Her reticulocyte count is 4.2%. The serum haptoglobin is 3 mg/dL. Serum chemistries show total protein 7.9 g/dL, albumin 3.8 g/dL, alkaline phosphatase 49 U/L, AST 81 U/L, ALT 27 U/L, total bilirubin 4.3 mg/dL, and direct bilirubin 0.8 mg/dL. Hemoglobinuria is detected on urinalysis. Which of the following underlying conditions is she most likely to have?

a. Multiple myeloma
b. Systemic lupus erythematosus
c. Hepatitis C infection
d. Hereditary spherocytosis
e. Vitamin B_{12} deficiency

38. A 42-year-old man known to be infected with HIV for the past 10 years has had abdominal pain for the past 7 days. Physical examination reveals abdominal distension with diffuse tenderness and absent bowel sounds. An abdominal CT scan reveals a mass lesion involving the small intestine. He is taken to surgery, and an area of bowel obstruction in the ileum is removed. Gross examination of the specimen shows a near-encircling firm white mass 10 cm long and 3 cm in greatest depth that infiltrates through the wall of the bowel. Which of the following neoplasms is this man most likely to have?

a. Plasmacytoma
b. Hodgkin lymphoma, lymphocyte predominant type
c. High-grade B-cell lymphoma
d. Metastatic adenocarcinoma
e. Adenocarcinoma

39. A 31-year-old healthy man incurs blunt force trauma to the abdomen in a motor vehicle accident. On physical examination, he has upper abdominal tenderness. An abdominal CT scan reveals a splenic hematoma. At laparotomy, a splenectomy is performed. Following splenectomy, which of the following peripheral blood morphologic findings is most likely to be present?

a. Tear drop cells
b. Elliptocytes
c. Target cells
d. Macro-ovalocytes
e. RBC inclusions

40. A 12-year-old girl is noted to have increasing facial distortion for the past 8 months from a lesion involving her jaw. On physical examination, she has a right mandibular mass. A biopsy is performed and on microscopic examination reveals a monotonous pattern of small noncleaved lymphocytes. Cytogenetic analysis of these cells shows t(8;14). Infection with which of the following organisms is most likely to be associated with development of this girl's mass lesion?

a. Adenovirus
b. Cytomegalovirus (CMV)
c. Epstein-Barr virus
d. Hepatitis C virus
e. HIV

41. Two teenage siblings in the same family are noted to have frequent nosebleeds and easy bruising from even minor trauma. Both have had menorrhagia since menarche. One girl's CBC shows Hb 14 g/dL, MCV 90 fL, platelet count 242,000/μL, and WBC count 7,720/μL. Her prothrombin time

is 12 seconds and partial thromboplastin time 25 seconds. Platelet function studies show decreased aggregation in response to adenosine diphosphate, collagen, epinephrine, and thrombin. Which of the following disorders are these siblings most likely to have?
a. Hemophilia A
b. Antithrombin III deficiency
c. Glanzmann thrombasthenia (GT)
d. Bernard-Soulier syndrome
e. von Willebrand disease (VWD)

42. A 52-year-old man has been chronically fatigued for the past year. A physical examination yields no abnormal findings. A CBC shows Hb 10.8 g/dL, MCV 104 fL, platelet count 239,000/μL, and WBC count 7,720/μL. His peripheral blood smear shows normal WBC morphology and RBCs with mild poikilocytosis and a few target cells. His serum vitamin B_{12} is 644 pg/mL and folate 2.8 ng/mL. His serum haptoglobin is 151 mg/dL. DCT and indirect Coombs test (ICT) are negative. Which of the following underlying conditions is most likely to explain his findings?
a. Chronic lymphocytic leukemia
b. Peptic ulcer disease
c. Lead poisoning
d. Chronic alcohol abuse
e. Hereditary spherocytosis

43. A 46-year-old man has had multiple episodes of painful red nodules on his skin from dermal venous thrombosis as well as abdominal pain from mesenteric vein thrombosis over the past year. He notes passing darker urine. Laboratory studies show Hb 9.4 g/dL, MCV 100 fL, platelet count 300,000/μL, and WBC count 8,800/μL. His RBCs show increased sensitivity to complement lysis. Flow cytometry is most likely to show reduction in which of the following markers on his RBCs?
a. CD4
b. CD19
c. CD33
d. CD55
e. CD68

44. A 4-year-old male child born by surrogacy was having recurrent pneumonia requiring hospitalization. He was not thriving well. His family history was not significant. His blood parameter showed normal CBC. Serology for HIV was negative. His immunological profile revealed:

Lymphocyte subset analysis showed:

	%	cells/micl	Reference range
CD16+/CD56+ cells (NK-cells)	41.18	713.16	61-510/uL
CD3 positive cells (T-cells)	42.23	756.13	850-4,300/uL
CD4 positive cells	14.91	266.91	500-2,700/uL
CD8 positive cells	25.39	454.53	200-1,800/uL

Contd...

Contd...

	%	cells/micL	Reference range
CD3+TCR α/β positive	82.6	625.56	600-4,300/uL
CD3+TCR γδ positive	16.6	125.51	27-960/uL
CD19 positive cells (B-cells)	10.66	184.60	180-1,300/uL

Immunoglobulin profile showed:
- Immunoglobulin IgA < 10 mg/dL (66–436)
- Immunoglobulin IgG < 75 mg/dL (791–1643)
- Immunoglobulin IgM 641 mg/dL (20–200)
- Immunoglobulin IgE 0.1 IU/mL (0–60)

What is the diagnosis?
a. CVID
b. X-linked agammaglobulinemia
c. Hyper IgM syndrome
d. Transient hypogammaglobulinemia of infancy.

45. An elderly gentleman had surgery for fracture femur and was given low molecular weight heparin as post-operative prophylaxis. On admission his CBC showed Hb of 13.2 g/dL, WBC count of 5,000/cumm and platelet count of 2,50,000/cumm. Coagulation parameters were normal at admission, but after a week later CBC showed Hb of 13 g/dL, WBC count of 6,000/cumm and platelet count dropped to 1,00,000/cumm and coagulation parameters being normal. He developed sudden weakness of right arm. What is the most likely cause of his findings?
a. ITP
b. DIC
c. Drug induced thrombocytopenia
d. TTP

46. A 25-year-old man presented with sudden onset of fever, abdominal pain, tachycardia, and nausea. On evaluation he had temperature of 102°F, Pulse of 90/min, RR 22/min and BP 100/60 mm Hg. He was having icterus and mild splenomegaly. CBC showed Hb of 9.0 g/dL, MCV of 99 fL, WBC count of 8,000/cumm and platelet count of 210,000/cumm. His reticulocyte count is 0.1% and PS showed small RBC's which lack central pallor. Which of the following most likely initiated this man's acute illness?
a. Parvovirus infection
b. Quinacrine use
c. Exposure to cold
d. Transfusion therapy

47. A 35-year-old man presented with worsening arthritis and bilateral pedal edema for the past 6 months. On examination he had bilateral fine crepts. Chest X-ray showed cardiomegaly and pulmonary edema. CBC showed Hb of 13.0 g/dL, MCV of 86 fL, WBC count of 11,000/cumm and platelet count of 2,75,000/cumm. His serum iron was 406 microgram/mL with TIBC of 0 microgram/mL and ferritin 830 ng/mL. Which of the following is the most likely diagnosis?
a. Beta thalassemia
b. Anemia of chronic disease
c. Polycythemia vera
d. Hereditary hemochromatosis
e. AIH

ANSWERS WITH EXPLANATIONS

1. Ans. d. Numerous plasma cells

Ref: WJM. 1996;164(6):514.

To summarize, this patient has anemia, renal failure, albumin/globulin (AG) reversal, lytic lesion in bone with bone pain, and active infection (pneumonia). So the likely diagnosis is multiple myeloma. Acute leukemia will not have AG reversal and lytic bone lesion is rare, so option e is incorrect. Nodular aggregates of small lymphocytes and Reed-Sternberg cells are characteristically seen in CLL and Hodgkin lymphoma, which are also unlikely diagnoses because of the absence of lymphadenopathy, organomegaly, and moreover presence of lytic bone lesions. Scattered granulomas in bone marrow can be seen in many diseases, but they are never associated with lytic bone lesions.

Causes of bone marrow granuloma:
- *Malignant*:
  - Hodgkin lymphoma
  - Non-Hodgkin lymphoma
- *Infections*:
  - Tuberculosis
  - Histoplasma
  - Brucellosis
  - Typhoid fever
  - Q fever
  - Mycobacterium avium-intracellulare
  - EBV
  - CMV
  - HIV
- *Drugs*:
  - Procainamide
  - Sulfonamide
- Foreign body
- Sarcoidosis
- Idiopathic diffuse granulomatosis
- Connective tissue disorder (rare).

2. Ans. b. Hodgkin lymphoma

The characteristic CD15+ and CD30+ Reed-Sternberg cells are seen in Hodgkin lymphoma. Burkitt lymphoma will not have this type of immunophenotype and morphology. Mycosis fungoides is a T-cell neoplasm with CD4 positivity. Multiple myeloma also will not have this morphology and immunophenotype; in fact, it is very rare to have lymphadenopathy in myeloma.

Cat scratch disease is caused by *Bartonella henselae* and occurs after cat scratch. It commonly presents as tender, swollen lymph nodes near the site of the inoculating bite or scratch or on the neck and is usually limited to one side. This condition is referred to as regional lymphadenopathy and occurs 1–3 weeks after inoculation. Lymphadenopathy in CSD most commonly occurs in the arms, neck, or jaw, but may also occur near the groin or around the ear. Most patients also develop systemic symptoms such as malaise, decreased appetite, and aches. Other associated complaints include headache, chills, muscular pains, joint pains, arthritis, backache, and abdominal pain. It may take 7–14 days, or as long as 2 months, before symptoms appear. Most cases are benign and self-limiting, but lymphadenopathy may persist for several months after other symptoms disappear. The disease usually resolves spontaneously, with or without treatment, in 1 month.

3. Ans. b. From a close contact on a date

Ref: William's 8/e p1199-203

The clinical features of this patient suggest mononucleosis syndrome (Kissing disease) because of the presence of fever, tender lymphadenopathy, splenomegaly, mild pharyngitis, and presence of atypical lymphocytes. Congenital diseases will not present at this age. Hematologic abnormalities include a peripheral blood lymphocytosis, and more than 10% of the leucocytes in blood consist of atypical looking lymphomonocytes. EBV is an etiologic agent. The virus penetrates through the epithelium of the oropharynx. It replicates in the oropharyngeal epithelium cells and B-lymphocytes. The routine test to find out infectious mononucleosis is the Paul-Bunnell test, proving heterophilic antibodies. Other diagnostic tests include anti-EBV, viral capsid antigen (VCA)-IgM/IgG, anti-ÅA-IgM/IgG, and anti-EBNA-IgG.

4. Ans. d. 4+ ketonuria and 4+ proteinuria

Ref: Harrison 17/e p1179, 2977

The patient is having fever and high total leukocyte count (TLC) with left shift and high LAP score which is in favor of leukemoid reaction. The causes of a high LAP score are leukemoid reaction, chronic myeloid leukemia (CML) in accelerated phase/blastic phase (AP/BP), aplastic anemia, Hodgkin lymphoma, and polycythemia vera. Now in this case it cannot be CML because no evidence is suggestive of CML AP/BP, so option a is wrong. There is no evidence of autoimmune disease or any evidence of megaloblastic anemia, so options b and c are also wrong. Viridians streptococci are part of normal flora of the mouth; some species can cause dental caries. Transient bacteremia following eating, tooth-brushing, etc., can lead to infective endocarditis. Viridians streptococcal bacteremia occurs relatively frequently in neutropenic patients, particularly after bone marrow transplant or high-dose chemotherapy. Some may have high fever and sepsis. But this patient is actually having leukemoid reaction, so option e is also wrong. 4+ proteinuria and 4+ ketonuria mean diabetic ketoacidosis, which is a recognized cause of leukemoid reaction, and leukocytosis is commonly found. Causes of leukocytosis include:

- Hemorrhage
- *Drugs*:
  - Use of glucocorticoids
  - Use of granulocyte-colony stimulating factor (G-CSF) or related growth factors
  - All-transretinoic acid
- *Infections*:
  - *Clostridium difficile*
  - Tuberculosis
  - Pertussis
  - Infectious mononucleosis (lymphocyte predominant)
  - Visceral larva migrans (eosinophil predominant)
- Asplenia
- Diabetic ketoacidosis
- Organ necrosis
- Hepatic necrosis
- Ischemic colitis
- As a feature of Trisomy 21 in infancy (incidence of ~10%)
- As a paraneoplastic phenomenon (rare).

5. Ans. b. Red blood cell (RBC) Howell-Jolly bodies
Ref: William's 8/e p820

The postsplenectomy phase is characterized by the presence of leukocytosis, thrombocytosis, Howell-Jolly bodies, Pappenheimer bodies, target cells, and occasional acanthocytes. The most specific finding is the pitted RBCs in wet preparation. Target cells (means increased surface area) are almost always present. Nucleated RBCs are rarely seen on blood films after splenectomy, except in patients with hemolytic anemia. Options a and d are never seen in any type of postsplenectomy. The diagnosis of a postsplenectomy/hyposplenic blood picture can be made reliably by identifying Howell-Jolly bodies in routine Wright-Giemsa-stained blood. These are round basophilic bodies in RBCs that represent residual nuclear material from marrow nucleated RBC precursors that is usually culled out by the spleen. These do not occur in individuals with normally functioning splenic tissue and their presence indicates either (1) an asplenic state or (2) a hypofunctioning splenic tissue as might be seen in a patient with late-stage sickle cell anemia.

6. Ans. c. Group A *Streptococcus* infection
Ref: Harrison's 17/e p1172, 1298, 1543, 1556

Tender lymphadenopathy is not seen in malignancy so options a and b are wrong.

Option e is also wrong because brucellosis usually presents with high-grade fever with generalized lymphadenopathy and the peripheral blood shows high TLC with relative lymphocytosis, but this patient is having neutrophilic leukocytosis. Group A *Streptococcus* infection presents with sore throat and high-grade fever. Enlarged tender anterior cervical lymphadenopathy commonly accompanies exudative pharyngitis. In HIV disease, lymphadenopathy is seen in two settings: (1) acute HIV syndrome and (2) persistent generalized lymphadenopathy (PGL). Acute HIV syndrome is characterized by fever, pharyngitis, and lymphadenopathy (generalized). PGL is characterized by >1 cm lymphadenopathy in two or more extrainguinal sites for >3 months without an obvious cause. So in HIV disease, the lymphadenopathy is usually generalized.

7. Ans. b. Acute myelogenous leukemia (AML)

This diagnosis is very clear by the presence of blasts with Auer rods.

8. Ans. c. Systemic lupus erythematosus (SLE)
Ref: Cullis JO. Diagnosis and management of anaemia of chronic disease: current status. Br J Haematol. 2011;154(3):289-300.

The clinical and biochemical features are suggestive anemia of chronic inflammation. Diverticulosis may present with both chronic and acute blood loss, and both the conditions may show absent iron stores in bone marrow. So, this option is wrong as bone marrow iron stores are increased. Hepatitis C infections usually do not present with anemia; however, they may present with hemolytic anemia particularly after ribavirin therapy. Atrophic gastritis is the later and final stage of chronic autoimmune gastritis which presents with megaloblastic anemia due to the loss of parietal cells. In Fanconi anemia also, there will not be any increased marrow iron stores and age is unusual. This patient is having ACD, so option c is correct.

Anemia of chronic disease is the second most common cause of anemia worldwide and is seen in a variety of inflammatory, infective, and malignant diseases. It is typically normochromic and normocytic, characterized by low serum iron, decreased transferrin saturation, decreased bone marrow sideroblasts, and increased reticuloendothelial iron. The mechanisms that produce the anemia include impaired production of erythropoietin (EPO), blunted marrow erythroid response to EPO, iron-restricted erythropoiesis, and a diminished pool of EPO-responsive cells. Serum iron and transferrin saturation are both decreased in ACD and iron-deficiency, indicating limited iron supply to the erythron, butxx transferrin levels are increased in IDA, whereas in ACD they are normal or decreased. Serum transferrin receptor levels are increased in IDA. The ratio of serum transferrin receptor to the log of the serum ferritin has been proposed to be a useful tool in the diagnosis of ACD and particularly in differentiating ACD from IDA. A ratio <1 makes ACD likely, whereas ratio >2 suggests that iron stores are deficient. The rationale for the use of erythropoiesis-stimulating agents in ACD is based on the blunted EPO response seen in ACD, with lower serum levels of EPO detected than would be expected for the observed degree of anemia, together with the reduced sensitivity of erythroid progenitors to endogenous EPO seen in ACD. Parenteral iron over oral iron has also shown beneficial effects in correcting ACD. Treatment of the underlying inflammatory or malignant process associated with ACD will often result in improvement in the degree of anemia.

9. Ans. a. Chronic lymphocytic leukemia
Ref: William's 8/e p1516-18, 1532

The histology of lymph node in this patient is showing nodular aggregates of small, monomorphic cells which suggest the malignant nature of the pathology. So, the options c and e are wrong. Follicular lymphoma will have a variable mixture of centrocytes (small cleaved cells) and centroblasts (large noncleaved cells). Hodgkin lymphoma will have characteristic large Reed-Sternberg cells, so this option is also wrong. However, in this there is no mention whether there is any monoclonal B-cell (MBC) lymphocytosis, and moreover the TLC is also 7,230 (differential count is not mentioned). So the ideal answer should be small lymphocytic lymphoma (SLL).

Chronic lymphocytic leukemia/small lymphocytic lymphoma is a neoplasm of monomorphic small, round B-lymphocytes in the peripheral blood, bone marrow, and lymph nodes admixed with prolymphocytes and paraimmunoblasts expressing CD5 and CD23. The term SLL is restricted to cases with the tissue morphology and immunophenotype of CLL but without a leukemic component. Diagnosis of CLL requires 5×10^9/L or more peripheral blood MBCs with a CLL phenotype.

10. Ans. a. Myelofibrosis
Ref: Harrison's 17/e p471

Clinically, this patient is having massive splenomegaly without ascites (absent fluid wave/thrill), so the most likely answer would be myelofibrosis. Splenomegaly is absolutely not seen in sickle cell disease and hemochromatosis. In infectious mononucleosis, the splenomegaly is not massive. As he is not having ascites, portal hypertension is also unlikely. The causes of massive splenomegaly are:
- CML
- HCL
- Myelofibrosis
- Portal hypertension
- Chronic malaria
- Storage disorders.

Idiopathic myelofibrosis (IMF) is a bone marrow disease characterized by excessive production of reticulin and collagen fibers. Although fibrosis of bone marrow can be the outcome of numerous hematologic and nonhematologic conditions, the term IMF is commonly used in primary MF without a secondary cause. The clinical signs of IMF include splenomegaly due to extramedullary hematopoiesis; leukocytosis and thrombocytosis, with predisposition to thrombotic events, due to clonal cellular proliferation affecting mainly megakaryocytes and granulocytes; cytopenias, a later finding that worsens with the progression of fibrosis; and constitutional symptoms (e.g., fatigue, weight loss, low-grade fever, night sweats), most likely induced by abnormal levels of circulating cytokines.

11. Ans. c. Thrombotic thrombocytopenic purpura.
Ref: William's 8/e p2166, 2107

Presence of fever, renal failure, schistocytes in peripheral blood, and normal coagulation profile with a low platelet count goes in favor of TTP. Schistocytes can also be seen in disseminated intravascular coagulation (DIC), but the coagulation profile will be abnormal in DIC. In ITP and AIHA, schistocytes will not be seen. Trousseau syndrome is also known as migratory thrombophlebitis seen mostly in case of gastrointestinal (GI) malignancy. This case does not seem to be Trousseau syndrome because of the presence of low platelet count and schistocytes.

Thrombotic thrombocytopenic purpura is characterized by a pentad of thrombocytopenia, microangiopathic hemolytic anemia (MAHA), fluctuating neurological signs, renal impairment, and fever and has insidious onset. The revised diagnostic criteria for TTP state that TTP must be considered even in the presence of thrombocytopenia and MAHA alone, without the pentad being present. Consumption of platelets in platelet-rich thrombi results in thrombocytopenia. Mechanical fragmentation of erythrocytes during flow through partially occluded, high shear small vessels causes a MAHA. The combination of hemolysis and tissue ischemia produces elevated lactate dehydrogenase values, and this has diagnostic and therapeutic implications. In view of the high risk of preventable, early deaths in TTP, treatment with plasma exchange should be initiated as soon as possible, preferably within 4–8 hours, regardless of the time of day at presentation, if a patient presents with a MAHA and thrombocytopenia in the absence of any other identifiable clinical cause (BCSH guidelines, 2012).

12. Ans. e. Chronic lymphocytic leukemia
Ref: William's 8/e p1437-38

This patient has presented with 4 months' history of mild anemia, lymphocytic leukocytosis, generalized lymphadenopathy, and hepatosplenomegaly which suggest the possibility of CLL. He also has DCT positivity which is seen in CLL.

Patients with B-CLL/SLL have a 5–10% risk of developing autoimmune complications which primarily cause cytopenia. These autoimmune cytopenias can occur at any stage of CLL and do not have an independent prognostic significance. The most common autoimmune complication is AIHA with a lower frequency of immune thrombocytopenia and pure red cell aplasia (PRCA) and only rare patients with autoimmune granulocytopenia. The effect of autoimmune cytopenia on prognosis of patients with CLL remains uncertain. There could be multiple possible causes of cytopenia in CLL including bone marrow failure, hypersplenism, chemotherapy, sepsis, and autoimmunity, and the possibility of two or more causes occurring simultaneously requires careful clinical and laboratory assessment. ITP causes particular diagnostic difficulties. There is no sensitive and specific test for ITP to parallel the DAT in AIHA, and thrombocytopenia in CLL is more commonly due to splenomegaly and bone marrow failure secondary to infiltration by disease. In advanced disease, anemia usually occurs before thrombocytopenia, so isolated thrombocytopenia is more likely to be immune in origin.

13. Ans. b. Beta-thalassemia   *Ref: William's 8/e p691*

This patient is having microcytic hypochromic anemia (low MCV) though the blood picture is not mentioned. His marrow is showing a ME ratio of 1:4 which means that there is erythroid hyperplasia which is seen in hemolytic anemia. All the options mentioned are causes of hemolytic anemia, but the associated iron overload is seen only in cases of thalassemia. In fact, iron overload without blood transfusion is seen in thalassemia intermedia syndromes because of increased GI absorption. Disordered iron metabolism is less common in adult forms of alpha thalassemia.

Symptomatic G6PD-deficient patients are almost exclusively male, due to the X-linked pattern of inheritance, but female carriers can be clinically affected due to unfavorable lyonization, where random inactivation of an X-chromosome in certain cells creates a population of G6PD-deficient RBCs coexisting with normal RBCs. The G6PD/NADPH pathway is the *only* source of reduced glutathione in RBCs. Individuals with G6PD deficiency incur a higher risk of acute hemolysis when exposed to certain medications.

Most children and adults with hereditary spherocytosis have mild-to-moderate enlargement of the spleen, but other than assisting in the diagnosis, this is of little clinical significance. Jaundice alters the lipid composition of the RBC membrane, masking the RBC morphology, and reducing hemolysis, but iron overload and hypersplenism are less frequent in hereditary spherocytosis.

14. Ans. c. Numerous mature and immature myeloid cells

This patient presented with 4-month history of weakness, splenomegaly, and leukocytosis with left shift and two blasts with low LAP score which is suggestive of CML, so bone marrow will show panmyelosis with increased myeloid precursors. Bone marrow examination in CML helps in assessing the distribution patterns of megakaryocytes, degree of fibrosis, and number and distribution of blasts.

15. Ans. e. Transfusion therapy

The clinical picture of the patient fits more in an acute transfusion reaction. The etiologies of hemolysis are often categorized as acquired or hereditary. The common acquired causes of hemolytic anemia are autoimmunity, microangiopathy, and infection. Immune-mediated hemolysis, caused by antierythrocyte antibodies, can be secondary to malignancies, autoimmune disorders, drugs, and transfusion reactions. MAHA occurs when the RBC membrane is damaged in circulation, leading to intravascular hemolysis and appearance of schistocytes. Infectious agents such as malaria and babesiosis invade RBCs. Disorders of RBC enzymes, membranes, and hemoglobin cause hereditary hemolytic anemias. G6PD deficiency leads to hemolysis in the presence of oxidative stress. Hereditary spherocytosis is characterized by spherocytes, a family history, and a negative direct antiglobulin test (DAT). Sickle cell anemia and thalassemia are hemoglobinopathies characterized by chronic hemolysis.

Acute transfusion reactions present with adverse signs or symptoms during or within 24 hours of a blood transfusion. The most frequent reactions are fever, chills, pruritus, or urticaria, which typically resolve promptly without specific treatment or complications. Other signs occurring in a temporal relationship with a blood transfusion, such as severe shortness of breath, red urine, high fever, or loss of consciousness, may be the first indication of a more severe potentially fatal reaction. Transfusion reactions require immediate recognition, laboratory investigation, and clinical management. If a transfusion reaction is suspected during blood administration, then stop the transfusion and keep the intravenous line open with 0.9% sodium chloride (normal saline). The transfusion reactions may be early or late and may be hemolytic or nonhemolytic. Though the history of blood transfusion is not provided in the question, the clinical picture presented here fits best in the post-transfusion hemolytic reaction. PRCA usually does not present with high fever and jaundice. History of drug exposure is also important to rule out drug-induced hemolytic anemia.

Drug-induced immune hemolytic anemia (DIIHA) is rare and less common than drug-induced thrombocytopenia and leucopenia, and it can be mild or associated with acute severe hemolytic anemia and death. About 125 drugs have been implicated as the cause. The HA can be caused by drug-independent antibodies that are indistinguishable, in vitro and in vivo, from autoantibodies causing idiopathic warm type AIHA. More commonly, the antibodies are drug dependent (i.e., will only react in vitro in the presence of the drug). The most common drugs to cause DIIHA are antimicrobials (e.g., cefotetan, ceftriaxone, and piperacillin), which are associated with drug-dependent antibodies.

Cold agglutinins (CAs) are antibodies that agglutinate erythrocytes at an optimum temperature of 0–4°C. CA disease is diagnosed when the following criteria are met: chronic hemolysis, CA titer more than 64 at 4°C, and typical findings by the DAT. The typical DAT pattern is defined as a positive polyspecific test with a monospecific test, positive for complement protein C3d and negative (or occasionally weakly positive) for IgG. The reasonable criteria for initiating drug therapy are symptom-producing anemia, transfusion dependence, or disabling circulatory symptoms. The ischemic symptoms may sometimes be sufficiently disabling to justify therapy even if the hemolysis is fully compensated. Peripheral cyanosis can be managed by maintaining warm surroundings.

16. Ans. e. Myelodysplasia

Out of all the options, only myelodysplasia can lead to secondary AML. Secondary AML may arise from the previous clonal disorder of hematopoiesis, usually from myelodysplastic syndrome or from chronic myeloproliferative neoplasia or after exposure to a leukemogenic agent (previous chemotherapy or radiotherapy, some immunosuppressive drugs or environmental leukemogenic agents). Secondary origin of AML is associated with unfavorable prognosis, and it is not considered to be conventionally curable (with the exception of secondary acute promyelocytic leukemia). Patients with secondary AML are older and less commonly treated with curative intention than those with primary AML. According to cytogenetic findings, their prognosis is often worse. Complete hematologic remission is achieved with a low probability, relapse of the disease occurs frequently, and overall survival is worse in almost all prognostic subgroups.

17. Ans. b. Myeloproliferative disorder

Ref: William's 8/e p1896

Epstein-Barr virus infection usually presents in childhood with mononucleosis with presence of atypical lymphoid cells in peripheral smear. Thrombocytopenia is seen and not the thrombocytosis. Drug reaction will not have myeloid hyperplasia in marrow. Wiskott-Aldrich syndrome will have microthrombocytopenia, eczema, recurrent infections, T-cell deficiency, and increased risk of autoimmune and lymphoproliferative disorders. It usually presents in childhood. Megaloblastic anemia will have cytopenia, and moreover bone marrow will show megaloblastosis in erythroid lineages. Platelet dysfunction is known to occur in myeloproliferative neoplasms (MPNs).

Myeloproliferative neoplasms are clonal hematopoietic stem cell disorders characterized by proliferation of one or more myeloid cell lines (granulocytic, erythroid, megakaryocytic, and mast cells). Arterial thrombosis, which accounts for about 60% of events related to MPNs, includes ischemic stroke, acute myocardial infarction, and peripheral arterial occlusion. MPNs are also the most common cause of splanchnic venous thrombosis, accounting for approximately 50% of Budd-Chiari syndrome cases and 25% of portal vein thrombosis. MPNs associated with Budd-Chiari syndrome and portal vein thrombosis have certain unique features compared to classic MPNs, including the onset at a younger age, female predominance in PV, and the presence of normal blood counts, which sometimes renders the diagnosis of MPN quite challenging. Conversely, extreme thrombocytosis (i.e., platelets more than 1500,000/μL) can favor hemorrhagic rather than thrombotic manifestations in MPN. This paradox has been attributed to the possible occurrence of an acquired VWD due to an increased clearance by platelets of the large circulating VWF multimers. Even if platelet count is normal, the platelets are dysfunctional to a certain extent.

18. Ans. e. Microcytic anemia

Ref: William's 8/e p467, 545, 661

The first four types of anemias can be seen after drug ingestion, but the microcytic type of anemia is not caused by any type of drug. Many types of drugs are implicated in the precipitation of anemia in G6PD deficiency. Drugs causing macrocytic anemia are dihydrofolate reductase inhibitors, antimetabolites, anticonvulsants, oral contraceptive pills (OCPs), etc. Many drugs are also known to cause AIHA. Chloramphenicol is implicated in causing aplastic anemia.

19. Ans. e. G6PD deficiency

Ref: William's 8/e p656, 661

The clue to the diagnosis is the drug-induced hemolytic anemia with Heinz bodies and most importantly positive family history with only male persons being affected. G6PD deficiency is one of the most common enzyme deficiencies in humans. It is inherited as an X-recessive linked disorder. G6PD deficiency is polymorphic, with more than 300 variants. G6PD deficiency can present as neonatal hyperbilirubinemia. Persons with this disorder can experience episodes of brisk hemolysis in response to oxidative stresses or, less commonly, have chronic hemolysis. However, many individuals with G6PD deficiency are asymptomatic.

20. Ans. d. Idiopathic thrombocytopenic purpura

Ref: Harrison's 17/e p855

Autoimmune hemolytic anemia, chronic alcohol abuse, and myeloproliferative disorders are all associated with increase in spleen size. Repeated microinfarctions can destroy tissues having microvascular beds prone to sickling. The spleen is frequently lost within the first 18–36 months of life, causing increased risk of infections. Presence of splenomegaly rules out the diagnosis of IPT and aplastic anemia.

21. Ans. a. Hypersegmented neutrophils

This patient is having macrocytic anemia (high MCV) without any significant abnormal finding on examination, so the answer will be megaloblastic anemia. The etiology of the megaloblastic anemia is impaired DNA synthesis and assembly. The most common causes are vitamin B_{12} (cobalamin) or folic acid deficiencies. These substances are essential in the DNA synthesis pathway. The finding of significant macrocytosis (MCV > 100 fL) suggests the presence of megaloblastic anemia. Other causes of macrocytes are hemolysis with increased reticulocytes, liver disease, alcoholism, hypothyroidism, and aplastic anemia; however, the macrocytes in these conditions are round, not oval. If the MCV is over 120 fL, the patient is most likely to have megaloblastic anemia. The neutrophils may show hypersegmentation. The finding of one neutrophil with six lobes signifies megaloblastic anemia (normal neutrophils have—two to four lobes). Large or bizarre misshapen platelets are usually present.

22. **Ans. c. Hypochromasia** *Ref: William's 8/e p573*

This elderly gentleman is having microcytic anemia which could most likely be due to iron deficiency because of chronic GI blood loss. Fragmented RBCs, spherocytes, and nucleated RBCs are all associated with mild indirect hyperbilirubinemia (in this case, total bilirubin is normal). Howell-Jolly bodies are seen after splenectomy, and there is no history of splenectomy. In men and postmenopausal women, iron deficiency is most commonly caused by chronic bleeding from the GI tract. Anisocytosis is an early and prominent finding in iron deficiency, often detectable before significant microcytosis and hypochromia develop. RDW is a measure of anisocytosis and an increased RDW suggests a state of increased anisocytosis as seen in early iron deficiency anemia.

23. **Ans. b. Alpha-thalassemia** *Ref: William's 8/e p636, 694*

This patient presented with anemia at birth with microcytosis, nucleated RBCs, and anisopoikilocytosis in peripheral blood. Out of the options mentioned, hemoglobin E disease and sickle cell disease do not present at birth. G6PD and hereditary elliptocytosis can rarely present at birth. Hereditary elliptocytosis is uncommon in the neonatal period. Typically, elliptocytosis does not appear on the blood film until the patient is 4–6 months old. Occasionally, severe forms of hereditary elliptocytosis present in the neonatal period with severe, hemolytic anemia with marked poikilocytosis and jaundice. Alpha thalassemia is a frequent cause of stillbirth in Southeast Asia. Infants either are stillborn at 34–40 weeks of gestation or are born alive but die within the first few hours. Pallor, edema, and hepatosplenomegaly are seen.

24. **Ans. f. Hereditary hemochromatosis**
Ref: William's 8/e p593-94; Bacon BR. Diagnosis and management of hemochromatosis. Hepatology. 2011.

This patient is having arthropathy, normal Hb with high serum iron, TIBC, and serum ferritin with cardiomegaly and features of heart failure. All these features point toward hereditary hemochromatosis. The other most important differential diagnosis mentioned in the options is anemia of chronic disease, but this is not the answer as there is no anemia and serum iron and TIBC will be low. AIHA will have anemia and spherocytes in the peripheral smear. Beta-thalassemia does not present at this age. Pernicious anemia will present as macrocytic anemia. Hb value is not suggestive of polycythemia.

Hereditary hemochromatosis is a common condition in which excessive iron absorption leads to greatly increased body iron stores. The deposition of iron occurs in parenchymal cells of the liver, heart, pancreas, and other organs. In the majority of patients with overt hereditary hemochromatosis, the first symptoms develop between the ages of 30 and 60 years. Approximately 85–90% of patients who have inherited forms of iron overload are homozygous for the C282Y mutation in *HFE* gene. The clinical manifestations can include the triad of cirrhosis, diabetes, and skin pigmentation (so-called bronze diabetes). Liver biopsy is recommended to stage the degree of liver disease in C282Y homozygotes or compound heterozygotes if liver enzymes (ALT, AST) are elevated or if ferritin is >1,000 μg/L. If there is no family history but hereditary hemochromatosis is suspected, the most useful tests are fasting transferrin saturation and serum ferritin. The transferrin saturation (ratio of serum iron to iron-binding capacity) reflects increased absorption of iron, which is the underlying biological defect in hereditary hemochromatosis. A fasting transferrin saturation >45% is the most sensitive test for hereditary hemochromatosis, and it is unlikely if the ferritin is very high but the transferrin saturation is normal. Siblings of individuals with HH, or siblings of unaffected C282Y homozygotes, have at least a 25% chance of having the same genotype and a 50% chance of being a carrier for the *HFE* mutation.

25. **Ans. a. High LAP**

Ref: See explanation to Q. No. 4

This patient is having active pulmonary tuberculosis with high TLC and left shift in differential count suggestive of leukemoid reaction. So his LAP score will be high. In CML LAP score will be low, so option b is wrong. Peripheral smear is also not suggestive of any lymphoid malignancy, so option e will also be wrong. Elevated D-dimer is suggestive of DIC, but this patient is not having any feature of DIC such as low platelet or schistocytes on peripheral smear. Monoclonal gammopathy will have anemia and rouleaux formation in peripheral smear.

26. **Ans. c. Acute lymphoblastic leukemia (ALL)**

The morphological description of primitive cells in the bone marrow is suggestive of blasts which are positive for CD10 which gives the diagnosis of ALL.

In some studies, ALL has been subdivided into CD10 [the common acute lymphoblastic leukemia antigen (cALLa)] positive and CD10 negative. The majority of B-lineage ALL cases express CD10. In B-lineage ALL, the percentage of cells expressing CD10 decreases in more mature forms. A positive CD10 expression is associated with a favorable clinical outcome.

27. Ans. e. Hemolytic anemia

Presence of jaundice and anemia with nucleated RBCs in peripheral smear is highly suggestive of hemolytic anemia. IDA will have low MCV and pernicious anemia will have high MCV. Mild jaundice may be seen in pernicious anemia. ACD usually has normocytic normochromic anemia, but there will not be any icterus, so this option is also wrong. Sickle cell disease does not present at this age.

28. Ans. e. Increased serum erythropoietin

Ref: William's 8/e p829

This patient is having renal mass with high Hb which may be suggestive of some tumor of kidney which secretes erythropoietin and causes secondary polycythemia. Absolute erythrocytosis is seen in solitary renal cysts, polycystic renal disease, or hydronephrosis. In patients with pheochromocytoma/paraganglionoma with erythrocytosis, erythropoietin assays of serum and urine show higher than normal values which are due to increased EPO production by the tumor cells.

29. Ans. a. Aplastic anemia

This patient is having pancytopenia without hepatosplenomegaly and lymphadenopathy, so the options hereditary spherocytosis, MPN, large cell lymphoma, and ITP are all ruled out.

30. Ans. b. Mycosis fungoides

Ref: William's 8/e p1484, 1596-97

This patient is having generalized erythrodermatous lesions which are infiltrated by malignant T cells, so the answer is mycosis fungoides. Skin lesions in this disease show distinct stages from patch to plaque to nodule or diffuse erythroderma, and the lesions progress in the above sequence. They arise from mature helper T cells with the immunophenotype of CD3+CD4+CD45RO+CD8–. CD4 is a marker of mature T cells. CD7 is characteristically absent. Burkitt lymphoma and Hodgkin lymphoma will not show CD4 positivity. ALL is an immature lymphoid cell malignancy. HCL is also a B-cell malignancy. Moreover, skin involvement is not seen in all these malignancies. Skin lesions in HCL are cutaneous vasculitic type of lesions.

Various cutaneous lesions can be observed in patients with hematologic malignancies. Leukemia cutis is an infiltration of neoplastic leukocytes into the skin, presenting as deep red or purple plaques or nodules. Sweet's syndrome and pyoderma gangrenosum are the most common of the neutrophilic dermatoses. They are cutaneous disorders characterized pathologically by superficial or deep dermal infiltrates of normal appearing neutrophils with no evidence of sepsis.

31. Ans. c. Hairy cell leukemia

Ref: Hum Pathol. 2005;36:945

The patient has presented with pancytopenia with massive splenomegaly, and the characteristic TRAP (tartrate-resistant acid phosphatase) positive lymphocytes in the peripheral blood points toward the diagnosis of HCL. TRAP can be positive in HCL, mantle cell lymphoma (57%), splenic marginal zone lymphoma (some), primary mediastinal B cell lymphoma (54%), CLL/SLL (41%), and giant cells in giant cell tumor of bone and soft-tissue.

32. Ans. e. Elevated free erythrocyte protoporphyrin

Ref: William's 8/e p582, 765

This patient is having microcytic hypochromic anemia without hepatosplenomegaly with a low haptoglobin level (normal range 41–165 mg/dL) also suggestive of some hemolysis and RBCs showing basophilic stippling. The causes of basophilic stippling are:
- Sideroblastic anemia
- Lead poisoning (microcytic anemia)
- Arsenic poisoning
- Beta thalassemia (though some have questioned this)
- Alpha-thalassemia, hemoglobin H (HbH) disease
- Hereditary pyrimidine 5'-nucleotidase deficiency.

Thalassemia will have hepatosplenomegaly. So, the only option left is chronic lead poisoning. Anemia of chronic lead poisoning is mild in adults but is frequently severe in children. The RBCs are normocytic and slightly hypochromic (because of coexistent iron deficiency). Basophilic stippling may be fine or coarse. Young cells are more likely to be stippled. Lead poisoning can be detected by erythrocyte or free protoporphyrin levels, principally zinc protoporphyrin level. This test cannot differentiate between iron-deficiency and lead poisoning.

33. Ans. d. Langerhans cell histiocytosis (LCH)

Ref: Weitzman S, Egeler RM. Langerhans cell histiocytosis: update for the pediatrician. Curr Opin Pediatr. 2008;20(1):23-9.

The characteristic macrophage like cells with CD1a positivity and presence of Birbeck granule points toward the diagnosis of LCH.

Langerhans cell histiocytosis, a disorder of antigen-presenting cells, is the most common disorder of the mononuclear phagocytic system. The disease varies widely in clinical presentation from localized involvement of a single bone to a widely disseminated life-threatening disease. In LCH, the pathologic LCH cells appear to be in an arrested state of activation and/or differentiation. LCH cells are prevented from leaving their peripheral tissue sites, where they accumulate and express inflammatory chemokines, resulting in their own recruitment and retention as well as that of other inflammatory cells including T lymphocytes. The classical radiologic finding is a punched-out lytic lesion in bone. Biopsy is necessary to confirm the diagnosis.

34. Ans. a. Non-Hodgkin lymphoma (NHL)

This elderly lady is having a cold type of AIHA with significant weight loss with just palpable splenomegaly which points toward the diagnosis of NHL, particularly B-cell type. AIHA can be classified based on the characteristics of the autoantibody. Warm autoantibodies have optimum affinity for RBCs at 37°C. In contrast, cold autoantibodies have optimum affinity for RBCs at lower temperatures. AIHA associated with CLL is usually of the warm type. Waldenström's macroglobulinemia is the most common lymphoproliferative disorder associated with cold AIHA.

35. Ans. d. Missense

This patient is having sickle cell disease which is caused by a point mutation leading to change of glutamic acid by valine at 6th position in the beta chain of hemoglobin. The genetic disorder is due to the mutation of a single nucleotide, from a GAG to GTG codon mutation. This is normally a benign mutation, causing "no" apparent effects on the secondary, tertiary, or quaternary structure of hemoglobin. What it does allow for, under conditions of low oxygen concentration, is the polymerization of the HbS itself. Point mutations can be of these types:
- *Silent mutations*: Which code for the same (or a sufficiently similar) amino acid
- *Missense mutations*: Which code for a different amino acid
- *Nonsense mutations*: Which code for a stop codon and can truncate the protein.

36. Ans. d. HIV-1 RNA of 80,000 copies/mL

Ref: William's 8/e p1188

This patient is a case of primary central nervous system (PCNS) lymphoma and approximately 75% have far advanced disease, with median CD4+ count <50/μL and a prior history of AIDS. Radiographic scanning reveals relatively large mass lesions (2–4 cm) with ring enhancement. Pathologically, all such lymphomas are of the DLBCL type (immunoblastic type) and are uniformly associated with EBV infection in malignant cells. Detection of EBV DNA in CSF may be used as diagnostic criteria for the diagnosis of PCNS lymphoma.

37. Ans. b. Systemic lupus erythematosus

Ref: Giannouli S. Anemia in systemic lupus erythematosus: from pathophysiology to clinical assessment. BMJ. 2005.

Clinically, this patient is having hemolytic anemia with intravascular hemolysis and features of SLE (presence of rash). In some AIHA, the hemolysis can be intravascular. The major hematological manifestations of SLE are anemia, leucopenia, thrombocytopenia, and antiphospholipid syndrome. AIHA may manifest in SLE patients at the time of diagnosis or within the first year of the disease. Anemia is found in approximately 50% of patients, with ACD being the most common form. Overt AIHA is characterized by an elevated reticulocyte count, low haptoglobin levels, increased indirect bilirubin concentration, and a positive DCT, which have been noted in up to 10% of patients with SLE. The AIHA in SLE patients is seldom severe and rarely fatal as prednisolone is usually sufficient in controlling hemolysis.

38. Ans. c. High-grade B-cell lymphoma

Ref: Williams 8/e; Hoffman 6/e

The malignancy most likely to be present in a patient with HIV disease is high-grade B-cell lymphoma of the immunoblastic type. In the GI tract, it can present with obstruction. GI tract involvement is seen in 25% of cases. All other options mentioned do not have an increased incidence in case of HIV disease. AIDS-related lymphoma can be divided into three types on the basis of areas of involvement: (1) systemic NHL, (2) primary central nervous system lymphoma (PCNSL), and (3) primary effusion lymphomas (body cavity lymphoma). Histologically, the most common variants are diffuse, large B-cell lymphoma and small, noncleaved cell lymphoma, including Burkitt and/or Burkitt-like lymphoma. Treatment involves chemotherapy regimens combined with highly active antiretroviral therapy.

39. Ans. e. RBC inclusions

Ref: De Porto. Assessment of splenic function. EJCMID, 2010:29;1465–73.

Various RBC inclusions and structural changes can be seen in RBCs post splenectomy. Hematological methods reflect the capacity of the spleen to phagocytose deviant erythrocytes and to facilitate an environment wherein erythrocytes rid themselves of solid waste material. Large amounts of thrombocytes and leukocytes normally reside in the spleen. Circulating thrombocyte- and leukocyte counts can either be increased or decreased, indicative of hyposplenism in a patient with a dysfunctional spleen (for example, thrombocytosis in asplenia and thrombopaenia associated with splenomegaly). One of the first methods available to evaluate splenic function was the detection of erythrocytes containing Howell–Jolly bodies. Other abnormalities that can be seen on peripheral blood smears of patients with absent or diminished splenic function are pitted RBCs, acanthocytes (spur cells), target cells (codocytes: erythrocytes with a pattern of central staining, a ring of pallor and an outer ring of staining), haemoglobin remnants (Heinz bodies), siderocytes and iron granulocytes (Pappenheimer bodies).

40. Ans. c. Epstein-Barr virus

Presence of mandibular mass, small noncleaved cells, and t(8;14) points toward the diagnosis of Burkitt lymphoma of the endemic type which is always associated with EBV. The particular epidemiological features of Burkitt lymphoma initiated the search for a virus as the causative agent and led to the discovery of EBV by Epstein and coworkers in 1964. The finding that EBV is a transforming virus that is present in nearly every Burkitt lymphoma cell had strongly supported EBV's role as a tumor virus in the development of Burkitt lymphoma. While EBV is associated with 98% of endemic Burkitt lymphoma, it is also seen in 20% of sporadic cases and 30–40% of HIV-associated cases.

41. Ans. c. Glanzmann thrombasthenia

Ref: Hoffman 6/e p1995

In Bernard-Soulier syndrome, the platelet will not show any aggregation in the presence of ristocetin and normal aggregation with all other agonists and reverse is seen in case of GT, so the answer is GT. Hemophilia A is usually not present in females and AT-III deficiency is present with thrombosis. VWD will have prolonged activated partial thromboplastin time (aPTT), and platelet function test will be normal.

Glanzmann thrombasthenia is a rare autosomal recessive disorder characterized by qualitative or quantitative abnormalities of the platelet membrane glycoprotein (GP) IIb/IIIa. Physiologically, this platelet receptor normally binds several adhesive plasma proteins, and this facilitates attachment and aggregation of platelets to ensure thrombus formation at sites of vascular injury. The lack of resultant platelet aggregation in GT leads to mucocutaneous bleeding whose manifestation may be clinically variable, ranging from easy bruising to severe and potentially life-threatening hemorrhages.

Bernard-Soulier syndrome is a severe bleeding disease due to a defect of GPIb/IX/V, a platelet complex that binds the von Willebrand factor. It is usually transmitted as a recessive trait with giant platelets and severe bleeding tendency.

42. Ans. d. Chronic alcohol abuse *Ref: William's 8/e p545*

This patient is having long-standing macrocytic anemia with target cells without any significant finding on examination. There is no evidence of CLL on peripheral smear examination without any lymphocytosis. Chronic lead poisoning will lead to hemolytic anemia and anemia is usually of the microcytic hypochromic type. Peptic ulcer disease will have microcytic anemia owing to chronic blood loss leading to iron-deficiency. There is no evidence of hemolysis with normal DCT/ICT, so option e is also wrong. Chronic alcohol abuse can have folate and thiamine deficiency. The normal serum folate levels are 6–20 ng/mL (13.5–45.3 nmol/L). RBC folate less than 100 ng/mL is considered as deficient. Measurement of RBC folate gives a better idea about tissue folate stores than serum folate levels and is preferred. Folate deficiency does not usually produce neurological problems but vitamin B_{12} deficiency does. Folate and B_{12} deficiency can be present at the same time. If B_{12} deficiency is treated with folate by mistake, the symptoms of anemia may lessen, but the neurological problems can become worse. Alcohol interferes with the absorption of folate.

43. Ans. d. CD55

This patient is having anemia and hemoglobinuria with mesenteric vein thrombosis which is highly suggestive of paroxysmal nocturnal hemoglobinuria (PNH), so the option is d. Hemolysis in PNH results from the increased susceptibility of PNH erythrocytes to complement-mediated lysis, due to a reduction, or absence, of two important glycophosphatidylinositol (GPI)-anchored complement regulatory membrane proteins CD55 and CD59. Thrombosis—the leading cause of death in PNH—occurs in up to 40% of patients. Venous thrombosis in PNH can occur anywhere, with the abdominal veins (hepatic, portal, splenic, and mesenteric) and the cerebral veins being the most common sites. Patients with a large PNH cell population (60% of granulocytes) seem to be at the greatest risk for thrombosis. The Ham test and the sucrose hemolysis test (sugar water test) were two of the first assays used to diagnosis PNH. Both assays are performed on erythrocytes and discriminate PNH cells from normal cells on the basis of their greater sensitivity to the hemolytic action of complements. These assays are relatively insensitive and nonspecific. Flow cytometric analysis of granulocytes is the best way to diagnose PNH.

44. Ans. c. Hyper IgM syndrome

The hyper IgM syndromes are a group of rare inherited immune deficiency disorders characterized by impairment of immunoglobulin isotype switching resulting from defects in the CD40 ligand/CD40 signaling pathway. Diagnosis of hyper-IgM syndrome is suspected based on clinical criteria, including recurrent sinopulmonary infections, chronic diarrhea, and lymphoid hyperplasia. Serum Ig levels are measured; normal or elevated serum IgM levels and low levels or absence of other immunoglobulins support the diagnosis. Flow cytometry testing of CD40 ligand expression on T-cell surfaces should be done. When possible, the diagnosis is confirmed by genetic testing. Immunoglobulin replacement therapy should be initiated on diagnosis and will largely correct the clinical consequences of humoral immunodeficiency. The mainstay of corrective therapy is bone marrow transplantation.

45. **Ans. c. Drug induced thrombocytopenia**

Ref: Hoffman's 6/e p1913-18

He has heparin-induced thrombocytopenia. In about 5% of patients exposed to any kind of heparin, antibodies develop to a complex of platelet factor 4 with heparin, and in 5-14 days there is a marked drop in platelet count. The feared complication is thrombosis ('white clot' syndrome), which can be arterial or venous, and in this patient a thrombotic stroke is likely to have occurred. Low molecular weight heparin or Fondaparinux are less likely to have this complication, but still can occur. Most patients with HIT have moderate thrombocytopenia. The median platelet count nadir is approximately 60,000/cumm; for 90% of patients, the platelet count nadir is greater than 20,000/cumm. The treatment is to avoid any kind of heparin and use DTIs (Direct Thrombin Inhibitors) if clinically anti-coagulation is needed.

46. **Ans. a. Parvovirus infection**

Ref: Hoffman's 6/e p 599

The findings in this case are typical of hereditary spherocytosis with superadded parvovirus infection. Parvovirus B19 infects erythroid precursors and can lead to an aplastic crisis in persons with hemoglobinopathies. The hemoglobinopathy impairs the marrow ability to respond to the stress of the acute infection. Most HS patients have either mild to moderate anemia or no anemia at all. Some patients of non-dominant HS can have very severe anemia. MCV of HS cells is low normal or slightly low and the MCHC is usually increased (>35 g/dL). The finding of an MCHC greater than 35.4 g/dL combined with RDW less than 14% is an excellent screening test for HS. Usually there are associated features of hemolysis like high LDH, elevated indirect bilirubin and reticulocytosis. But in case of Parvovirus infection there can be reticulocytopenia. This infection (erythema infectiosum, fifth disease) manifests with fever, chills, lethargy, malaise, nausea, vomiting, abdominal pain with occasional diarrhea, respiratory symptoms, muscle and joint pain and a maculopapular rash on face (slapped cheek appearance). The virus selectively affects erythroid precursors and inhibits their growth.

47. **Ans. d. Hereditary hemochromatosis**

Ref: Hoffman's 6/e p445-47

Hereditary hemochromatosis results from increased iron absorbtion with markedly increased iron stores. The iron accumulation in tissues results in manifestations such as hepatomegaly, skin pigmentation, diabetes mellitus, heart disease, arthritis, and hypogonadism.

SECTION 10
Novel Therapies

44. Novel Therapies

CHAPTER 44

Novel Therapies

1. **Caplacizumab is used for:**
   a. Thrombotic thrombocytopenic purpura (TTP)
   b. Paroxysmal nocturnal hemoglobinuria (PNH)
   c. Hemophilia
   d. Antiphospholipid antibody syndrome

2. **Ravulizumab is used for:**
   a. Thrombotic thrombocytopenic purpura
   b. Paroxysmal nocturnal hemoglobinuria
   c. Hemophilia
   d. Antiphospholipid antibody syndrome

3. **Emicizumab is used for:**
   a. Thrombotic thrombocytopenic purpura
   b. Paroxysmal nocturnal hemoglobinuria
   c. Hemophilia
   d. Antiphospholipid antibody syndrome

4. **Fostamatinib is used for:**
   a. Immune thrombocytopenia (ITP)
   b. Chronic myeloid leukemia (CML)
   c. Mastocytosis
   d. Eosinophilia

5. **True about blinatumomab is:**
   a. Antibody conjugated to the cytotoxin calicheamicin
   b. Antibody conjugated to bacterial or plant toxin
   c. Bispecific antibody
   d. Antibody active against both B and T cells

6. **Tocilizumab is an:**
   a. Interleukin-2 (IL-2) receptor antibody
   b. IL-4 receptor antibody
   c. IL-6 receptor antibody
   d. IL-22 receptor antibody

7. **Ruxolitinib is used in:**
   a. Polycythemia vera
   b. Myelofibrosis
   c. Acute graft-versus-host disease (GVHD)
   d. All of the above

8. **Crizanlizumab is used in:**
   a. Multiple myeloma
   b. Hodgkin lymphoma
   c. Peripheral T-cell lymphoma
   d. Mantle cell lymphoma
   e. Sickle cell anemia

9. **L-glutamine therapy is useful for:**
   a. Immune thrombocytopenia
   b. Sickle cell disease
   c. Aplastic anemia
   d. Hemophilia

10. **What is the mechanism of action of voxelotor?**
    a. Molecules targeting hemolysis-induced vasculopathy
    b. Agents that modulate the abnormal vascular tone
    c. Molecules that prevent sickling
    d. Molecules specifically interfering with sickle cell–endothelial adhesive mechanisms
    e. Antioxidant agent

11. **Idelalisib is used in all, except:**
    a. Relapsed CLL
    b. Relapsed follicular B cell
    c. Chronic lymphocytic leukemia with 17p deletions
    d. Acute myeloid leukemia
    e. All of the above

12. **Differentiation syndrome is seen with:**
    a. Enasidenib   b. Idelalisib
    c. Alemtuzumab   d. Blinatumomab
    e. Daratumumab

13. **Crizotinib is used for:**
    a. Anaplastic large cell lymphoma
    b. Cutaneous T-cell lymphoma
    c. Natural killer (NK)–T-cell lymphoma
    d. Angioimmunoblastic T-cell lymphoma

14. **Vorinostat is a:**
    a. IDH1 inhibitor
    b. Histone deacetylase (HDAC) inhibitor
    c. JAK-STAT (Janus kinase/signal transducers and activators of transcription) inhibitor
    d. IKROS inhibitor

15. **Bevacizumab is used for:**
    a. Peripheral T-cell lymphoma, not otherwise specified
    b. Anaplastic large cell lymphoma, primary systemic type
    c. Angioimmunoblastic T-cell lymphoma
    d. Hepatosplenic T-cell lymphoma

16. **Siplizumab is a monoclonal antibody against:**
    a. CD2
    b. CD3
    c. CD4
    d. CD5

17. **Emapalumab is used for the treatment of:**
    a. Hemophagocytic lymphohistiocytosis
    b. Paroxysmal nocturnal hemoglobinuria
    c. Sézary syndrome
    d. Multiple myeloma
    e. Mantle cell lymphoma

18. **Which of the following is a telomerase inhibitor?**
    a. Imetelstat
    b. Roxadustat
    c. Luspatercept
    d. Idelalisib

19. **The drug used of reversal of dabigatran-induced bleeding is:**
    a. Idarucizumab
    b. Adalimumab
    c. Bezlotoxumab
    d. Daclizumab
    e. Natalizumab

20. **Brentuximab vedotin (BV) in not indicated for:**
    a. Relapsed anaplastic large cell lymphoma
    b. Cutaneous large cell lymphoma
    c. Relapsed CD30 expressing mycosis fungoides
    d. Refractory CD30 expressing diffuse large B-cell lymphoma (DLBCL)

21. **All are notable side effects associated with BV, except:**
    a. Progressive multifocal leukoencephalopathy
    b. Infusional toxicity
    c. Myelosuppression
    d. Cerebral hemorrhage

22. **All are BiTE (Bispecific T cell Engager) antibodies, except:**
    a. Blinatumomab
    b. Ipilimumab
    c. Panitumumab
    d. Cetuximab

23. **Check-point inhibitors are targeted against all of the following, except:**
    a. Cytotoxic T-lymphocyte-associated protein 4 (CTLA-4)
    b. Programmed death-1 (PD-1)
    c. Programmed death-ligand 1 (PDL1)
    d. CD28

24. **All are used in treatment of hemophilia A, except:**
    a. Mononine
    b. Emicizumab
    c. Eloctate
    d. Adynovate

25. **Plerixafor acts by binding to:**
    a. CXCR4
    b. Stromal cell-derived factor 1 (SDF1)-alpha
    c. C-X-C motif chemokine 12 (CXCL)-12
    d. C-C chemokine receptor type 5 (CCR5)

26. **True about asciminib is:**
    a. Mechanism of action is similar to that of imatinib
    b. Not effective in T315I mutation
    c. It cannot be combined with other TKI inhibitors
    d. It is an allosteric inhibitor
    e. All of the above

27. **Mechanism of action of daratumumab includes all, except:**
    a. Complement-dependent cytotoxicity
    b. Proteasome inhibition
    c. Antibody-dependent cellular toxicity
    d. Antibody-dependent cellular phagocytosis

28. **Patients on daratumumab need monitoring for all of the following, except:**
    a. Serial two-dimensional (2D) echo monitoring for the risk of cardiomyopathy
    b. Baseline Rh and Kell typing
    c. Infusion-related allergic reactions
    d. Interference in response assessment by serum protein electrophoresis due to daratumumab detection in protein electrophoresis assay

29. **The 2019 Nobel Prize for Medicine to William Kaelin, Sir Peter Ratcliffe, and Gregg Semenza was given for the discovery of:**
    a. The discovery of Philadelphia chromosome and identification of BCR-ABL as a therapeutic target in CML
    b. The discovery of hypoxia inducible factor alpha (HIF 1 alpha) and its role in adaptation to oxygen availability
    c. The discovery of arsenic trioxide as a therapeutic agent in acute promyelocytic leukemia
    d. Their work on gene therapy in hemophilia

30. **Identify the correct disease and CAR-T cell target combination:**
    a. Chronic lymphocytic leukemia: CD5
    b. Acute myeloid leukemia: CD 125
    c. Multiple myeloma: B-cell maturation antigen (BCMA)
    d. Diffuse large B-cell lymphoma: CD 45

31. **True regarding tazemetostat:**
    a. Is an EZH2 inhibitor
    b. Used in patients with relapsed or refractory (R/R) follicular lymphoma
    c. Second primary malignancy can occur
    d. All of the above

32. **Magrolimab is a:**
    a. Anti-CD52 monoclonal antibody
    b. Anti CD47 monoclonal antibody
    c. Anti-CD56 monoclonal antibody
    d. Anti-CD200 monoclonal antibody

33. **Tafasitamab is recommended for:**
    a. Immune thrombocytopenia
    b. Diffuse large B cell lymphoma

c. Acute myeloid leukemia
d. Paroxysmal nocturnal hemoglobinuria

34. Selinexor acts by:
a. Inhibiting exportin
b. Inhibiting vascular endothelial growth factor
c. Inhibiting RANK1
d. Inhibiting signaling lymphocytic activation molecule family member 7 (SLAMF7)

35. True about selinexor is:
a. Parenteral administration
b. Most common toxicity is gastrointestinal
c. Hypoglycemia common
d. None of the above

36. Which of the following JAK-2 inhoibitor is best suited for patient with myelofibrosis with thrombocytopenia?
a. Momelotinib
b. Ruxolitinib
c. Fedratinib
d. Pacritinib

37. Anlotinib inhibits:
a. Vascular endothelial growth factor receptor
b. Fibroblast growth factor receptor
c. Platelet-derived growth factor receptors
d. c-kit
e. All of the above

38. Ulocuplumab acts by inhibiting:
a. CXCR4
b. PDGFRA
c. PDGFRB
d. VEGF
e. All of the above

39. Moxetumomab pasudotox is a drug approved for HCL. What is the devastating side effect seen with the drug?
a. HUS
b. Arrhythmia
c. Thrombosis
d. Bone marrow aplasia

40. Which of the following is a newly approved drug for high risk myelodysplastic syndrome (MDS)?
a. Pevonedistat
b. Venetoclax
c. Magrolimab
d. Cedazuridine

ANSWERS WITH EXPLANATIONS

1. Ans. a. Thrombotic thrombocytopenic purpura (TTP)

Ref: Scully M. Caplacizumab treatment for acquired thrombotic thrombocytopenic purpura. N Engl J Med. 2019;380:335-46.

In acquired TTP, an immune-mediated deficiency of the von Willebrand factor (VWF) cleaving protease ADAMTS13 allows unrestrained adhesion of VWF multimers to platelets and microthrombosis, which result in thrombocytopenia, hemolytic anemia, and tissue ischemia. Caplacizumab, an anti-VWF factor humanized, bivalent immunoglobulin (Ig) fragment, inhibits interaction between VWF multimers and platelets by binding to A1 domain of VWF. Treatment with caplacizumab is associated with faster normalization of the platelet count, a lower incidence of TTP-related deaths, recurrence of TTP, or a thromboembolic event. Since caplacizumab interferes with VWF, a key protein in hemostasis, it is associated with mucocutaneous bleeding similar to that observed in patients with von Willebrand disease.

2. Ans. b. Paroxysmal nocturnal hemoglobinuria

Ref: Roth A. Ravulizumab in patients with paroxysmal nocturnal hemoglobinuria. Blood Adv. 2018;2:2176-85.

Ravulizumab is a long-acting C5 complement inhibitor. After eculizumab, ravulizumab has been approved for PNH. Compared to eculizumab, ravulizumab is noninferior, with no patients undergoing a transfusion and all patients having similar incidence of hemolysis. The benefit is that ravulizumab achieves similar outcomes while being administered only once every 8 weeks, while eculizumab needs to be given once every 2 weeks.

3. Ans. c. Hemophilia

Ref: Weyand AC. New therapies for hemophilia. Blood. 2019;133(5):389-98.

Hemophilia A is characterized by impaired or absent expression of factor VIII (FVIII). It has long been managed *via* direct factor replacement. Functionally, FVIII acts as a cofactor for factor IXa and allows activation of factor X, which, in combination with factor V, generates thrombin. Emicizumab, a bispecific monoclonal antibody that acts as a substitutive therapy for hemophilia A, has been approved for patients with and without inhibitors. It is capable of recognizing and binding to two distinct antigenic targets simultaneously. It binds factors IXa and X, resulting in spatial approximation and activation of factor X, thereby mimicking the actions of FVIII. Emicizumab enhances the generation of factor Xa and does so by behaving like constantly activated factor VIIIa. The presence of antifactor VIII antibodies (inhibitors) impacts neither the mechanism nor the efficacy by which emicizumab functions. The US Food and Drug Administration (FDA) has approved emicizumab as prophylaxis to prevent or reduce the frequency of bleeding episodes in adult and pediatric patients with hemophilia A with or without FVIII inhibitors. The half-life of emicizumab is approximately 28 days. It is given subcutaneously once per week. The most common adverse events experienced are injection-site reaction, hematoma, bruising, erythema, induration, pruritus, or rash and rarely thrombotic microangiopathy and thromboembolism.

4. Ans. a. Immune thrombocytopenia (ITP)

Ref: Bussel J. Fostamatinib for the treatment of adult persistent and chronic ITP. Am J Hematol. 2018;93(7):921-30.

Fostamatinib is an oral spleen tyrosine kinase (SYK) inhibitor that received FDA approval for the treatment of chronic ITP in adults. SYK signaling is a critical step in phagocytosis of Fc receptor-bound, antibody-coated platelets, and blockade with fostamatinib has shown favorable results. Fostamatinib has a unique mechanism of action, dissimilar to other approved ITP therapies, and has produced responses in patients who had relapsed or not responded to thrombopoietin-receptor agonists (TPO-RAs) (eltrombopag), rituximab, and/or splenectomy.

5. Ans. c. Bispecific antibody

Ref: Kantarjian H. Blinatumomab versus chemotherapy for advanced acute lymphoblastic leukemia. N Engl J Med. 2017;376:836-47.

Blinatumomab is a bispecific antibody that redirects host cytotoxic T cells to cancer cells that express cluster of differentiation 19 (CD19) on their surface. Blinatumomab contains the variable domains of a CD19 antibody and a CD3 antibody, which are joined by a nonimmunogenic linker. On binding to CD19, the cytotoxic T cells become activated and induce cell death via the pore-forming perforin system. Inotuzumab ozogamicin is the antibody conjugated to the cytotoxin calicheamicin, which is a potent cytotoxic compound that induces double-strand DNA breaks. Immunotoxins are proteins that consist of two primary components: a targeting moiety for cell binding and a bacterial or plant toxin that is internalized and causes cell death. Moxetumomab pasudotox is an immunotoxin.

Alemtuzumab is a humanized monoclonal antibody against CD52. CD52 is expressed in 30–60% of leukemia cases, including B and T *acute lymphocytic leukemia* (ALL) and acute myeloid leukemia (AML). CD52 expression is particularly high on T-cell prolymphocytic leukemia (T-PLL), Sézary syndrome, ALL, chronic lymphocytic leukemia (CLL), and AML, which is the reason why it was selected as therapeutic target despite not having a clear role in the pathogenesis of these conditions.

6. Ans. c. IL-6 receptor antibody

Ref: Le RQ. Tocilizumab for treatment of CAR-T cell induced CRS. Oncologist. 2018.

Tocilizumab is a humanized monoclonal antibody against both the soluble and membrane-bound IL-6 receptors. Tocilizumab demonstrates impressive efficacy in the management of chimeric antigen receptor T (CAR-T) cell-related cytokine release syndrome (CRS). Tocilizumab does not attenuate symptoms of neurotoxicity and is currently not FDA approved for the treatment of CAR-T cell-related encephalopathy syndrome.

Cytokine release syndrome in the setting of CAR-T cell therapy manifests as a wide constellation of symptoms with multiorgan involvement. CRS can vary from a mild, self-limited course to a life-threatening systemic inflammatory response which, in severe cases, may be associated with manifestations similar to those seen in hemophagocytic lymphohistiocytosis (HLH). Tocilizumab, an antihuman IL-6 receptor antibody, has become a widely accepted pharmacologic intervention of first choice in severe CRS based on the observation of elevated levels of inflammatory cytokines, most notably IL-6 and interferon (IFN)-γ.

7. Ans. d. All of the above

Ref: Hofmann 7/e

Ruxolitinib, the Janus kinase (JAK) 1 and 2 inhibitor, and has demonstrated effectivity in reducing splenomegaly and constitutional symptoms in patients with primary myelofibrosis and in those with polycythemia vera resistant or intolerant to hydroxyurea. Ruxolitinib exerts its anti-JAK activity by competitive inhibition of the ATP-binding catalytic site of the kinase domain. Ruxolitinib has also been found to be effective in acute and chronic GVHD. Ruxolitinib reduces the proliferation of T-effector cells and mediates suppression of proinflammatory cytokine production.

8. Ans. e. Sickle cell anemia

Ref: Ataga KI. Crizanlizumab for the prevention of pain crises in sickle cell disease. N Engl J Med. 2017;376:429-39.

In patients with sickle cell disease (SCD), crizanlizumab therapy results in a significantly lower rate of sickle cell-related pain crises. The prevention of crises could minimize or prevent tissue and organ damage and decrease the subsequent risk of death among patients with SCD. Vaso-occlusion and crises are caused by the adhesion of sickle erythrocytes and leukocytes to the endothelium, which results in vascular obstruction and tissue ischemia. P-selectin is found in storage granules of resting endothelial cells and platelets and is rapidly transferred to the cell membrane on activation of the cell during processes such as inflammation. P-selectin that is expressed on the surface of the endothelium mediates abnormal rolling and static adhesion of sickle erythrocytes to the vessel surface. The upregulation of P-selectin in endothelial cells and platelets contributes to the cell—cell interactions that are involved in the pathogenesis of vaso-occlusion and sickle cell-related pain crises.

Crizanlizumab is a humanized monoclonal antibody that binds to P-selectin and blocks its interaction with P-selectin glycoprotein ligand 1.

9. Ans. b. Sickle cell disease

Ref: Nijhara Y. l-Glutamine in sickle cell disease. N Engl J Med. 2018;379(3):226-35.

Oxidative stress contributes to the complex pathophysiology of SCD. Oral therapy with pharmaceutical-grade L-glutamine (glutamine) has been shown to increase the proportion of the reduced form of nicotinamide adenine dinucleotides (NADs) in sickle cell erythrocytes, which probably reduces oxidative stress and could result in fewer episodes of sickle cell-related pain. Glutamine is involved in glutathione metabolism since it preserves nicotinamide adenine dinucleotide phosphate (NADPH) levels required for glutathione recycling, and it is the precursor for NAD and arginine.

10. Ans. c. Molecules that prevent sickling

Ref: Vichinsky E. A phase 3 randomized trial of voxelotor in sickle cell disease. NEJM 2019;381(6):509-19.

Voxelotor is a novel hemoglobin S polymerization inhibitor. It increases hemoglobin's affinity for oxygen, thereby blocking polymerization and the subsequent sickling of red blood cells (antisickling agent). By increasing hemoglobin, voxelotor may reduce the likelihood of strokes in patients with SCD.

11. Ans. d. Acute myeloid leukemia

Ref: Miller BW. FDA approval: idelalisib monotherapy for the treatment of patients with follicular lymphoma and small lymphocytic lymphoma. Clin Can Res. 2015;21(7):1525-9.

The phosphoinositide 3-kinase (PI3K) plays a major role in many aspects of cellular biology and is often hyperactivated in human cancers. The targeted inhibition of PI3K-delta is designed to preserve PI3K signaling in normal, non-neoplastic cells. Idelalisib is a novel, selective inhibitor of phosphoinositide-3-kinase-delta (PI3Kδ kinase), which is active in the signaling pathways of B-cell malignancies. Idelalisib also inhibits cell-signaling receptors [e.g., B-cell receptor, CXCR4/5 (C-X-C chemokine receptor type 4) chemokine receptors] that are involved in the migration of B cells to the lymph nodes and bone marrow. Idelalisib inhibits ATP binding, which results in apoptosis and thereby decreases proliferation of malignant B cells and primary tumor cells. It is an oral kinase inhibitor that is approved for use in combination with rituximab in relapsed or refractory CLL and as monotherapy for relapsed follicular B cell and small lymphocytic lymphoma. It has also been approved in the European Union as first-line therapy for poor-prognosis CLL with 17p deletions or *TP53* mutations and in patients unsuitable for chemoimmunotherapy.

12. Ans. a. Enasidenib

Ref: Stein EM. Enasidenib in mutant IDH2 relapsed or refractory acute myeloid leukemia. Blood. 2017;130(6):722-31.

The enzymes isocitrate dehydrogenase 1 and 2 (IDH1 and IDH2) are part of the cell metabolism—the citric acid cycle or tricarboxylic acid (TCA) cycle. IDH1 is in the cytoplasm and IDH2 is in the mitochondria. Mutant IDH enzymes convert a Krebs cycle intermediate, α-ketoglutarate, into 2-hydroxyglutarate (oncometabolite). About 20% of AML cases involve mutations in IDH1 or IDH2. Ivosidenib has been approved for patients with AML with an IDH-1 and enasidenib has been approved for patients with AML when the patients have a mutation in the *IDH-2* gene. Vorasidenib is an orally available pan-inhibitor of both IDH1 and IDH2.

Isocitrate dehydrogenase inhibitors can lead to differentiation syndrome, similar to that seen with all-trans retinoic acid (ATRA) in APL. Differentiation syndrome is a potentially deadly complication with the use of IDH inhibitors in AML. IDH-differentiation syndrome appears to have a later onset, with a median of 30 days, as compared to 10–12 days for differentiation syndrome in patients with APL. The treatment is same as that for ATRA-induced differentiation syndrome.

13. Ans. a. Anaplastic large cell lymphoma

Ref: Mossé YP. Targeting ALK with crizotinib in pediatric anaplastic large cell lymphoma. J Clin Oncol. 2017;35(28):3215-21.

Crizotinib is an oral selective small molecule tyrosine kinase inhibitor (TKI) which targets anaplastic lymphoma kinase (ALK), hepatocyte growth factor receptor (HGFR, c-Met), and ROS1 tyrosine kinases. Crizotinib demonstrates potent growth inhibitory activity and induces apoptosis in tumor cell lines exhibiting ALK fusion events or *ALK* or *MET* gene amplification. Antitumor efficacy is dose dependent. Crizotinib, in an adenosine triphosphate (ATP)-competitive manner, binds to and inhibits ALK kinase and ALK fusion proteins. The ALK gene rearrangements can be detected in tumor specimens using immunohistochemistry, reverse transcription polymerase chain reaction (RT-PCR) of the complementary DNA (cDNA), and fluorescence *in situ* hybridization (FISH). The *ALK* gene is expressed in > 50% of anaplastic large cell lymphomas (ALCLs). Although most patients with ALK-positive ALCL respond well to anthracycline-based chemotherapy, relapses do occur (5-year failure-free survival 60%) and require salvage therapy, generally with poor outcomes.

14. Ans. b. Histone deacetylase (HDAC) inhibitor

Ref: Siegel D. Vorinostat in solid and hematologic malignancies. J Hemat Oncol. 2009;2:31.

Alterations in tumor suppressor genes or oncogenes are not always due to mutations. They may also be due to transcriptional regulation by epigenetic mechanisms, including DNA methylation or demethylation and/or histone acetylation or deacetylation. The balance between histone acetylation and deacetylation is usually well-regulated, but the balance is often upset in cancers. Vorinostat and belinostat are HDAC inhibitors which broadly inhibits all zinc-dependent HDAC enzymes. By inhibiting the enzymatic activity of HDAC, they cause the accumulation of acetylated histones and other proteins, thus inducing cell cycle arrest and/or apoptosis of transformed cells. HDAC inhibitors are a relatively new class of anticancer agents that play important roles in epigenetic or nonepigenetic regulation, inducing death, apoptosis, and cell cycle arrest in cancer cells.

15. Ans. c. Angioimmunoblastic T-cell lymphoma

Ref: Hyseni KF. Bevacizumab. Oncologist. 2010;15(8):819-25.

Vascular endothelial growth factor A (VEGF) is a potent proangiogenic growth factor that stimulates the proliferation, migration, and survival of endothelial cells. The interaction of VEGF with its receptors leads to endothelial cell proliferation and new blood vessel formation (angiogenesis). VEGF is an important target of anticancer therapy. Bevacizumab, is an antivascular endothelial growth factor (anti-VEGF) monoclonal antibody, and is useful in angioimmunoblastic T-cell lymphoma (AITL), as it is characterized by the overexpression of angiogenic factors, such as VEGF and prominent proliferation of high endothelial venules. Bevacizumab binds VEGF and prevents the interaction of VEGF to its receptors [Fms-related tyrosine kinase 1 (Flt-1) and kinase insert domain receptor (KDR)] on the surface of endothelial cells and inhibits angiogenesis.

16. Ans. a. CD2

Siplizumab is an anti-CD2 monoclonal antibody. CD2 is an adhesion molecule highly expressed on activated T cells and NK cells and on the majority of cells from patients with T-cell lymphoma and leukemia. Siplizumab eliminates both CD4+ and CD8+ T cells and NK cells without affecting B cells. Siplizumab has been used in conditioning regimens for hematopoietic cell transplantation and tolerance induction with combined kidney-bone marrow transplantation. Siplizumab-based tolerance induction regimens deplete T cells globally while enriching regulatory T cells (T-regs) early post-transplantation.

17. Ans. a. Hemophagocytic lymphohistiocytosis

Ref: Al-Salama ZT. Emapalumab: first global approval. Drugs. 2019;79(1):99-103.

Emapalumab is an anti-interferon gamma (IFNγ) antibody used for the treatment of HLH. IFNγ is a cytokine secreted by cells of the immune system to help regulate immune functions. It is produced by NK and NK-T cells, as well as by helper T-cells and cytotoxic T-lymphocytes in response to specific pathogens. High levels of IFNγ lead to macrophage activation and an overproduction of proinflammatory cytokines, which can cause severe tissue damage and organ failure. Emapalumab inhibits the interaction of IFNγ with its cognate receptor on T-cells, thereby neutralizing IFNγ activity. Patients with HLH generally have a poor prognosis and there is considerable morbidity and mortality, largely related to persistent HLH, intercurrent infections, or organ failure. Conventional therapy may contribute to these problems due to its myelosuppressive or broadly immunosuppressive effects, which is not there with emapalumab. The recommended starting emapalumab dose is 1 mg/kg as an intravenous infusion over 1 hour twice per week. The most common adverse reactions occurring in ≥20% of patients were infections, hypertension, infusion-related reactions, and pyrexia.

18. Ans. a. Imetelstat

Ref: Vasko T. Telomeres and telomerase in hematopoietic dysfunction: prognostic implications and pharmacological interventions. Int J Mol Sci. 2017:18;2267.

Imetelstat is a telomerase inhibitor targeting cells with short telomere lengths and hyperactive telomerase. Telomeres and telomerases are thought to be critical in maintaining normal hematopoiesis. Consecutive shortening of telomeres is thought to lead to reduction of mitotic capacity and ultimately lead to apoptosis. Telomerase hyperactivity can extend this natural limit of mitotic divisions and may promote disease evolution. It has been shown that MDS patient cells have significantly shorter telomeres than those of healthy controls and that high telomerase activity is linked to disease risk. Patients treated with telomerase inhibitor, imetelstat, have shown transfusion independence in low-risk MDS patients who have not responded to erythropoietin stimulating agents. The use of the telomerase inhibitor imetelstat in patients with essential thrombocythemia or myelofibrosis as well as the use of dendritic cell-based telomerase vaccination in AML patients with complete remissions are promising examples for antitelomerase-targeted strategies in hematologic malignancies.

19. Ans. a. Idarucizumab

Ref: Pollack CV. Idarucizumab for dabigatran reversal. N Engl J Med. 2017;377:431-41.

Idarucizumab is a humanized monoclonal antibody fragment that binds specifically to dabigatran. It has been proved to reverse rapidly, effectively, and consistently anticoagulant activity in dabigatran-treated patients. A single 5 g dose of idarucizumab is sufficient in 98% of the patients, and reversal is maintained for 24 hours in most patients. Idarucizumab is effective for dabigatran reversal among patients who have uncontrolled bleeding or will be undergoing urgent surgery.

20. Ans. d. Refractory CD30 expressing diffuse large B-cell lymphoma (DLBCL)
Ref: Garnock-Jones KP. Brentuximab vedotin: a review of its use in patients with Hodgkin lymphoma and systemic anaplastic large cell lymphoma following previous treatment failure. Drugs. 2013;73:371-81.

Brentuximab vedotin is FDA approved for upfront (advanced stage) or relapsed classical Hodgkin lymphoma and upfront or relapsed CD30 expressing T-cell lymphomas in view of significant overall and progression-free survival benefit with BV containing versus conventional CHOP regimen. Although phase 2 data has shown benefit of using BV in relapsed CD30 expressing DLBCL, it is not approved for this indication at present.

21. Ans. d. Cerebral hemorrhage
Ref: Richardson NC. Brentuximab vedotin in first-line treatment of peripheral T-cell lymphoma. Oncologist. 2019;24:180-7.

Notable toxicities of BV use are progressive multifocal leukoencephalopathy, infusional toxicity, myelosuppression, serious or life-threating infections, serious dermatological toxicity, and embryo-fetal toxicity. Cerebral hemorrhage is not a notable side effect.

22. Ans. b. Ipilimumab
Ref: Sentman AM. Bispecific T cell engagers for cancer immunotherapy. Immunol Cell Biol. 2015;93:290-6.

Bispecific T cell engager antibodies are members of bispecific class of antibodies. These can engage with tumor antigen (e.g., CD19) on one side and with T cell antigen (e.g., CD3) on the other, thereby directing the normal T cells of the body to act against the tumor antigen. Blinatumomab is expressed against CD19, and cetuximab and panitumumab are directed against epidermal growth factor receptor (EGFR). Ipilimumab is a check-point inhibitor and does not belong to BiTE class of antibody.

23. Ans. d. CD28
Ref: Darvin P. Immune checkpoint inhibitors: recent progress and potential biomarkers. Exp Mol Med. 2018;50:165.

Immune system is normally kept under check by controlling T-cell-mediated attack on other cells. Checkpoint inhibitors work by releasing this natural brake on the immune system so that T cells recognize and attack tumors. This therapy is called immune checkpoint blockade because the molecules that act as a brake on immune cells—the checkpoint—are blocked by the drug. Checkpoint inhibitors mount antitumor immune responses by interrupting coinhibitory signaling pathways and promote immune-mediated elimination of tumor cells. Pembrolizumab and nivolumab are directed against PD1. Ipilimumab is directed against CTLA-4, and avelumab and atezolizumab against PDL1. Although CD28 is a targetable check-point, no monoclonal antibodies have been developed against it so far.

24. Ans. a. Mononine
Ref: Balkaransingh P, Young G. Novel therapies and current clinical progress in hemophilia A. Ther Adv Hematol. 2018;9:49-61.

Major limitation in hemophilia treatment is related to short half-life of FVIII. Various techniques have been used to prolong its circulation in blood, which include fusion of Fc region of monomeric IgG to FVIII molecule that leads to its bypassing lysosomal degradation (eloctate) or using pegylated FVIII (adynovate). Recently, BiTE technology is being used whereby the molecule (emicizumab) acts as activated FVIII molecule binding FIXa on one variable region and FX on other, thereby helping in generation of Tenase complex. Mononine is recombinant FIX. Nonfactor alternatives, such as emicizumab, and the anticoagulant inhibitors, such as fitusiran and concizumab, offer a dramatic reduction in treatment burden for patients with or without inhibitors.

25. Ans. a. CXCR4
Ref: Fricker S. Physiology and pharmacology of plerixafor. Transfus Med Hemother. 2013;40(4):237-45.

Plerixafor is used for stem cell mobilization in patients undergoing stem cell transplantation. It antagonizes CXCR4 chemokine receptor and blocks its binding to its cognate ligand SDF-1 alpha (also known as CXCL-12) that results in mobilization of CD34 stem cells into peripheral blood.

26. Ans. d. It is an allosteric inhibitor
Ref: Hughes TP. Asciminib in chronic myeloid leukemia after ABL kinase inhibitor failure. N Engl J Med. 2019;381:2315-26.

Asciminib is a potent and specific BCR-ABL1 inhibitor with a novel allosteric mechanism of action targeting the ABL1 myristoyl pocket. It acts on a site different from that of ATP-binding-site TKIs, hence is not affected by the known mutations of the ATP pocket that actually render the current TKIs ineffective, providing potential for both monotherapy and combination therapy with ATP-binding-site TKIs. Asciminib targets both native and mutated BCR-ABL1, including the gatekeeper T315I mutant. Asciminib is also active in heavily pretreated patients with CML who have resistance to or develop unacceptable side effects from TKIs, including patients in whom ponatinib has failed and those with a T315I mutation.

27. Ans. b. Proteasome inhibition
Ref: Tzogani K. EMA Review of daratumumab for the treatment of adult patients with multiple myeloma. Oncologist. 2018;23(5):594-602.

Daratumumab is an IgG1κ human monoclonal antibody that binds to the CD38 protein expressed at a high level on the surface of myeloma cells, as well as other cell types and tissues at various levels. Daratumumab inhibits the in vivo growth of CD38-expressing tumor cells and has the potential to bind to all Fc receptors (FcγRs), inducing antibody-dependent cell-mediated cytotoxicity, complement-dependent cytotoxicity, and antibody-dependent cellular phagocytosis, resulting in high tumor-cell lysis. Binding of daratumumab to CD38 also mediates cell apoptosis and modulated enzymatic activities of CD38, inhibiting cyclase enzyme activity and stimulating hydrolase activity.

28. Ans. a. Serial two-dimensional (2D) echo monitoring for the risk of cardiomyopathy

Ref: Tzogani K. EMA Review of daratumumab for the treatment of adult patients with multiple myeloma. Oncologist. 2018;23(5):594-602.

Being a monoclonal antibody, infusion reactions can occur and have to be managed with premedication and close observation. It is an IgG kappa antibody and can appear as a small spike in serum protein electrophoresis and immune fixation electrophoresis assays. It is known to interfere with blood cross-matching and Rh and Kell typing, so prior crossmatching should be done before initiating the drug and this can be helpful in managing transfusion-related issues.

29. Ans. b. The discovery of hypoxia inducible factor alpha (HIF 1 alpha) and its role in adaptation to oxygen availability

Ref: The Nobel Prize in Physiology or Medicine 2019. NobelPrize.org. Nobel Media AB 2019.

The Nobel Prize in Physiology or Medicine 2019 was awarded jointly to William G Kaelin Jr, Sir Peter J Ratcliffe, and Gregg L Semenza for their discoveries of "how cells sense and adapt to oxygen availability". This discovery formed the basis of roxadustat, a member of a new therapeutic class, HIF prolyl hydroxylase inhibitors, for the treatment of anemia of chronic kidney disease.

30. Ans. c. Multiple myeloma: B-cell maturation antigen (BCMA)

Ref: Raje N. Anti-BCMA CAR T-cell therapy bb2121 in relapsed or refractory multiple myeloma. NEJM. 2019;380:1726-37.

Chimeric antigen receptor T-cell therapy has emerged as a novel treatment that has the potential for long-term disease control in some hematologic cancers, with anti-CD19 CAR T-cell therapies showing efficacy in patients with leukemia or lymphoma. BCMA is a member of the tumor necrosis factor superfamily of proteins that is primarily expressed by malignant and normal plasma cells and some mature B cells, making it a potential target for multiple myeloma.

31. Ans. d. All of the above

Tazemetostat, an EZH2 inhibitor (histone methyl-transferase inhibitor), has been approved for adult patients with relapsed or refractory (R/R) follicular lymphoma whose tumors are positive for an EZH2 mutation. The most common (≥20%) adverse reactions include fatigue, upper respiratory tract infection, musculoskeletal pain, nausea and abdominal pain. Serious adverse reactions occur in 30%, most often from infection. Second primary malignancy is the most common reason for treatment discontinuation (2% of patients).

32. Ans. b. Anti-CD47 monoclonal antibody

Magrolimab is a monoclonal antibody against CD47 and a macrophage checkpoint inhibitor that is designed to interfere with recognition of CD47 by the SIRPα receptor on macrophages, thus blocking the "don't eat me" signal used by cancer cells to avoid being ingested by macrophages. Magrolimab is being used in previously untreated acute myeloid leukemia and high risk MDS patients who are ineligible for intensive chemotherapy, including patients with TP53-mutant AML. This drug is especially important for patients with TP53 mutations, which are associated with poor outcomes and limited response to existing treatment options.

33. Ans. b. Diffuse large B cell lymphoma

Ref: Zinzani PL, Rodgers T, Marino D, et al. RE-MIND study: Comparison of tafasitamab + lenalidomide (L-MIND) vs lenalidomide monotherapy (real-world data) in transplant-ineligible patients with relapsed/refractory diffuse large B-cell lymphoma)

Tafasitamab is a humanized Fc-engineered CD19-directed monoclonal antibody that potentiates antibody-dependent cell-mediated cytotoxicity and antibody-dependent cellular phagocytosis. It has been approved for relapsed/refractory DLBCL. The RE-MIND study compared real-world response data from patients receiving lenalidomide monotherapy with findings from patients who received the investigational combination of tafasitamab and lenalidomide.

34. Ans. a. Inhibiting exportin

Ref: Jhaveri K. Selinexor for Refractory Multiple Myeloma. N Engl J Med. 2019;381(20):197

Exportin 1 (XPO1) is responsible for the nuclear export of innumerous cargo proteins, including nearly all tumor suppressor proteins and several oncoproteins. In MM, XPO1 is overexpressed resulting in enhanced transport of tumor suppressor proteins out of the nucleus and allowing immune surveillance evasion by cancer cells and escape from cell-cycle regulation. Selinexor is the first-in-class selective inhibitor of XPO1, forcing the nuclear retention and activation of tumor suppressor proteins, trapping IκBα in the nucleus to suppress NF-κB activity, and reducing oncoprotein mRNAs translation. Ultimately, it causes a selective induction of apoptosis in malignant cells, sparing normal cells. Thus, selinexor appears as a promising treatment for MM patient's refractory to all of the previously mentioned classes of drugs.

35. Ans. d. None of the above

Ref: Peterson T. Selinexor: A First-in-Class Nuclear Export Inhibitor for Management of Multiply Relapsed Multiple Myeloma. Ann Pharmacother. 2020 Jun;54(6):577-82

Common adverse reactions reported in at least 20% of patients include nausea, fatigue, decreased appetite, diarrhea, peripheral neuropathy, upper respiratory tract infection decreased weight, cataract and vomiting. Grade 3-4 laboratory abnormalities (≥10%) are thrombocytopenia, lymphopenia, hypophosphatemia, anemia hyponatremia and neutropenia. The recommended selinexor dose is 100 mg orally once weekly in combination with bortezomib and dexamethasone.

36. Ans. d. Pacritinib

Pacritinib is a selective JAK2 inhibitor that has been shown to reduce spleen size in patients who have anemia and thrombocytopenia.

37. Ans. e. All of the above

Anlotinib is a new, orally administered tyrosine kinase inhibitor that targets vascular endothelial growth factor receptor (VEGFR), fibroblast growth factor receptor (FGFR), platelet-derived growth factor receptors (PDGFR), and c-kit. Anlotinib exerts inhibitory effects on tumor growth and angiogenesis. Anlotinib also exerts anti-leukemia function by inhibiting SETD1A/AKT-mediated DNA damage response and highlights a novel mechanism underlying anlotinib in the treatment of MLL-rearranged AML.

38. Ans. a. CXCR4

Ref: Cancilla D. Targeting CXCR4 in AML and ALL. Front Oncol. 2020;10:1672.

The CXCR4 receptor (Chemokine C-X-C motif receptor 4) is highly expressed in different hematological malignancies. The CXCR4 ligand (CXCL12) stimulates CXCR4 promoting cell survival and proliferation, and may contribute to the tropism of leukemia cells. Therefore, strategies targeting CXCR4 may constitute an effective therapeutic approach. Ulocuplumab is a fully human IgG4 anti-CXCR4 antibody. Ulocuplumab inhibits CXCL12 mediated CXCR4 activation-migration of cells. Plerixafor (CXCR4 antagonist) has also been tested as a chemosensitizing agent in patients with AML or ALL.

39. Ans. a. HUS

Ref: Dhillon S. Moxetumomab Pasudotox: First Global Approval. Drugs, 2018

Moxetumomab pasudotox, an anti-CD22 recombinant immunotoxin, has been developed for the treatment of hairy cell leukaemia. Moxetumomab pasudotox is composed of the Fv fragment of an anti-CD22 monoclonal antibody fused to a 38 kDa fragment of Pseudomonas exotoxin A, PE38. The Fv portion of moxetumomab pasudotox binds to CD22, a cell surface receptor expressed on a variety of malignant B-cells, thereby delivering the toxin moiety PE38 directly to tumour cells. Once internalized, PE38 catalyzes the ADP ribosylation of the diphthamide residue in elongation factor-2 (EF-2), resulting in the rapid fall in levels of the anti-apoptotic protein myeloid cell leukemia 1 (Mcl-1), leading to apoptotic cell death. It is approved for the treatment of adults with relapsed or refractory hairy cell leukemia who received at least two prior systemic therapies, including treatment with a purine nucleoside analogue. The most common serious adverse events are hemolytic uremic syndrome (HUS), grade 3 or 4 infections patients, pyrexia and capillary leak syndrome.

40. Ans. d. Cedazuridine

Ref: Garcia-Manero G. Oral cedazuridine/decitabine for MDS and CMML: a phase 2 pharmacokinetic/pharmacodynamic randomized crossover study. Blood, 2020

Pevonedistat selective NEDD8 inhibitor, Venetoclax a BCL-2 inhibitor, Magrolimab: anti-CD47 antibody used in combination with azacytidine in intermediate- to very high-risk MDS are in phase 3 trial. Oral HMA may be inactivated by cytidine deaminase (CDA) in the gastrointestinal tract. Cedazuridine (ced) is an oral CDA inhibitor shown to increase HMA exposure after oral administration. A phase 2 RCT with oral ced/decitabine and intravenous decitabine for patients with advanced MDS or CMML indicates similar pharmacokinetic profiles and similar OS. Based on the results, the US FDA has granted priority review of ced/decitabine.

SECTION 11

Drugs and Miscellaneous

45. Drugs
46. Miscellaneous

CHAPTER 45

Drugs

1. Which of the drugs is contraindicated as intrathecal injection?
   a. Cytarabine
   b. Methotrexate
   c. Amphotericin
   d. Vincristine

2. Which of the following is not an alkylating agent?
   a. Treosulfan
   b. Cyclophosphamide
   c. Cytarabine
   d. Melphalan

3. Increased risk of thrombus with L-asparaginase is due to:
   a. Protein C and S deficiency
   b. Decreased fibrinogen level
   c. Antithrombin III deficiency
   d. Reduced factor IX level

4. After intrathecal injection of methotrexate, the patient develops headache and neck rigidity. The diagnosis is:
   a. Chemical meningitis
   b. Central nervous system (CNS) relapse
   c. Postlumbar puncture headache
   d. Bacterial meningitis

5. Ruxolitinib acts by inhibiting:
   a. JAK1
   b. JAK2
   c. MPL
   d. BCR-ABL
   e. Both JAK1 and JAK2

6. Eltrombopag is useful in:
   a. Myelodysplastic syndrome
   b. Chronic immune thrombocytopenic purpura (ITP)
   c. Paroxysmal nocturnal hemoglobinuria (PNH)
   d. Myelofibrosis (MF)

7. Mechanism of action of eltrombopag involves:
   a. Similar to endogenous thrombopoietin (TPO)
   b. Through TPO receptor
   c. Through JAK/STAT pathway
   d. Through JAK inhibition

8. Bortezomib acts by:
   a. Proteasome inhibition
   b. Lysosome inhibition
   c. Ribosome inhibition
   d. Microsome inhibition

9. Side effects of bortezomib include all, *except*:
   a. Thrombocytopenia
   b. Peripheral neuropathy
   c. Diarrhea
   d. Seizures

10. Lenalidomide is used in:
    a. Multiple myeloma (MM)
    b. Myelodysplastic syndrome
    c. Mantle cell lymphoma
    d. All of the above

11. Which drug is effective for T315I positive chronic myeloid leukemia?
    a. Imatinib
    b. Dasatinib
    c. Nilotinib
    d. Ponatinib
    e. None of the above

12. Bendamustine is used in:
    a. Follicular lymphoma
    b. Chronic lymphocytic leukemia (CLL)
    c. Multiple myeloma
    d. All of the above

13. True regarding vincristine are all, *except*:
    a. Never given intrathecal
    b. Is an antimetabolite
    c. Causes peripheral neuropathy
    d. No dose modification required in renal failure

14. The following are the side effects of daunorubicin, *except*:
    a. Vesicant
    b. Cardiotoxicity
    c. Cerebellar symptoms
    d. All of the above

15. True regarding cyclophosphamide is:
    a. Cardiotoxicity can develop
    b. SIADH (syndrome of inappropriate antidiuretic hormone secretion) can occur
    c. No dose adjustment required in hepatic failure
    d. All of the above

16. Mechanism of action of intravenous immunoglobulins (IVIg) is:
    a. Blockade of Fc receptors
    b. Anticytokine effects
    c. Inhibition of complement activation
    d. Neutralization of autoantibodies
    e. All of the above

17. The dose of anti-D for treatment of ITP is:
   a. 25 µg/kg
   b. 50 µg/kg
   c. 75 µg/kg
   d. 100 µg/kg

18. True about zoledronate are all, *except*:
   a. Osteonecrosis of jaw
   b. Dose modification required in renal failure
   c. Non-nitrogen-containing bisphosphonates
   d. All are true

19. True about mercaptopurine are all, *except*:
   a. Inhibits purine synthesis
   b. Specific for the S phase of the cell cycle
   c. Should be given with milk
   d. Dose reduction required in thiopurine methyl-transferase (TPMT) deficiency

20. True about the methotrexate are all, *except*:
   a. High doses of folic acid rescue are used
   b. Dose reduction required in pleural effusion
   c. Excreted through kidneys
   d. Glucarpidase is useful in toxicity
   e. Lung toxicity can develop

21. Mechanism by which resistance to high-dose chemotherapy develops is:
   a. Reduced drug uptake by the tumor cell
   b. Enhanced drug efflux
   c. Increased repair of drug-induced damage to DNA or other critical tumor cell targets enhanced intracellular metabolism or detoxification of the chemotherapeutic agent
   d. Overexpression of the target gene product for a specific drug
   e. All of the above

22. True regarding the use of high-dose melphalan for multiple myeloma are all, *except*:
   a. Maximum tolerated dose is 200 mg/m²
   b. Mucositis is the dose-limiting toxicity
   c. Alveolitis can develop
   d. Renal failure is a contraindication for its use

23. Eculizumab is used in the treatment of:
   a. Myelodysplastic syndrome
   b. Idiopathic myelofibrosis
   c. Paroxysmal nocturnal hemoglobinuria
   d. Mantle cell lymphoma

24. Curative treatment for hemolytic paroxysmal nocturnal hemoglobinuria is:
   a. Steroids
   b. Danazol
   c. Eculizumab
   d. Allogenic stem cell transplant

25. Which of the following drugs can cause agranulocytosis?
   a. Olanzapine
   b. Chloramphenicol
   c. Risperidone
   d. Clozapine
   e. Levetiracetam

26. Omalizumab is used in the treatment of:
   a. Bronchial asthma
   b. Small cell lung cancer
   c. Immune thrombocytopenic purpura
   d. Rheumatoid arthritis

27. Which of the following is not a part of fetal warfarin syndrome (teratogenic effect of warfarin)?
   a. Hydrocephaly
   b. Microcephaly
   c. Mental retardation
   d. Blindness
   e. Macroophthalmia

28. Which of the following vitamin K antagonists has the longest plasma half-life?
   a. Warfarin
   b. Acenocoumarol
   c. Phenindione
   d. Fluindione
   e. Phenprocoumon

29. Which of the following anticoagulants does not require co-administration of low molecular weight heparin at the start, in the management of acute pulmonary or deep vein thrombosis?
   a. Dabigatran
   b. Edoxaban
   c. Rivaroxaban
   d. Idarucizumab
   e. Warfarin

30. True regarding receptors associated with tyrosine kinase activity is:
   a. They are integral membrane proteins
   b. Ligand-induced cross-linking
   c. Tyrosine kinase domains are located in their cytoplasmic tails
   d. SRC, is the prototype for an important family receptor with tyrosine kinase activity
   e. All of the above

ANSWERS WITH EXPLANATIONS

1. Ans. d. Vincristine *Ref: William's 8/e p288, 289, 293*
- Intrathecal cytarabine is usually well-tolerated, but neurological side effects have been reported (seizures, alterations in mental status).
- Vincristine administered inadvertently into the cerebrospinal fluid causes acute neurologic dysfunction, coma, and death.
- Methotrexate can be given intrathecally.
- Liposomal amphotericin B is administered intrathecally at 0.006 mg/kg weekly for the treatment of coccidial meningitis.

2. Ans. c. Cytarabine *Ref: Tripathi 5/e p759-60*

The classification of chemotherapeutic drug is:
- Alkylating agents:
  - *Nitrogen mustards*: Mechlorethamine (mustine HCl)
  - Cyclophosphamide, ifosfamide
  - Chlorambucil
- Antimetabolites:
  - Folate antagonists:
    - Methotrexate
  - Purine antagonists:
    - 6-Meracaptopurine
    - 6-Thioguanine
    - Azathioprine
    - Fludarabine
    - Cladribine
    - Clofarabine
    - Nelarabine
      - Pentostatin (2′-deoxycoformycin)
  - Pyrimidine antagonists:
    - 5-Fluorouracil
    - Cytarabine
    - Gemcitabine
    - 5-Azacyticline
- Vinca alkaloids:
  - Vincristine
  - Vinblastine
  - Vindesine
  - Vinorelbine
- Taxanes:
  - Paclitaxel
  - Docetaxel
- Epipodophyllotoxin:
  - Etoposide
  - Temoside
- Camptothecin analogs:
  - Topotecan
  - Irinotecan
- Antibiotics:
  - Actinomycin D (dactinomycin)
  - Daunorubicin (rubidomycin)
  - Doxorubicin
  - Mitoxantrone
  - Epirubicin
  - Idarubicin
  - Bleomycin
  - Mitomycin C
  - Mithramycin (plicamycin)
- Miscellaneous:
  - Hydroxyurea
  - Procarbazine
  - L-asparaginase
  - Cisplatin
  - Carboplatin.

3. Ans. c. Antithrombin III deficiency
Ref: Haematologica. 2008;93(10):1488-94.

L-asparaginase-induced deficiency of antithrombin-III is responsible for the increased risk of sinovenous thrombosis.

4. Ans. a. Chemical meningitis *Ref: William's 8/e p298*
- A possible complication of intrathecal methotrexate could be acute arachnoiditis.
- Chronic toxicities include dementia, motor deficits, seizures, and coma.
- Rarely, these neurotoxicities develop hours after intrathecal drug administration.
- More commonly, they occur in the days or weeks after initiation of intrathecal treatment and are most often seen in patients with active meningeal leukemia.
- Leucovorin is ineffective in reversing or preventing these toxicities.
- This patient is having clinical evidence of meningitis as he is having headache and neck rigidity. It cannot be bacterial meningitis as there is no history of fever. Postlumbar puncture headache is also unlikely as there is presence of neck rigidity.
- As the patient developed symptoms after intrathecal treatment and these symptoms were not present before, so CNS relapse is also unlikely.

5. Ans. e. Both JAK1 and JAK2 *Ref: Hoffman 6/e p1070*

Ruxolitinib is a kinase inhibitor which selectively inhibits Janus-associated kinases (JAKs)—JAK1 and JAK2. JAKs mediate the signaling pathway of cytokines and growth factors for hematopoiesis and immune function. In MF, the dysregulation of the JAK1 and JAK2 signaling leads to impaired hematopoiesis and immune function. Ruxolitinib modulates the cytokine-stimulated signaling through the inhibition of JAK1 and JAK2. Anti-JAK therapy and ruxolitinib, in particular, are an important advance in the treatment of MF and should be considered in patients who are symptomatic without limiting cytopenias. Currently, there is not sufficient evidence to indicate that ruxolitinib possesses the ability to correct pathologic features in the bone marrow, induce cytogenetic/molecular remissions, modify the natural history and progression of disease, or significantly alter survival in MF. It is indicated for the treatment of symptomatic intermediate- or high-risk MF. Ruxolitinib has demonstrated promising efficacy in reducing splenomegaly and MF-related symptoms. However, ruxolitinib did not demonstrate disease-modifying potential and is not considered a curative therapeutic option. Adverse events associated with ruxolitinib are primarily hematologic, with thrombocytopenia and anemia being the most common toxicologic events identified.

6. Ans. b. Chronic ITP *Ref: Hoffman 6/e p1888*

Eltrombopag is indicated for adult chronic ITP to increase platelet counts in splenectomized patients who are refractory to first-line treatments (e.g., corticosteroids and immunoglobulins). It has also been approved to increase platelet counts in thrombocytopenic patients with chronic hepatitis C virus (HCV) infection to allow the initiation and maintenance of interferon-based therapy.

7. Ans. b. Through TPO receptor

Ref: Hoffman 6/e p1888

Thrombopoietin is the main cytokine involved in regulation of megakaryopoiesis and platelet production, and is the endogenous ligand for the thrombopoietin receptor (TPO-R). Eltrombopag interacts with the transmembrane domain of the human TPO-R and initiates signaling cascades similar but not identical to that of endogenous thrombopoietin, inducing proliferation and differentiation of megakaryocytes from bone marrow progenitor cells.

8. Ans. a. Proteasome inhibition

Ref: Hoffman 6/e p795-6

The ubiquitin-proteasome pathway is responsible for degradation of the majority of regulatory proteins in eukaryotic cells, including proteins that control cell-cycle progression, apoptosis, and DNA repair and therefore play an essential role in maintaining normal cellular homeostasis. Proteasome inhibition has been extensively explored as a therapeutic strategy in MM, and proteasome inhibitors now form a cornerstone of antimyeloma therapy. By inhibiting the proteasome, bortezomib acts through multiple mechanisms to suppress tumor survival pathways and to arrest tumor growth, tumor spread, and angiogenesis. Bortezomib directly induces apoptosis of tumor cells, inhibits the activation of NF-κB in cells and in the tumor microenvironment, reduces adherence of myeloma cells to bone marrow stromal cells, blocks production and intracellular signaling of IL-6 in myeloma cells, stops the production and expression of proangiogenic mediators, and overcomes defects in apoptotic regulators, such as Bcl-2 overexpression and alterations in tumor suppressor p53. Bortezomib has also been associated with increased bone formation and osteoblastic activity, and decreased bone resorption and osteoclastic activity.

9. Ans. d. Seizures *Ref: Hoffman 6/e p795-6*

The most commonly reported (>20%) adverse reactions overall are nausea (52%), diarrhea (52%), fatigue (39%), peripheral neuropathies (35%), thrombocytopenia (33%), constipation (30%), vomiting (29%), and anorexia (21%). 8% of patients experienced a grade 4 thrombocytopenia and neutropenia (2%). Once the symptoms of the toxicity have resolved, bortezomib treatment may be reinitiated at a 25% reduced dose (1.3 mg/m^2 reduced to 1.0 mg/m^2; 1.0 mg/m^2 reduced to 0.7 mg/m^2).

10. Ans. d. All of the above *Ref: Hoffman 6/e p795-6*

In multiple myeloma, lenalidomide is given 25 mg orally daily on days 1–21 of a 28-day cycle. In myelodysplastic syndrome, transfusion-dependent, deletion 5q abnormality, low or intermediate-1 risk: 10 mg orally once daily. In 2013, the US Food and Drug Administration (FDA) approved lenalidomide for the treatment of patients with mantle cell lymphoma whose disease has relapsed or progressed after two prior therapies. The recommended dose and schedule for lenalidomide is 25 mg orally once daily on days 1–21 of repeated 28-day cycles.

11. Ans. d. Ponatinib *Ref: Hoffman 6/e p993*

The indication of ponatinib is in the treatment of adult patients with T315I-positive chronic myeloid leukemia (chronic phase, accelerated phase, or blast phase) or T315I-positive Philadelphia chromosome positive acute lymphoblastic leukemia (Ph+ ALL).

12. Ans. d. All of the above *Ref: Hoffman 6/e p788*

The FDA has approved bendamustine in follicular lymphoma and CLL. Recent studies have shown it to be effective in relapsed and refractory multiple myeloma also. Bendamustine is a chemotherapeutic agent that displays a unique pattern of cytotoxicity compared with conventional alkylating agents. It has both alkylating and antimetabolite properties. The alkylating agent properties are similar to those seen with cyclophosphamide, chlorambucil, and melphalan, and the benzimidazole ring is similar to cladribine. Molecular analyses have revealed that bendamustine differs from other alkylating agents in its mechanism of action. Differences have been observed in regard to its effects on DNA repair and cell cycle progression. Moreover, bendamustine can induce cell death through both apoptotic and nonapoptotic pathways, thereby retaining activity even in cells without a functional apoptotic pathway. Bendamustine has demonstrated significant efficacy in patients with indolent lymphomas and CLL, including in patients with disease refractory to conventional alkylating agents and rituximab. The toxicity profile of bendamustine is also superior to that of conventional alkylating agents.

13. Ans. b. Is an antimetabolite   *Ref: Hoffman 6/e p789*

Vinca alkaloids act as antimicrotubule agents that block mitosis by arresting cells in the metaphase. These drugs act by preventing the polymerization of tubulin to form microtubules as well as by inducing depolymerization of formed tubules. Inadvertent administration of vincristine by the intrathecal route is nearly always fatal and a medical emergency. Neurotoxicity involves peripheral, autonomic, and central neuropathy. It is the primary and dose-limiting toxicity of vincristine. Most side effects are dose related and reversible, but neurotoxicity can persist for months after discontinuation of therapy in some patients, and in rare cases may be disabling. Peripheral neuropathy is the most common type of neuropathy and develops in almost all patients. Loss of deep tendon reflexes, peripheral paresthesias, pain, and tingling can occur. If therapy is prolonged or high doses are administered, wrist and foot drop, ataxia, a slapping gait, and difficulty in walking can occur. Cranial nerve toxicities may lead to vocal cord paresis or paralysis (hoarseness, weak voice), ocular motor nerve dysfunction (ptosis, strabismus), bilateral facial nerve palsies, or jaw pain. Severe jaw pain can occur within a few hours of the first dose of vincristine. Autonomic neuropathy results in constipation (which can be severe), abdominal pain, urinary retention, and paralytic ileus. Central neuropathy includes headache, malaise, dizziness, seizures, mental depression, psychosis, and SIADH. No dose modifications are indicated in renal failure. In hepatic impairment, the dose modification is according to bilirubin levels (1 mg/dL = 17.1 μmol/L).

Bilirubin (μmol/L)	Vincristine dose
<25	100%
26–50	50%
>50	25%

14. Ans. c. Cerebellar symptoms   *Ref: Hoffman 6/e p789*

Daunorubicin is an anthracycline antibiotic which damages DNA by intercalating between base pairs resulting in uncoiling of the helix, ultimately inhibiting DNA synthesis and DNA-dependent RNA synthesis. Tissue necrosis may be caused by extravasation of anthracyclines. These agents may bind to DNA and recycle locally to cause a progressive slough of tissue or ulceration over several weeks, requiring excision and skin grafting. Flare reaction is a painless local reaction along the vein or near the intact injection of anthracyclines. It is characterized by immediate red blotches, streaks, and local wheals, probably due to histamine release. Cardiotoxicity is thought to be due to free radical damage as myocardial tissue is susceptible to these highly reactive species. Anthracycline cardiotoxicity may present with early or late effects. Early cardiotoxic effects are not dose related and may present from mild ECG changes to life-threatening arrhythmias. These events may occur during or immediately after a single dose of anthracycline treatment. Late cardiotoxic effects, which are dose-related and clinically the most important type of cardiotoxic effect, present as reduced left ventricular ejection fraction (LVEF) or symptomatic congestive heart failure and typically occur weeks to years after completion of treatment. LVEF changes are related to the total cumulative dose, are irreversible, and are refractory to medical therapy. Daunorubicin dose modification is required in renal and hepatic dysfunction. Neuropathy can develop in 13% cases, but cerebellar symptoms do not develop.

15. Ans. d. All of the above   *Ref: Hoffman 6/e p789*

Cyclophosphamide is an alkylating agent of the nitrogen mustard type. An activated form of cyclophosphamide, phosphoramide mustard, alkylates or binds to DNA. Its cytotoxic effect is mainly due to cross-linking of strands of DNA and RNA and to inhibition of protein synthesis. Cardiac toxicity may occur in patients receiving high-dose cyclophosphamide. High dose can be defined as 60 mg/kg daily or 120–270 mg/kg over a few days. The mechanism may involve direct injury to the endothelium by phosphoramide mustard, an active metabolite of cyclophosphamide. Unlike anthracyclines, cyclophosphamide-induced cardiotoxicity does not appear to be cumulative. In contrast to anthracycline-induced cardiomyopathy which occurs months to years after cumulative doses of anthracyclines, cyclophosphamide-induced cardiotoxicity occurs much earlier. Toxicity has ranged from minor, transient ECG changes and asymptomatic elevation of cardiac enzymes at a total dose of 100 mg/kg to fatal myocarditis and myocardial necrosis at total doses ranging upward from 144 mg/kg delivered over 4 days. Hemorrhagic cystitis may occur in up to 40% of patients (especially children) on long-term or high-dose cyclophosphamide therapy. The mechanism may involve direct injury to the urothelium by acrolein, an active metabolite of cyclophosphamide. Hemorrhagic cystitis can develop within a few hours (early onset HC) or be delayed several weeks (late-onset HC). SIADH may occur in patients receiving cyclophosphamide, resulting in hyponatremia, dizziness, confusion or agitation, and unusual tiredness or weakness. This syndrome is more common with doses >50 mg/kg and may be aggravated by administration of large volumes of fluids to prevent hemorrhagic cystitis. No dose adjustment is required in hepatic dysfunction. In severe renal dysfunction, dose reduction is required.

16. Ans. e. All of the above
Ref: Hoffman 6/e p1887

The effectiveness of IVIg as an immunomodulator is probably dependent on a range of mechanisms including: (1) blockade of Fc receptors, (2) anticytokine effects, (3) inhibition of complement activation, (4) enhanced clearance of endogenous pathogenic autoantibodies via the FcR receptor, (5) neutralization of autoantibodies, (6) neutralization of superantigens, and (7) downregulation of T- or B-cell function. IVIg prevents attachment of the antibody to the platelet, therefore preventing premature destruction by the spleen. Human immunoglobulin (IVIg) is a pooled blood product collected from 100 to 100,000 donors. It is composed of mostly IgG, but contains smaller amounts of all Ig subtypes. The dose of 1 g/kg/day for 1–2 days appears to be the optimal dose. Typically, IVIg is administered over several hours, at rates from 0.03 to 0.13 mL/kg/min.

17. Ans. c. 75 µg/kg
Ref: Hoffman 6/e p1887

Intravenous infusion of anti-D into a D-positive recipient leads to antibody coating of circulating erythrocytes that are cleared primarily by the spleen. This immune-mediated clearance of sensitized erythrocytes occupies the reticuloendothelial system (RES) and allows survival of antibody-coated platelets. There is immunologic blockade of Fc receptors (FcR) within the RES, so antibody-coated platelets spared as FcR are blocked by antibody (anti-D) coated RBC. This can result in mild hemolysis seen with anti-D use. The dose of anti-D is 75 µg/kg single dose.

18. Ans. c. Non-nitrogen-containing bisphosphonates
Ref: Hoffman 6/e p1334-7

Bisphosphonates are synthetic analogs to inorganic pyrophosphates found within the bone matrix that, unlike natural pyrophosphates, are resistant to hydrolysis by phosphatases found in the blood. Bisphosphonates inhibit bone resorption by suppressing osteoclast activity. They are widely used in the management of lytic bone lesions in patients with MM, in the treatment and prevention of osteoporosis, in the treatment of moderate-to-severe hypercalcemia, and in the therapy of certain other bone diseases. Bisphosphonates appear to inhibit bone resorption by suppressing osteoclast activity. Clinically, this translates into fewer lytic bone lesions and fewer skeletal events (e.g., pathologic fracture) in patients with MM. Zoledronic acid inhibits osteoclastic activity and induces osteoclast apoptosis. It also blocks the osteoclastic resorption of mineralized bone and cartilage through its binding to bone. It also inhibits the increased osteoclastic activity and skeletal calcium release induced by various stimulatory factors released by tumors. There are two main classes of bisphosphonates: non-nitrogen-containing and nitrogen-containing. Etidronate and clodronate are non-nitrogen-containing bisphosphonates. Pamidronate, zoledronic acid, ibandronate, and risedronate are examples of nitrogen-containing bisphosphonates. The recommended dose of zoledronate in patients with myeloma and metastatic bone lesions from solid tumors for patients with creatinine clearance greater than 60 mL/min is 4 mg infused over no less than 15 minutes every 3–4 weeks.

Baseline creatinine clearance (mL/min)	Zoledronate recommended dose
>60	4 mg
50–60	3.5 mg
40–49	3.3 mg
30–39	3 mg
<30	Withhold

Zoledronate is excreted intact primarily via the kidney, and the risk of adverse reactions, in particular renal adverse reactions, may be greater in patients with impaired renal function. Osteonecrosis of the jaw (ONJ) has been reported predominantly in cancer patients treated with intravenous bisphosphonate. While on treatment, these patients should avoid invasive dental procedures if possible. For patients who develop ONJ while on bisphosphonate therapy, dental surgery may exacerbate the condition. Atypical subtrochanteric and diaphyseal femoral fractures have been reported in patients receiving bisphosphonate therapy. Patients may experience thigh or groin pain weeks to months before presenting with a completed femoral fracture. Hypocalcemia has been reported in patients treated with Zoledronate. Patients should be supplemented with calcium and vitamin D.

19. Ans. c. Should be given with milk
Ref: William's 8/e p289-91

Mercaptopurine is a purine antagonist. It is a prodrug that is converted intracellularly to thioinosine monophosphate (TIMP) by the enzyme hypoxanthine-guanine phosphoribosyl transferase (HGPRT). TIMP inhibits purine synthesis. TIMP is sequentially metabolized to thioguanine monophosphate (TGMP) and then to thioguanosine triphosphate (TGTP). The cytotoxic effect of mercaptopurine is a result of the incorporation of these nucleotides into DNA. Mercaptopurine is an immunosuppressant. It is specific for the S phase of the cell cycle. Mercaptopurine-induced hepatotoxicity is most common when doses exceed 2.5 mg/kg/day. Milk decreases the bioavailability of 6-MP, because it is inactivated by high concentration of xanthine oxidase in milk. TPMT is involved in the metabolism of mercaptopurine and subject to genetic polymorphism, with heterozygous individuals having intermediate and homozygous mutant individuals having very low TPMT activity. Patients with ALL are often treated with 6-mercaptopurine, and those with homozygous deficiency in TPMT enzyme activity have an extreme sensitivity to this drug as a result of the accumulation of higher cellular concentrations of thioguanine nucleotides. Unless TPMT-deficient patients are treated with 10- to 15-folds lower doses of these medications, they develop profound hematopoietic toxicity that precludes the administration of other chemotherapies and can be fatal.

20. Ans. a. High doses of folic acid rescue are used
Ref: William's 8/e p286-9; Internet

Methotrexate is a folate antagonist. Tetrahydrofolate is the active form of folic acid required for purine and thymidylate synthesis. Folic acid is reduced to tetrahydrofolate by dihydrofolate reductase (DHFR). The cytotoxicity of methotrexate results from three actions: (1) inhibition of DHFR, (2) inhibition of thymidylate, and (3) alteration of the transport of reduced folates. Inhibition of DHFR results in a deficiency of thymidylate and purines and therefore a decrease in DNA synthesis, repair, and cellular replication. The affinity of DHFR to methotrexate is far greater than its affinity for folic acid or dihydrofolic acid; therefore, large doses of folic acid given simultaneously will not reverse the effects of methotrexate. However, leucovorin calcium, a derivative of tetrahydrofolic acid, may block the effects of methotrexate if given shortly after the methotrexate since it does not require DHFR for activation. Methotrexate exits slowly from third space compartments resulting in prolonged half-life and unexpected toxicity. In patients with significant third space accumulation, the fluid should be removed prior to treatment and methotrexate levels should be monitored. If the fluid cannot be drained prior to therapy, a dose reduction is appropriate. For rescue leucovorin dose, PO/IV/IM 10–25 mg/m² every 6 hours for approximately 8–10 doses is used, starting 24 hours after the start of methotrexate infusion, for leucovorin doses >25 mg, administer IV. Methotrexate-induced hepatotoxicity can be seen with both high- and low-dose methotrexate and can be life-threatening. Methotrexate-induced pulmonary toxicity can be acute, subacute, or chronic. Patients who experience pulmonary toxicity will often develop this within the first year of methotrexate therapy, but it can occur much earlier or much later. High-dose methotrexate-induced renal failure is a medical emergency because methotrexate is mainly eliminated by the kidneys. Renal damage is due to precipitation of methotrexate in the tubules and to tubule injury. Drug precipitation can often be prevented by hydration and alkalization of the urine. Hydration produces a high urine output and lowers the concentration of methotrexate in the tubular fluid; alkalization of the urine increases the solubility of methotrexate. During the recovery period, sustained methotrexate levels may result in substantial bone marrow and gastrointestinal toxicity. Dose modifications are required in hepatic and renal dysfunction. Glucarpidase (carboxypeptidase-G2) is a recombinant bacterial enzyme that inactivates extracellular methotrexate to 2,4-diamino-N10-methylpteroic acid (DAMPA). Glucarpidase can rapidly lower serum methotrexate levels by >95% within 15 minutes of administration.

21. Ans. e. All of the above
Ref: Housman G. Drug Resistance in Cancer: An Overview. Cancers. 2014;6:1769-92.

High-dose chemotherapy is not uniformly successful because many types of cancer in humans harbor small populations of tumor cells that are intrinsically resistant to treatment or acquire resistance during therapy. High-dose chemotherapy may also fail because the incremental increase in drug doses possible with hematopoietic cell support is insufficient to either produce lethal tumor cell damage or result in sufficient concentrations at all sites of the tumor. Multiple factors impair the efficacy of high-dose chemotherapy.

22. Ans. d. Renal failure is a contraindication to its use
Ref: K Sweiss. Melphalan 200 mg/m² in patients with renal impairment is associated with increased short-term toxicity but improved response and longer treatment-free survival. BMT. 2016;51:1337-41.

The dose-limiting toxicities of high-dose melphalan (MEL) are mucositis and sinusoidal obstruction syndrome (SOS). Gastrointestinal mucosal injury limits both the escalation of drug dose >200 mg/m² as a single agent and its use at doses >140 mg/m² with other agents that produce severe gastrointestinal tract toxicity. SOS has been observed, especially when high-dose MEL has been combined with other high-dose alkylating agents. High-dose MEL can produce diffuse pulmonary alveolitis; it also can stimulate inappropriate antidiuretic hormone secretion in the high-dose chemotherapy setting. Because of the limited renal excretion of MEL, high-dose therapy has been used in patients with MM and significantly compromised kidney function (creatinine clearance < 40 mL/min); no evidence of alterations in half-life or AUC were demonstrated, although the performance status of such patients may enhance their toxicity profile. The lack of any major effect of renal dysfunction on the clearance of high-dose MEL has been confirmed, and a patient with MM with renal failure can undergo autologous stem cell transplant with high-dose melphalan.

23. Ans. c. Paroxysmal nocturnal hemoglobinuria
Ref: William's 8/e p528

The clinical features of PNH result from the lack of one or more glycosylphosphatidylinositol (GPI)-linked proteins that protect cells from complement-mediated attack. Two such proteins—CD55 and CD59—are absent from PNH erythrocytes, platelets, and other blood cells. Eculizumab is a recombinant humanized monoclonal antibody that was designed to block the activation of terminal complement components. It binds specifically to the terminal complement protein C5, inhibiting its cleavage into C5a and C5b, thereby preventing the release of the inflammatory mediator C5a and the formation of the cytolytic pore C5b–C9. Eculizumab is safe and well-tolerated in patients with PNH. This antibody against terminal complement protein C5 reduces intravascular hemolysis, hemoglobinuria, and the need for transfusion, with an associated improvement in the quality-of-life in patients with PNH.

24. Ans. d. Allogeneic stem cell transplant
Ref: William's 8/e p529

Paroxysmal nocturnal hemoglobinuria is a rare clonal blood disorder that manifests with hemolytic anemia, bone marrow failure, and thrombosis. Many of the clinical manifestations of the disease result from complement-mediated intravascular hemolysis. Allogeneic bone marrow transplantation is the only curative therapy for PNH. Eculizumab, a monoclonal antibody that blocks terminal complement activation, is highly effective in reducing hemolysis, improving quality-of-life, and reducing the risk for thrombosis in PNH patients.

25. Ans. b. Chloramphenicol   *Ref: William's 7/e p420*

Chloramphenicol is the most notorious drug documented to cause aplastic anemia.

26. Ans. a. Bronchial asthma   *Ref: Harrison's 18/e p2112*

Omalizumab is blocking antibody that neutralizes circulating IgE without binding to cell-bound IgE and thus inhibits IgE-mediated reactions.

27. Ans. e. Macro-ophthalmia
Ref: Mehndiratta S, Suneja A, Gupta B, Bhatt S. Fetotoxicity of warfarin anticoagulation. Arch Gynecol Obstet. 2010;282:335-7.

Fetal warfarin syndrome (FWS) can induce blindness via optic nerve atrophy. Microphthalmia rather than macrophthalmia is associated with FWS.

FWS often results in:
- Skeletal system abnormalities (e.g., nasal ridge hypoplasia, short limbs, scoliosis, stippled epiphyses). These are seen after exposure to warfarin in the first trimester.
- CNS abnormalities (e.g., microcephaly, optic nerve atrophy hydrocephaly). These are seen after exposure to warfarin in the second and third trimesters. They lead to mental retardation, blindness, deafness, and seizures.
- Cardiac abnormalities (e.g., coarctation of the aorta, patent ductus arteriosus).
- Low birth weight
- Bleeding

28. Ans. e. Phenprocoumon

Phenprocoumon has the longest plasma t½ (approximately 5–6 days). The t½ of the other vitamin K antagonists (VKAs) are:
- Warfarin 40 hours
- Fluindione 31 hours
- Phenindione 5–10 hours
- Acenocoumarol 8–11 hours

29. Ans. c. Rivaroxaban

Only the anti-Xa inhibitors rivaroxaban and apixaban do not require co-administration of low molecular weight heparin (LMWH). Based on data from randomised studies, the dose of these 2 drugs can be halved after 6 months of therapy to reduce the risk of recurrence. There was, however, no significant difference in major bleeding between the standard and lower doses.

Dabigatran, edoxaban, and warfarin require a minimum of 5 days LMWH prior to starting therapy. LMWH should only be stopped when the INR is ≥2.

Idarucizumab is a monoclonal antibody used for the reversal of dabigatran.

30. Ans. e. All of the above
Ref: Du Zhenfang. Mechanisms of receptor tyrosine kinase activation in cancer. Molecular Cancer. 2018;17:58.

Receptor tyrosine kinases (RTKs) are a subclass of tyrosine kinases that are involved in mediating cell-to-cell communication and controlling a wide range of complex biological functions, including cell growth, motility, differentiation, and metabolism. All RTKs share a similar protein structure comprised of an extracellular ligand binding domain, a single transmembrane helix, and an intracellular region that contains a juxtamembrane regulatory region, a tyrosine kinase domain (TKD) and a carboxyl (C⁻) terminal tail. Dysregulation of RTK signaling leads to many human diseases, especially cancer. RTKs are generally activated by receptor-specific ligands. Growth factor ligands bind to extracellular regions of RTKs, and the receptor is activated by ligand-induced receptor dimerization and/or oligomerization. Tyrosine kinase inhibitors (TKIs) attach with RTKs ATP-binding site for ATP and hitherto reduce tyrosine kinase phosphorylation, thus hampering the growth of cancer cells. TKIs can either be monoclonal antibodies that compete for the receptor's extracellular domain or small molecules that inhibit the tyrosine kinase domain and prevent conformational changes that activate RTKs. Progression of cancer is related to aberrant activation of RTKs due to mutation, excessive expression, or autocrine stimulation.

CHAPTER 46

Miscellaneous

1. **For primary hemochromatosis the treatment of choice is:**
   a. Iron chelation therapy
   b. Phlebotomy
   c. Hydroxyurea
   d. Allogenic bone marrow transplant

2. **Most common symptom or manifestation of hyperviscosity syndrome is:**
   a. Thrombosis
   b. Bleeding
   c. Headache
   d. Breathlessness

3. **All of the following can be used in the treatment of hypercalcemia, *except*:**
   a. Calcitonin
   b. Calcitriol
   c. Zoledronate
   d. Steroids

4. **Heinz bodies are seen in all, *except*:**
   a. Acute oxidant-induced hemolysis
   b. Hereditary persistence of fetal hemoglobin (HPFH)
   c. Acute hemolysis in G6PD deficiency
   d. Unstable Hb, postsplenectomy

5. **High hemoglobin with elevated serum erythropoietin (EPO) levels is seen in all, *except*:**
   a. Cyanotic congenital heart disease
   b. Pseudo or relative polycythemia
   c. Renal artery stenosis
   d. Renal cell carcinoma

6. **A positive direct Coombs test (DCT) is characteristically seen in all, *except*:**
   a. Hemolytic disease of newborn
   b. Delayed hemolytic transfusion reaction
   c. Warm autoimmune hemolytic anemia (AIHA)
   d. Hemorrhagic disease of newborn

7. **Which one is the first stage of grief in patient who is recently told to have poor prognosis acute leukemia?**
   a. Anger
   b. Denial
   c. Depression
   d. Acceptance

8. **Transfused red cells have survival of:**
   a. 30 days
   b. 60 days
   c. 90 days
   d. 120 days

9. **Which of the following is not associated with hyposplenism?**
   a. Celiac disease
   b. Inflammatory bowel disease (IBD)
   c. Sickle cell disease
   d. Hodgkin lymphoma

10. **Which of the following is commonly seen 2 weeks postsplenectomy?**
    a. Increase in platelet count of up to $1,000 \times 10^9/L$
    b. Monocytosis
    c. Disseminated intravascular coagulation
    d. Postsplenectomy overwhelming sepsis

11. **Which of the following statements is correct about postsplenectomy infection?**
    a. Prophylaxis with oral penicillin 250 mg is recommended for life
    b. Patient should not travel to malaria endemic area
    c. Inactivated vaccines are not useful in preventing infections
    d. Patients should be monitored for viral infections particularly herpes

12. ***Plasmodium vivax* infects which of the following?**
    a. Mature RBC
    b. Young RBC
    c. RBC of all ages
    d. None of the above

13. **Congenital dyserythropoietic anemia type II (CDA II) is characterized by all, *except*:**
    a. Lysis with autologous serum
    b. Autosomal recessive
    c. Splenectomy is useful in transfusion dependency
    d. Positive Ham test

14. **Lymphoblasts cannot be easily differentiated from which type of these cells?**
    a. Monocyte
    b. Myeloblast
    c. Myelocyte
    d. Mature lymphocyte

15. **Auer rods are seen only in:**
    a. Monoblast and myeloblast
    b. Lymphocyte and lymphoblast
    c. Monoblast and lymphoblast
    d. Lymphocyte and lymphoblast

16. **Slide preparation for cell count in cerebrospinal fluid (CSF) should be done as soon as possible because the cells degenerate within how much time?**
    a. 2 hours
    b. 12 hours
    c. 24 hours
    d. After 24 hours

17. **Clotting in the CSF may be seen due to:**
    a. Increased protein
    b. Increased fibrinogen
    c. Increased glucose concentration
    d. Bacteria
    e. Both a and b

18. **Xanthochromia in CSF indicates:**
    a. Increased WBCs   b. RBCs
    c. Presence of bacteria
    d. Traumatic lumbar puncture

19. **Blood sample in newborn is usually taken from:**
    a. Heel
    b. Toe
    c. Finger
    d. Ear lobe

20. **Clots present in blood sample will give an:**
    a. Increased cell count
    b. Decreased cell count
    c. Normal cell count
    d. No effect

21. **Which of the following increases the erythrocyte sedimentation rate (ESR) most?**
    a. Fibrinogen
    b. Prothrombin
    c. Factor VIII
    d. Factor IX

22. **The most important factor determining an ESR is:**
    a. Plasma concentration
    b. Platelet aggregation
    c. Red blood cells
    d. White blood cells

23. **Using an ocular of 10X, with a low power objective, the magnification of the object will be:**
    a. 10 times
    b. 100 times
    c. 1,000 times
    d. 400 times

24. **If the ESR is performed 24 hours after collection, then it will be:**
    a. Higher than freshly drawn sample
    b. Lower than freshly drawn sample
    c. Same as freshly drawn sample
    d. No effect

25. **The ESR can be affected by all, *except*:**
    a. Fraction of anticoagulant in blood
    b. Level of fibrinogen in the blood
    c. Position of tube
    d. Temperature
    e. High blood sugar

26. **The angle used to prepare a good blood smear slide is:**
    a. 10°
    b. 30°
    c. 45°
    d. 15°

27. **The leukemia which involves both the erythroid precursors and granulocytic precursors:**
    a. Monocytic leukemia
    b. Erythroleukemia
    c. Myelogenous leukemia
    d. Eosinophilic leukemia

28. **In acute lymphoblastic leukemia:**
    a. t(12;21) indicates good prognosis
    b. t(12;21) indicates poor prognosis
    c. t(9;22) indicates good prognosis
    d. t(1;19) indicates good prognosis

29. **Philadelphia chromosome is seen with which type of leukemia?**
    a. Chronic myeloid leukemia
    b. Chronic myelomonocytic leukemia
    c. Chronic lymphocytic leukemia
    d. Acute erythroid leukemia

30. **A 60-year-old patient is diagnosed to have multiple myeloma. Skeletal survey showed lytic lesions in skull and vertebrae. Urine examination showed Bence-Jones proteins. What are these Bence-Jones proteins?**
    a. IgA antibody
    b. IgM antibody
    c. Light chains
    d. IgG antibody

31. **All of the following are X-linked disease, *except*:**
    a. Fabry's disease
    b. G6PD deficiency
    c. von Willebrand disease
    d. Hemophilia A

32. **What is the recommended cleaner for removing oil from microscope lens?**
    a. Xylene
    b. Commercial lens cleaner
    c. Benzene
    d. Distilled water
    e. 20% alcohol

33. The computed tomography scan of the skull shown below is suggestive of:

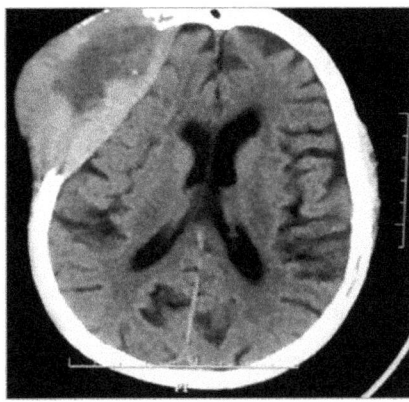

a. CNS aspergillosis
b. CNS leukemia
c. Plasmacytoma
d. Primary CNS lymphoma

34. The bone marrow examination of a patient showed gelatinous transformation of the marrow. The most probable clinical condition would be:
a. A 14 years-old-girl with petechial rash for 2 days, without fever hepatosplenomegaly or lymphadenopathy
b. An 18-years-old girl with weight of 30 kg and BMI 14.6
c. A 52 years old male high white cell count, splenomegaly and JAK-2 positive
d. A 40-years old male patient who presented with pancytopenia after accidental exposure to radiation injury

35. Schumm test was historically done to detect:
a. Haptoglobin
b. Methaemalbumin
c. Carboxyhaemoglobin
d. Hemopexin

36. Pseudolymphoma may be produced by all, *except*:
a. Cyclosporine
b. Primidone
c. Lithium
d. Phenytoin

37. Serum Vitamin B12 levels are increased in:
a. Pernicious anemia
b. Di Guglielmo's disease
c. Chronic myeloid leukemia
d. Hereditary orotic aciduria

38. Peripheral smear in a patient post-splenectomy can have all of the following, *except*:
a. Howell Jolly bodies
b. Heinz bodies
c. Target cells
d. Döhle bodies

39. Waldeyer's Ring includes of all the following, *except*:
a. Faucial tonsils
b. Adenoids
c. Lingual tonsils
d. Submandibular nodes

40. Leucocyte alkaline phosphatase score is diminished in:
a. Sickle cells anemia
b. Polycythemia vera
c. Paroxysmal nocturnal hemoglobinuria
d. Hodgkins lymphoma

41. Which of the following neoplasms does not qualify for myeloid/lymphoid neoplasms with eosinophilia and gene rearrangement:
a. Neoplasms PDGFR rearrangement
b. Neoplasms FGFR1 rearrangement
c. Neoplasms with PCM1-JAK2 rearrangement
d. Chronic eosinophilic leukemia

42. Thymoma is associated with all the following, *except*:
a. Cushing's syndrome
b. Hypergammaglobulinemia
c. Myasthenia gravis
d. Pernicious anemia

43. Plummer Vinson syndrome is associated with all the following, *except*:
a. Angular stomatitis
b. Splenomegaly
c. Clubbing
d. Post cricoid webs

44. Crow-Fukase syndrome includes all the following, *except*:
a. Monoclonal plasma cell proliferative disorder
b. Castelman's disease
c. Osteosclerotic bone lesions
d. Thrombocytopenia

45. TEMPI syndrome is characterized by all the following, *except*:
a. Telangiectasia
b. Polyneuropathy
c. Monoclonal gammopathy
d. Intrapulmonary shunting

46. Which of the following is not true about Donath-Landsteiner syndrome:
a. Increased haptoglobin
b. IgG antibody mediated process
c. Precipitated by exposure to cold
d. Not a cold agglutinin disease

SECTION 11 | Drugs and Miscellaneous

47. Henoch–Schönlein purpura is characterized by all the following, *except*:
   a. IgA vasculitis
   b. Thrombocytopenia
   c. Palpable purpura
   d. Abdominal pain

48. Which of the statement is false?
   b. Normal plasma cells are usually CD38 bright, CD19+, CD56-
   c. CD38 and ZAP-70 are poor prognostic markers in CLL.
   d. Sezzary cells are often CD7-, CD26-, CD25+/-
   e. Marginal zone lymphoma often shows positivity for CD23, CD5 and CD11c.

49. Hypocupremia is seen in:
   a. Osteoporosis
   b. Celiac disease
   c. Cardiovascular disease
   d. Colon cancer
   e. All of the above

50. Deficiency of Vitamin B12 and folic acid have the similar symptoms, *except*:
   a. Glossitis
   b. Neurological symptoms
   c. Muscle wasting
   d. Dizziness

51. Which of the following is a considered a high-risk organ for Langerhans cell histiocytosis?
   a. Spleen
   b. Bone
   c. Skin
   d. Lymph nodes

52. Langerhans cell histiocytosis that impacts skin, bone and the pituitary would be termed:
   a. High-risk
   b. Single-system
   c. Multisystem
   d. Moderate-risk

53. All medicines among following have proven to be effective in relapsed/refractory multisystem Langerhan cell histiocytosis (MS-LCH), *except*:
   a. Trametinib
   b. Vemurafenib
   c. Dabrafenib
   d. Sunitinib

54. Which of the following is true regarding Covid-19 infection?
   a. Monocytes and endothelial cells are infected
   b. Intravascular thrombosis can occur
   c. Bleeding is rare
   d. All of the above

55. All of the following are true regarding Covid-19 infection, *except*:
   a. Neutropenia
   b. Lymphopenia
   c. Thrombocytopenia
   d. Anemia

56. The most common site of thrombosis in Covid-19 infection is:
   a. Stroke
   b. Myocardial infarction
   c. Pulmonary embolism
   d. Mesenteric vein thrombosis

57. Eltrombopag should not be taken with:
   a. Iron
   b. Calcium
   c. Zinc
   d. Magnesium
   e. All of the above

58. Which of the following is not a feature of TAFRO syndrome?
   a. Anasarca
   b. Fever
   c. Organomegaly
   d. M protein

59. All can be used in haemophilia A patients with inhibitors presented with acute bleed, *except*:
   a. Recombinant factor VII
   b. Activated prothrombin complex concentrates
   c. Antifibrinolytic agents
   d. Emicizumab

60. Which of the following is incorrect about BPDCN (Blatic plasmacytoid dendritic cell neoplasm)?
   a. It involves skin, bone marrow, lymph nodes and other extramedullary organs
   b. Tagraxofusp is FDA approved for BPDCN
   c. Tagraxofusp targets CD 123
   d. Universally positive for CD4, CD56, and CD123 and frequently positive for CD 36, CD38, CD43, CD303, TCL 1, Tdt and positive for CD 34.

61. Which of the following is true about SNAPS?
   a. It includes patients whose diagnostic test are negative for APS but have suspected APS clinically
   b. It includes patients having SLE and APS
   c. It includes cases of primary APS only
   d. It includes primary APS, secondary APS, and catastropic APS

62. Differentiation syndrome is found associated with all of the following, *except*:
   a. Arsenic trioxide   b. ATRA
   c. Ivisidenib and enasidenib
   d. Giltertinib
   e. None of the above

ANSWERS WITH EXPLANATIONS

1. Ans. b. Phlebotomy Ref: William's 8/e p594

2. Ans. b. Bleeding

Hyperviscosity syndrome classically refers to a combination of clinical symptoms and physical findings, with laboratory documentation of an increased serum viscosity, as measured by Ostwald viscometry.

Symptoms are related to impairment of blood flow in microcirculation of the central and peripheral nervous system. Symptoms include headache, dizziness, vertigo, nystagmus, hearing loss, visual impairment, somnolence, coma, and seizure. Other possible findings could be mucosal hemorrhage, such as epistaxis, gingival and gastric bleeding, and congestive heart failure.

Causes of hyperviscosity syndrome are:
- Increased plasma Ig, especially IgM, less commonly IgA, IgG, or light chain.
- Increased cellular blood components (typically WBCs and RBCs), e.g., in leukemias, polycythemia, essential thrombocytosis, and the MDS.
- Normal relative serum viscosity ranges from 1.4 to 1.8 centipoise. Symptoms usually are not seen at value <4 units.
- Clinical symptoms generally are related to the triad of mucosal bleeding, visual changes, and neurologic symptoms. The tendency to bleed is the most common symptom of hypervicocity syndrome. Neurological manifestations are referred to as Bings-Neel syndrome. Treatments for immediate relief of symptoms are plasmapheresis and leukapheresis/phlebotomy.

3. Ans. b. Calcitriol Ref: Harrison's 18/e p594

Therapies for severe hypercalcemia are:

Treatment	Onset of action	Duration of action	Advantages	Disadvantages
Hydration with saline	Hours	During infusion	Rehydration invariably needed	Volume overload
Forced diuresis saline plus loop diuretics	Hours	During treatment	Rapid action	Volume overload, cardiac decompensation, intensive monitoring, electrolyte disturbance
Phosphonates				
Pamidronate	1–2 days	10–14 days to weeks	High potency, intermediate onset of action	Fever in 20% hypophosphatemia, hypocalcemia, hypomagnesemia, rarely jaw necrosis
Zoledronate	1–2 days	>3 weeks	Same as for pamidronate (may last longer)	Same as pamidronate above
Calcitonin	Hours	1–2 days	Rapid onset of action, useful as adjunct in severe hypercalcemia	Rapid tachyphylaxis
Special use therapies				
Phosphate (oral)	24 hours	During use	Chronic management (with hypophosphatemia); low toxicity if P < 4 mg/dL	Limited use except as adjuvant or chronic therapy
Glucocorticoids	Days	Days, weeks	Oral therapy, antitumor agents	Active only in certain malignancies vitamin D excess and sarcoidosis, steroid side effects
Dialysis	Hours	During use and 24–48 hours afterward	Useful in renal failure, onset of effect in hours, can immediately reverse life-threatening hypercalcemia	Complex procedure, reserved for extreme or special circumstances

4. Ans. b. Hereditary persistence of fetal hemoglobin (HPFH) Ref: Dacie and Lewis 10/e p315-316

Heinz, in 1890, was the first to describe in detail inclusions in red cells developing as a result of the action of acetylphenyl hydrazine on the blood. There are other compounds viz. nitro and amino compounds, as well as inorganic oxidizing agents such as potassium chlorate.

Causes of Heinz body formation are:
- Unstable hemoglobin
- G6PD deficiency
- Acute oxidant-induced hemolysis, e.g., chemical poisoning, drug intoxication.

In unstable hemoglobin, they are not seen in freshly withdrawn samples (needs 24–48 hours of incubation). In case of chemical or drug intoxication, they are seen postsplenectomy or if the dose is massive. Spleen helps in removing the RBCs with Heinz bodies.

5. Ans. b. Pseudo or relative polycythemia Ref: William's 8/e p823-30

High Hb with elevated serum EPO level means secondary polycythemia which can further be divided into appropriate and inappropriate category.

Appropriate: Appropriate secondary erythrocytosis occurs in response to increased erythropoietin (EPO)

levels resulting from sustained hypoxia. The common causes are:
- High-altitude polycythemia
- Smokers polycythemia
- Hemoglobin with increased affinity for oxygen
- Pulmonary or cardiac disease
- Sleep apnea syndrome
- Polycythemia.

Inappropriate: Erythropoiesis is being stimulated by EPO-producing tumors or in response to EPO or other simulators of erythropoiesis. Examples are:
- Renal cell carcinoma
- Chuvash polycythemia
- Postrenal transplantation erythrocytosis
- Brain tumors
- Hepatoma
- Endocrine disorders, e.g. pheochromocytomas, aldosterone-producing adenomas, Bartter syndrome, and dermoid cyst of the ovary.

Apparent or relative polycythemia is merely a mild absolute polycythemia accentuated by compensatory reduction in plasma volume. The main clinical associations are obesity, hypertension, and smoking.

6. Ans. d. Hemorrhagic disease of newborn
Ref: William's 8/e p807, 2296, 787, Wikipedia

Hemolytic disease of newborn is predominantly associated with Rh alloimmunization. Other causes are ABO incompatibility, maternal alloantibodies, as well as red cell enzyme and membrane defects.

Direct antiglobulin test is positive in delayed hemolytic transfusion reaction and should be done on fresh blood sample.

AIHA will classically have DCT positive.

Hemorrhagic disease of newborn is a coagulation disturbance in newborns due to vitamin K deficiency. Most common sites of bleeding are the umbilicus, mucus membranes, gastrointestinal tract, circumcision, and venipunctures.

7. Ans. b. Denial
Ref: Elisabeth Kübler-Ross. Death and Dying book. 1969

Kubler-Ross developed five-stage model for grief:
- *1st stage*: Denial
- *2nd stage*: Anger
- *3rd stage*: Bargaining
- *4th stage*: Depression
- *5th stage*: Acceptance.

8. Ans. b. 60 days
Ref: Hoffman 5/e p2426

Transfused red cells have shorter survival than normal red cells (mean of 60 days instead of 120 days, unless specially prepared neocytes are used).

9. Ans. d. Hodgkin lymphoma
Ref: Hoffman 6/e p2259-60

The causes of hyposplenism are:
- Congenital asplenia or hyposplenia may be associated with the severe cyanotic congenital heart disease
- Acquired hyposplenism:
  - Infarction in sickle cell disease
  - Systemic lupus erythematosus
  - Rheumatoid arthritis
  - Sarcoidosis
  - Systemic vasculitis
  - IBD (ulcerative colitis)
  - Amyloidosis
  - Chronic graft versus host disease
  - Mastocytosis
- Congenital and acquired immune deficiency.

10. Ans. a. Increase in platelet count of up to 1,000 × 10^9/L
Ref: Hoffbrand 5/e p365

Complications of splenectomy
- *Immediate postoperative complications*:
  - Bleeding
  - Subphrenic abscesses
- *Delayed complications*:
  - Overwhelming postsplenectomy infections
  - Thrombocytosis with a risk of thromboembolic incidents.

In the immediate postoperative period in uncomplicated splenectomy patients, the platelet count rises steeply to a maximum of usually 600–1,000 10^9/L with a peak at 7–12 days. In a number of patients, the thrombocytosis persists indefinitely after splenectomy. Although a reactive thrombocytosis is not usually associated with thromboembolic problems, it may sometimes cause pulmonary thromboembolism.

Postsplenectomy changes

Red cell changes: Appearance of Howell-Jolly bodies, siderotic granules, and target cell vacuoles. Some patients may show irregularly contracted or crenated, acanthocytic red cells. Reticulocytes usually increase and occasionally RBCs may also be seen. No alteration in red cell survival.

Leukocyte changes: Rise in total leukocyte count. A neutrophilic leukocytosis in the immediate postoperative phase and in majority later replaced by significant and permanent increase in both lymphocytes and monocytes.

Platelet changes: Thrombocytosis is transitory and falls to normal values over next 1-2 months but occasional large and bizarre platelets can be seen.

Immunological effects: Fall in IgM fraction is commonly found. IgG levels do not change while IgA and IgE levels increase.

Overwhelming postsplenectomy infections does not occur in first 2 weeks postsplenectomy. Disseminated intravascular coagulation occurs usually in the immediate (<1 week) postoperative phase.

11. Ans. a. Prophylaxis with oral penicillin 250 mg is recommended for life
Ref: Hoffbrand 5/e p365

Postoperatively lifelong prophylactic antibiotics should be advocated in all cases, but if not possible, antibiotics should be given for at least 2 years and for children up to 16 years where there is underlying impaired immune function. Oral penicillin 250 mg BD or erythromycin 250 mg BD. When travelling to tropical countries, asplenic patients are at increased risk of severe *Plasmodium* infection and antimalarial prophylaxis should be given. Inactivated vaccines like *Pneumococcal*, meningococcal, and Hib vaccine should ideally be given at least 2–3 weeks prior to splenectomy if possible for maximal immune response. In asplenic patients, there is no risk of viral infection as viral infections are controlled by innate or adaptive cell-mediated immunity and not by humoral immunity and spleen is only involved in humoral immunity.

12. Ans. b. Young RBC
Ref: William's 8/e p770

P. vivax invades only young red cells, whereas *P. falciparum* attacks both young and old RBCs.

13. Ans. a. Lysis with autologous serum
Ref: William's 8/e p514, 517

Main features of congenital dyserythropoietic anemia types are:

	Light microscopy	Electron microscopy	Serology	Inheritance
Type I	Most erythroid cells abnormal; double nuclei internuclear chromatic bridges	Widened nuclear pores, spongy appearance of the heterochromatin invasion by the cytoplasm containing various organelles	No serologic abnormalities	AR
Type II	Mature stage erythroblasts with two or more nuclei, lobulated nuclei, Karyorrhexis, Pseudo-Gaucher cells	ER cisternae lining the inner surface of the red cell plasma membrane	Cells, containing the HEMPAS antigen are lysed by 30% of acidified normal sera; increased agglutinability and lysis with anti-"i" auto-antibodies	AR
Type III	Giant erythroblasts, up to 50 µg in diameter, with up to 12 nuclei, basophilic stippling	Clefts and blebs within nuclear areas, some iron-filled mitochondria, autophagic vacuoles and myelin figures in the cytoplasm	None	AD (not all cases)

There are no specific treatments for type II CDA. Splenectomy is indicated in the transfusion-dependent cases.

14. Ans. b. Myeloblast
Ref: Hoffman's 6/e p961-3

There are some special characteristics of lymphoblast and myeloblast. Lymphoblasts are small to intermediate in size and have scant, agranular cytoplasm. Myeloblasts have relatively large cytoplasm, more opened chromatin, and prominent nucleoli. But still no pathologist can surely differentiate between lymphoblast and myeloblast, just based on morphology.

15. Ans. a. Myeloblast and monoblast
Ref: Dacie and Lewis 10/e p330

16. Ans. a. 2 hours
Ref: Stokes BO. Principles of cytocentrifugation. Lab Med. 2004;35(7):434-7.

The cytospin preparation of CSF should be processed within few hours of collection as delay may lead to denaturation of cells/blasts.

17. Ans. e. Both a and b

Clot formation is always abnormal and is often due to increased level of proteins, especially fibrinogen. When protein level is more than 1,000 mg/dL, clot formation will most likely occur, but may occur at low levels as well. Some clots are fine and may appear as thin film or "scum" on the surface of CSF. This type of clot is also called pellicle which is composed of fibrinogen and WBCs. In bacterial meningitis, pellicle forms in short time; in TB meningitis, web-like clot (pellicle) forms after 12–24 hours; and in neurosyphilis, there is incomplete clot.

18. Ans. b. RBCs

Xanthochromia (yellow color) in CSF is examined in centrifuged sample and looking into the supernatant. It can be seen as spillover in case of very high serum bilirubin levels (>15 mg/dL). With this exception, xanthochromia in a freshly spun sample is evidence of preexistent blood in subarachnoid space.

19. Ans. a. Heel

Ref: Book of WHO guidelines on drawing blood samples.

Venipuncture is the procedure of choice in term neonates; however, it requires an experience and trained phlebotomist. If trained phlebotomist is not available, physician needs to draw the sample. Selection of a site for capillary sampling depends on the age and weight of the child.

Condition	Heel prick	Finger prick
Age	Birth to 6 months	Over 6 months
Weight	From 3 to 10 kg	More than 10 kg
Placement of lancet	On the medial or lateral plantar surface	On the side of ball of finger perpendicular to the lines of fingerprint
Recommended finger	NA	2nd and 3rd finger; avoid thumb and index finger because of calluses and avoid little finger because of thin skin

20. Ans. b. Decreased cell count

Ref: Dacie and Lewis 10/e p3

If the sample for cell count contains clot, the cell counts will be decreased as the blood clot also contains various cells such as RBCs, WBCs, and platelets.

21. Ans. a. Fibrinogen *Ref: Dacie and Lewis 10/e p599*

In ESR, the principle is based on the rate of fall of red cells. It depends on the difference in specific gravity of red cells and plasma. Red cell rouleaux fall more rapidly than single cell. The all-important rouleaux formation and red cell clumping that are associated with increased ESR are mainly controlled by the concentration of fibrinogen, immunoglobulins, and other acute-phase reactants (haptoglobin, ceruloplasmin, alpha1-antitrypsin, alpha1-acid glycoprotein, and C-reactive protein). It is retarded by albumin.

22. Ans. c. Red blood cells *Ref: Dacie and Lewis 10/e p599*

Erythrocyte sedimentation rate is dependent on various physiologic and pathologic factors including hemoglobin concentration, ratio of plasma proteins, serum lipid concentration, and plasma Ph. The process of erythrocyte sedimentation is described in three phases: aggregation, precipitation, and packing; aggregation is the most influential phase in determining the outcome of the test. There are two main factors, which may influence the aggregation process: high molecular weight components of the plasma and RBC structure. Normally, RBCs have negative charges and repel each other; while, many plasma proteins have positive charges and neutralize the surface charges of erythrocytes, which promote the aggregation. ESR is directly proportionate to the mass of erythrocyte, but inversely related to the area of its surface. Macrocytes sediment more rapidly than normal cells and microcytes.

23. Ans. b. 100 times

Magnification in microscope means enlargement of image. The magnification of microscope is given by:

M (microscope) = M (objective lens) × M (eye piece).

	Objective lens	Ocular lens (eye piece)	Total magnification
Scanning	4×	10×	40×
Low power	10×	10×	100×
High power dry	40×	10×	400×
High power oil	100×	10×	1,000×

24. Ans. b. Lower than freshly drawn sample

Ref: Dacie and Lewis 10/e p595-9

Conditions associated with decrease in ESR are abnormally shaped RBCs (sickle cells, spherocytosis) and technical factors [short ESR tubes, low room temperature, delay in test performance (>2 hours), clotted blood samples, excess anticoagulant, bubbles in tubes].

25. Ans. e. High blood sugar

Ref: Dacie and Lewis 10/e p595-9

Refer to explanation for Q. No. 22.

26. Ans. b. 30° *Ref: Dacie and Lewis 10/e p60*

The spreader should be placed in front of the blood or marrow drop at an angle of 30° and spreaded in forward direction to prevent crushing of cells between the edges.

27. Ans. b. Erythroleukemia *Ref: William's 7/e p1192*

In erythroleukemia, there is increase in both erythroid precursors and myeloblasts. Spontaneous growth of leukemic erythroid clonogenic cells is a feature of the disease and these cells are periodic acid-Schiff (PAS) positive. These cell features include glycophorin A, spectrin, carbonic anhydrase I, ABH blood group antigens, or other antigens that occur on early erythroid precursors.

28. Ans. a. t(12;21) indicates good prognosis

Ref: Hoffman's 6/e p941-5

The presence of TEL-AML1 translocation is associated with an excellent prognosis, with event free survival rates of approximately 90%. The presence of Philadelphia chromosome is associated with extremely poor prognosis, similarly E2A-PBX1 and mixed lineage leukemia fusion genes abnormalities are also associated with poor prognosis.

29. Ans. a. Chronic myeloid leukemia
Ref: Hoffman's 6/e p981

Chronic myeloid leukemia is defined by the presence of translocation 9;22. This translocation can be detected by routine cytogenetics, FISH, or RT-PCR in the order of increasing sensitivity.

30. Ans. c. Light chains
Ref: Hoffman's 5/e p1342

A Bence-Jones protein is a monoclonal globulin protein or immunoglobulin light chain found in the urine, with a molecular weight of 22–24 kDa.

31. Ans. c. von Willebrand disease
Ref: Hoffman's 6/e p582

von Willebrand disease is inherited as an autosomal dominant disease in majority, and rest all diseases are X linked (Fabry's disease, Hemophilia A, and G6-PD deficiency).

32. Ans. b. Commercial lens cleaner
Ref: Dacie and Lewis 10/e p707

After use of optics, wipe the immersion objective with lens tissue, absorbent paper, soft cloth, or medical cotton wool. For cleaning oil, toluene or a solution of 40% petroleum ether, 40% ethanol, and 20% ether is used.

33. Ans. c. Plasmacytoma
Ref: Madan S, Kumar S. Review: extramedullary disease in multiple myeloma. Clin Adv Hematol Oncol 2009;7:802-04

The computed tomography scan of head is showing involvement of right frontal bone by plasmacytoma with extensive bone destruction. The lesion has an exophytic component and reveals multiple areas of calcifications along its periphery. The other three mentioned diseases primarily involve CNS parenchyma and not the skull bone. Multiple myeloma is a neoplastic disorder of plasma cells. Plasma cell neoplasms can present as a single lesion (solitary plasmacytoma) or as multiple lesions (multiple myeloma). Solitary plasmacytomas can occur in bone (plasmacytoma of bone), or in soft tissues (extramedullary plasmacytoma). The bone lesions are due to monoclonal or malignant plasma cell infiltration.

34. Ans. b. An 18-years-old girl with weight of 30 kg and BMI 14.6
Ref: Jain R. Gelatinous transformation of bone marrow: a study of 43 cases. Indian J Pathol Microbiol 2005;48:1-3

The bone marrow biopsy showing gelatinous transformation of the marrow can be seen in a patient with anorexia nervosa. Gelatinous transformation of bone marrow is a rare event characterized by fat cell necrosis, loss of hematopoietic cells and deposition of extracellular gelatinous mucopolysaccharides, particularly hyaluronic acid. This gelatinous substance stains for Alcian Blue at pH 2.5. The common causes of gelatinous transformation of bone marrow are anorexia nervosa, acquired immunodeficiency syndrome, alcoholism, carcinomas, leukemias, lymphomas and chemotherapeutic agents. The other cases presented include ITP, myelofibrosis and post RT bone marrow aplasia, which are usually not associated with gelatinous transformation of the marrow. Anorexia nervosa is an eating disorder characterized by an abnormally low body weight, an intense fear of gaining weight and a distorted perception of weight.

35. Ans. b. Methaemalbumin
Ref: Barbara J. Bain, in Dacie and Lewis Practical Haematology, 12/e 2017

The Schumm test is a blood test that uses spectroscopy to determine significant levels of methaemalbumin in the blood. A positive result could indicate intravascular hemolysis. The Schumm test was named for Otto Schumm, a German chemist who lived in the early 20th century. A positive test result occurs when the haptoglobin binding capacity of the blood is saturated, leading to heme released from cell free hemoglobin to bind to albumin.

36. Ans. c. Lithium
Ref: Magro CM, Daniels BH, & Crowson AN. Drug induced pseudolymphoma. Seminars in Diagnostic Pathology 2018;35(4):247–59.

The spectrum of atypical cutaneous lymphocytic infiltrates of the skin is broad especially in regard to the various subtypes of primary cutaneous lymphoma. A common cause of atypical cutaneous lymphoid infiltrates that can resemble B and T cell lymphoma is the drug induced pseudolymphoma.

37. Ans. c. Chronic myeloid leukemia
Ref: Ermens AA, Vlasveld LT, Lindemans J. Significance of elevated cobalamin (vitamin B12) levels in blood. Clin Biochem. 2003;36(8):585-90.

Elevated levels of serum cobalamin may be a sign of a serious, even life-threatening, disease. Hematologic disorders like chronic myelogeneous leukemia, promyelocytic leukemia, polycythemia vera and also the hypereosinophilic syndrome can result in elevated levels of cobalamin. Not surprisingly, a rise of the cobalamin concentration in serum is one of the diagnostic criteria for the latter two diseases. The increase in circulating cobalamin levels is predominantly caused by enhanced production of haptocorrin. Several liver diseases like acute hepatitis, cirrhosis, hepatocellular carcinoma and metastatic liver disease can also be accompanied by an increase in circulating cobalamin. This phenomenon is predominantly caused by cobalamin release during hepatic cytolysis and/or decreased cobalamin clearance by the affected liver.

38. Ans. d. Döhle bodies
Ref: Barbara J. Bain, in Dacie and Lewis Practical Haematology, 12/e 2017

Döhle bodies are small, round or oval, pale blue-grey structures usually found at the periphery of the neutrophil. They consist of ribosomes and endoplasmic reticulum. They are seen in bacterial infections but also following tissue damage including burns, in inflammation, following administration of G-CSF, in neutrophilic leukaemoid reactions and during pregnancy. There is also a benign inherited condition known as May—Hegglin anomaly with a similar but not identical morphological structure; in this condition, the inclusions tend to be larger and angular and occur in all types of leucocyte except lymphocytes. Similar inclusions are seen in related conditions, referred to collectively as MYH9-related disorders.

39. Ans. d. Submandibular nodes

Ref: Hellings P, Jorissen M, Ceuppens JL. The Waldeyer's ring. Acta Otorhinolaryngol Belg. 2000;54(3):237-41

Waldeyers ring named after Heinrich Wilhelm Gottfried Waldeyer-Hartz. The palatine tonsils, nasopharyngeal tonsil (adenoid) and lingual tonsil constitute the major part of Waldeyer's ring or nasal-associated lymphoid tissue (NALT), with the tubal tonsils and lateral pharyngeal bands as less prominent components. The lymphoid tissue of Waldeyer's ring is located at the gateway of the respiratory and alimentary tract and belongs to the mucosa-associated lymphoid tissue (MALT).

40. Ans. c. Paroxysmal nocturnal hemoglobinuria

Ref: Barbara J Bain, in Dacie and Lewis Practical Haematology, 12/e 2017

Normal Range: 10 to 100. In normal individuals, it is rare to find any neutrophils with a score of 3, and a score of 4 should not be present. There is some physiological variation in LAP scores. Newborn babies, children and pregnant women have high scores, and pre-menopausal women have, an average, scores one-third higher than those of men. In pathological states, the most significant diagnostic use of the NAP score is in CML. In the chronic phase of the disease, the score is almost invariable low, usually zero. Transient increases may occur with inter-current infection. In myeloid blast transformation or accelerated phase, the score rises. Low scores are also commonly found in paroxysmal nocturnal haemoglobinuria (PNH) and the very rare condition of hereditary hypophosphatasia. There are many causes of raised NAP score, notably in the neutrophilia of infection, polycythaemia vera, leukaemoid reactions, and Hodgkin's disease. In aplastic anaemia, the NAP score is high, but it falls if PNH supervenes. With the greater use of cytogenetic and molecular genetic techniques to confirm the diagnosis of CML, the NAP score is needed much less often.

41. Ans. d. Chronic eosinophilic leukemia

Ref: WHO Book 2017

Chronic Eosinophilic leukemia is under myeloproliferative neoplasms category.

42. Ans. b. Hypergammaglobulinemia

43. Ans. c. Clubbing

Plummer–Vinson syndrome is a rare disease characterized by difficulty swallowing, iron-deficiency anemia, glossitis, cheilosis and esophageal webs. Treatment with iron supplementation and mechanical widening of the esophagus generally provides an excellent outcome.

44. Ans. d. Thrombocytopenia *Ref: WHO Book 2017*

POEMS syndrome also known as osteosclerotic myeloma; Crow-Fukase syndrome is a paraneoplastic syndrome associated with a plasma cell neoplasm, usually characterized by fibrosis and osteosclerotic changes in bone trabeculae, and often with lymph node changes resembling the plasma cell variant of Castleman disease. The POEMS acronym stands for polyneuropathy, organomegaly, endocrinopathy, mono clonal gammopathy, and skin changes, but these components are not all required for diagnosis; in many cases, not all are present.

45. Ans. b. Polyneuropathy *Ref: WHO Book 2017*

TEMPI syndrome is a paraneoplastic syndrome associated with a plasma cell neoplasm. The acronym stands for telangiectasias, elevated erythropoietin and erythrocytosis, monoclonal gammopathy, perinephric fluid collection, and intrapulmonary shunting included in the WHO classification as a provisional category of plasma cell neoplasm. The reported patient age range is 35-58 years, and it occurs in both men and women.

46. Ans. a. Increased haptoglobin

Ref: Barbara J Bain, in Dacie and Lewis Practical Haematology, 12/e, 2017

Paroxysmal cold hemoglobinuria (PCH) also known as Donath-Landsteiner syndrome is an autoimmune hemolytic anemia featured by complement-mediated intravascular hemolysis after cold exposure.

Infectious agents are implicated in the acute form of PCH. Viral agents include measles, mumps, Epstein-Barr virus, cytomegalovirus, varicella-zoster virus, influenza virus, and adenovirus. Non-viral agents include Mycoplasma pneumoniae and Haemophilus influenzae. Chronic relapsing PCH is classically associated with syphilis, as well as hematological malignancies including non-Hodgkin lymphoma and myeloproliferative neoplasms. For intravascular hemolysis, the laboratory parameters include increased serum free hemoglobin, lactate dehydrogenase, unconjugated bilirubin, and reduced haptoglobin. Urine tests may show elevated hemoglobinuria and hemosiderinuria in chronic cases. Reticulocytosis may not be apparent in the acute phase or when there is viral-induced myelosuppression.

47. Ans. b. Thrombocytopenia

Henoch–Schönlein purpura (HSP), also known as IgA vasculitis, is characterized by the "classic triad" of

Purpura, arthritis and abdominal pain. The platelet count may be raised, and distinguishes it from diseases where low platelets are the cause of the purpura, such as idiopathic thrombocytopenic purpura and thrombotic thrombocytopenic purpura.

48. **Ans. d. Marginal zone lymphoma often shows positivity for CD23, CD5 and CD11c**

Ref: WHO Book 2017

Marginal zone lymphomas are usually CD5 negative. CD5 positive neoplasms include CLL and mantle cell lymphoma.

49. **Ans. e. All of the above**

Common causes of hypocupremia include malabsorption disorders (celiac disease, Crohn disease, colon cancer), loss in nephrotic syndrome, copper chelation, zinc ingestion, cardiac failure. Hypocupremia may result in bone marrow failure.

50. **Ans. b. Neurological symptoms**

Production of S-adenosyl methionine from methionine requires methyl-cobalamin as a cofactor, so neurological symptoms are seen commonly in vitamin B12 deficiency, and not in folate deficiency.

51. **Ans. a. Spleen**

Ref: Jezierska M. Langerhans cell histiocytosis in children. Postepy Dermatol Alergol. 2018; 35(1): 6–17.

Multisystem LCH may have two forms, either with or without organ involvement. Low-risk organs include the skin, bones, lymph nodes, and the pituitary gland, whereas high-risk organs include bone marrow, liver, spleen and the lungs.

52. **Ans. c. Multisystem LCH**

Ref: Jezierska M. Langerhans cell histiocytosis in children. Postepy Dermatol Alergol. 2018;35(1):6–17

Treatment of LCH is based on where LCH cells are found in the body and whether the LCH is low-risk or high-risk. LCH is described as single-system disease or multisystem disease, depending on how many body systems are affected:
- **Single-system LCH**: LCH is found in one part of an organ or body system or in more than one part of that organ or body system. Bone is the most common single place for LCH to be found followed by skin.
- **Multisystem LCH**: LCH occurs in two or more organs or body systems or may be spread throughout the body. Multisystem LCH is less common than single-system LCH.

53. **Ans. d. Sunitinib**

Ref: Lee LH. Blood Advances 2020;4(4):717-27

Genomic alterations resulting in activation of the mitogen-activated protein kinase pathway are a key molecular pathogenic feature of the histiocytic neoplasms and in LCH usually involve activating mutations in BRAF and MAP2K1. Targeted therapy with BRAF V600E–specific inhibitors has demonstrated significant responses in adults and children with LCH.

Dabrafenib and vemurafinib are specific inhibitor of BRAFV600E. Trametininb is a MEK inhibitor. Sunitinib malate is a novel oral multitargeted tyrosine kinase inhibitor with antitumor and antiangiogenic activities.

54. **Ans. d. All of the above**

Ref: Rahi S. Hematologic disorders associated with COVID-19: a review. Ann Hematol 2021

Severe acute respiratory syndrome coronavirus 2 (Covid-19) infects monocytes and endothelial cells leading to a complex downstream cascade, cytokine storm, and eventual intravascular thrombosis. Cytokine storm and IL-6 in particular are particularly elevated in COVID-19 compared to other septic conditions, and these are upregulate multiple thrombogenic pathways. Prophylactic anticoagulation is vital in patients with Covid-19, as its effect on the coagulation system is associated with significant morbidity and mortality. The disease can cause both arterial and venous thromboses, especially pulmonary embolism and pulmonary microthrombi. A high index of suspicion is indispensable in recognizing these complications, and timely institution of therapeutic anticoagulation is vital in treating them. Bleeding is rare unlike in DIC.

55. **Ans. a. Neutropenia** *Ref: Rahi S. Hematologic disorders associated with COVID-19: a review. Ann Hematol 2021*

Covid-19 invades human cells by binding to the angiotensin-converting enzyme 2 (ACE-2) receptor, which is primarily found in the lungs, heart, and gastrointestinal tract. These receptors are also expressed on the surface of lymphocytes. Consequently, SARS-CoV-2 may bind directly to these cells and cause lysis. Infection also results in the production and release of multiple inflammatory cytokines. Covid-19-associated immune dysregulation leads to neutrophil production and lymphocyte apoptosis. Thus, neutrophilia coincides with lymphopenia. Neutrophilia by itself is associated with Covid-19 disease progression, increased risk of acute respiratory distress syndrome (ARDS), and death. Covid-19 causes lymphopenia, neutrophilia, anemia and thrombocytopenia.

56. **Ans. c. Pulmonary embolism**

Pulmonary embolism and deep vein thrombosis are the most frequently noted thrombotic events in Covid-19, with initial reports noting an incidence of 20% to 30% in critically ill patients, leading to acute right ventricular dysfunction and cor pulmonale. By autopsy, microthrombi have been identified in several extrapulmonary organs, but at a much lower frequency than pulmonary involvement.

57. Ans e. All of the above

Eltrombopag is known to interact with polyvalent cations in certain foods, drinks and medicines. This interaction can significantly impair the absorption of eltrombopag into the body. Polyvalent cations to be avoided include calcium, aluminium, iron, magnesium, selenium and zinc as these can significantly reduce the absorption of eltrombopag. Eltrombopag must be administered at least 2 hours before or 4 hours after polyvalent cation-containing antacids, dairy products (or any foods, drinks, or medicines containing ≥50 mg calcium) and other products containing polyvalent cations, such as mineral supplements.

58. Ans. d. M protein

Ref: Igawa. TAFRO Syndrome Hematol Oncol Clin North Am. 2018

TAFRO syndrome is a newly recognized variant of idiopathic multicentric Castleman disease (iMCD) that involves a constellation of syndromes: thrombocytopenia (T), anasarca (A), fever (F), reticulin fibrosis (R), and organomegaly (O). Thrombocytopenia and severe anasarca accompanied by relatively low serum immunoglobulin levels are characteristic clinical findings of TAFRO syndrome that are not present in iMCD-not otherwise specified (iMCD-NOS). Lymph node biopsy is recommended to exclude other diseases and to diagnose TAFRO syndrome, which reveals characteristic histopathological findings similar to hyaline vascular-type CD. TAFRO syndrome follows a more aggressive course, compared with iMCD-NOS, and there is no standard treatment.

59. Ans. d. Emicizumab

Ref: Hoffmann 6/e p 2031

A novel therapeutic approach has recently been reported based on the use of a conformational replica of FVIII, Emicizumab. This humanized, bispecific antibody binds both FIX and FX forming a thrombin-generation complex. This complex, in vitro and in vivo, elicits thrombin formation independent of the FVIII levels and, most importantly, the presence of an inhibitor to FVIII. A recent clinical trial showed a strong reduction of spontaneous bleeding in patients with hemophilia A with or without inhibitors. No use in acute bleed in haemophilia A with inhibitors.

60. Ans. d. Universally positive for CD4, CD56, and CD123 and frequently positive for CD36, CD38, CD43, CD303, TCL 1, Tdt and positive for CD34

Ref: Yun S. Survival outcomes in blastic plasmacytoid dendritic cell neoplasm by first-line treatment and stem cell transplant. Blood advances, 2020

BPDCN is characterized by common involvement of skin, bone marrow (BM), lymph node (LN), spleen, and other extramedullary organs and by its unique immunophenotype that is universally positive for CD4, CD56, and CD123; frequently positive for CD36, CD38, CD43, CD45RA, TCL1, TCF4, CD303/BDCA-2, and TdT; and negative for CD34, CD3, CD13, CD16, CD19, CD20, lysozyme, and MPO. Of note, there is a small subset of cases showing CD4 or CD56 negativity; however, it should not be excluded when 2 or more PDC-associated markers (CD123, TCL1, BDCA2, CD2AP, TCF4) are expressed. Tagraxofusp is FDA approved for BPDCN Tagraxofusp targets CD123.

61. Ans. a. It includes patients whose diagnostic test are negative for APS but have suspected APS clinically

Ref: Hoffman 7/e, p2088

SNAPS also known as seronegative APS includes patients whose diagnostic test are negative for APS but have suspected APS clinically.

62. Ans. e. None of the above

Ref: Gasparovic L. Incidence of differentiation syndrome associated with treatment regimens in acute myeloid leukemia: A systematic review of the literature. J Clin Med 2020

Differentiation syndrome (DS) is a potentially fatal adverse drug reaction caused by the so-called differentiating agents such as all-trans retinoic acid (ATRA) and arsenic trioxide (ATO), used for remission induction in the treatment of acute promyelocytic leukemia (APL). More recently, two clinical trials of isocitrate dehydrogenase (IDH)-inhibitor drugs for the treatment of relapsed/refractory IDH2-mutated (non-M3) AML unexpectedly observed DS as an adverse event, thereby identifying the IDH-inhibitors (enasidenib and ivosidenib) as potentially differentiating agents.

SECTION 12 Self-Assessment

47. Self-Assessment

CHAPTER 47

Self-Assessment

1. SELF-ASSESSMENT

1. Average life span of platelets is:
   a. 3–5 days   b. 7–10 days
   c. 12–15 days   d. 16–20 days

2. Pseudothrombocytopenia is due to:
   a. Ethylenediaminetetraacetic acid (EDTA)
   b. Heparin
   c. Citrate
   d. All of the above

3. Heparin-induced thrombocytopenia is due to antibodies against:
   a. Platelet factor 1 (PF1)   b. PF2
   c. PF3   d. PF4

4. Heparin-induced thrombocytopenia with thrombosis should be treated with:
   a. Low doses of heparin   b. Warfarin
   c. Platelet transfusion   d. None of the above

5. In thrombotic thrombocytopenic purpura (TTP):
   a. Prothrombin time (PT) is prolonged
   b. Activated partial thromboplastin time (APTT) is prolonged
   c. Both are prolonged
   d. None of the above

6. Autosomal hemophilia is the term used for:
   a. Type 2A von Willebrand disease (vWD)
   b. Type 2B vWD
   c. Type 2M vWD
   d. Type 2N vWD

7. In factor XIII deficiency:
   a. PT is prolonged
   b. APTT is prolonged
   c. Thrombin time (TT) is prolonged
   d. All of the above are prolonged
   e. None of the above is prolonged

8. Combined factor deficiency commonly seen is:
   a. Factor V and VII   b. Factor V and VIII
   c. Factor V and IX   d. Factor V and X

9. 1 mg of protamine neutralizes:
   a. 1 units of heparin   b. 10 units of heparin
   c. 100 units of heparin   d. 200 units of heparin

10. After allogeneic stem cell transplantation, neutrophil engraftment occurs after:
   a. 10–12 days   b. 18–20 days
   c. 26–28 days   d. 34–36 days

11. Acute graft-versus-host disease (GVHD) usually does not involve:
   a. Skin   b. Liver
   c. Kidney   d. Colon

12. Autologous transplant is not done for:
   a. Lymphoma
   b. Myeloma
   c. Acute myeloid leukemia (AML)
   d. Aplastic anemia

13. Treatment of choice for Philadelphia chromosome positive acute lymphoblastic leukemia (Ph + ALL) is:
   a. Imatinib
   b. Hyper-CVAD (hyperfractionated cyclophosphamide, vincristine, doxorubicin, and dexamethasone) chemotherapy
   c. Autologous transplant
   d. Allogeneic transplant

14. Treatment of choice for 20-year-old aplastic anemia patient is:
   a. Cyclosporine
   b. Antithymocyte globulin
   c. Autologous bone marrow transplantation (BMT)
   d. Allogeneic BMT

15. Eltrombopag is for:
   a. Paroxysmal nocturnal hemoglobinuria (PNH)
   b. Immune thrombocytopenic purpura (ITP)
   c. Hodgkin's lymphoma
   d. Non-Hodgkin's lymphoma

16. Graft-versus-host disease risk is high if donor inoculum contains large numbers of:
   a. Regulatory T-cells   b. Cytotoxic T-cells
   c. B-cells   d. Neutrophils

17. Veno-occlusive syndrome post-transplant includes all, *except*:
   a. Weight gain   b. Ascites
   c. Hepatomegaly   d. Decreased urine output

18. Primary hemophagocytic lymphohistiocytosis (HLH) is due to defect in:
   a. Cytotoxic T cells
   b. Natural killer (NK) cells
   c. Macrophages
   d. All of the above

19. Diagnostic criteria for HLH include all, *except*:
   a. Splenomegaly
   b. Cytopenias
   c. Hemophagocytosis
   d. Hypocellular bone marrow

20. Ferritin for the diagnosis of HLH should be more than:
   a. 500 µg/L
   b. 2,000 µg/L
   c. 5,000 µg/L
   d. 10,000 µg/L

21. The least common cause of thrombocytopenia in pregnancy is:
   a. Gestational thrombocytopenia
   b. Eclampsia/HELLP (hemolysis, elevated liver enzymes, and a low platelet count) syndrome
   c. Immune thrombocytopenia
   d. All have equal frequency

22. True about gestational thrombocytopenia is:
   a. Usually mild to moderate thrombocytopenia
   b. No previous history
   c. Typically occurs in 3rd trimester
   d. May recur in subsequent pregnancy
   e. All of the above

23. False about gestational thrombocytopenia is:
   a. Incidental finding
   b. Diagnosis of exclusion
   c. No previous history
   d. Cause fetal thrombocytopenia

24. Gestational thrombocytopenia accounts for _____ of cases of thrombocytopenia in pregnancy.
   a. 70–80%   b. 50–60%
   c. 30–40%   d. 10–20%

25. Diagnostic test for immune thrombocytopenia (ITP) is:
   a. Antiplatelet antibody testing
   b. Bone marrow biopsy
   c. Thrombopoietin levels
   d. All of the above   e. None of the above

26. The drug most effective in HLH is:
   a. Cyclophosphamide   b. Etoposide
   c. Melphalan   d. Ifosfamide

27. Mutation associated with Waldenström macroglobulinemia is:
   a. MYD88 L265P
   b. C-X-C chemokine receptor type 4 (CXCR4)
   c. Both of the above
   d. None of the above

28. Cytogenetic abnormalities associated with Waldenström macroglobulinemia include all, *except*:
   a. Deletion 13q14   b. Deletion 17p13
   c. Deletion 6q   d. Deletion 7p

29. Khorana score is used for:
   a. Deep vein thrombosis
   b. Chronic lymphocytic leukemia
   c. Myelofibrosis
   d. Hairy cell leukemia

30. Cancer patients with incidentally diagnosed DVT should:
   a. Not be treated
   b. Treated with low-molecular-weight heparin (LMWH) for 3 months
   c. Treated with LMWH for 6 months
   d. Treated life-long with LMWH

Ans.	1. b	2. a	3. d	4. d	5. d	6. d
	7. e	8. b	9. c	10. a	11. c	12. d
	13. d	14. d	15. b	16. b	17. d	18. d
	19. d	20. a	21. c	22. e	23. d	24. a
	25. e	26. b	27. c	28. d	29. a	30. c

2. SELF-ASSESSMENT

1. Post-hepatitis marrow failure is commonly seen due to: *Ref: Harrison 6/e p664*
   a. Hepatitis A
   b. Hepatitis C
   c. Hepatitis G
   d. None of the above

2. Which is not a feature of PNH? *Ref: Harrison p664*
   a. Due to *PIG-A* (phosphatidylinositol N-acetylglucosaminyltransferase subunit A) gene mutation
   b. Cells are deficient in glycosylphosphatidylinositol (GPI)-linked proteins
   c. Never associated with myelodysplastic syndrome
   d. Thrombosis can be one of the presentation

3. Most common mutation in Fanconi's anemia is: *Ref: Harrison p665*
   a. Fanconi anemia subtype FANC D
   b. FANC A
   c. FANC B
   d. FANC L

4. Incorrect for dyskeratosis congenital: *Ref: Harrison p665*
   a. Mucous membrane leukoplasia
   b. Hyperpigmentation
   c. Abnormal nails
   d. None of the above
   e. All of the above

5. For very severe aplastic anemia ANC should be: *Ref: Harrison p666*
   a. 0
   b. $<50/mm^3$
   c. $<200/mm^3$
   d. $<100/mm^3$

6. Chronic cyclosporine toxicity includes all, *except*: *Ref: Harrison p667*
   a. Hypertension
   b. Seizure
   c. Myocardial infarction
   d. *Pneumocystis carinii* infection

7. Which statement is correct? *Ref: Hoffman 5/e p348,350*
   a. TAR (thrombocytopenia with absent radius) syndrome has normal thumb
   b. In Fanconi's anemia, when radii are absent, thumb is preserved
   c. Barth syndrome is related to platelet
   d. None of the above

8. Clastogenic agent is:
   a. Mitomycin d
   b. Dystrophic epidermolysis bullosa (DEB)
   c. Cyclosporine
   d. Antithymocyte globulin (ATG)

9. Prevention of transfusion-associated graft-versus-host disease (TA-GVHD) is by use of:
   a. Directed donation
   b. Irradiated blood products
   c. Leukodepleted blood products
   d. Storage for 4 hours at room temperature before transfusion

10. Corrected Count Increment (CCI) term is used for:
   a. Neutrophil recovery
   b. Red blood cell (RBC) recovery
   c. Platelet recovery
   d. Eosinophil recovery in hypereosinophilic syndrome

11. The mutation in cytomegalovirus (CMV) genes which lead to resistance to ganciclovir include all, *except*:
   a. UL97
   b. UL54
   c. UL27
   d. UL47

12. Drug effective against UL54 mutation is:
   a. Ganciclovir
   b. Cidofovir
   c. Maribavir
   d. None of the above

13. Drugs effective against cytomegalovirus include all, *except*:
   a. Leflunomide
   b. Artesunate
   c. Sirolimus
   d. Hydroxyurea

14. True about letermovir is:
   a. Target the pUL56
   b. Most potent
   c. Narrow antiviral effect
   d. Daily dose is 480 mg
   e. All of the above

15. Least specific test for the diagnosis of acute promyelocytic leukemia is:
   a. Karyotyping
   b. Fluorescence in situ hybridization (FISH)
   c. Polymerase chain reaction (PCR)
   d. Nuclear staining by anti-progressive multifocal leukoencephalopathy (anti-PML) monoclonal antibodies

16. QTc following arsenic therapy should not be allowed to increase more than:
   a. 400 milliseconds
   b. 450 milliseconds
   c. 500 milliseconds
   d. 550 milliseconds

17. Not true regarding central nervous system (CNS) prophylaxis in acute promyelocytic leukemia is:
   a. Restricted to patients with white blood cell (WBC) counts $>10 \times 10^9/L$ at presentation
   b. Should be done in those who have had a CNS hemorrhage
   c. Should be postponed after the achievement of complete remission (CR)
   d. Should be done in patients who develop headache after starting treatment

18. What percentage of acute myeloid leukemia (AML) are constituted by acute promyelocytic leukemia?
   a. <5%
   b. 5–10%
   c. 15–20%
   d. 25–30%

19. Which is a checkpoint inhibitor?
   a. Ipilimumab
   b. Pembrolizumab
   c. Avelumab
   d. Atezolizumab
   e. All of the above

20. Which of the following drug is not used in hemophagocytic lymphohistiocytosis?
   a. Vincristine
   b. Dexamethasone
   c. Etoposide
   d. Cyclosporine

21. The virus most commonly causing hemophagocytic lymphohistiocytosis is:
   a. Human immunodeficiency virus (HIV)
   b. Epstein-Barr virus (EBV)
   c. Cytomegalovirus (CMV)
   d. Herpes simplex virus (HSV)

22. Which of the following is not used in hemophagocytic lymphohistiocytosis?
   a. Intravenous immunoglobulin (IVIG)
   b. Rituximab
   c. Tocilizumab
   d. Granulocyte colony-stimulating factor (G-CSF)

23. Familial hemophagocytic lymphohistiocytosis (HLH) is:
   a. Autosomal recessive
   b. Autosomal dominant
   c. Sex-linked recessive
   d. Sex-linked dominant

24. Which is not a feature of HLH?
   a. Bicytopenia
   b. Hypotriglyceridemia
   c. Hypofibrinogenemia
   d. Coagulopathy

25. True about HLH are all, *except*:
   a. Accumulation of lymphocytes
   b. Increase in mature macrophages
   c. Increased NK cell activity
   d. All of the above

26. Parameters which were not present in HLH 94 and were added in HLH 2004 diagnostic criteria are all, *except*:
   a. Hypofibrinogenemia
   b. Low or absent NK-cell activity
   c. Ferritin ≥500 mg/L
   d. Soluble CD25 (i.e., soluble IL-2 receptor) ≥2,400 U/mL

27. Extensive inflammatory infiltrate with poor antitumor immune response is seen in:
   a. Marginal zone lymphoma
   b. Lymphocyte-depleted Hodgkin's lymphoma
   c. Plasmablastic lymphoma
   d. Small lymphocytic lymphoma

28. Programmed death-ligand 1/2 (PD-L1/L2) overexpression is caused by gene amplification at:
   a. Chromosome 9p24.1
   b. Chromosome 11p22.1
   c. Chromosome 13q24.1
   d. Chromosome 14q22.1
   e. Chromosome 17p22.1

29. Hodgkin-Reed-Sternberg (HRS) cells originate from:
   a. Germinal center
   b. Pregerminal center
   c. Postgerminal center
   d. Not known

30. True about Hodgkin-Reed-Sternberg cells is:
   a. They downregulate their major histocompatibility complex I (MHC I) and MHC II expression
   b. Secrete Chemokine (C-C motif) ligand 5 (CCL5) and migration inhibitory factor (MIF) that attract macrophages
   c. Secrete CCL17 and CCL22 that recruit immunosuppressive regulatory T cells (Tregs)
   d. All of the above

Ans.	1. d	2. c	3. b	4. d	5. c	6. c
	7. a	8. b	9. b	10. c	11. d	12. c
	13. d	14. e	15. a	16. c	17. d	18. b
	19. e	20. a	21. b	22. d	23. a	24. b
	25. c	26. a	27. b	28. a	29. a	30. d

3. SELF-ASSESSMENT

1. Following syndromes are associated with AML all, *except*:
Ref: Harrison p677
a. Down's syndrome
b. Kostmann syndrome
c. Ataxia telangiectasia
d. Fanconi's anemia
e. None of the above

2. Acute promyelocytic leukemia (APML) is commonly associated with:
a. Gum hypertrophy
b. Disseminated intravascular coagulation (DIC)
c. Chloroma
d. None of the above

3. Extramedullary involvement is commonly seen in:
a. AML-M1
b. AML-M3
c. AML-M7
d. AML-M4

4. Tumor lysis syndrome is characterized by all, *except*:
a. Hyperkalemia
b. Hypokalemia
c. Hyperuricemia
d. Hyperphosphatemia

5. Which one is considered favorable marker in AML?
a. t (6;9)
b. inv (3)
c. Monosomal 7
d. inv 16

6. High-dose cytarabine has side effects all, *except*:
a. Hepatitis
b. Cerebellar dysfunction
c. Renal dysfunction
d. Vomiting

7. Imatinib shows specificity for all, *except*:
Ref: Harrison p685
a. Platelet-derived growth factor receptor (PDGFR) receptor
b. BCR-ABL
c. Janus-associated Kinase-2 (JAK-2)
d. Kit tyrosine kinase

8. Philadelphia positivity is commonly seen in all cases of B-cell acute lymphoblastic leukemia (ALL) all, *except*:
a. Elderly
b. Mixed phenotype acute leukemia
c. CD 10 + ALL
d. Patients with central nervous system (CNS) disease

9. Which cytogenetic abnormality is associated with mucosa-associated lymphoid tissue (MALT) lymphoma?
a. t(11:14)
b. t(11:18)
c. t(14:18)
d. t(8:14)

10. IPI (International Prognostic Index) includes all, *except*:
a. Age
b. Ann arbor stage
c. Performance status
d. Number of node involvement

11. Not correct for polycythemia vera:
a. Splenomegaly may be presenting sign
b. JAK-2 v617 is seen in >90% of patients
c. Aquagenic pruritus is a distinguishing feature
d. Hypertension is not seen

12. Tear drop cells are seen commonly in:
a. Chronic myelogenous leukemia (CML)
b. Myelofibrosis
c. Polycythemia
d. Essential thrombocytosis

13. Nonmalignant cause of myelofibrosis are all, *except*:
a. Human immunodeficiency virus (HIV) infection
b. Tuberculosis
c. Hypoparathyroidism
d. Hyperparathyroidism

14. Massive splenomegaly is not seen in:
a. Myelofibrosis
b. Polycythemia vera
c. Essential thrombocytosis
d. CML

15. All are causes of reactive thrombocytosis all, *except*:
a. Iron deficiency anemia (IDA)
b. Surgery
c. Essential thrombocytosis
d. Hemorrhage

16. t(15:19) is seen in:
a. Chronic myeloid leukemia (CML)
b. Chronic neutrophilic leukemia (CNL)
c. Chronic lymphocytic leukemia (CLL)
d. Chronic eosinophilic leukemia (CEL)

17. Hasford system is related with:
a. Hodgkin's disease
b. Non-Hodgkin's lymphoma (NHL)
c. Chronic myeloid leukemia
d. Cutaneous lymphoma

18. Donor lymphocyte infusion is commonly indicated for:
a. AML
b. ALL
c. NHL
d. CML

19. Following are common side effects of imatinib all, *except*:
a. Skin rashes
b. Leg edema
c. Diarrhea
d. Renal dysfunction

20. In CML, BCR-ABL transcript seen is:
a. p230
b. p190
c. p210
d. p240

21. Brentuximab vedotin acts by:
a. Inhibiting tubulin
b. Inhibiting deoxyribonucleic acid (DNA) polymerase
c. Inhibiting DNA synthetase
d. Inhibiting DNA methylation

22. Peripheral neuropathy is caused by all, *except*:
a. Bortezomib
b. Brentuximab vedotin
c. Vinblastine
d. All of the above

23. The most promising target antigen for CAR-T cell approaches in classical Hodgkin's lymphoma is:
a. CD30
b. CD15
c. Programmed cell death protein 1 (PD-1)
d. CD25

24. Pembrolizumab acts by:
a. Blocking binding of PD-1 to cell surface
b. Blocking binding of PD-L1 to cell surface
c. Blocking binding of PD-1 to PD-L1
d. Blocking binding of PD-1 to CD30

25. Which infection can increase the expression of PD-1 on HRS cell surface?
a. HIV
b. CMV
c. EBV
d. HSV

26. The bispecific antibody for Hodgkin's lymphoma targets:
a. CD30/CD16
b. CD30/CD15
c. CD15/CD16
d. CD15/CD25

27. High-dose methotrexate is defined as dose more than:
a. 500 mg/m^2
b. 1,000 mg/m^2
c. 1,500 mg/m^2
d. 5,000 mg/m^2

28. Which of the following drug should not be given simultaneously with high-dose methotrexate?
a. Pantoprazole
b. Trimethoprim and sulfamethoxazole
c. Diclofenac
d. Leucovorin
e. All of the above

29. Glucarpidase acts by eliminating:
a. Extracellular methotrexate
b. Intracellular methotrexate
c. Both intracellular and extracellular methotrexate
d. Depends upon the pH of blood

30. Which route is not recommended for leucovorin administration?
a. Oral
b. Intravenous
c. Intramuscular
d. Intrathecal
e. Any of the above can be used

Ans. 1. e   2. b   3. d   4. b   5. d   6. c
      7. c   8. d   9. b   10. d 11. d 12. b
      13. c 14. c 15. c 16. b 17. c 18. d
      19. d 20. c 21. a 22. d 23. a 24. c
      25. c 26. a 27. a 28. e 29. a 30. d

4. SELF-ASSESSMENT

1. Staging of multiple myeloma includes all, *except*:
   a. Globulin
   b. Albumin
   c. b2 microglobulin
   d. None

2. Waldenström's macroglobulinemia is characterized by all, *except*:
   a. Lymphadenopathy
   b. Organomegaly
   c. Hypercalcemia
   d. Hyperviscosity

3. Seligmann disease is:
   a. Gamma heavy chain disease
   b. Alpha heavy chain disease
   c. Mu heavy chain disease
   d. Light chain disease

4. Plasma cell leukemia should have:
   a. <1,000/µL plasma cell on peripheral smear
   b. 1,000–2,000/µL
   c. >2000/µL
   d. None of the above

5. Hyperviscosity is commonly seen with which paraprotein?
   a. Immunoglobulin M (IgM)
   b. IgG
   c. IgA
   d. IgD

6. Spherocytes in the blood film are a feature of which one of the following?
   a. Thalassemia major
   b. Autoimmune hemolytic anemia (AIHA)
   c. PNH
   d. Glucose-6-phosphate dehydrogenase (G6PD) deficiency

7. Which one of the following is a feature of a chronic extravascular hemolysis?
   a. Raised serum conjugated bilirubin
   b. Low reticulocyte count
   c. Gallstones
   d. Hypocellular marrow

8. All of the followings are the inherited causes of hemolytic anemia all, *except*:
   a. Hereditary spherocytosis (HS)
   b. G6PD deficiency
   c. PNH
   d. Pyruvate kinase (PK) deficiency

9. Which one of the following is not true about autoimmune hemolytic anemia?
   a. Can complicate patients of lymphomas and leukemia
   b. Can be caused by drugs
   c. Can be caused by pernicious anemia
   d. Is associated with positive Coombs test

10. Tear drop cells are seen in all of the following all, *except*:
    a. Myelofibrosis
    b. Thalassemia major
    c. Megaloblastic anemia
    d. HS

11. Hemolytic anemia associated with venous thrombosis in:
    a. Autoimmune hemolytic anemia
    b. Hereditary spherocytosis
    c. Paroxysmal nocturnal hemoglobinuria
    d. Paroxysmal cold hemoglobinuria (PCH)

12. Thrombotic thrombocytopenic purpura consists of all of the following all, *except*:
    a. Fever
    b. Thrombocytopenia
    c. Neurological symptoms
    d. Bleeding

13. Microangiopathic hemolytic anemia is caused by all of the following all, *except*:
    a. Sepsis
    b. Prosthetic heart valves
    c. Hemangioma
    d. Methyldopa

14. Ribavirin causes hemolysis by:
    a. Antibody mediated
    b. Complement mediated
    c. Adenosine triphosphate (ATP) depletion
    d. None of the above

15. Which one is not a cause of intravascular hemolysis?
    a. Sepsis
    b. PNH
    c. ABO incompatibility
    d. HS

16. Hydroxyurea should not be used in:
    a. Coinheritance of alpha-thalassemia
    b. Sickle hemoglobin (HbS)-beta thalassemia
    c. Compound heterozygous forms of HbSC
    d. Can be used in all these

17. Lifespan of sickled erythrocytes is:
    a. 15–20 days
    b. 40–45 days
    c. 70–75 days
    d. 90–95 days

18. Which of the following is not the complication of sickle hepatopathy?
    a. Intrahepatic cholestasis
    b. Cirrhosis
    c. Sinusoidal obstruction syndrome
    d. All of the above

19. Hydroxyurea in sickle cell disease acts by:
    a. Increasing fetal hemoglobin (HbF)
    b. Decreasing white blood cells
    c. Decreasing endothelial adhesion
    d. Decreasing chronic inflammation
    e. All of the above

20. Which of the following is an adverse prognostic marker in AML?
   a. t(6;9)(p23;q34)
   b. inv(3)(q21q26.2)
   c. Mutated RUNX1
   d. Mutated ASXL1
   e. All of the above

21. True about midostaurin is:
   a. Effective in FLT3-ITD (fms-like tyrosine kinase 3 internal tandem duplication) high allelic ratio
   b. Effective in FLT3-ITD low allelic ratio
   c. Effective in FLT3-TKD high allelic ratio
   d. Effective in FLT3-TKD low allelic ratio
   e. All of the above

22. CPX 351 (liposomal cytarabine-daunorubicin) is a liposomal formulation of cytarabine and daunorubicin at a fixed ratio of:
   a. 2:1 M
   b. 3:1 M
   c. 4:1 M
   d. 5:1 M

23. Combined deficiency of factor V (FV) and factor VIII (FVIII) is due to:
   a. Defective synthesis from DNA
   b. Defective transport from endoplasmic reticulum to Golgi body
   c. Defective secretion from cell
   d. All of the above

24. CPX 351 is a liposomal formulation of:
   a. Cytarabine and daunorubicin
   b. Cytarabine and idarubicin
   c. Cytarabine and mitoxantrone
   d. Cytarabine and doxorubicin

25. Which of the following drug is not used in acute myeloid leukemia (AML)?
   a. Venetoclax
   b. Dasatinib
   c. Enasidenib
   d. Entospletinib
   e. All of the above used

26. Which of the following is not age-related clonal hematopoiesis?
   a. DNA methyltransferase 3 alpha (DNMT3a)
   b. Tet methylcytosine dioxygenase 2 (TET2)
   c. ASXL Transcriptional Regulator 1 (ASXL1)
   d. Fms-like tyrosine kinase 3 (FLT3)

27. Rituximab was approved for use in lymphoma in:
   a. 1997
   b. 2000
   c. 2003
   d. 2006

28. What percentage of AML cases are acute promyelocytic leukemia (APL)?
   a. 5–10%
   b. 10–20%
   c. 20–30%
   d. 30–40%

29. Rapid diagnosis of APL can be made by:
   a. Fluorescence in situ hybridization (FISH)
   b. Karyotyping
   c. Polymerase chain reaction (PCR)
   d. Immunofluorescence for PML protein

30. Treatment of choice for low-risk APL is:
   a. All-trans retinoic acid (ATRA) plus arsenic trioxide (ATO)
   b. ATRA plus daunorubicin
   c. ATO plus daunorubicin
   d. Any of the above

Ans.	1. a	2. c	3. b	4. c	5. a	6. b
	7. c	8. c	9. c	10. d	11. c	12. d
	13. d	14. c	15. d	16. a	17. a	18. c
	19. e	20. e	21. e	22. d	23. b	24. a
	25. e	26. d	27. a	28. a	29. d	30. a

5. SELF-ASSESSMENT

1. Hereditary spherocytosis is due to the defect in:
   a. Ankyrin
   b. Band 3
   c. Protein 4.2
   d. All of the above

2. Target cells are formed due to:
   a. Increase in surface area due to lipid gain
   b. Decrease in surface area due to lipid loss
   c. Weakening of skeletal protein
   d. All of the above

3. Membrane loss in the form of microvesicles is the characteristic feature of:
   a. Stomatocytes
   b. Echinocytes
   c. Acanthocytes
   d. Microspherocytes

4. South-east Asian ovalocytosis is due to defect in:
   a. Ankyrin
   b. Band 3
   c. Protein 4.2
   d. Protein 4.1

5. In HS, there is loss of:
   a. Horizontal connections
   b. Vertical connections
   c. Both connections
   d. Variable connections

6. Pincer-like red cells are seen in deficiency of:
   a. Ankyrin
   b. Band 3
   c. Protein 4.2
   d. Protein 4.1

7. The characteristic RBC indices in HS are:
   a. Low mean corpuscular volume (MCV), increased mean corpuscular hemoglobin concentration (MCHC), increased red cell distribution width (RDW)
   b. Low MCV, increased MCHC, decreased RDW
   c. High MCV, increased MCHC, increased RDW
   d. High MCV, increased MCHC, decreased RDW

8. Incubation increases the sensitivity of osmotic fragility test by:
   a. Overhydration of the cell
   b. Dehydration of the cell
   c. Increasing the loss of surface area
   d. Increasing the MCV

9. Instrument used in measuring osmotic gradient in HS is:
   a. Osmocytometer
   b. Spherocytometer
   c. Ektacytometer
   d. Viscometer

10. The most sensitive and specific screening test for HS is:
    a. Cryohemolysis test
    b. Pink test
    c. Glycerol lysis test
    d. Eosin-5′-maleimide (EMA) binding test

11. Which of the following is not a myeloproliferative disorder?
    a. Chronic neutrophilic leukemia
    b. Chronic eosinophilic leukemia/hypereosinophilic syndrome
    c. Chronic myelomonocytic leukemia
    d. Myeloproliferative disease, unclassifiable

12. Which of the following are risk factors for thrombosis in polycythemia vera?
    a. Age 60 years
    b. History of previous thrombosis
    c. High rate of phlebotomy
    d. Both a and b

13. Risk of transformation to AML in patients of polycythemia vera treated with phlebotomy is:
    a. <1%
    b. 1–3%
    c. 3–5%
    d. 5–8%

14. The most common cause of mortality in polycythemia vera is:
    a. Bleeding
    b. Thrombosis
    c. Progression to myelofibrosis
    d. Transformation to AML

15. ECLAP (European Collaboration on Low-dose Aspirin in Polycythemia Vera) study is related to:
    a. Polycythemia vera
    b. Myelofibrosis
    c. Hypereosinophilic syndrome
    d. AML

16. Which of the following statement about JAK2 mutation in essential thrombocythemia (ET) is correct?
    a. Patients with ET who have JAK2 mutation have a higher median hemoglobin concentration and neutrophil count than those who lack the mutation
    b. They may have more thromboembolic events
    c. They may require more cytoreductive therapy
    d. All of the above
    e. None of the above

17. In CML t(9;22) results from:
    a. Long-arm of chromosome 9 to short-arm of chromosome 22
    b. Long-arm of chromosome 9 to long-arm of chromosome 22
    c. Short-arm of chromosome 9 to short-arm of chromosome 22
    d. Short-arm of chromosome 9 to long-arm of chromosome 22

18. IRIS (Insulin Resistance Intervention after Stroke) trial compared:
    a. Hydroxyurea with imatinib
    b. Cytarabine with imatinib
    c. Interferon with imatinib
    d. Interferon and cytarabine with imatinib

19. Which of the following is not a good risk cytogenetic factor in myelodysplastic syndrome (MDS)?
   a. –Y
   b. del 5q
   c. del 20q
   d. Inv 16

20. Gold standard for diagnosis of CML is:
   a. Leukocyte alkaline phosphatase (LAP) score
   b. Cytogenetics
   c. Fluorescence in situ hybridization (FISH)
   d. Reverse transcription polymerase chain reaction (RT-PCR)

21. True about combined deficiency of factors VIII and V is:
   a. Presents with severe bleeding
   b. Sex-linked recessive disease
   c. Due to defects in *LMAN1* and *MCFD2* genes
   d. All of the above

22. The Leyden phenotype of hemophilia B is characterized by:
   a. Severe hemophilia A in childhood that becomes mild after puberty
   b. Mild hemophilia A in childhood that becomes severe after puberty
   c. Severe hemophilia B in childhood that becomes mild after puberty
   d. Severe hemophilia A and B in childhood that become mild after puberty

23. The incidence of hemophilia A is:
   a. 1 in 5,000 live male births
   b. 1 in 10,000 live male births
   c. 1 in 15,000 live male births
   d. 1 in 20,000 live male births

24. The cause of decreased risk of bleeding in severe hemophilia A may be:
   a. Factor V Leiden
   b. Protein C deficiency
   c. Prothrombin *G20210A* gene variant
   d. All of the above

25. The inhibitors develop in------of patients with severe hemophilia A.
   a. 5%
   b. 15%
   c. 25%
   d. 35%

26. Symptomatic hemophilia A can develop in females because of:
   a. X-chromosome inactivation resulting in low levels of factor VIII
   b. Mating between an affected male and a carrier female producing homozygous disease
   c. Loss of an X-chromosome in Turner syndrome
   d. All of the above

27. Obligate carrier in hemophilia is defined as:
   a. Mother of more than one hemophilic son
   b. Daughter of a patient with hemophilia
   c. All of the above
   d. None of the above

28. Patients with high responder inhibitors have:
   a. Increase in antibody titer after each exposure
   b. Response begins within 2–3 days
   c. Peaks at 7–21 days
   d. May persist for years in the absence of re-exposure
   e. All of the above

29. Inhibitor development is least common with:
   a. Large deletions
   b. Nonsense mutations
   c. Inversions
   d. Small deletions
   e. Missense mutations

30. According to the CANAL (Concerted Action on Neutralizing Antibodies in severe hemophilia A) study, one of the following is not a risk factor for inhibitor development:
   a. Family history of inhibitors
   b. High-risk gene mutation present
   c. Intensive treatment at first episode
   d. Starting treatment with factor at early age

Ans.	1. d	2. a	3. d	4. b	5. b	6. b
	7. a	8. c	9. c	10. d	11. c	12. d
	13. b	14. b	15. a	16. d	17. b	18. d
	19. d	20. b	21. c	22. c	23. a	24. d
	25. c	26. d	27. c	28. e	29. e	30. d

6. SELF-ASSESSMENT

1. The following is not the feature of Fanconi's anemia:
   a. Short stature
   b. Hypopigmented spots and Café-au-lait spots
   c. Abnormality of thumbs
   d. Macrocephaly
   e. Hypogonadism

2. The most common malignancy in Fanconi's anemia is:
   a. AML
   b. Squamous cell carcinoma of the head and neck
   c. Genitourinary malignancy
   d. Skin cancers

3. Peak age of presentation of Fanconi's anemia is:
   a. Less than 1 year
   b. 1–5 years
   c. 5–15 years
   d. 15–20 years
   e. More than 20 years

4. Triad of dyskeratosis congenita include all, *except*:
   a. Anemia
   b. Hyperpigmented rash
   c. Nail dystrophy
   d. Mucosal leukoplakia

5. Dyskeratosis congenita is inherited as:
   a. X-linked recessive trait
   b. Autosomal dominant trait
   c. Autosomal recessive trait
   d. All of the above

6. Treatment of choice for dyskeratosis congenita is:
   a. Androgens
   b. Growth factors
   c. Androgens, growth factors, and supportive care
   d. Stem cell transplantation

7. True about Shwachman-Diamond syndrome are, *except*:
   a. Usually presents in infancy
   b. Endocrine pancreatic insufficiency
   c. Bone marrow failure
   d. Skeletal anomalies

8. True about Shwachman-Diamond syndrome are:
   a. Conversion mutations which recombine portions of the pseudogene and *SBDS* gene, resulting in a dysfunctional *SBDS* gene
   b. Autosomal recessive disorder
   c. It is a ribosomopathy
   d. All of the above

9. Bone marrow involvement in CLL is:
   a. Stage 0
   b. Stage 1
   c. Stage 3
   d. Stage 4

10. Stage of most common presentation of CLL is:
    a. Stage 0 (lymphocytosis)—25%
    b. Stages I to II (lymphadenopathy, organomegaly)—50%
    c. Stages III to IV (anemia, thrombocytopenia)—25%
    d. All stage have equal frequency of presentation

11. The median survival from the time of diagnosis in stage III and IV CLL patients is:
    a. 10 months
    b. 20 months
    c. 30 months
    d. 40 months

12. Autoimmune phenomena seen in CLL are all, *except*:
    a. Coombs positive autoimmune hemolytic anemia
    b. Idiopathic thrombocytopenic purpura
    c. Pure red cell aplasia
    d. Rheumatoid arthritis

13. Cytogenetic abnormalities seen in CLL are all, *except*:
    a. Trisomy 12
    b. 14q+
    c. del 13q14
    d. 11p deletion

14. Indications for treatment in CLL are all, *except*:
    a. Symptomatic anemia and/or thrombocytopenia
    b. Repeated episodes of infection
    c. Severe insect hypersensitivity
    d. Autoimmune hemolytic anemia and/or thrombocytopenia that are poorly responsive to corticosteroid therapy
    e. del 17p

15. Adverse prognostic features in CLL are all, *except*:
    a. ZAP 70
    b. CD38
    c. Unmutated immunoglobulin Vh genes
    d. del 13q14

16. Treatment of choice for patients with localized (stage I) small lymphocytic lymphoma (SLL) is:
    a. Observation
    b. Localized radiation therapy
    c. Chemotherapy
    d. Chemotherapy plus localized radiation therapy

17. Patients with del(17p) or del(11q) are at high risk because of:
    a. Not responding adequately to initial treatment
    b. Relapsing soon after achieving remission
    c. Requiring treatment early
    d. All of the above

18. Regarding alemtuzumab therapy in CLL, all are true, *except*:
   a. Single agent alemtuzumab results in overall response and complete remission (CR) rates of approximately 83% and 24%, respectively
   b. A survival benefit has not been demonstrated
   c. Effective when maximum lymph nodes <5 cm in diameter
   d. Can deplete bone marrow leukemic clone and achieve minimal residual disease (MRD) negativity
   e. All are true

19. Which of the following drug is not used in CLL?
   a. Mitoxantrone
   b. Pentostatin
   c. Fludarabine
   d. All are used

20. Alemtuzumab is effective in CLL with chromosome 17p deletion because it:
   a. Acts through IP3/mToR (phosphoinositide 3-kinase-AKT-mammalian target of rapamycin) pathway
   b. Acts through heat shock proteins
   c. Acts through p53 pathway of apoptosis
   d. Bypasses p53 pathway of apoptosis

21. Antibodies are most commonly directed against the following domain in factor VIII inhibitors:
   a. A2 domain
   b. C2 domain
   c. A3 domain
   d. C1 domain

22. Cryoprecipitate contains......times more factor VIII compared to fresh frozen plasma.
   a. 10
   b. 30
   c. 50
   d. 100

23. Intravenous administration of 0.5 IU/kg of body weight of factor VIII will increase circulating factor VIII levels by:
   a. 0.5 IU/dL
   b. 1 IU/dL
   c. 1.5 IU/dL
   d. 2 IU/dL

24. The usual dose of epsilon aminocaproic acid is:
   a. 25–50 mg/kg per dose every 6 hours
   b. 50–75 mg/kg per dose every 6 hours
   c. 75–100 mg/kg per dose every 6 hours
   d. 100–125 mg/kg per dose every 6 hours

25. Patients with factor IX inhibitors have:
   a. Increased risk of nephrotic syndrome
   b. Increased risk of anaphylaxis
   c. Poor response to immune tolerance induction
   d. All of the above

26. What percent of patients with hemophilia A do not have a family history of bleeding?
   a. 10%
   b. 20%
   c. 30%
   d. 40%

27. How many patients of hemophilia A have severe disease?
   a. 10–20%
   b. 20–30%
   c. 30–40%
   d. 50–60%

28. Which of the following is not a feature of differentiation syndrome?
   a. Pulmonary infiltrates
   b. Fever
   c. Hypotension
   d. Acute renal failure
   e. Seizures

29. True about pseudotumor cerebri in APL are all, *except*:
   a. Observed in children
   b. Characterized by headache
   c. Papilledema
   d. Caused by ATO

30. Most common side effect of eculizumab is:
   a. Loose stools
   b. Vomiting
   c. Cough
   d. Headache

Ans.
1. d	2. b	3. c	4. a	5. d	6. d
7. b	8. d	9. a	10. b	11. b	12. d
13. d	14. e	15. d	16. b	17. d	18. e
19. d	20. d	21. b	22. d	23. b	24. c
25. d	26. c	27. d	28. e	29. d	30. d

7. SELF-ASSESSMENT

1. Acute myeloid leukemia has been associated with:
   a. Trisomy 21
   b. Fanconi's anemia
   c. Bloom's syndrome
   d. All of the above

2. The minimum number of blasts required for diagnosis of AML with t(8;21)(q22;q22) are:
   a. 10%
   b. 20%
   c. 30%
   d. None of the above

3. Good risk AML include all, *except*:
   a. t(8;21)(q22;q22)
   b. inv(16)(p13.1q22)
   c. APL with t(15;17)(q22;q12) with DIC
   d. All of the above

4. AML with t(8;21)(q22;q22) is associated with:
   a. CEFB-MYH11
   b. RUNX1-RUNX1T1
   c. MLLT3-MLL
   d. All of the above

5. WHO classification of AML includes the following major categories all, *except*:
   a. AML with recurrent genetic abnormalities
   b. AML with myelodysplasia-related features
   c. Relapsed and refractory AML
   d. Therapy-related AML
   e. AML, not otherwise specified

6. True about AML with t(8;21)(q22;q22) are:
   a. Blasts with long thin Auer rods
   b. Presence of c-KIT (receptor tyrosine kinase) mutations is an adverse prognostic feature
   c. Patients can have transcripts of the RUNX1-RUNX1T1 detected by RT-PCR even in patients who have been in remission for many years
   d. All of the above

7. Patients with AML with inv(16)(p13;q22) have:
   a. FAB M4Eo phenotype
   b. Occurs in younger patients
   c. Can present as an extramedullary myeloid sarcoma
   d. All of the above

8. Which of the following AML has favorable prognosis among these?
   a. AML with t(9;11)(p22;q23)
   b. AML with t(6;9)(p23;q34)
   c. AML with inv(3)
   d. AML with del 7q

9. True about AML with mutations in fms-like tyrosine kinase 3 (FLT3) are all, *except*:
   a. Seen in 30–40% of patients with AML and normal cytogenetics
   b. Often present with high white blood cell (WBC) counts
   c. The presence of a FLT3 mutation can overcome the favorable effects of NPM1) and CEBPA mutations
   d. High-dose cytarabine is the preferred treatment

10. True about AML with minimal differentiation is:
    a. There are no cytoplasmic granules or Auer rods
    b. They cannot be differentiated from ALL based upon morphology
    c. The blasts are negative for the myeloperoxidase (MPo) or Sudan black B (SBB) reactions
    d. Most cases express CD15 and CD65

11. Acute myeloid leukemia without maturation has the following features all, *except*:
    a. At least 20% of the blasts stain for MPO and/or SBB (3% not 20%)
    b. Many cases express antigens of early hematopoiesis [e.g., CD34, CD38, (human leukocyte antigen–DR isotype) HLA-DR]
    c. They express one or more myeloid-associated antigens (e.g., CD13, CD33, CD117)
    d. Markers of granulocytic maturation (e.g., CD15, CD65) are not expressed in most cases

12. The goal of induction chemotherapy is:
    a. To rapidly restore normal bone marrow function
    b. To decrease the minimal residual disease
    c. To prevent the relapse
    d. All of the above

13. After achieving remission following induction therapy, the number of blasts left in body is:
    a. No blast left
    b. 10^3 blasts left
    c. 10^6 blasts left
    d. 10^9 blasts left

14. The best induction therapy for AML is:
    a. Double induction with 3 + 7 regimen
    b. Single induction with 3 + 7 regimen
    c. Induction using high-dose cytarabine
    d. Using granulocyte colony-stimulating factor (G-CSF) as priming therapy followed by induction with 3 + 7

15. Cerebrospinal fluid (CSF) to evaluate for CNS involvement in AML is recommended for all, *except*:
    a. Patients with a high WBC count (>100,000/µL) at the time of diagnosis
    b. Patients with a monoblastic phenotype
    c. CD56 positivity
    d. AML M7

16. Eastern Cooperative Oncology Group (ECOG) 3 performance status is:
    a. Fully ambulatory and able to carry out light work
    b. Up and about >50% of waking hours
    c. Confined to bed >50% of waking hours
    d. Completely disabled, totally confined to bed

17. A "monosomal karyotype" is:
    a. Defined as at least two autosomal monosomies
    b. Is a single autosomal monosomy in the presence of one or more structural cytogenetic abnormalities
    c. Is associated with unfavorable risk disease than a complex karyotype
    d. All of the above

18. True regarding abnormalities in the *nucleophosmin* (*NPM1*) gene in AML are:
a. Found in approximately 50% of patients with de novo normal karyotype AML
b. NPM1 mutations have been associated with improved outcomes in both adults and children with AML
c. The concurrence of FLT3 mutations negates the positive effect of NPM1 mutations
d. All of the above

19. False regarding *CEBPA* gene mutation is:
a. Found in approximately 10% of patients with newly diagnosed AML
b. Longer median overall survival
c. Its effect is independent of other high-risk molecular features
d. Prognosis is similar whether patient has two copies of the mutation or single allele CEBPA mutation

20. Older patients with AML have poor prognosis because:
a. Poorer performance status
b. Higher incidence of multidrug resistance
c. Lower percentage of favorable cytogenetics
d. Lower CR rates, shorter remission durations, and shorter median overall survival
e. All of the above

21. Cytogenetic abnormalities that are closely associated with AML and are not seen in MDS are:
a. Chromosomal deletion
b. Chromosomal gain
c. Chromosomal loss
d. Balanced translocations

22. Patients with a "good risk MDS" can have:
a. Normal karyotypes b. -Y
c. del(5q) d. del(20q)
e. All of the above

23. The 5q-syndrome is a distinctive type of primary MDS that primarily occurs in:
a. Median age at diagnosis is 68 years
b. Female predominance of 7:3
c. Presents with refractory macrocytic anemia and normal or elevated platelet counts
d. Absence of significant neutropenia
e. All of the above

24. RPS14 (ribosomal protein S14), required for the maturation of 40S ribosomal subunits, is implicated in the genesis:
a. 5q-syndrome
b. MDS/MPN syndrome
c. MDS with trisomy 8
d. MDS with del 7
e. All of the above

25. The following is not true of 5q-syndrome:
a. Lenalidomide is the treatment of choice
b. Median survival is 63 months
c. Hypomethylating agents are highly effective
d. Infection and bleeding are unusual

26. Which of the following mutation is present in primary HLH?
a. PRF1 b. UNC13D
c. RAB27A d. LYST
e. All of the above

27. Emapalumab is used for:
a. Hemophagocytic lymphohistiocytosis (HLH)
b. Paroxysmal nocturnal hemoglobinuria
c. Immune thrombocytopenia
d. Mantle cell lymphoma

28. Emapalumab is an:
a. Anti-interleukin-2 antibody
b. Anti-interleukin-6 antibody
c. Anti-tumor necrosis factor-α antibody
d. Anti-interferon gamma antibody

29. Platelet microparticles are identified by:
a. Microscopy
b. Flow cytometry
c. Next generation sequencing (NGS)
d. Polymerase chain reaction (PCR)

30. Cause of bleeding in antiphospholipid syndrome is:
a. Thrombocytopenia
b. Acquired thrombocytopathy
c. Acquired factor VIII inhibitor
d. Acquired prothrombin deficiency
e. All of the above

Ans.
1. d   2. d   3. d   4. b   5. c   6. d
7. d   8. a   9. d   10. d   11. a   12. a
13. d   14. b   15. d   16. c   17. d   18. d
19. d   20. e   21. d   22. e   23. e   24. a
25. c   26. e   27. a   28. d   29. b   30. e

8. SELF-ASSESSMENT

1. **Definitive hematopoiesis begins in:**
   a. Liver
   b. Yolk sac
   c. Aorta-gonad-mesonephros (AGM) region (Around aorta)
   d. Spleen

2. **Essential properties of hematopoietic stem cells include all, *except*:**
   a. Self-renewal
   b. Ability to differentiate
   c. Transdifferentiation
   d. High proliferative capacity

3. **Which of the following growth factors/cytokines are not of potential clinical value to stimulate hematopoiesis?**
   a. Thrombopoietin
   b. Erythropoietin
   c. Granulocyte-macrophage colony-stimulating factor (GM-CSF)
   d. Interleukins

4. **Earliest hemoglobin to appear is:**
   a. Portland
   b. Gower 1
   c. Gower 2
   d. Hemoglobin F (HbF)

5. **Division occurs up to which stage of erythroid development?**
   a. Proerythroblast
   b. Early normoblast
   c. Intermediate normoblast
   d. Late normoblast

6. **Primary granules are seen first in which stage of myeloid development?**
   a. Myeloblast
   b. Myelocyte
   c. Band
   d. Promyelocyte

7. **Which of the following is the constituent of azurophilic granules in myeloid development?**
   a. Esterase
   b. Major basic protein
   c. MPO
   d. Elastase

8. **Basophils are characteristically stained by which cytochemistry?**
   a. MPO
   b. Acid phosphatase
   c. Toluidine blue
   d. PAS

9. **Germinal center B-cells are characterized by:**
   a. B-cell lymphoma 2 (BCL2)
   b. BCL6
   c. FMC7
   d. CD34

10. **Paracortical areas are most rich in:**
    a. Memory B-cells
    b. Naïve B-cells
    c. Plasma cells
    d. T-cells

11. **Cortical thymocytes are characterized by:**
    a. CD1a positivity
    b. CD 3 positivity
    c. CD 4 positivity
    d. CD 8 positivity

12. **The color of Dhole bodies in neutrophil:**
    a. Blue
    b. Violet
    c. Magenta
    d. Red

13. **Transient leukemia of Down's syndrome develops in:**
    a. Fetal liver
    b. Bone marrow
    c. Thymus
    d. Placenta

14. **True about transient leukemia of Down's syndrome is:**
    a. Transient leukemia of Down's syndrome should be defined as the presence of a GATA1 mutation together with a peripheral blood blast percentage >10%
    b. GATA1 mutation(s) are not leukemogenic in cells that are not trisomic for chromosome 21
    c. Blast count assessment after the 1st week of life may underestimate the prevalence of disease as the blast percentage often falls rapidly after birth
    d. All of the above

15. **True about primary HLH is:**
    a. Genetic defect is the most common cause
    b. All children should be treated with HLH protocol
    c. All children should undergo allogeneic stem cell transplant
    d. All of the above

16. **True about HLH in adults is:**
    a. Genetic defect is the most common cause
    b. All adults should be treated with HLH protocol
    c. All adults with HLH should undergo allogeneic stem cell transplant
    d. None of the above

17. **Risk factor for early death in transient leukemia of Down's syndrome is:**
    a. Hyperleukocytosis
    b. Liver disease
    c. Preterm delivery
    d. All of the above

18. **True about light-chain deposition disease is:**
    a. Light-chain deposition is seen along tubular basement membrane
    b. Amyloid deposition of immunoglobulin light chains
    c. Deposition is restricted to kidneys only
    d. Stain with Congo red on kidney biopsy
    e. All of the above

19. Which of the following is accurate regarding the use of heparin in patients with venous thromboembolism (VTE)?
   a. Heparin is contraindicated in pregnant women with VTE
   b. In patient with deep vein thrombosis (DVT), low-molecular-weight heparin is less effective than ultrafractionated heparin
   c. The maximum time for which heparin can be given is 3 months
   d. Adequacy of therapy with heparin is determined by an activated partial thromboplastin time (aPTT) of 1.5–2 times baseline

20. CD146 is the marker of:
   a. Eosinophils
   b. Mast cells
   c. Basophils
   d. Dendritic cells
   e. Endothelial cells

21. CD11c is the marker of:
   a. Eosinophils
   b. Mast cells
   c. Basophils
   d. Dendritic cells
   e. Endothelial cells

22. Daratumumab-specific immunofixation reflex assay (DIRA) is used:
   a. To identify patients who will develop allergic reaction to daratumumab
   b. To identify those patients who will show response to daratumumab
   c. To identify interference of crossmatching of red blood cells by daratumumab
   d. To exclude daratumumab as the cause of monoclonal band in patients on this drug

23. True about romiplostim is:
   a. Steroids are synergistic with romiplostim
   b. If patient has not responded to eltrombopag, then he is unlikely to respond to romiplostim
   c. Is less potent than eltrombopag
   d. All of the above

24. Frozen plasma is used for:
   a. Treatment or prophylaxis of thromboembolism in antithrombin, protein C, and protein S deficiencies
   b. Heparin resistance (antithrombin III deficiency) in a patient requiring heparin
   c. Therapy of acute angioedema or preoperative prophylaxis in hereditary C1-inhibitor deficiency
   d. All of the above

25. Which of the following parameter is not directly measured by Coulter counter instrument?
   a. Total leukocyte count
   b. Differential leukocyte count
   c. Mean corpuscular volume
   d. Reticulocyte count

26. Coulter is based on the principle of:
   a. Impedance measurements
   b. Flow cytometry
   c. Magnetic twisting cytometry
   d. Viscoelastometry

27. Gray-zone lymphomas are intermediate between:
   a. Diffuse large B-cell lymphoma (DLBCL) and Hodgkin lymphoma
   b. Hodgkin lymphoma and primary mediastinal B-cell lymphoma
   c. Hodgkin lymphoma and anaplastic large-cell lymphoma
   d. DLBCL and Burkitt lymphoma

28. What percent of AML patients have BCR-ABL mutation?
   a. None
   b. 1%
   c. 5%
   d. 10%

29. Villalta scoring system is used for:
   a. DVT risk scoring
   b. Post-thrombotic syndrome diagnosis
   c. Bleeding risk with newer oral anticoagulants
   d. Risk assessment of recurrent thrombosis

30. Elotuzumab is a monoclonal antibody against:
   a. SLAMF7 (surface antigen CD319)
   b. Interleukin 2
   c. Interleukin 6
   d. Cytokine receptor-like factor 2 (CRLF2)

Ans.
1. c   2. c   3. d   4. a   5. c   6. d
7. c   8. c   9. a   10. d   11. a   12. a
13. a   14. d   15. d   16. d   17. d   18. a
19. d   20. e   21. d   22. d   23. d   24. d
25. c   26. a   27. a   28. b   29. b   30. a

9. SELF-ASSESSMENT

1. All of the following are good prognostic factors in CLL all, *except*:
   a. Cd 38 positivity
   b. ZAP 70 positivity
   c. TLC >100,000/mm^3
   d. Unmutated phenotype

2. Most common cytogenetic abnormality in CLL:
   a. del13q14
   b. del17p
   c. t(9;22)
   d. del11q22

3. Which of the following explain the lymphocytosis in CLL?
   a. Response to cytokines
   b. Balanced chromosomal translocations
   c. Upregulation of antiapoptotic gene
   d. Shortened cell cycle time

4. Monoclonal B-cell lymphocytosis is characterized by:
   a. Lymphocytosis >5,000 cell/mm^3
   b. CLL phenotype
   c. Young patients
   d. Lymph nodes are always involved

5. Not a classical feature of CLL immunophenotype:
   a. CD19
   b. CD23
   c. CD5
   d. Bright immunoglobulin

6. Prolymphocytic transformation is marked by all, *except*:
   a. Worsening cytopenias
   b. Increasing splenomegaly
   c. Appearance of increased numbers of "prolymphocytes" in the peripheral blood
   d. Development of marrow fibrosis

7. Autoantibodies against red cells in CLL are:
   a. IgG
   b. IgM
   c. IgA
   d. IgE

8. Richter syndrome develops in:
   a. ALL
   b. CLL
   c. Huntington disease (HD)
   d. Diffuse large B-cell lymphoma (DLBCL)

9. Not true about CLL:
   a. Insect bite hypersensitivity
   b. Caused by ionizing radiation
   c. Can have AIHA
   d. ZAP 70 is surrogate for immunoglobulin heavy (IGH) mutation

10. Elotuzumab is used for the treatment of:
   a. Multiple myeloma
   b. T-cell lymphoma
   c. Hairy-cell leukemia
   d. Anaplastic lymphoma kinase (ALK)-positive anaplastic large-cell lymphoma

11. Williams trait is:
   a. High-molecular-weight kininogens deficiency
   b. Hageman factor deficiency
   c. Factor XIII deficiency
   d. Prothrombin deficiency

12. Matutes score is used for the diagnosis of:
   a. Hairy-cell leukemia
   b. Chronic lymphocytic leukemia (CLL)
   c. T-Large granular lymphocytic leukemia
   d. Primary central nervous system (CNS) lymphoma

13. Thrombocytopenia is frequently seen with which type of von Willebrand disease:
   a. Type 2A
   b. Type 2B
   c. Type 2M
   d. Type 2N

14. Platelet poor plasma is defined as plasma with platelets less than:
   a. 1,000/μL
   b. 5,000/μL
   c. 10,000/μL
   d. 20,000/μL

15. Lenalidomide is used for:
   a. Marginal zone lymphoma
   b. Mantle cell lymphoma
   c. Follicular lymphoma
   d. CLL
   e. All of the above

16. True about myeloid reconstitution syndrome is:
   a. Similar to immune reconstitution inflammatory syndrome
   b. Develops in parallel with neutrophil recovery from aplasia
   c. Can present as fever and progression of preexisting inflammatory response
   d. All of the above

17. CD200 positivity is seen in:
   a. CLL
   b. Marginal zone lymphoma
   c. Lymphoplasmacytic lymphoma
   d. Mantle cell

18. Not required in diagnosis of chronic myelomonocytic leukemia (CMML):
   a. Increased blasts
   b. Monocytosis
   c. Myeloid dysplasia
   d. Myeloproliferation

19. Not included in current World Health Organization (WHO) classification is:
a. CMML-0
b. CMML-1
c. CMML-2
d. CMML-3

20. The following is not of prognostic value in CMML:
a. Blast counts
b. Karyotype
c. Age of patient
d. Monocyte counts

21. Not true about juvenile myelomonocytic leukemia (JMML):
a. Organomegaly is uncommon
b. Pathogenesis involves renin-angiotensin system (RAS) pathway
c. Farnesyltransferase inhibitors are potential therapies
d. Hemoglobin F (HbF) level is of prognostic value

22. Not true about AML:
a. Incidence increases with increasing age
b. BCR-ABL positive AML is a WHO defined entity
c. Minimum requirement for diagnosis of acute monocytic leukemia (AML-M5b) is more than 80% monoblasts and promonocytes
d. AML-M7 commonly has dry marrow aspirates

23. Poorest prognostic factor in ALL among these is:
a. Early T precursor ALL
b. Male sex
c. t 1:19 (TCF3-PBX1)
d. High blast percentage at diagnosis

24. Drug not used in treatment of AML:
a. Sorafenib
b. Clofarabine
c. Panobinostat
d. Nelarabine

25. Not a poor prognostic feature in AML:
a. Monoallelic CEBPA (CCAAT/enhancer-binding protein alpha) mutation
b. FLT-3 low allelic ratio internal tandem duplication (ITD) mutation
c. DNMT3a mutation
d. TP53 mutation

26. Not true for PNH:
a. Can be a congenital disease
b. Thrombosis is common in hemolytic paroxysmal nocturnal hemoglobinuria (PNH)
c. PNH clone size determines clinical severity
d. Extravascular hemolysis does not occur

27. Not true for acquired aplastic anemia:
a. Diagnosis requires low marrow cellularity
b. 5-year event-free survival (EFS) is nearly 35% after hATG-CSA (antithymocyte globulin-cyclosporine A) therapy
c. Allogeneic stem cell transplantation is preferred for patients younger than 40 years of age
d. Thyroid peroxidase (TPO) receptor agonists do not have a role in young patients

28. Not true about thalassemia:
a. Iron deficiency is not seen in thalassemia trait subjects
b. Thalassemia intermedia usually have two defective beta globin genes
c. HbF levels can be >90% in thalassemia intermedia
d. Iron overload is an important prognostic factor for allogeneic transplant outcome

29. Hemoglobin E (HbE) disease is diagnosed on Hb HPLC (high performance liquid chromatography) by:
a. Increased Hb F
b. Increased Hb A2
c. Decreased Hb A
d. Decreased Hb E

30. Thalassemia trait is differentiated from iron deficiency on complete blood count (CBC) by:
a. Normal red blood cell distribution width (RDW)
b. More severe microcytosis
c. Higher number of target cells
d. Lower hematocrit

Ans.	1. b	2. a	3. c	4. b	5. d	6. d
	7. a	8. b	9. b	10. a	11. a	12. b
	13. b	14. c	15. e	16. d	17. a	18. a
	19. d	20. d	21. a	22. c	23. a	24. d
	25. a	26. d	27. d	28. a	29. b	30. a

10. SELF-ASSESSMENT

1. Monocytosis in CML is associated with:
   a. p210
   b. p190
   c. p230
   d. p220

2. Accelerated phase of CML is characterized by all, *except*:
   a. Thrombocytosis > 450,000
   b. Blast count 10–19% in peripheral smear (PS) or bone marrow (BM)
   c. Clonal cytogenetic evolution
   d. Persistent thrombocytopenia unrelated to therapy

3. Which of the following are recognized complications in essential thrombocytosis?
   a. Acute leukemia
   b. Erythromelalgia
   c. Thrombosis
   d. All of the above

4. The marrow fibrosis is reflected by all peripheral blood findings all, *except*:
   a. Nucleated RBC
   b. Presence of immature myeloid cells
   c. Microcytic hypochromic blood
   d. Tear drop cells

5. Molecular abnormality seen most commonly in polycythemia vera is:
   a. JAK2 V617F
   b. BCR-ABL
   c. *MLL* gene rearrangements
   d. CEBPA mutations

6. Parts of the physical examination will be most helpful in ruling out causes of secondary erythrocytosis all, *except*:
   a. Musculoskeletal
   b. Cardiac
   c. Respiratory
   d. Abdominal

7. CML is associated with all, *except*:
   a. Abnormal chromosome
   b. High neutrophil alkaline phosphatase
   c. An oncogenic fusion protein
   d. Huge spleen

8. Translocation t(9;22) in a primitive hematopoietic stem cell results in the all, *except*:
   a. A constitutively activated tyrosine kinase
   b. Solely responsible for the malignant phenotype
   c. Targeted inhibition of the BCR-ABL tyrosine kinase is the basis for modern treatment of CML
   d. Can be seen in all myeloproliferative neoplasm

9. Janus-associated Kinase-2 (JAK2) mutation causes cellular proliferation which is due to a:
   a. Cytokine mediation
   b. Hypersensitivity of progenitor cells to erythropoietin and thrombopoietin
   c. Reactive marrow hyperplasia
   d. Stimulation of viral oncogene

10. Which among the following is the most common tumor associated with neurofibromatosis in a child?
   a. Juvenile myelomonocytic leukemia
   b. Acute lymphoblastic leukemia
   c. Acute monocytic leukemia
   d. Acute myeloid leukemia

11. Not true for immune thrombocytopenia:
   a. Can be T cell mediated
   b. Steroid is first-line treatment
   c. Spleen is the common site of platelet destruction
   d. Splenomegaly is usually seen

12. Not a useful therapy in immune thrombocytopenia (ITP):
   a. Rituximab
   b. Dapsone
   c. Recombinant human thrombopoietin
   d. Romiplostim

13. Not true of blood component therapy:
   a. Platelets are stored at 22°C in a shaker to avoid clumping
   b. Shelf-life of platelet concentrates is 5 days
   c. Blood group matching is always needed for selection of platelet units
   d. Half-life of transfused platelets is 24 hours

14. Not true for transfusion:
   a. Nonhemolytic febrile transfusion reactions can be avoided by proper crossmatching of blood
   b. Anaphylaxis may not always be avoidable even by using blood unit matched at extended blood group antigens
   c. Transfusion-related acute lung injury (TRALI) can largely be prevented by using blood and plasma from previously untransfused males and nonparous female donors
   d. Leukocyte filters can prevent HLA alloimmunization in chronically transfused patients

15. Not true for lymphoma:
   a. These are neoplasms of mature/peripheral lymphocytes
   b. B-cell lymphomas are commoner than T-cell lymphomas
   c. Hodgkin's lymphoma is a disease of uncertain cell lineage
   d. Natural killer (NK) cell lymphomas are always EBV driven

16. Not true for anemia of chronic disease:
   a. Microcytic to normocytic
   b. Serum total iron binding capacity (TIBC) is low usually
   c. Serum hepcidin is low
   d. Serum ferritin is usually elevated

17. Not true for BCR-ABL:
   a. Product of translocation between chromosome 9 and 22
   b. Can be seen in elderly ALL
   c. Dasatinib is one of the targeted therapies
   d. Can be seen in atypical chronic myeloid leukemia (CML)

18. The dose of imatinib in children is:
   a. 200–240 mg/m^2
   b. 260–340 mg/m^2
   c. 350–380 mg/m^2
   d. 380–440 mg/m^2

19. Pink test is used for the diagnosis of:
   a. Amyloidosis
   b. Hereditary spherocytosis
   c. Congenital dyserythropoietic anemia
   d. Pure red cell aplasia

20. Most common cytogenetic abnormality in CLL:
   a. Del 13q14
   b. Del 17p
   c. t(9;22)
   d. Del 11q22

21. Basophilia in AML is usually associated with:
   a. t(9;11)
   b. t(6;9)
   c. t(1;22)
   d. inv 16

22. Monoclonal B-cell lymphocytosis is characterized by:
   a. Lymphocytosis >5,000 cell/mm^3
   b. CLL phenotype
   c. Involving young patients
   d. Always involvement of lymph nodes

23. Which among the following is the most common hematological malignancy associated with neurofibromatosis in a child?
   a. Juvenile myelomonocytic leukemia
   b. Acute lymphoblastic leukemia
   c. Childhood myelodysplastic syndrome
   d. AML

24. Paracortical areas are rich in:
   a. Memory B cells
   b. Naïve B cells
   c. Plasma cells
   d. T cells

25. Which hemostatic process is defective in Bernard-Soulier syndrome?
   a. Vasoconstriction
   b. Platelet adhesion
   c. Platelet secretion
   d. Platelet aggregation

26. Which one of the following is not a feature of δβ (Delta Beta) thalassemia?
   a. Leads to an increased percentage of HbF
   b. Leads to an increased percentage of hemoglobin A2
   c. Usually results from deletion of the δ and β genes
   d. Even when homozygous, may lead to the phenotype of thalassemia intermedia

27. Autoantibodies against red cells in CLL are:
   a. IgG
   b. IgM
   c. IgA
   d. IgE

28. A higher mortality rate in sickle cell anemia does not correlate with:
   a. Higher white cell count
   b. A lower percentage of HbF
   c. Coexisting α thalassemia trait
   d. Previous cerebrovascular accident

29. Not true regarding the normal blood count during infancy is:
   a. The reticulocyte count is very high 1 week after birth
   b. The cord blood Hb is approximately 17 g/dL
   c. The neutrophil count is normally lower than the lymphocyte count in children
   d. The lower limit of Hb during childhood is 11 g/dL

30. False statement regarding thrombosis during pregnancy is:
   a. Heparin does not cross the placenta
   b. The hypercoagulable state associated with pregnancy resolves within 24 hours of delivery
   c. Plasma level of factors VII, VIII, X, fibrinogen, and von Willebrand factor (vWF) levels are increased
   d. Women with thrombophilia may suffer from recurrent fetal loss

---

Ans.
1. b	2. a	3. d	4. c	5. a	6. a
7. b	8. d	9. b	10. d	11. d	12. c
13. c	14. a	15. c	16. c	17. d	18. b
19. b	20. a	21. b	22. b	23. a	24. d
25. b	26. b	27. a	28. c	29. a	30. b

11. SELF-ASSESSMENT

1. Following is a myeloid marker:
   a. CD3
   b. CD10
   c. CD13
   d. CD19

2. Most common type of congenital leukemia is:
   a. ALL
   b. AML
   c. CLL
   d. CML

3. Which of the following cytogenetic abnormality is associated with spontaneous remission of leukemia?
   a. Monosomy 5
   b. Trisomy 18
   c. Trisomy 21
   d. Monosomy 7

4. Basophilia in AML is associated with:
   a. t(9;11)
   b. t(6;9)
   c. t(1;22)
   d. FLT3-ITD (fms-like tyrosine kinase 3 internal tandem duplication) mutations

5. Which of the following cytogenetic abnormality associated with leukemia/lymphoma is incorrect?
   a. t(8;14), Burkitt lymphoma
   b. t(15;17) M3
   c. t(9;22) CML
   d. t(9;20) ALL

6. Block PAS positivity is usually seen in:
   a. B-cell acute lymphoblastic leukemia (B-ALL)
   b. *T*-lymphoblastic leukemia/lymphoma (T-ALL)
   c. Natural killer (NK) leukemia
   d. Large granular lymphocyte (LGL)

7. Which is not a poor prognostic factor for ALL?
   a. Hyperdiploidy
   b. t(9;22)
   c. Age >12 years
   d. t(4;11)

8. High apoptotic tumor cell death is characteristic of:
   a. Follicular lymphoma
   b. Burkitt lymphoma
   c. DLBCL
   d. CLL

9. Central nervous system involvement is more common in:
   a. ALL
   b. AML
   c. CML
   d. CLL

10. Which of the following is a bad prognostic cytogenetic marker in MDS?
   a. Del 20q
   b. Del 5q
   c. Del y
   d. Del 7q

11. MDS 5q-syndrome is characterized by all, *except*:
   a. Marked megakaryocytic dysplasia
   b. Female preponderance
   c. Normal platelet count
   d. Microcytic anemia

12. The likely cause of neonatal anemia with raised reticulocyte count and positive direct Coombs test is:
   a. Beta thalassemia
   b. Fetomaternal bleed
   c. Hemolytic disease of the newborn
   d. Alpha thalassemia

13. True regarding folate deficiency during pregnancy is:
   a. Folate requirements are stable during pregnancy
   b. Is the most common cause of anemia in pregnancy
   c. Folate fortification of food is usually associated with a reduction in the incidence of neural tube defects
   d. Folic acid at a dose of 5 mg/day is recommended for all women in the peripartum period

14. Following statements are true about the direct antiglobulin test, *except*:
   a. It is useful for crossmatching of recipient and donor blood
   b. It detects agglutination of antibody-coated red cells
   c. It is positive in hemolytic disease of the newborn
   d. It may detect complement on the surface of red cells

15. Which of the following is not a feature of acute gut graft-versus-host disease (GVHD)?
   a. Crypt abscesses
   b. Luminal apoptosis
   c. Gut ulcerations
   d. Gut strictures

16. The Indian blood group system is carried on:
   a. CD 34
   b. CD 35
   c. CD 44
   d. CD 45

17. Absence of which blood group system resists red blood cell (RBC) lysis in 2M urea: *Ref: Hoffman 7/e*
   a. MNS blood group
   b. Kidd blood group
   c. Diego blood group
   d. Duffy blood group

18. True about anti-A and anti-B antibodies in ABO blood group system is: *Ref: Hoffman 7/e*
   a. Anti-A and anti-B antibodies are produced in response to bacteria
   b. They are present at the time of birth
   c. Are mostly immunoglobulin G (IgG) type
   d. All of the above

19. Until what stage neutrophil precursors can divide: *Ref: Hoffman 7/e p321*
   a. Myeloblast
   b. Promyelocyte
   c. Myelocyte
   d. Metamyelocyte

20. Granulocyte-colony stimulating factor receptor (G-CSFR) is expressed on: *Ref: Hoffman 7/e p323*
   a. Myelocytes
   b. Platelets
   c. Lymphocytes
   d. Endothelial cells
   e. All of the above

21. Acute myeloid leukemia (AML) associated with mutations in the *Runx1* gene:
 a. AML with t(8;21)
 b. AML with inv16
 c. AML with t(6;9)
 d. AML with t(11;17)

22. Emergency granulopoiesis is mediated by:
 a. Runx1
 b. C/EBP-beta (Cebpb CCAAT/enhancer binding protein-beta)
 c. Transforming growth factor (TGF)-beta
 d. MicroRNA (miR)-223

23. What percentage of bone marrow (BM) cells do megakaryocytes constitute?
 a. 0.1%
 b. 1%
 c. 2%
 d. 5%

24. Sponge model is used to define the homeostatic mechanism of: *Ref: Hoffman 7/e p340*
 a. Neutrophil regulation
 b. Platelet regulation
 c. Erythrocyte regulation
 d. Eosinophil regulation

25. What percentage of patients with clinical Fanconi's anemia do not show increased chromosome breakage when tested with diepoxybutane (DEB) or mitomycin C (MMC)?
 a. None
 b. Less than 5%
 c. 10–15%
 d. 15–20%

26. The most common *FANC* gene mutation in Fanconi's anemia is:
 a. FANCA
 b. FANCB
 c. FANCD1
 d. FANCD2

27. What percentage of Fanconi's anemia patients does not have physical abnormalities?
 a. Less than 10%
 b. 15%
 c. 30%
 d. 40%

28. The syndrome of refractory sideroblastic anemia with vacuolization of BM precursors is known as:
 a. Pearson syndrome
 b. McCune–Albright syndrome
 c. Cartilage-hair hypoplasia syndrome
 d. Barth syndrome
 e. Cohen syndrome

29. Mutations in the *ELANE* gene results in:
 a. Kostmann syndrome
 b. Holt-Oram syndrome
 c. Dyskeratosis congenita
 d. Noonan syndrome
 e. Thrombocytopenia with absent radii syndrome

30. The dose of horse antithymocyte globulin (ATG) in aplastic anemia is:
 a. 20 mg/kg/day for 4 days
 b. 30 mg/kg/day for 4 days
 c. 40 mg/kg/day for 4 days
 d. 50 mg/kg/day for 4 days

Ans.	1. c	2. b	3. c	4. b	5. d	6. a
	7. a	8. b	9. a	10. d	11. d	12. a
	13. c	14. a	15. d	16. c	17. b	18. a
	19. c	20. e	21. a	22. b	23. a	24. b
	25. c	26. a	27. c	28. a	29. a	30. c

12. SELF-ASSESSMENT

1. WHO diagnostic criteria for multiple myeloma includes all, *except*:
   a. M protein in serum
   b. M protein in urine
   c. Marrow plasma cell >30%
   d. Organ damage

2. Known case of amyloidosis presents with prolonged PT, aPTT, and normal TT. Most likely diagnosis is:
   a. Acquired factor V deficiency
   b. Acquired factor X deficiency
   c. Acquired dysfibrinogenemia
   d. Acquired hypofibrinogenemia

3. Plasmablasts show positivity for:
   a. Neuron-specific enolase (NSE)
   b. MPO
   c. SBB
   d. Para-aminosalicylic acid (PAS)

4. Which of the following is not true about multiple myeloma?
   a. Background staining in PS
   b. Rouleaux formation
   c. Circulating plasmacytoid cells
   d. Reduced erythrocyte sedimentation rate (ESR)

5. Good prognostic cytogenetic in multiple myeloma is:
   a. t(11;14)   b. 17p13 deletion
   c. t(4;14)   d. t(14;16)

6. Dutcher bodies are:
   a. Intracytoplasmic   b. Intranuclear
   c. Intramitochondrial d. Extracellular

7. The least common monoclonal Ig ("M protein") is:
   a. IgG   b. IgA
   c. IgM   d. IgD

8. Not true about monoclonal gammopathy of undetermined significance (MGUS):
   a. 1% per year transformation to multiple myeloma (MM)
   b. Cytogenetic abnormalities different from that seen in MM
   c. M protein <3 g/dL
   d. No disease-related symptoms

9. M spike can be seen in all, *except*:
   a. Lymphoplasmacytic lymphoma
   b. Multiple myeloma
   c. Mycosis fungoides
   d. CLL

10. A patient is found to have multiple lytic bone lesions with increased plasma cells including immature forms in bone marrow examination. No M spike is seen on serum protein electrophoresis. The next best investigation is:
   a. Serum/urine immunofixation
   b. Free light chain assay
   c. Plasma cell labeling index
   d. Immunohistochemistry

11. Cell surface glycosyl phosphatidylinositol (GPI)-anchored proteins absent on paroxysmal nocturnal hemoglobinuria (PNH) blood cells are:
   a. CD55 and CD59   b. CD14 and CD16
   c. CD24 and CD48   d. All of the above

12. True about PNH is:
   a. Approximately 25% of patients with PNH have significant marrow aplasia
   b. Esophageal spasm are more common in patients with large PNH populations (>60% of granulocytes)
   c. Thrombosis occurs in approximately 40% of PNH patients
   d. Myelodysplastic syndrome (MDS) and AML are the most common malignancies to evolve from PNH
   e. All of the above

13. True about eculizumab is:
   a. Monoclonal antibody against C5
   b. Effective in reducing intravascular hemolysis
   c. Not effective in reducing extravascular hemolysis
   d. Reduces the risk of thrombosis
   e. All of the above

14. True about benign ethnic neutropenia are all, *except*:
   a. It is the most common form of neutropenia
   b. There is increased susceptibility to infection
   c. Bone marrow is able to produce enough normally functioning cells when needed
   d. More common in African descents and some ethnic groups in the Middle East
   e. None of the above

15. True about hepcidin is:
   a. Inflammation decreases plasma hepcidin through interleukin-6 (IL-6)
   b. Bone morphogenetic protein 6 (BMP6) is the endogenous regulator of hepcidin synthesis
   c. Transmembrane protease serine 6 (TMPRSS6) activates BMP6 induction of hepcidin synthesis
   d. Hemolysis increases circulating hepcidin concentration
   e. All of the above

16. The receptor for hepcidin is on:
   a. Transferrin
   b. Ferroportin
   c. Divalent metal transporter 1 (DMT1)
   d. Hemojuvelin
   e. All of the above

17. Iron overload increases the risk of infection with:
   a. *Vibrio vulnificus*   b. *Listeria monocytogenes*
   c. *Yersinia enterocolitica* d. *Candida*
   e. All of the above

18. True about iron deficiency anemia is:
   a. High percent transferrin saturation
   b. Low ferritin
   c. High hepcidin
   d. All of the above

19. Definition of refractoriness to oral iron therapy is:
   a. Less than 1 g/dL hemoglobin increase after 4 weeks of oral iron therapy
   b. Less than 2 g/dL hemoglobin increase after 4 weeks of oral iron therapy
   c. Less than 1 g/dL hemoglobin increase after 2 weeks of oral iron therapy
   d. Less than 2 g/dL hemoglobin increase after 2 weeks of oral iron therapy

20. True about the currently available intravenous iron formulations is:
   a. They consist of iron-carbohydrate complexes
   b. There is slow release of the iron
   c. Total replacement dose in just one or two infusions
   d. Premedication is not needed
   e. All of the above

21. True about transferrin is:
   a. It has two binding sites for iron, one at each of its two terminals
   b. It is tested by estimating the difference between the total iron content of serum before and after the addition of a saturating concentration of iron
   c. In normal individuals, it is only one-third saturated (30%)
   d. In patients with iron overload, it is usually completely saturated (100%)
   e. All of the above

22. Pyridoxine responsive anemia is seen in which mutation?
   a. 5-Aminolevulinic acid synthase (ALAS2) mutation
   b. SLC25A38 mutation
   c. Glutaredoxin 5 (GLRX5) mutation
   d. SLC19A2 mutation

23. Thiamine-responsive megaloblastic anemia syndrome results from mutation in:
   a. ALAS2
   b. SLC25A38
   c. GLRX5
   d. SLC19A2

24. True about anemia associated with isoniazid is:
   a. It causes sideroblastic anemia after 1–10 months of therapy
   b. Ring sideroblasts are seen in the marrow
   c. It occur only in slow acetylators of isoniazid
   d. Anemia can be fully reversed by coadministration of pyridoxine
   e. All of the above

25. Sideroblastic anemia can result from:
   a. Deficiency of both copper and zinc
   b. Overload of both copper and zinc
   c. Copper overload and zinc deficiency
   d. Copper deficiency and zinc overload

26. Macrocytosis without megaloblastosis is seen in:
   a. Reticulocytosis   b. Liver disease
   c. Aplastic anemia   d. Hypoxemia
   e. All of the above

27. Which of the following statements is not true?
   a. The combined use of homocysteine and methylmalonic acid levels can differentiate cobalamin from folate deficiency
   b. Normal levels of methylmalonic acid and homocysteine rule out clinically significant cobalamin deficiency with virtually 100% certainty
   c. Normal homocysteine levels suggest that megaloblastic anemia is not caused by folate deficiency
   d. Serum homocysteine concentrations are elevated in both cobalamin deficiency and folate deficiency
   e. All are true

28. Total gastrectomy leads to cobalamin deficiency in about:
   a. 3 months   b. 6 months
   c. 12 months   d. 4 years

29. The thalassemia mutations common in Asian Indians are all, *except*:
   a. Intervening sequence-1 (IVS-1), position 5 (G → C)
   b. 619-bp deletion
   c. Codons 8/9, frameshift (++G)
   d. Codons 41/42, frameshift (–CTTT)
   e. Codon 39, nonsense (CAG → TAG)

30. True about deferoxamine are all, *except*:
   a. Isolated from cultures of *Streptomyces pilosus*
   b. Half-life of 8–10 hours
   c. Dose is 20–60 mg/kg/day
   d. Can cause visual and auditory impairments

Ans.
1. c	2. b	3. a	4. d	5. a	6. b
7. d	8. b	9. c	10. a	11. d	12. e
13. e	14. b	15. b	16. b	17. e	18. b
19. a	20. e	21. e	22. a	23. d	24. e
25. d	26. e	27. e	28. d	29. e	30. b

13. SELF-ASSESSMENT

1. Following are the features of hairy cell leukemia (HCL), *except*:
a. Splenomegaly
b. Pancytopenia
c. Tartrate resistant acid phosphatase (TRAP) positivity
d. Leukocytosis

2. B symptoms in Hodgkin disease is defined as:
a. Weight loss more than 10% in 3 months
b. Generalized lymphadenopathy
c. Drenching night sweats
d. Erythroderma

3. Which of the following is not true regarding epidemiology of non-Hodgkin lymphoma?
a. It is more frequent after solid organ transplantation
b. It is associated with hepatitis C infection
c. Incidence is decreasing in Western Europe
d. It may be associated with malaria

4. A 60-year-old man presents with headache and anemia. Investigation revealed an IgM paraprotein of 30 g/L. What is the most likely diagnosis?
a. Burkitt lymphoma
b. Follicular lymphoma
c. Mycosis fungoides
d. Lymphoplasmacytic lymphoma

5. Which is the single most valuable investigation in diagnosis of non-Hodgkin lymphoma?
a. Computed tomography (CT) scan
b. Fine needle aspiration cytology (FNAC)
c. Flow cytometry
d. Lymph node biopsy

6. Which of the following is not associated with development of NHL?
a. *Helicobacter pylori*
b. Cytomegalovirus (CMV)
c. Epstein-Barr virus (EBV)
d. Human T-lymphotropic virus 1 (HLV-1)

7. Which of the following is true regarding lymphoplasmacytic lymphoma?
a. Associated with neuropathy
b. Plasmapheresis is rarely useful in cases of acute hyperviscosity syndrome as IgM is largely extravascular
c. The bone marrow is infrequently involved
d. Treatment should be started as soon as possible

8. Which of the following lymphoma has poorest prognosis?
a. DLBLC
b. Anaplastic large-cell lymphoma (ALCL)
c. Blastoid variant of mantle cell lymphoma
d. Burkitt lymphoma

9. Classical RS cell is seen in:
a. Nodular lymphocyte predominant Hodgkin lymphoma (NLPHL)
b. Lymphocyte predominant
c. Nodular sclerosis
d. Mixed cellularity

10. Which variant has best prognosis?
a. Lymphocyte predominant
b. Lymphocyte depletion
c. Mixed cellularity
d. NLPHL

11. The indications of splenectomy in thalassemia major are:
a. A large spleen
b. RBC alloimmunization
c. Age more than 12 years
d. Transfusion requirements of more than 180–200 mL/kg/y of packed RBCs
e. All of the above

12. True about thalassemia intermedia are all, *except*:
a. Constitutes 10% of patients with homozygous β-thalassemia
b. Many patients develop progressive iron overload even without transfusion
c. Higher incidence of extramedullary hematopoiesis than thalassemia major
d. Chelation in nontransfused patients is not indicated
e. Higher risk of thromboembolism

13. Thalassemia intermedia phenotype develops because of:
a. Less severe defect in β-globin chain synthesis
b. A decrease in α-globin chain synthesis
c. A decrease in β-globin chain synthesis
d. An increase in γ-globin chain synthesis
e. All of the above

14. In α^+-thalassemia trait, the number of dysfunctional α genes is:
a. One   b. Two
c. Three   d. Four

15. The α-thalassemia associated with mental retardation are encoded on:
a. Chromosomes 16 and X
b. Chromosomes 8 and 22
c. Chromosomes 10 and 12
d. Chromosomes 14 and 17

16. True about sickle cell-hemoglobin C (HbSC) are all, *except*:
a. Hemoglobin c (HbC) increase hemoglobin S (HbS) concentration from 40% (in HbAS) to 50% (in HbSC)
b. Heterozygotes of HbA with HbC are largely asymptomatic, whereas HbSC disease is clinically milder than hemoglobin SS (HbSS) disease
c. HbSC heterozygotes represent about a third of sickle cell disease (SCD) cases

d. Homozygous HbCC individuals behave like HbSS
e. Crystals of HbC are sometimes present in oxygenated RBCs

17. Which of the following is the cause of chronic hereditary nonspherocytic hemolytic anemia?
a. Pyrimidine 5′ nucleotidase-1 deficiency
b. Pyruvate kinase deficiency
c. Hexokinase
d. Adenosine deaminase hyperactivity
e. All of the above

18. True about spherocytes in hereditary spherocytosis is:
a. They lack central pallor
b. Their mean cell diameter is decreased
c. They appear more intensely hemoglobinized
d. All of the above
e. None of the above

19. Molecular defect in hyperimmunoglobulin E syndrome is:
a. Integrin beta-2 (ITGB2) mutation
b. CYBA mutation
c. Immunoglobulin variable heavy (IGVH) mutation
d. Signal transducer and activator of transcription 3 (STAT3) mutation

20. Percentage of myelofibrosis or essential thrombocythemia patients having calreticulin (CALR) mutation is:
a. 5%
b. 15%
c. 25%
d. 35%

21. The most common mutation seen in chronic neutrophilic leukemia:
a. CSF3R (colony stimulating factor 3 receptor)
b. KIT D816V
c. Tet methylcytosine dioxygenase 2 (TET2)
d. CREB-binding protein (CREBBP)

22. Chromosomal evolution is seen in what percent of chronic myeloid leukemia (CML) chronic phase patients who progress to blast crises?
a. 80–85%
b. 60–65%
c. 40–45%
d. 20–25%

23. How many patients with de novo MDS have isolated monosomy 7 or del 7?
a. 5%
b. 10%
c. 20%
d. 30%

24. True about loss of the Y chromosome is:
a. Observed in 10% of patients with MDS
b. Seen in 7% of older adult males without MDS
c. Patients with MDS with loss of Y chromosome who achieve complete hematologic remission regain the Y chromosome in their marrow cells
d. All of the above

25. True about haptoglobin is:
a. It binds free hemoglobin in plasma
b. Haptoglobin-hemoglobin complex is removed by reticuloendothelial system
c. Used to evaluate intravascular hemolysis
d. All of the above

26. True regarding red blood cell distribution width (RDW) is:
a. Elevated with increased variability in red blood cell (RBC) size and shape
b. RDW-CV is about 11–15%
c. RDW-SD is less influenced by mean corpuscular volume (MCV)
d. All of the above

27. Red blood cell distribution width is elevated in all, *except*:
a. Iron-deficiency anemia
b. Hereditary sideroblastic anemia
c. Thalassemia major
d. Thalassemia minor
e. All of the above

28. Hemoglobin A2 is elevated in:
a. β-thalassemia
b. Megaloblastic anemia
c. Thyrotoxicosis
d. All of the above

29. True about hemoglobin S (HbS) solubility test is:
a. Positive when HbS >30% and negative when HbS <20%
b. False negative with severe anemia
c. False positive with cryoglobulinemia
d. Positive results should be confirmed by another method
e. All of the above

30. Soluble transferrin receptor levels are increased in:
a. Erythroid hypoplasia
b. Iron-deficiency
c. Inflammation
d. All of the above

Ans.	1. d	2. c	3. c	4. d	5. d	6. b
	7. a	8. c	9. d	10. d	11. d	12. d
	13. e	14. a	15. a	16. d	17. e	18. d
	19. d	20. d	21. a	22. a	23. c	24. d
	25. d	26. d	27. d	28. d	29. e	30. b

14. SELF-ASSESSMENT

1. Which of the following stain is done to diagnose mast cell disease?
   a. Reticulin stain
   b. Cyclin D1
   c. Cytoplasmic CD3
   d. Tryptase stain

2. Bone marrow flow cytometry in a 14-year-old male child with acute leukemia showed HLADR (human leukocyte antigen – DR isotype) -ve, CD11+, CD13+, CD33+, CD14 -ve, CD41 -ve, and glycophorin –ve. What is the possible diagnosis?
   a. AML-M2
   b. APML
   c. AML-M7
   d. AML M6

3. The molecular abnormality in PNH directly involves the following protein:
   a. Glycophorin-A
   b. Delay activating factor
   c. Glycosylphosphatidylinositol
   d. Complement C4 binding protein

4. What is detected by indirect Coombs test?
   a. Antibodies in serum
   b. Antibodies in plasma
   c. Antibodies on RBC surface
   d. Antigen on RBC surface

5. Normal HbF value at the age of 1 year is:
   a. 1%
   b. Less than 1%
   c. 2%
   d. 5%

6. Monitoring of unfractionated heparin therapy is done by:
   a. APTT alone
   b. PT alone
   c. APTT and PT
   d. APTT and TT

7. Which of the following coagulation test will be prolonged in a case of congenital hypofibrinogenemia?
   a. APTT
   b. PT
   c. Both PT and APTT
   d. Clot solubility

8. Which of the following is not a feature of pure red cell aplasia (PRCA)?
   a. Anemia
   b. Splenomegaly
   c. Reduction in erythroid series of cells in bone marrow aspirate
   d. Lymphoid aggregates in bone marrow biopsy

9. Splenomegaly may be found with all, *except*:
   a. Autoimmune myelofibrosis
   b. CLL
   c. Kala-azar
   d. HCL

10. Most common congenital red cell membrane disorder is:
   a. Spherocytosis
   b. Elliptocytosis
   c. Pyropoikilocytosis
   d. Stomatocytosis

11. AML M6 is best described by all of the following, *except*:
   a. Bone marrow blast count > 20%
   b. Bone marrow erythroid cells > 50%
   c. t(8;21)
   d. Erythroid dysplasia

12. Following are the recognized associations, *except*:
   a. Thalassemia trait and microcytosis
   b. HS and gallstone
   c. PNH and reticulocytosis
   d. HCL and marrow fibrosis

13. All are true for HCL, *except*:
   a. Bone marrow fibrosis
   b. TRAP positivity
   c. Progressive pancytopenia
   d. CD20 negativity

14. Extravascular hemolysis is best characterized by all, *except*:
   a. Increased lactate dehydrogenase (LDH)
   b. Splenomegaly
   c. Jaundice
   d. Increased plasma hemoglobin

15. In acute leukemia, gating of blasts by flow cytometry is best done by using:
   a. CD34
   b. CD45
   c. Side scatter (SSC)
   d. Forward scatter (FSC)

16. Low APTT is seen in:
   a. DIC
   b. Deep vein thrombosis (DVT)
   c. Factor VIII deficiency
   d. Factor VII deficiency

17. Which of the following is used for estimation of APTT?
   a. Platelet rich plasma
   b. Platelet poor plasma
   c. Whole blood
   d. Serum

18. Normal APTT values are seen in:
   a. Factor X deficiency
   b. Factor XIII deficiency
   c. Factor XII deficiency
   d. Acute liver disease

19. Which of the following occurs as result of splenectomy?
   a. Neutropenia
   b. Thrombocytopenia
   c. Target cells
   d. Toxic granules

20. Cobalamin deficiency is characterized by all of the following, *except*:
   a. Angular cheilosis
   b. Glossitis
   c. Cognitive impairment
   d. Jaundice, conjugated

21. Fibrin degradation product (FDP) or D-Dimer may cause prolongation of APTT by:
   a. Inhibition of thrombin-mediated conversion of fibrinogen to fibrin
   b. Conversion of plasminogen to plasmin
   c. Inhibition of platelet aggregation
   d. Inhibition of fibrin crosslinking by factor XIII

22. Which of following organ is a primary site of hematopoiesis in a fetus before 20 weeks of gestation?
   a. Spleen
   b. Liver
   c. Bone marrow
   d. Lung

23. Thalassemia major is characterized by all of following, *except*:
   a. Splenomegaly
   b. Microcytic hypochromic anemia
   c. Presence of target cells in peripheral blood picture
   d. Increased osmotic fragility

24. JAK2 mutation is seen in:
   a. Polycythemia vera
   b. ITP
   c. CML
   d. CMML

25. A 15-year-old male child presented with gum bleeding and thrombocytopenia of one day duration. He was diagnosed to have acute leukemia. Most likely he is suffering from:
   a. AML-M5a   b. AML M7
   c. AML M3   d. ALL

26. Euglobulin lysis time is prolonged in:
   a. Hypofibrinogenemia
   b. Factor XIII deficiency
   c. DIC   d. Myocardial infarction

27. Direct Coombs test detects all of the following, *except*:
   a. Antibody on red cell surface
   b. Antigen on red cell surface
   c. Coating of RBC by complement C3
   d. Adsorption of immune complex on RBC membrane

28. All the statement are *true* of PNH, *except*:
   a. It is an acquired clonal disorder
   b. Jaundice is common presenting feature
   c. Complement is activated via alternate or classical pathway
   d. All PNH cells are sensitive to complement lysis

29. The genetic defect in PNH is:
   a. Somatic mutation   b. Translocation
   c. Deletion   d. Trisomy

30. The MPO is:
   a. Located in primary and secondary granules of neutrophils
   b. A lipophilic dye
   c. Inhibited by heparin
   d. Not seen in eosinophilic granules

Ans.	1. d	2. b	3. c	4. a	5. b	6. a
	7. c	8. b	9. a	10. a	11. c	12. c
	13. d	14. d	15. b	16. b	17. b	18. b
	19. d	20. d	21. a	22. b	23. d	24. a
	25. c	26. d.	27. b	28. d	29. a	30. a

15. SELF-ASSESSMENT

1. **Leukocyte alkaline phosphatase activity is found in:**
   a. Neutrophils   b. Eosinophils
   c. Myeloblasts   d. Monocytes

2. **Zap 70 is a marker used for:**
   a. CML   b. CLL
   c. AML   d. MCL

3. **Which of the following lymphoma shows cyclin D1 positivity?**
   a. Mantle cell   b. Follicular
   c. Small lymphocytic   d. Marginal zone

4. **Microcytosis is seen in:**
   a. Beta-thalassemia
   b. Depletion of body iron stores without anemia
   c. Hereditary elliptocytosis
   d. Hypothyroidism

5. **Platelet life span is normal in:**
   a. ITP   b. DIC
   c. Hypersplenism   d. TTP

6. **A 5-year-old child presents with jaundice and pallor off and on since birth. Examination reveals mild splenomegaly. Which of the following will you consider?**
   a. Autoimmune hemolytic anemia
   b. HS
   c. PNH
   d. Aplastic anemia

7. **Very high reticulocyte count is seen in:**
   a. Acute hemorrhage
   b. PRCA
   c. Beta-thalassemia
   d. Hemoglobin E (HbE) disease

8. **Bone biopsy is indicated in:**
   a. NHL   b. ALL
   c. Megaloblastic anemia   d. DIC

9. **Bone marrow aspiration is not indicated in:**
   a. Myelofibrosis
   b. AML
   c. Multiple myeloma
   d. Leishmaniasis

10. **Spherocytes in peripheral smear may be seen in all, *except*:**
    a. AIHA   b. HS
    c. PK deficiency   d. Post-transfusions

11. **Basophilic stippling is seen in all, *except*:**
    a. Thalassemia major
    b. Thalassemia minor
    c. Lead poisoning
    d. Untreated iron-deficiency

12. **Nonspecific esterase stains the following, *except*:**
    a. Platelets   b. Promyelocytes
    c. Monocytes   d. Lymphocytes

13. **Acid phosphates stain the:**
    a. Neutrophil   b. B-lymphocyte
    c. T-lymphocyte   d. Monocytes

14. **Blasts have oil red O positive vacuoles in:**
    a. ALL-L1   b. ALL-L2
    c. ALL-L3   d. NK-cell leukemia

15. **The following has good prognosis in AML:**
    a. NPM mutation   b. FLT3 mutations
    c. Trisomy 7   d. BCR-ABL

16. **In CLL, the following has a good prognosis:**
    a. Immunoglobulin heavy chain variable (IgVH) mutation present
    b. CD38 present
    c. IgVH mutation absent
    d. ZAP 70 present

17. **A 45-year-old patient has TLC of 2 lakhs with 95% mature looking lymphocytes. The following is a close differential diagnosis (D/D):**
    a. Mantle cell lymphoma with spill
    b. HCL
    c. Prolymphocytic leukemia
    d. Tuberculosis

18. **Monocytosis is seen in:**
    a. Leishmaniasis
    b. Parvovirus infection
    c. Acute bacterial infection
    d. Poststeroid therapy

19. **Reactive eosinophilia is seen in all, *except*:**
    a. Hodgkin's disease   b. ALL
    c. Filariasis   d. CMV

20. **A 6-year-old male child presents with swelling of knee joints and history of prolonged bleeding from injury. The following test would help in diagnosis, *except*:**
    a. Bleeding time   b. PT
    c. APTT   d. Clot retraction

21. **Anticoagulant of choice for coagulation studies is:**
    a. EDTA   b. Trisodium citrate
    c. Heparin   d. Hirudin

22. **Cryoprecipitate is used in all, *except*:**
    a. F IX deficiency
    b. vWF deficiency
    c. Fibrinogen deficiency
    d. VIII deficiency

23. All of the following have a high risk for thrombosis, *except*:
   a. Protein C deficiency
   b. Antithrombin (AT) deficiency
   c. High homocysteine E
   d. Glycoprotein IIb/IIIa (GPIIb IIIa) deficiency

24. Platelet aggregation with ADP is absent in:
   a. Afibrinogenemia
   b. Bernard-Soulier syndrome
   c. vWD
   d. Hemophilia A

25. Half-life of F XIII is:
   a. 8 hours
   b. 12 hours
   c. 24 hours
   d. 21 days

26. Serum iron maybe reduced in:
   a. Anemia of chronic disorder
   b. Thalassemia major
   c. Multiple transfused aplastic anemia
   d. Hemochromatosis

27. Direct Coombs test maybe positive in:
   a. Immediate post-transfusion
   b. Thalassemia major
   c. HS
   d. PNH

28. Polycythemia vera has the following, *except*:
   a. Low partial pressure of oxygen (PAO_2)
   b. JAK mutation
   c. High red cell mass
   d. Normal crythroprothesis

29. Common causes of myelofibrosis are following, *except*:
   a. Tuberculosis
   b. Hodgkin's disease
   c. Metastatic carcinoma (Ca)
   d. Leishmaniasis

30. Leukoerythroblastosis is seen in all, *except*:
   a. Metastatic Ca in bone
   b. Hereditary spherocytic anemia
   c. Myelofibrosis
   d. Aplastic anemia

Ans.	1. a	2. b	3. a	4. a	5. c	6. a
	7. a	8. a	9. a	10. c	11. d	12. d
	13. c	14. c	15. a	16. a	17. a	18. a
	19. d	20. d	21. b	22. a	23. d	24. a
	25. d	26. a	27. a	28. a	29. d	30. d

16. SELF-ASSESSMENT

1. As per WHO criteria, acute leukemia is diagnosed when blast percentage is more than:
   a. 10%
   b. 20%
   c. 30%
   d. 40%

2. HbE is seen most often in:
   a. Assam
   b. Punjab
   c. Nagpur
   d. Jaipur

3. CD34 is a marker for:
   a. Angiogenesis
   b. T-lymphocytes
   c. B-lymphocyte
   d. Myeloblast

4. NK-cells are positive for:
   a. CD19
   b. CD56
   c. CD20
   d. CD25

5. Inversion 16 is seen in:
   a. AML-M2
   b. AML-M4
   c. AML-M6
   d. ALL

6. t8:14 is seen in:
   a. Lymphoma
   b. ALL
   c. AML-M1
   d. AML-M3

7. Microcytic hypochromic cells are seen:
   a. Sideroblastic anemia
   b. Hypothyroidism
   c. Liver disease
   d. Aplastic anemia

8. 5Q of abnormality is diagnostic for:
   a. ALL
   b. AML
   c. MDS
   d. CLL

9. Parvovirus B_{19} infection is associated with:
   a. PRCA
   b. ET
   c. Polycythemia vera
   d. MDS

10. The following is true of essential thrombocythemia:
    a. Splenomegaly is not a feature
    b. Asymptomatic patients with platelet counts of more 1,500,000/mm³ need treatment
    c. Low-dose aspirin is contraindicated
    d. C-reactive protein is raised

11. Leukostasis is most often seen in:
    a. AML
    b. Non-Hodgkin's lymphoma
    c. Acute lymphoblastic leukemia
    d. Chronic myeloid leukemia

12. Plasma homocysteine levels are elevated by a deficiency of:
    a. Vitamin A
    b. Vitamin B_6
    c. Folic acid
    d. Vitamin C

13. In therapy of AML, the following is true of high-dose cytosine arabinoside:
    a. It causes ATRA syndrome
    b. It is used as induction therapy for acute promyelocytic leukemia (AML-M3)
    c. It can cause chemical conjunctivitis
    d. It has no role in consolidation therapy

14. The diagnosis of polycythemia vera is supported by:
    a. Splenomegaly
    b. Renal mass
    c. High serum erythropoietin
    d. Hypoxia

15. In a 75-year-old man with CLL, treatment is indicated when:
    a. Lymphocyte count is more than 50,000/mm³
    b. Hemoglobin is less than 9 g/dL
    c. Two groups of lymph nodes are involved
    d. Spleen is palpable more than 3 cm

16. Which of the following is not true in *Plasmodium falciparum* malaria?
    a. May be complicated by severe anemia
    b. May be complicated by jaundice
    c. Is always sensitive to chloroquine
    d. May coexist with vivax malaria in the same patient

17. A patient with sickle cell anemia should avoid the following:
    a. Swimming
    b. Dehydration
    c. Pneumococcal immunization
    d. Early antibiotics for respiratory infection

18. Which of the following may constitute high risk during surgery?
    a. Beta-thalassemia minor
    b. Hemoglobin S homozygous
    c. Hemoglobin Punjab
    d. Hemoglobin E trait

19. A syngeneic (identical twin) is the ideal donor for bone marrow transplantation in the following conditions, for the reasons mentioned:
    a. Thalassemia major, as there is no GVHD
    b. Relapse acute lymphoblastic leukemia, for more graft versus leukemia effect
    c. Aplastic anemia, as there is neither graft rejection nor GVHD
    d. Sickle cell anemia, as no prior chemotherapy for conditioning is needed

20. In polycythemia vera, the best therapy is:
    a. Regular phlebotomy, to keep hematocrit less than 45% (0.45)
    b. Intermittent busulfan
    c. Interferon
    d. Aspirin 500 mg/day

21. A child with acute ITP presents with gastrointestinal bleeding. The blood group is O negative. The best treatment option is:
   a. Intravenous immunoglobulin
   b. Splenectomy
   c. Anti-D injection
   d. Pulse dexamethasone

22. The following are true of childhood acute lymphoblastic leukemia:
   a. Presence of Tel-AML1 fusion [t(12;21)] suggests a poor prognosis
   b. Survival is best in patients with hyperdiploidy (chromosome number >50)
   c. An initial total leucocyte count more than 50,000/mm^3 suggests a good prognosis
   d. Testicular involvement at diagnosis is found in more than 10% cases

23. Spherocytes are seen in large number in:
   a. G6PD deficiency
   b. Aplastic anemia
   c. ABO incompatibility
   d. Megaloblastic anemia

24. All of the followings are suggestive of intravascular hemolysis, *except*:
   a. Increased plasma hemoglobin
   b. Increased reticulocyte count
   c. Increased haptoglobin
   d. Hemoglobinuria

25. The most common cause of thrombocytopenia in a newborn is:
   a. Immune mediated   b. Liver dysfunction
   c. Blood loss   d. DIC

26. All of the followings are the features of PNH, *except*:
   a. Frontal bossing   b. Dark colored urine
   c. Deep vein thrombosis   d. Thrombocytopenia

27. One unit/kg of factor IX concentrate raises plasma level by:
   a. 1%   b. 2%
   c. 3%   d. 5%

28. Which of the following is not true for PRCA?
   a. Idiopathic PRCA usually respond to immunosuppressive drugs
   b. Parvovirus infection can result in PRCA
   c. Resection of thymoma usually reverse the disease
   d. Progress to leukemia is very common

29. Which is not a late effect of treatment for childhood ALL?
   a. Cataract
   b. Bone disorders
   c. Obesity
   d. Restrictive lung disease

30. Epstein-Barr virus is not associated with:
   a. Nasopharyngeal carcinoma
   b. HCL
   c. Oral hairy leukoplakia
   d. Leiomyosarcoma in young people with acquired immunodeficiency syndrome (AIDS)

Ans.	1. b	2. a	3. d	4. b	5. b	6. a
	7. a	8. c	9. a	10. b	11. a	12. c
	13. c	14. a	15. b	16. c	17. b	18. b
	19. c	20. a	21. a	22. b	23. c	24. c
	25. d	26. a	27. a	28. d	29. d	30. b

17. SELF-ASSESSMENT

1. Which of the following finding is not true in visceral leishmaniasis?
   a. Lymphadenopathy
   b. Positive leishmanin test in most cases
   c. Thrombocytopenia
   d. Splenomegaly

2. In G6PD deficiency, hemolysis is induced by:
   a. Levamisole
   b. Dapsone
   c. Chloromycetin
   d. Erythromycin

3. Kostmann syndrome is characterized by:
   a. Pure red cell aplasia
   b. Severe neutropenia
   c. Thrombocytopenia
   d. Pancytopenia

4. Thalassemia control has been most successful in:
   a. USA
   b. Cyprus
   c. Iraq
   d. Thailand

5. Major cause of death in patients with thalassemia major is secondary to:
   a. Endocrinopathies
   b. Cardiomyopathy
   c. Liver failure
   d. Aplastic crisis

6. Thrombosis in neonates is mostly due to:
   a. Protein C and protein S deficiency
   b. Antithrombin III deficiency
   c. Liver dysfunction
   d. Catheter related

7. Penicillin prophylaxis following splenectomy should be given for:
   a. Life long
   b. Up to 20 years of age
   c. 3 years following splenectomy
   d. 5 years following splenectomy

8. Conventional cytogenetics is of not much help in which disorder?
   a. MDS
   b. Aplastic anemia
   c. Acute leukemia
   d. Chronic leukemias

9. Which of the following is not a favorable cytogenetic marker in AML?
   a. t (9:22)
   b. t (15:17)
   c. t (8:21)
   d. Inv 16

10. Following anticoagulants can be used in patients with heparin-induced thrombocytopenia, *except*:
    a. Argatroban
    b. Low-molecular-weight heparin (LMWH)
    c. Lepirudin
    d. Danaparoid

11. Corrected reticulocyte count corrects for:
    a. Differences in blood volume
    b. Differences in hematocrit
    c. Differences in hemoglobin
    d. Differences in red cell number

12. Advantages of LMWH are:
    a. More specific anti-Xa activity
    b. Broader activity
    c. Shorter half-life
    d. Easier to reverse

13. Hematopoiesis in the fetus starts in the:
    a. Liver at 12 weeks
    b. Liver at 6 weeks
    c. Bone marrow 8 weeks
    d. Yolk sac 4 weeks

14. Relative anemia is associated with:
    a. Increased plasma volume
    b. Prematurity
    c. Microcytic but normochromic anemia
    d. Elevated reticulocyte count

15. Following are associated with poor prognosis in CLL, *except*:
    a. ZAP 70 by flow cytometry
    b. Mutated IgVH
    c. Raised β2 microglobulin
    d. Trisomy 12

16. Lymphocytosis is unusual for a diagnosis of:
    a. Follicular lymphoma
    b. Splenic lymphoma with villus lymphocytes (SLVL)
    c. Mantle cell lymphoma
    d. HCL

17. Congenital dyserythropoietic anemia type 2 (CDA type II) is characterized by all, *except*:
    a. Lysis with autologous serum
    b. Autosomal recessive
    c. Splenectomy is useful in transfusion dependency
    d. Positive HEMPAS (hereditary erythroblastic multinuclearity associated with positive acidified serum)

18. Drug of choice for candidiasis in neutropenic patient is:
    a. Fluconazole
    b. Itraconazole
    c. Ketoconazole
    d. Amphotericin B

19. Waldenström macroglobulinemia is characterized by all, *except*:
    a. IgG paraprotein
    b. IgM paraprotein
    c. Renal dysfunction is uncommon
    d. Hyperviscosity

20. Major molecular response after Imatinib therapy in CML is best described by:
    a. 2 log reduction in BCR-ABL
    b. 3 log reduction in BCR-ABL
    c. 4.5 log reduction in BCR-ABL
    d. 3.5 log reduction in BCR-ABL

21. True about osmotic fragility are all, *except*:
   a. Incubation for 24 hours at 37°C enhance assay sensitivity
   b. Normal test excludes hereditary spherocytosis
   c. Flow cytometry for band 3 using eosin-5-maleimide (EMA) is more sensitive
   d. Decreased osmotic fragility seen in sickle cell disease
   e. All of the above

22. True about complements is:
   a. Reduced C4 with or without reduced C3 is seen in lupus
   b. Reduced C3 with normal C4 is seen in sepsis
   c. Elevated C3 and/or C4 implies an acute-phase response
   d. C3 and C4 when measured together examine both classical and alternative complement pathways
   e. All of the above

23. Mean platelet volume is increased in all, *except*:
   a. Wiskott-Aldrich syndrome
   b. Bernard-Soulier syndrome
   c. Myosin heavy chain 9 (MYH9) disorders
   d. Immune thrombocytopenia

24. Peak levels of desmopressin after subcutaneous or intranasal administration is achieved after:
   a. 10–30 minutes
   b. 60–90 minutes
   c. 3–4 hours
   d. 6 hours

25. True regarding performing minor surgeries in liver dysfunction are:
   a. Prophylactic intervention is rarely required with prothrombin time-international normalized ratio (PT-INR) <2
   b. Complete PT-INR correction is less likely to be achieved with fresh-frozen plasma
   c. Fresh-frozen plasma should not be given to all patients with prolonged PT-INR
   d. All of the above

26. The major function of red pulp of the spleen is:
   a. Phagocytosis
   b. Hematopoiesis
   c. Immunoregulation
   d. Antibody production
   e. All of the above

27. The most common cause of anemia in human immunodeficiency virus (HIV) disease is:
   a. Decreased RBC production
   b. Increased RBC destruction
   c. Chronic blood loss
   d. Decreased nutritional intake

28. Which of the following is not used in the treatment of HIV-associated immune thrombocytopenia?
   a. Steroids
   b. Intravenous immunoglobulin (IVIG)
   c. Anti-RhD
   d. All can be used

29. True about parvovirus B_{19} infection are all, *except*:
   a. In normal children, this infection usually is not associated significantly with hematologic abnormalities
   b. In patients with hemolytic anemias, it can cause aplastic crisis
   c. Can be associated with transient erythroblastopenia of childhood
   d. All of the above

30. Which of the following infection can cause pancytopenia?
   a. *Mycobacterium tuberculosis*
   b. *Histoplasma capsulatum*
   c. *Leishmania donovani*
   d. Mucor
   e. All of the above

Ans.	1. b	2. b	3. b	4. b	5. b	6. d
	7. a	8. b	9. a	10. b	11. b	12. a
	13. b	14. a	15. b	16. d	17. a	18. d
	19. a	20. b	21. b	22. e	23. a	24. b
	25. d	26. a	27. a	28. d	29. c	30. e

18. SELF-ASSESSMENT

1. The cause of elevated vitamin B_{12} levels is:
a. An increase in plasma vitamin B_{12} by liberation from liver
b. A quantitative deficiency or lack of affinity of transcobalamin for vitamin B_{12}
c. An increase in transcobalamin because of lack of clearance
d. All of the above

2. True about elevated vitamin B_{12} levels are all, *except*:
a. Is mostly asymptomatic
b. Associated with solid tumors
c. Associated with myeloproliferative neoplasms
d. Can manifest as vitamin B_{12} deficiency
e. All are true

3. True about coagulation abnormalities in cyanotic congenital heart diseases are all, *except*:
a. About 40% patients have coagulation abnormalities
b. There is increased risk of postoperative bleeding
c. Blood samples should be collected in 1:2 ratio of 3.8% sodium citrate to blood
d. The coagulation abnormalities usually are corrected after surgical repair of the heart defect
e. If surgery is not possible, the coagulopathy may be treated by correction of polycythemia to a hematocrit level of 60%

4. True about celiac disease is:
a. Is due to gluten sensitivity
b. Aberrant intestinal T-cell immune response leads to injury of the mucosa of the small intestine
c. More common in children and adolescents
d. There is failure to thrive, weight loss, and nutritional deficiency
e. All of the above

5. The nutritional deficiency seen in celiac disease is:
a. Iron-deficiency
b. Folic acid deficiency
c. Vitamin B_{12} deficiency
d. All of the above

6. All are true about passenger lymphocyte syndrome, *except*:
a. It is a graft-versus-host reaction
b. Antibodies are made by recipient B cells
c. Anti-RhD is the most common type of antibody
d. All of the above

7. True about lead poisoning is:
a. Decreased activity of pyrimidine 5-nucleotidase
b. Decreased activity of δ-aminolevulinic acid dehydratase
c. Decreased activity of ferrochelatase
d. All of the above

8. The complication of using prothrombin complex concentrates is:
a. Disseminated intravascular coagulation
b. Thrombotic complications
c. Anaphylaxis
d. All of the above

9. Volume of fresh-frozen plasma used to prevent bleeding is:
a. 10–20 mL/kg
b. 20–30 mL/kg
c. 30–40 mL/kg
d. 40–50 mL/kg

10. One unit of cryoprecipitate for every 10 kg of body weight increases plasma fibrinogen by approximately:
a. 20 mg/dL
b. 30 mg/dL
c. 40 mg/dL
d. 50 mg/dL

11. True about cirrhosis of liver are all, *except*:
a. There is increased risk of bleeding
b. There is increased risk of thrombosis
c. Recombinant factor VIIa can be used
d. All are true

12. Which of the following is not true about dabigatran?
a. It inhibits both free and fibrin-bound thrombin
b. It has a half-life of 12–14 hours
c. Preferred for patients with mechanical heart valves
d. All are true

13. Idarucizumab is used for reversal of the activity of:
a. Rivaroxaban
b. Dabigatran
c. Edoxaban
d. Apixaban

14. Macrophage activation syndrome is associated with:
a. Lymphoma
b. Genetic defects
c. Tuberculosis
d. Still's disease

15. Deep vein thrombosis in pregnancy should be treated with:
a. Aspirin
b. Warfarin
c. Dabigatran
d. Low-molecular-weight heparin
e. Low-molecular-weight heparin and aspirin

16. Secondary HLH with highest mortality is seen in:
a. EBV-associated HLH
b. Malignancy-associated HLH
c. HIV-associated HLH
d. Tuberculosis-associated HLH

17. Eosin-5-maleimide binding test for hereditary spherocytosis is dependent on binding of EMA to:
a. Band 3 protein
b. Protein 4.2
c. Protein 4.1
d. Ankyrin

18. Eosin-5-maleimide binding test is done by:
  a. Flow cytometry
  b. Osmotic fragility
  c. SDS-PAGE electrophoresis
  d. High-performance liquid chromatography

19. True about splenectomy for hereditary spherocytosis are all, *except*:
  a. There is increased lifespan of the red cells to near normal
  b. The osmotic fragility becomes normal
  c. There is increased risk of thrombosis
  d. All are true

20. Hemolysis is caused by all, *except*:
  a. Dapsone
  b. Sulfasalazine
  c. Menadiol
  d. Phenazopyridine
  e. Paracetamol

21. True about Zieve syndrome is:
  a. Intravascular hemolysis
  b. Seen mainly in alcoholics
  c. Spherocytes are seen
  d. None of the above
  e. All of the above

22. False about congenital dyserythropoietic anemia type II is:
  a. Inheritance is autosomal dominant
  b. Electron microscopy shows double membrane
  c. HAM test is positive
  d. Bone marrow shows more than 10% binucleate erythroblasts

23. Mechanism of action of antithymocyte globulin (ATG) in aplastic anemia is:
  a. T-cell depletion by complement-mediated lysis
  b. Direct stimulation of T-regulatory cells
  c. Reduced apoptosis and Fas expression on CD34+ bone marrow cells
  d. Destruction of activated cytotoxic T lymphocytes by Fas-mediated apoptosis
  e. All of the above

24. H score is used as a probability criteria for:
  a. Deep vein thrombosis
  b. Hereditary spherocytosis
  c. HLH
  d. Antiphospholipid antibody syndrome

25. True about antibodies to RhD antigen are all, *except*:
  a. Antibodies to RhD antigen are naturally occurring antibodies
  b. Antibodies to the RhD antigen occur as a result of transfusion or pregnancy in individuals who are RhD negative
  c. The RhD antigen is highly immunogenic
  d. RhD negative components may be given to RhD-positive recipients without any risk of immunization

26. Which of the following blood product does not require irradiation?
  a. Random donor platelets
  b. Single donor platelets
  c. Buffy coat
  d. Frozen plasma
  e. Granulocyte transfusion

27. Irradiation of blood components is not needed in:
  a. HIV/AIDS (acquired immunodeficiency syndrome)
  b. Congenital humoral deficiency disorders
  c. Solid organ transplantation
  d. All of the above

28. Indefinite irradiation is indicated for all, *except*:
  a. Hodgkin lymphoma
  b. Purine nucleoside analogues
  c. Active chronic GVHD
  d. Autologous stem cell transplant
  e. All of the above

29. Cryoprecipitate is a source of all, *except*:
  a. Fibrinogen
  b. von Willebrand factor (vWF)
  c. Factor VIII
  d. Factor IX
  e. Factor XIII

30. Which of the following is an Rh antigen?
  a. C
  b. c
  c. D
  d. E
  e. All of the above

Ans.
1. d	2. e	3. c	4. e	5. d	6. b
7. a	8. d	9. a	10. d	11. d	12. c
13. b	14. d	15. d	16. a	17. b	18. a
19. a	20. b	21. e	22. a	23. e	24. c
25. a	26. d	27. d	28. d	29. d	30. e

19. SELF-ASSESSMENT

1. **Fedratinib is used for:**
   a. Chronic myeloid leukemia
   b. Myelofibrosis
   c. Langerhans histiocytosis
   d. Mantle cell lymphoma

2. **Erythrodontia (red teeth) is a feature of:**
   a. Congenital erythropoietic porphyria
   b. Congenital *dyserythropoietic* anemia type III
   c. Leukocyte adhesion deficiency
   d. Hereditary sideroblastic anemia

3. **Functional independence score is used for:**
   a. Thalassemia
   b. Hemophilia
   c. Primary CNS lymphoma
   d. Chronic GVHD

4. **Factor V deficiency is associated with:**
   a. Factor VII (FVII) deficiency
   b. FVIII deficiency
   c. FX deficiency
   d. FII deficiency

5. **Age of a blood donor should be between:**
   a. 18 and 65 years
   b. 18 and 58 years
   c. 18 and 60 years
   d. 16 and 58 years

6. **The ratio of blood: anticoagulant-preservative solution in blood-collected bag is:**
   a. 100:14
   b. 100:16
   c. 100:15
   d. 100:13

7. **Major crossmatch comprises interaction between:**
   a. Patient red cells and donor serum
   b. Patient serum and patient red cells
   c. Donor red cells and patient serum
   d. Donor red cells and donor serum

8. **A "microaggregate" blood filter (BT set) has an approximate filter screen size of:**
   a. 170 μm
   b. 40 μm
   c. 15 μm
   d. 8 μm
   e. None of the above

9. **Which of the following is not true for nucleic acid test (NAT) of donated blood?**
   a. It helps in detecting the blood donor during the window period of an infection
   b. It detects the DNA or RNA of viruses such as hepatitis B virus (HBV), HIV, and hepatitis C virus (HCV)
   c. It is a mandatory test to be done on donated blood
   d. It can detect the occult HBV infections in blood donors

10. **All of the following are true about Direct Coombs test (DCT)-negative autoimmune hemolytic anemia (AIHA), *except*:**
    a. Cases where the number of IgG molecules attached to the RBCs are less than the detection limit of the test
    b. Cases where AIHA is due to IgA type autoantibody
    c. These cases behave like warm AIHA
    d. Steroid therapy is contraindicated in these cases

11. **Which of the following is not the complication of ABO-incompatible hematopoietic stem cell transplantation?**
    a. Pure red cell aplasia
    b. Passenger lymphocyte syndrome
    c. Delayed engraftment
    d. Transfusion-associated graft-versus-host disease (TA-GVHD)

12. **All are true about immature platelet fraction (IPF), *except*:**
    a. High levels indicate increased platelet production
    b. MYH9-related disorder should be considered when IPF is >40%
    c. Levels are decreased in immune thrombocytopenic purpura (ITP)
    d. The normal level is 1–5%

13. **The International Society on Thrombosis and Haemostasis (ISTH) score for disseminated intravascular coagulation (DIC) includes all of the following parameters, *except*:**
    a. Activated partial thromboplastin time (aPTT)
    b. PT
    c. Platelet counts
    d. Fibrinogen

14. **Post-transplant cyclophosphamide is widely used for which type of allogeneic stem cell transplant?**
    a. Matched-sibling donor transplant
    b. Matched-unrelated donor transplant
    c. Haploidentical donor transplant
    d. Mismatched sibling donor transplant

15. **All of the following are features of hyperhemolysis, *except*:**
    a. High reticulocyte count
    b. Post-transfusion hemoglobin less than pretransfusion hemoglobin
    c. Most common in alloimmunized sickle cell disease patients
    d. Indirect hyperbilirubinemia

16. **Tisagenlecleucel is a:**
    a. Monoclonal antibody
    b. Chimeric antigen receptor T cell therapy
    c. BTK inhibitor
    d. None of the above

17. **Hydroxyurea is commonly used in all of the following, *except*:**
    a. Sickle cell disease
    b. Thalassemia major
    c. Myelofibrosis
    d. Thalassemia intermedia

18. **A six antigen human leukocyte antigen (HLA) match in a sibling allogeneic transplant tests for all of the following, *except*:**
    a. HLA A
    b. HLA B
    c. HLA C
    d. HLA DR

19. **High-titer inhibitors in hemophilia A patients is defined as a level of:**
    a. 5-10 BU
    b. >5 BU
    c. >1 BU
    d. >10 BU

20. **Time line for defining chronic ITP is thrombocytopenia for:**
    a. >3 months
    b. >6 months
    c. >9 months
    d. >12 months

21. **Which of the following are causes of a raised mean corpuscular hemoglobin concentration (MCHC)?**
    a. Hereditary spherocytosis
    b. Cold agglutinins
    c. Hypercholesterolemia
    d. All of the above

22. **Which of the following is true for cold agglutinin disease monospecific DCT?**
    a. IgG-, C3d+
    b. IgG+, C3d-
    c. IgG-, C3d-
    d. IgG+, C3d+

23. **Which of the following drugs is used in sickle cell disease?**
    a. L-Glutamine
    b. Hydroxyurea
    c. Crizanlizumab
    d. All of the above

24. **In smoldering myeloma, which one of the following is a myeloma defining event?**
    a. Bone marrow plasma cell >60%
    b. Involved light chain is to uninvolved light chain ratio of >100
    c. More than one focal lesion on magnetic resonance imaging (MRI) studies
    d. All of the above

25. **MR4.5 in chronic myeloid leukemia is defined as a real-time quantitative polymerase chain reaction (RQ-PCR) for BCR-ABL of:**
    a. <0.1%
    b. <0.01%
    c. <0.001%
    d. <0.0032%
    e. <0.0045%

26. **What is the cell of origin of hairy cell leukemia?**
    a. Germinal center cell
    b. Memory B cell
    c. Marginal zone B cell
    d. Pre germinal center cell

27. **Erythropoietin is produced by which cells:**
    a. Podocytes of glomerulus
    b. Interstitial fibroblastic cells of kidney
    c. Endothelial cell of glomerular capillaries
    d. Intercalated cells of proximal tubules of the kidney

28. **Upshaw-Schulman syndrome is:**
    a. Atypical hemolytic uremic syndrome (HUS)
    b. Congenital thrombotic thrombocytopenic purpura (TTP)
    c. Heparin-induced thrombocytopenia
    d. Acquired TTP

29. **Mushroom-shaped (or "pincered") red cells are seen in hereditary spherocytosis:**
    a. Band 3 defect
    b. Ankyrin deficiency
    c. Spectrin defect
    d. Protein 4.2 defect

30. **McLeod phenotype is characteristically associated with which type of the RBCs:**
    a. Elliptocyte
    b. Echinocyte
    c. Acanthocyte
    d. Pyropoikilocyte

31. **Which blood group has the lowest levels of vWF?**
    a. A
    b. B
    c. O
    d. AB

32. **The dose of rituximab in RCHOP is:**
    a. 275 mg/m^2
    b. 375 mg/m^2
    c. 475 mg/m^2
    d. 575 mg/m^2

33. **Antifungal effective against mucormycosis is:**
    a. Clotrimazole
    b. Voriconazole
    c. Posaconazole
    d. Itraconazole

34. **Alemtuzumab is a monoclonal antibody against:**
    a. CD33
    b. CD13
    c. CD52
    d. CD22

35. **Alemtuzumab can lead to reactivation of:**
    a. HBV
    b. HCV
    c. Cytomegalovirus
    d. Epstein-Bar virus

36. **Leukemia with 11q23 abnormality has worst prognosis in:**
    a. Infants
    b. Children
    c. Adolescents
    d. Adults

37. **11q23 abnormality is seen in:**
    a. B-cell acute lymphoblastic leukemia
    b. T-cell acute lymphoblastic leukemia
    c. Acute myeloid leukemia
    d. Mixed phenotype acute leukemia
    e. All of the above

38. **The red cell membrane contains carbohydrates: lipids:proteins in the ratio of:**
    a. 1:4:6
    b. 1:2:3
    c. 1:3:5
    d. 1:3:8

39. **All are glycosylphosphatidylinositol (GPI)-linked structures, *except*:**
    a. CD157
    b. CD24
    c. CD71
    d. CD99

40. **In t(v;11) (qn;q23), the v stands for:**
    a. 4
    b. 6
    c. 9
    d. All of the above
    e. None of the above

41. **Incidence of acute myeloid leukemia (AML) with inv(16):**
    a. 5%
    b. 15%
    c. 20%
    d. 25%

42. **True for AML with CBFB- MYH11 are all, *except*:**
    a. Marrow shows a variable number of eosinophils
    b. Myelomonocytic leukemia
    c. Monoblasts shows nonspecific esterase reactivity
    d. Mutations of KIT are uncommon in this subtype

43. **Not in favorable risk category of AML as per 2017 ELN risk stratification?**
    a. t(8;21)
    b. Mutated NPM1 without FLT3 ITD
    c. Biallelic mutated CEBPA
    d. Wild type NPM1 without FLT3-ITD

44. **Which of the following is true for relapse rate in favorable risk AML with chemotherapy without allogeneic HSCT?**
    a. 20%
    b. 40%
    c. 60%
    d. 80%

45. **A newly diagnosed Case of AML demonstrates positivity of blasts by flow cytometry for CD19 in addition to CD34, MPO, CD13 and HLA DR. The most likely cytogenetic abnormality associated with this immunophenotype is:**
    a. t(6;9)
    b. t(8;21)
    c. t(16;16)
    d. t(15;17)

46. **Which of the following is not expected in AML with t(6;9) (p23;q34); DEKNUP214?**
    a. Thrombocytosis
    b. Basophilia
    c. Multilineage dysplasia
    d. Pancytopenia

47. **All are true for AML with mutated NPM1, *except*:**
    a. Strong association with acute monocytic leukaemia
    b. Multilineage dysplasia can be seen in 25% of cases
    c. NPM1 immunohistochemistry can be done on marrow biopsy
    d. Usually associated with a complex karyotype

48. **True about Sanger sequencing is:**
    a. Commonly used to detect base-level DNA sequence alterations
    b. Automated systems perform sequencing of PCR-amplified templates using fluorescent dye terminators
    c. Difficult to resolve more complex insertion/deletion events and cannot detect large deletions or amplifications
    d. Cannot reliably distinguish allelic nature of heterozygous changes (e.g., biallelic versus compound heterozygote) without specialized techniques
    e. All of the above

49. **True about next-generation sequencing are all, *except*:**
    a. Massively parallel sequencing of DNA with applications spanning targeted gene panels to whole exome and genome sequencing; efficient detection of single base changes and small insertion/deletion events
    b. Ability to multiplex many samples per run with sample indexing
    c. Can resolve complex small insertion/deletion events and often distinguish precise nature of heterozygous mutation variants
    d. Web application interfaces allow direct visualization of analyzed data and sequence variants
    e. Sensitivity is equal to that of Sanger method

50. **True about ALK+ T-cell anaplastic large-cell lymphoma is:**
    a. t(2;5) is the major cytogenetic abnormality
    b. FISH or RT-PCR for NPM1-ALK mRNA is diagnostic
    c. ALK protein detection by immunohistochemistry is also diagnostic
    d. All of the above

51. Constitutive activation of MEK-MAP kinase pathway signaling leads to:
   a. Hairy cell leukemia
   b. Langerhans cell histiocytosis
   c. Erdheim-Chester disease
   d. All of the above

52. Which test by flow cytometry will help in further confirmation of diagnosis?
   a. DHR assay by flow cytometry
   b. CD11c and CD18 on neutrophils
   c. CD40L expression (CD154) by flow cytometry
   d. Perforin by flow cytometry

53. Which parameter is considered as bad prognosis in childhood ALL?
   a. Hyperdiploidy
   b. t(1;19) (q23 ;p13.3); TCF3-PBX1(E2A- PBX1)
   c. t(12; 21) (p13;q22); ETV6-RUNX1(TEL-AML1)
   d. Intrachromosomal amplification of chromosome 21 (iAMP21)

54. Which one of the following is a wrong statement regarding 6-mercaptopurine?
   a. Mercaptopurine is a prodrug that must first be activated to form thioguanine nucleotides (TGNs), of which 6-thioguanine triphosphate (6-TGTP) is the major active metabolite
   b. Initial dose of mercaptopurine should be reduced in individuals who are known to lack thiopurine S-methyltransferase (TPMT)
   c. Nudix hydrolase 15 (NUDT15) deficiency do not need 6 MP dose modification
   d. Individuals with homozygous deficiency of TPMT or NUDT15 enzyme typically require 10% or less of the standard mercaptopurine oral suspension dosage.

55. Which of the following drugs does not cause neutrophilia?
   a. Epinephrine
   b. Glucocorticoids
   c. G-CSF
   d. Alkylating agents

56. Which of the following is not a part of diagnostic criteria for Erdheim-Chester disease (ECD)?
   a. Activating mutations in ECD are BRAFV600E, MAPK pathway, CSF1R
   b. Symmetric diaphyseal and metaphyseal osteosclerosis in the legs on PET scan
   c. Touton giant cells and lipid laden histiocytes on histopathology
   d. Staining positive for CD1a and negative for CD68, CD163

57. Patient aged 65 years presents with opthalmoplegia, ataxia, peripheral neuropathy and IgM protein on electrophoresis which is the likely diagnosis in the patient?
   a. CANOMAD
   b. POEMS
   c. Bing Neel syndrome
   d. TAFRO syndrome

58. Which of the following is not a FLT3 inhibitor?
   a. Sorafenib
   b. Quizartinib
   c. Gilteritinib
   d. Glasdegib

59. CART T cell therapy approved for MM is:
   a. Tisagenlecleucel
   b. Axicabtagene ciloleucel
   c. Lisocabtagene maraleucel
   d. Idecabtagene vicleucel

60. Which of the following is not a feature of POEMS syndrome?
   a. Extravascular volume overload
   b. Polyneuropathy
   c. Monoclonal plasma cell proliferative disorder
   d. Thrombocytopenia

61. Which of the following drugs is known as a keratinocyte growth factor?
   a. Everolimus
   b. Sirolimus
   c. Palifermin
   d. Benzydamine

62. Which of the following is not a cause of reactive thrombocytosis?
   a. Burns
   b. Metastatic Cancer
   c. Hyposplenism
   d. CML

63. In the human body, iron is found in the largest amount in:
   a. Macrophages in reticuloendothelial system
   b. Hemoglobin
   c. Myoglobin
   d. Enzymes

64. As per the WHO, what is the absolute monoclonal lymphocyte count required to diagnose chronic lymphocytic leukemia?
   a. $\geq 5 \times 10^9/L$
   b. $< 5 \times 10^9/L$
   c. $1 \times 10^9/L$
   d. $10 \times 10^9/L$

65. All are tyrosine kinase inhibitors used in chronic myeloid leukemia, *except*:
   a. Dasatinib
   b. Bosutinib
   c. Ponatinib
   d. Ibrutinib

66. Which of the following is not true about caplacizumab?
   a. It is humanized bivalent nanobody which targets A1 domain of VWF
   b. It inhibits autoantibody formation in TTP
   c. Time to normalization of platelet count was shortened by it in the Hercules trial
   d. It also reduces risk of death and complications caused by thrombotic events and organ damage.

67. MASCC scoring for febrile neutropenia does not include which of the following?
   a. Presence or abscence of hypotension
   b. Presence or abscence of COPD
   c. Solid tumour or hematological malignancy without previous fungal infection
   d. Use of steroids

68. Regarding Magrolimab which of the following is true?
   a. It is a monoclonal antibody against CD 47
   b. It inhibits a protein that works as a "do not eat me" signal used by cancer cells to avoid being ingested by macrophages
   c. It is an investigational agent for AML who are ineligible for induction chemotherapy
   d. All of the above

69. Which of the following is not true about antibody drug conjugate (ADCs)?
   a. Includes antibody conjugated to cytotoxic agent
   b. GO is an ADC against CD33
   c. Brentuximab Vedotin is ADC against CD30
   d. Inotuzumab ozogamicin and Moxetumomab pasudotox are active against CD22 and both are used in hairy cell leukemia

70. Which of the following is incorrect about Covid-19 coagulopathy?
   a. Covid-19 coagulopathy is same as DIC
   b. Pulmonary involvement is more common in Covid-19 coagulopathy than DIC
   c. Thrombocytopenia is more common in DIC than Covid-19
   d. Fibrinogen levels are found increased in Covid-19 coagulopathy rather than decreased

---

Ans.					
1. b	2. a	3. b	4. b	5. b	6. b
7. c	8. a	9. c	10. d	11. d	12. c
13. a	14. c	15. a	16. b	17. b	18. c
19. b	20. b	21. d	22. a	23. d	24. d
25. d	26. b	27. c	28. b	29. a	30. c
31. c	32. b	33. c	34. c	35. c	36. a
37. e	38. a	39. c	40. d	41. a	42. d
43. d	44. b	45. b	46. a	47. d	48. e
49. e	50. d	51. d	52. c	53. d	54. c
55. d	56. d	57. a	58. d	59. d	60. d
61. c	62. d	63. a	64. a	65. d	66. b
67. d	68. d	69. d	70. a		

20. SELF-ASSESSMENT

1. All of these are associated with prolonged APTT except:
   a. Factor XII deficiency
   b. Factor XI deficiency
   c. Factor VII deficiency
   d. HMWK deficiency

2. Which of these are not associated with prolonged thrombin time?
   a. Vitamin K deficiency
   b. Heparin contamination
   c. Fibrinogen abnormalities
   d. Liver disease

3. Which of these bleeding disorder is not associated with normal screening coagulation profile?
   a. Von Willebrand's disease
   b. Glanzman's thrombasthenia
   c. Factor XI deficiency
   d. Factor XIII deficiency

4. Which of these is/are not LAIP marker in MRD evaluation of B ALL?
   a. CD38
   b. CD73
   c. CD123
   d. CD34

5. Which of these molecular abnormality is not associated with ALL?
   a. t(9;22)(q34.1;q11.2)
   b. t(1;22)(p13.3;q13.1)
   c. t(v;11q23.3)
   d. t(1;19)(q23;p13.3)

6. Which of these is true about Burkitt's lymphoma?
   a. Predominantly a disease of lymphnodes
   b. It is an indolent disease
   c. Molecular abnormality is translocation of MYC
   d. Annexin A1 is the most specific immunophenotypic marker

7. ETP ALL is characterised by all, except:
   a. Negative for CD8 and CD1a
   b. Lacks expression of CD7
   c. CD5 is negative or dim
   d. Express one or more myeloid/stem cell markers

8. Sézary syndrome is characterised by all, except:
   a. Absolute Sézary cell count ≥1,500/µL
   b. Erythroderma
   c. Lymphadenopathy
   d. Clonal "T" cells in skin, lymph node, peripheral blood

9. FISH panel for multiple myeloma does not include:
   a. del13
   b. del11q
   c. t(11;14)
   d. 1p abnormality

10. All are true about factor VIII inhibitors, except:
    a. Develops in one third of severe hemophilia A patients
    b. Bethesda assay is used for measuring titer
    c. Develops after 50 exposure days
    d. Leads to decreased in vivo recovery of factor VIII

11. Which of these is not true about CLL?
    a. Monoclonal B cell count of ≥5,000/µL
    b. Dim expression of B cell antigens
    c. Peripheral blood sample is preferred for MRD
    d. Most common leukemia of adults

12. Which of these is not a GPI anchor protein used for PNH testing by flow cytometry?
    a. CD157
    b. CD24
    c. CD33
    d. CD14

13. Which of these is new confirmed entity in 2016 WHO classification?
    a. AML with mutated NPM1
    b. AML with BCR-ABL1
    c. AML with mutated RUNX1
    d. All of the above

14. Which of these disease is caused by ADAMTS 13 deficiency?
    a. Hemolytic uremic syndrome
    b. Thrombotic thrombocytopenic purpura
    c. Idiopathic thrombocytopenic purpura
    d. None of the above

15. MDS with ring sideroblasts mandates:
    a. Ring sideroblasts ≥15% with SF3B1 mutation
    b. Ring sideroblasts ≥5% with SF3B1 mutation
    c. None of the above
    d. Either of the above

16. The following is true for treatment for EBV associated lymphoproliferative disorder post HSCT:
    a. Donor lymphocyte infusion (DLI) or EBV specific T cells from donor can help
    b. Chemotherapy for lymphoma is needed
    c. Rituximab can prevent
    d. All of the above

17. Brentuximab vedotin is recommended in Hodgkin lymphoma in:
    a. Upfront
    b. Relapsed/refractory
    c. Maintenence
    d. All of the above

18. Covid-19 infection leads to:
    a. Lymphocytosis
    b. Neutrophilia
    c. Thrombocytosis
    d. Basophilia

19. Khorana score consists of which of the components:
a. Type of cancer, ANC, weight
b. Site of cancer, Hb, platelet count and BMI
c. BMI, hemoglobin, platelet count
d. Height, hemoglobin, previous DVT

20. As per ISTH guidelines for COVID thrombosis, which is not recommended?
a. PT, D-Dimer, fibrinogen monitoring is recommended
b. Maintain platelet count > 50,000/cumm and PT-INR <1.5, fibrinogen >2 g/L in bleeding patients
c. LMWH for minimum of 3 months is recommended therapeutic anticoagulation of choice
d. No extended anticoagulation is required even in patients at low risk of bleeding

21. Which of the following vaccine is a recombinant subunit vaccine?
a. Covishield   b. Covaxin
c. Sputnik V   d. Moderna

22. HDAC inhibitors are used in all of the following diseases, *except*:
a. Cutaneous T cell lymphoma
b. Multiple myeloma
c. PTCL- NOS
d. CLL

23. All of the following are indications for irradiated blood products, *except*:
a. Allo HSCT patients up to > 6 months post-transplant until ALC > 1,000 and free of active chronic GVHD and are off immunosuppression
b. Auto HSCT recipients until 3 months post-transplant (6 months if TBI in conditioning)
c. Patients with Hodgkin's lymphoma
d. Patients treated with Fludarabine, bendamustine, ATG, alemtuzumab
e. None of the above

24. T regulatory cells express all, *except*:
a. CD4   b. CD25
c. FoxP3   d. CD123

25. True about thrombin are all *except*:
a. Activates factor XI and XII
b. Inhibits factors V and VIII
c. Potent inducer of platelet adhesion and aggregation
d. Has proinflammatory effect

26. Franklin disease is:
a. Mu heavy chain disease
b. Gamma heavy chain disease
c. Alpha heavy chain disease
d. Delta heavy chain disease

27. DIPSS scoring system is used for:
a. Primary amyloidosis
b. Primary myelofibfosis
c. Multiple myeloma
d. Myelodysplastic syndrome

28. Proapoptotic BH3-only protein subfamily includes all, *except*:
a. BIM   b. BID
c. NOXA   d. PUMA
e. MCL

29. *ETNK1*, which catalyzes the conversion of ethanolamine to phophoethanolamine, is recurrently mutated in?
a. Atypical CML
b. CMML
c. Systemic mastocytosis with eosinophilia
d. All of the above

30. Increased bleeding and decreased vWF is associated with blood group:
a. A   b. B
c. AB   d. O

Ans.
1. c 2. a 3. c 4. d 5. b 6. c
7. b 8. a 9. b 10. c 11. c 12. c
13. a 14. b 15. b 16. d 17. d 18. b
19. b 20. d 21. a 22. d 23. e 24. d
25. b 26. b 27. b 28. e 29. d 30. d

21. SELF-ASSESSMENT

1. A 48-year-old female patient, with history of rheumatoid arthritis presented with moderate splenomegaly and severe anemia. Her peripheral smear examination revealed increased lymphocytes. The immunophenotypic analysis revealed these cells to be positive for CD2, CD3, CD8, CD57, CD16 and alpha-beta TCR-positive, and abnormally decreased expression of CD5. Most likely diagnosis is:
   a. T-cell prolymphocytic leukemia
   b. T-cell large granular lymphocytic leukemia
   c. Adult T-cell leukaemia/lymphoma
   d. Hepatosplenic T-cell lymphoma
   e. Sézary syndrome

2. Oligoclonal or clonal expansions of T-LGLs can be observed in a variety of situations. Which among the underlying conditions are associated with T-large granular lymphocytosis?
   a. Post-transplant lymphoproliferative disorder
   b. Hairy cell leukemia
   c. Rheumatoid arthritis
   d. CLL
   e. All of these

3. Which of the following is not the advantage of limiting the donor exposure in neonatal transfusions?
   a. Reduced risk of TTI's
   b. Reduced risk of immunomodulation
   c. Optimal utilization of resources
   d. Improved overall outcome in pediatric cardiac surgery

4. Which of the following is not true about "Neonatal alloimmune thrombocytopenia" (NAIT)?
   a. This is due to the antibodies against platelets antigen
   b. The antibodies are mostly against HPA-1a or 5b
   c. Multiple platelets transfusion to mother during pregnancy may cause generation of these antibodies.
   d. Often random platelets are used to treat the newborn in resource poor settings

5. Parent's donation should not be used to transfuse the neonates due to the fact:
   a. It has higher risk of TTI's
   b. It possesses the risk of TA-GVHD
   c. Promotes replacement donation
   d. All of the above

6. A donor, after donating 450 mL of whole blood, complained of pain in the arm the next day which aggravated on movement. He reported to an emergency next day who where a surgeon performed a fasciotomy on the arm to improve the symptoms. Which of the following of adverse donor reaction or event did the donor encountered?
   a. Vasovagal reaction
   b. Haematoma
   c. Compartment syndrome
   d. Median nerve injury

7. Collection of blood or blood components from a person who has recovered from an infection (usually viral) and using that blood to treat some other person suffering from the same infection is called as:
   a. Convalescent blood therapy
   b. Immunotherapy
   c. Cellular therapy
   d. Biotherapy

8. Which of the following is a "Major" ABO incompatibility in case of random platelets units transfusion in neonates?
   a. RDP: O, Neonate: A
   b. RDP: A, Neonate: AB
   c. RDP: A, Neonate: B
   d. RDP: A, Neonate: O

9. A "polyspecific Direct Agglutinin test" positive means:
   a. The plasma of the patient has come significant antibodies
   b. The red cell of the patient is coated with IgG type of antibody only
   c. The plasma of the patient has autoantibodies
   d. The red cell of the patient is coated with IgG type of antibody and complement

10. Red blood cells exchange is not indicated in following conditions:
   a. Severely polycythemia patient with the risk of thrombosis
   b. Thalassemia
   c. Severe sickle cells anemia
   d. Methemoglobinemia

11. "Neocyte-gerocyte" exchange is a form of RBC exchange which involves:
   a. Removal of denser "old" RBCs and replace with "young" donor reticulocyte rich donor cells
   b. Collection of cells from thalassemia patients
   c. Collection of blood from young adults
   d. Collection of RBC from children

12. Which of the following is not an advantage of use of citrate as anticoagulant in apheresis?
   a. Chelates positively charged calcium ions
   b. Blocks calcium dependent clotting factors reaction
   c. Provides systemic anticoagulation
   d. It can also cause thrombocytopenia

13. "DAT negative" AIHA means:
   a. IgA induced AIHA
   b. IgG induced AIHA
   c. C3d induced AIHA
   d. Both IgG and C3d induced AIHA

14. Which of the following organism is not screened routinely on the donated blood units?
   a. HIV
   b. HBV
   c. HCV
   d. CMV

15. Most common cause of fever during or after transfusion is:
   a. Hemolytic transfusion reaction
   b. Non-hemolytic transfusion reaction
   c. Allergic reaction
   d. Transfusion transmitted infection

16. NAT testing on donated blood signifies following:
   a. Molecular screening for HIV, HBV and HCV
   b. Molecular screening for Malaria and Syphilis
   c. Molecular screening of newer infections in the blood
   d. Molecular screening of all possible infection in blood

17. All of the following leads to therapy related AML, *except*:
   a. Alkylating agents
   b. Topoisomerase II inhibitors
   c. Topoisomerase I inhibitors
   d. Radiation exposure

18. Which of the following is not true entity under 2016 WHO classification of AML and related neoplasms?
   a. AML with mutated NPM1
   b. AML with BCR-ABL1
   c. AML with mutated CEBPA
   d. Acute basophilic leukemia

19. Prerequisite for the diagnosis of acute basophilic leukemia include:
   a. Presence of hyperbasophilia (HB) (absolute basophil count exceeding 1,000/micl of peripheral blood, present for over at least 8 weeks)
   b. Percentage of basophils must be ≥40% of total leukocytes
   c. Basophils must belong to the malignant clone
   d. All of the above

20. Inhibitor of NEDD8-activating enzyme is:
   a. Pevonedistat
   b. Glasdegib
   c. Imetelstat
   d. Vorinostat

Ans. 1. b.   2. e.   3. d.   4. c.   5. d.   6. c.
      7. a.   8. d.   9. d.   10. b. 11. a. 12. c.
      13. a. 14. d. 15. b. 16. a. 17. c. 18. b.
      19. d. 20. a.

SECTION 13: Tables

48. Tables

Chapter 48: Tables

1. Hemoglobin levels to diagnose anemia (WHO criteria).

Ref: WHO, UNICEF, UNU. Iron deficiency anaemia: assessment, prevention and control, a guide for programme managers. Geneva, World Health Organization, 2001

Pregnant women	11 g/dL
Nonpregnant women (15 years of age and above)	12 g/dL
Men (15 years of age and above)	13 g/dL

2. Ann Arbor staging system—four stages.

Ref: Carbone PP. Report of the committee on Hodgkin disease staging classification. Cancer Res. 1971

Stage I:	Involvement in a single lymph node region or single extralymphatic site
Stage II:	Involvement of two or more lymph node regions on the same side of the diaphragm; localized contiguous involvement of only one extralymphatic site and lymph node region (stage IIE)
Stage III:	Involvement of lymph node regions on both sides of the diaphragm, may include spleen
Stage IV:	Disseminated involvement of one or more extralymphatic organs with or without lymph node involvement

3. Risk factors for central nervous system (CNS) involvement in NHL-7 points.

- High IPI score
- Extranodal sites involved
- Raised LDH level
- Age more than 60 years
- Specific involvement of the following organs: bone marrow, testis, paranasal sinuses, Waldeyer ring
- Low albumin level
- Retroperitoneal glands

(IPI: International Prognostic Index; NHL-7: non-Hodgkin lymphoma-7; LDH: lactate dehydrogenase).

4. Monoclonal antibodies in NHL.

Antibody	Antigen
Rituximab	CD20
Alemtuzumab	CD52
Epratuzumab	CD22
Apolizumab	HLA-DR
Ibritumomab (Y-90 conjugate)	CD20
Tositumomab (I-131 conjugate)	CD20
Immunotoxins	CD19, CD22
Ofatumumab	CD20
Lumiliximab	CD23

(HLA-DR: human leukocyte antigen-DR isotype; NHL: non-Hodgkin lymphoma).

5. Prognostic factors for follicular lymphoma: Follicular Lymphoma International Prognostic Index (FLIPI)—five points.

Ref: Solal-Ce'ligny P. Follicular Lymphoma International Prognostic Index. Blood. 2004

1. Age more than 60 years
2. Ann Arbor stage III/IV
3. Hemoglobin less than 12 g/dL
4. Serum lactate dehydrogenase elevated
5. Number of nodal areas involved: more than four sites.

6. Prognostic factors for aggressive non-Hodgkin lymphoma: International Prognostic Index (IPI)—five points.

Ref: Williams 8/e; Hoffman 6/e

1. Age more than 60 years
2. Ann Arbor stage III or IV
3. Increased lactate dehydrogenase concentration
4. Performance score more than 2
5. Involvement of more than one extranodal site.

7. Characteristic chromosomal translocations found in non-Hodgkin's lymphoma.

Type of lymphoma	Translocations
Burkitt's lymphoma	t(8;14)(q24;q32)
Burkitt's lymphoma	t(8;2)(p11/2;24)
Burkitt's lymphoma	t(8;22)(q24;q11)
Mantle cell lymphoma	t(11;14)(q24;q32)
Follicular lymphoma	t(14;18)(q32;q21)
Large B-cell lymphoma	t(3;4)(q27;q32)
T-cell anaplastic large-cell lymphoma	t(2;5)(p23;q35)

8. Hasenclever index—seven points.
Ref: Hasenclever D. A prognostic score for advance Hodgkin's disease. N Engl J Med. 1998

1. Age more than 45 years
2. Male gender
3. Serum albumin less than 40 g/L
4. Hemoglobin less than 10.5 g/dL
5. Stage IV disease
6. Leukocytosis (white cell count more than 15,000/μL)
7. Lymphopenia (less than 600/μL or < 8% of the white cell count).

9. Symptomatic multiple myeloma—three points.
Ref: WHO 2008

- M—protein in serum and/or urine
- Bone marrow (clonal) plasma cells or plasmacytoma
- Related organ or tissue impairment (end-organ damage, including bone lesions).

10. Berlin-Frankfurt-Münster Consortium risk classification of childhood acute lymphoblastic leukemia (ALL).
Ref: Childhood acute lymphoblastic leukemia ALL-BFM study group

Standard risk	Prednisone good response; no t(9;22)/BCR—ABL1 or t(4;11)/MLL-AF4; MRD negative on days 33 and 78
Medium risk	Prednisone good response; morphological remission on day 33; no t(9;22)/BCR-ABL1 or t(4;11)/MLL-AFF1; do not fulfill other standard or high risk criteria
High risk	Prednisone poor response; M2 or M3 marrow on day 33; presence of t(9;22)/BCR-ABL1 or t(4;11)/MLL-AFF1; MRD more than 0.1% on day 78

(MRD: minimal residual disease).

11. Diagnostic criteria for hemophagocytic lymphohistiocytosis (HLH).
Ref: Henter J. HLH-2004: Diagnostic and therapeutic guidelines for hemophagocytic lymphohistiocytosis. Pediatr Blood Cancer. 2006

- Familial disease/known genetic defect
- Clinical and laboratory criteria (5/8 criteria):
  - Fever
  - Splenomegaly
  - Cytopenia in two or more cell lines:
    - Hemoglobin less than 9 g/dL
    - Platelets less than 100,000/μL
    - Neutrophils less than 1,000/μL
  - Hypertriglyceridemia and/or hypofibrinogenemia:
    - Fasting triglycerides more than 3 mmol/L
    - Fibrinogen less than 150 mg/L
  - Ferritin more than 500 μg/L
  - Soluble CD25 (sCD25) more than 2,400 U/mL
  - Decreased or absent NK cell activity
  - Hemophagocytosis in bone marrow, CSF, or lymph nodes

(CSF: cerebrospinal fluid).

12. Glucksberg staging of acute graft-versus-host disease (GVHD).
Ref: Glucksberg H. Clinical manifestations of graft versus host disease in human recipients of marrow from HLA matched sibling donors. Transplantation. 1974

Stage	Skin	Liver (bilirubin)	Gut
1	Rash less than 25% BSA	2–3 mg/dL	Diarrhea 500–1,000 mL/day
2	Rash 25–50% BSA	3–6 mg/dL	Diarrhea 1,000–1,500 mL/day
3	Generalized erythroderma, more than 50% BSA	6–15 mg/dL	Diarrhea more than 1,500 mL/day
4	Desquamation and bullae	More than 15 mg/dL	Pain and ileus

(BSA: body surface area).

13. Clinical severity of Hemophilia A.

FVIII (units/dL)	Bleeding tendency
Less than 1	*Severe:* Spontaneous bleeding into joints, muscles, and internal organs
2–5	*Moderate:* Some "spontaneous" bleeds, bleeding after minor trauma
5–45	*Mild:* Bleeding only after significant trauma, surgery

(FVIII: factor VIII).

14. Diagnostic criteria in antiphospholipid syndrome.
Ref: Keeling D. Guidelines on the investigation and management of antiphospholipid syndrome. BJH. 2012

- Clinical criteria:
  - Thrombosis: Arterial, venous, or microvascular thrombosis in any tissue or organ
- Laboratory criteria:
  - Antiphospholipid antibody
  - IgG or IgM anticardiolipin antibodies at moderate or high concentration and/or
  - Lupus anticoagulant
- Pregnancy complications:
  - Unexplained death of morphologically normal fetus at or beyond 10 weeks of gestation
  - Three or more unexplained consecutive miscarriages before 10 weeks
  - One or more premature births of a morphologically normal fetus before 34 weeks of gestation due to pre-eclampsia, eclampsia, or severe placental insufficiency

15. WHO definition of chronic myeloid leukemia phases.
Ref: WHO Classification of Tumours of Haematopoietic and Lymphoid Tissues. 2008

Chronic phase: Peripheral blood blasts fewer than 10% in the blood and bone marrow.

Accelerated phase: Blasts 10–19% of white blood cells in peripheral and/or nucleated bone marrow cells; persistent thrombocytopenia (less than 100,000/μL) unrelated to therapy or persistent thrombocytosis (more than 1,000,000/μL) unresponsive to therapy; increasing white blood cells and spleen size unresponsive to therapy; cytogenetic evidence of clonal evolution.

Blast crisis: Peripheral blood blasts ≥20% of peripheral blood white blood cells or nucleated bone marrow cells; extramedullary blast proliferation; and large foci or clusters of blasts on bone marrow biopsy.

16. European LeukemiaNet definition of optimal response and failure to tyrosine kinase inhibitors (TKIs) as first-line treatment.

Ref: Adapted from: Baccarani M, European LeukemiaNet recommendations for the management of chronic myeloid leukemia. Blood. 2013

	Optimal response of TKI	Failure of TKI
Baseline	NA	
3 months	BCR-ABL1 ≤10% and/or Partial cytogenetic response CyR (Ph+ ≤35%)	Noncomplete hematological response and/or Ph+ >95%
6 months	BCR-ABL1 <1% and/or complete cytogenetic response (Ph+ 0)	BCR-ABL1 >10% and/or Ph+ >35%
12 months	BCR-ABL1 ≤0.1%	BCR-ABL1 >1% and/or Ph+ >0

(CyR: cytogenetic response; NA: not available).

17. The diagnosis of chronic lymphocytic leukemia (CLL) is established by the following criteria.

Ref: Oscier D. Guidelines on the diagnosis and management of chronic lymphocytic leukaemia. BJH. 2004; Hoffman 6/e

The presence in the peripheral blood of ≥5,000 monoclonal B lymphocytes/μL for the duration of at least 3 months. The clonality of the circulating B lymphocytes needs to be confirmed by flow cytometry.

The leukemia cells found in the blood smear are characteristically small, mature lymphocytes with a narrow border of cytoplasm and a dense nucleus lacking discernible nucleoli and having partially aggregated chromatin.

Chronic lymphocytic leukemia cells coexpress the CD5 antigen and B-cell surface antigens CD19, CD20, and CD23. The levels of surface immunoglobulin, CD20 and CD79b are characteristically low compared with those found on normal B cells. Each clone of leukemia cells is restricted to expression of either or immunoglobulin light chains.

Scoring system for the diagnosis of chronic lymphocytic leukemia (CLL):

Marker	1	0
CD5	Positive	Negative
CD23	Positive	Negative
SmIg	Weak	Strong
FMC7	Negative	Positive
CD22 or CD79b	Weak	Strong

Scores in CLL are usually more than 3, in other B-cell malignancies the scores are usually less than 3.

(SmIg: surface membrane immunoglobulin).

18. Rai classification divides chronic lymphocytic leukemia (CLL) into five stages.

Rai KR. Clinical staging of chronic lymphocytic leukemia. Blood. 1975

1. *Rai stage 0:* Lymphocytosis and no enlargement of the lymph nodes, spleen, or liver, and with near normal red blood cell and platelet counts.
2. *Rai stage I:* Lymphocytosis plus enlarged lymph nodes. The spleen and liver are not enlarged and the red blood cell and platelet counts are near normal.
3. *Rai stage II:* Lymphocytosis plus an enlarged spleen (and possibly an enlarged liver), with or without enlarged lymph nodes. The red blood cell and platelet counts are near normal.
4. *Rai stage III:* Lymphocytosis plus anemia, with or without enlarged lymph nodes, spleen, or liver. Platelet counts are near normal.
5. *Rai stage IV:* Lymphocytosis plus thrombocytopenia, with or without anemia, enlarged lymph nodes, spleen, or liver.

19. Binet staging for chronic lymphocytic leukemia (CLL).

Binet stage A: Fewer than three areas of lymphoid tissue are enlarged, with no anemia or thrombocytopenia.

Binet stage B: Three or more areas of lymphoid tissue are enlarged, with no anemia or thrombocytopenia.

Binet stage C: Anemia and/or thrombocytopenia are present.

20. Adverse prognostic factors in chronic lymphocytic leukemia (CLL).

- Diffuse pattern of bone marrow involvement
- Advanced age
- Male gender
- Deletions of chromosomes 17 or 11
- Increased levels of beta-2-microglobulin
- Lymphocyte doubling time of less than 6 months
- Increased fraction of prolymphocytes in the blood
- High proportion of CLL cells containing ZAP-70 (more than 20%) or CD38 (more than 30%)
- CLL cells with nonmutated gene for the immunoglobulin heavy chain variable region (IGHV)

(ZAP-70: Zeta-chain-associated protein kinase 70).

21. Indications for treatment in chronic lymphocytic leukemia (CLL).

- *Progressive marrow failure:* The development or worsening of anemia and/or thrombocytopenia
- Massive (>10 cm) or progressive lymphadenopathy
- Progressive splenomegaly
- Lymphocyte doubling time <6 months
- Systemic symptoms:
  - Weight loss more than 10% in previous 6 months
  - Fever more than 38°C for more than 2 weeks
  - Extreme fatigue
  - Night sweats
  - Recurrent infections
- Autoimmune cytopenias.

22. Definition of severity of aplastic anemia (AA).

Ref: Williams 8/e; Hoffbrands 7/e

Severe AA

Bone marrow cellularity less than 25%, or 25–50% with less than 30% residual hemopoietic cells.

And two out of three of the following:
1. Neutrophil count less than 500/μL
2. Platelet count less than 20,000/μL
3. Reticulocyte count less than 20,000/μL.

Very severe AA: As for severe AA but neutrophils less than 200/μL.

Nonsevere AA: Patients not fulfilling the criteria for severe or very severe aplastic anemia.

23. Response criteria (to immunosuppressive therapy) for severe aplastic anemia.

Ref: Marsh JCW. Guidelines for the diagnosis and management of aplastic anaemia. BJH. 2009

None	Still severe
Partial	• Transfusion independent • No longer meeting criteria for severe disease
Complete	• Hemoglobin normal for age • Neutrophil count more than 1,500/μL • Platelet count more than 150,000/μL

24. International Staging System (ISS) for multiple myeloma.

Ref: Greipp PR. International Staging System for Multiple Myeloma. JCO. 2005

Stage	Criteria	Median survival (in months)
I	Serum β2 microglobulin less than 3.5 mg/L and serum albumin more than 3.5 mg/dL	62
II	Neither I or III	45
III	Serum β2 microglobulin more than 5.5 mg/L	29

25. Risk stratification according to cytogenetics in myeloma.

Ref: WHO Classification of Tumours of Haematopoietic and Lymphoid Tissues. 2008

Standard risk	Hyperdiploidy, t(6;14), t(11;14)
High risk	t(4;14), t(14;16), t(14;20), del17p

26. Genetic risk stratification in acute myeloid leukemia (ELN).

Ref: Dohner H. Diagnosis and management of AML in adults: 2017 ELN recommendations from an international expert panel. Blood. 2017;129(4):424-47.

Favorable	• t(8;21)(q22;q22.1); RUNX1-RUNX1T1 • inv(16)(p13.1q22) or t(16;16)(p13.1;q22); CBFB-MYH11 • Mutated NPM1 without FLT3-ITD or with FLT3-ITD low • Biallelic mutated CEBPA
Intermediate	• Mutated NPM1 and FLT3-ITD high • Wild-type NPM1 without FLT3-ITD or with FLT3-ITD low (without adverse-risk genetic lesions) • t(9;11)(p21.3;q23.3); MLLT3-KMT2A • Cytogenetic abnormalities not classified as favorable or adverse
Adverse	• t(6;9)(p23;q34.1);DEK-NUP214 • t(v;11q23.3);KMT2Arearranged • t(9;22)(q34.1;q11.2);BCR-ABL1 • inv(3)(q21.3q26.2) or t(3;3)(q21.3;q26.2); GATA2, MECOM (EVI1) • del(5q); -7; -17/abn(17p) • Complex karyotype, monosomal karyotype • Wild-type NPM1 and FLT3 ITD high • Mutated RUNX1 • Mutated ASXL1 • Mutated TP53

27. WHO classification-based Prognostic Scoring System (WPSS) in myelodysplastic syndrome (MDS).

Variable	0	1	2	3
WHO classification	RA, RARS, 5q–	RCMD± RS	RAEB-1	RAEB-2
Karyotype	Good	Intermediate	Poor	
Transfusions	No	Regular		

Risk groups: very low (score = 0), low (score = 1), intermediate (score = 2), high (score = 3–4), very high (score = 5–6).

(RA: refractory anemia; RAEB: refractory anemia with excess blast; RARS: RA with ringed sideroblast; RCMD RS: refractory cytopenia with multilineage dysplasia and ringed sideroblast).

28. WHO diagnostic criteria for essential thrombocythemia.

Ref: WHO Classification of Tumours of Haematopoietic and Lymphoid Tissues. 2016

Major criteria	• Platelet count ≥ 450 × 10^9/L • Bone marrow biopsy showing proliferation mainly of the megakaryocyte lineage with increased numbers of enlarged, mature megakaryocytes with hyperlobulated nuclei. No significant left-shift of neutrophil granulopoiesis or erythropoiesis and very rarely minor (grade 1) increase in reticulin fibers • Not meeting WHO criteria for BCR-ABL1 +CML, PV, PMF, MDS, or other myeloid neoplasms • Presence of JAK2, CALR or MPL mutation
Minor criteria	Presence of a clonal marker (e.g., abnormal karyotype) or absence of evidence for reactive thrombocytosis

Diagnosis of essential thrombocythemia requires meeting all 4 major criteria or the first 3 major criteria and the minor criterion.

29. WHO diagnostic criteria for polycythemia vera

Ref: WHO Classification of Tumours of Haematopoietic and Lymphoid Tissues. 2016

Major criteria	• Hemoglobin > 16.5 g/dL (men), Hemoglobin > 16.0 g/dL (women), or Hematocrit > 49% (men), Hematocrit > 48% (women) or increased red cell mass • Bone marrow biopsy showing hypercellularity for age with trilineage growth (panmyelosis) including prominent erythroid, granulocytic and megakaryocytic proliferation with pleomorphic, mature megakaryocytes (differences in size) • Presence of JAK2 or JAK2 exon 12 mutation
Minor criteria	Subnormal serum erythropoietin level

Diagnosis of polycythemia vera requires meeting either all 3 major criteria, or the first 2 major criteria and the minor criterion.

30. WHO diagnostic criteria for chronic myelomonocytic leukemia.

Ref: WHO Classification of Tumours of Haematopoietic and Lymphoid Tissues. 2016

Persistent peripheral blood monocytosis >1 × 10^9/L, with monocytes accounting for >10% of the WBC count

Not meeting WHO criteria for BCR-ABL1 CML, PMF, PV, or ET

No evidence of PDGFRA, PDGFRB, or FGFR1 rearrangement or PCM1-JAK2 (should be specifically excluded in cases with eosinophilia)

<20% blasts in the blood and BM

Dysplasia in 1 or more myeloid lineages. If myelodysplasia is absent or minimal, the diagnosis of CMML may still be made if the other requirements are met

An acquired clonal cytogenetic or molecular genetic abnormality is present in hemopoietic cells

OR

The monocytosis (as previously defined) has persisted for at least 3 months

All other causes of monocytosis have been excluded

31. Characteristic features of peripheral blood smear.

Ref: Lynch EC. Peripheral blood smear: Clinical Methods: The History, Physical, and Laboratory Examinations. 3rd edition. Boston: Butterworths; 1990

The examination of blood films stained with Wright's stain provides important clues in the diagnosis of anemias and various disorders of leukocytes and platelets:

- The normal human red blood cells (RBCs) are biconcave-shaped disks (diskocytes) with a mean diameter of about 7.5 μm. Erythrocytes are slightly smaller than small lymphocytes. The hemoglobin of red cells is located peripherally, leaving an area of central pallor equal to approximately 30–45% of the diameter of the cells. Cells of normal size and hemoglobin content (color) are termed normocytic and normochromic.
- Larger than normal erythrocytes are termed macrocytes (diameter greater than 9 μm); small red cells are called microcytes (diameter less than 6 μm); and those with central pallor greater than 50% of the diameter are hypochromic.
- Abnormal variability in size is termed anisocytosis and abnormal variability in shape is called poikilocytosis.
- Significant differences among erythrocytes in the amount of central pallor are referred to as anisochromia. Polychromatophilia (also called polychromasia) means the erythrocytes have a blue-gray hue to the color of their cytoplasm. From a diagnostic standpoint, poikilocytosis has no specificity, but the recognition of specific forms of poikilocytes (irregularly shaped cells) often points to specific disorders.
- Spherocytes are round, densely staining red cells that lack central pallor and have a smaller diameter. In stomatocytes, the area of central pallor is elliptical rather than round, giving the cell the appearance of the opening of a mouth (stoma).
- Target cells (codocytes) have a centrally located disk of hemoglobin surrounded by an area of pallor with an outer rim of hemoglobin adjacent to the cell membrane giving the cell the appearance of a target. Leptocytes (or wafer cells) are thin, flat cells with the hemoglobin at the periphery of the cell.
- Sickle cells (drepanocytes) are elongated, sometimes crescent-shaped, erythrocytes with pointed ends.

- Elliptocytes (ovalocytes) range from slightly oval to elongated cigar-shaped forms. Teardrop erythrocytes (dacryocytes) are red cells with one end round and the other end more pointed.
- *Acanthocytes* have several (usually three to seven) irregularly spaced blunted projections from the margin of the cells. *Echinocytes* are also cells with cytoplasmic projections, but in contrast to acanthocytes, the projections are typically evenly spaced on the cell surface, more numerous (often 10–15), and frequently have sharper points.
- Schizocytes (schistocytes) are fragmented erythrocytes appearing in a variety of morphologic forms such as small triangular erythrocytes, helmet cells, and normal-size erythrocytes with two to three pointed surface projections (keratocytes or "horn cells"). Round erythrocytes with a single, elliptical or round surface defect are termed *bite cells.*
- Rouleaux formation denotes the stacking of erythrocytes, generally in a curving pattern.
- Morphologic identification of inclusion bodies within erythrocytes can be helpful clinically. Howell-Jolly bodies are purple spheres, usually about 0.5 μm in diameter, presenting singly, or rarely multiply, in the cytoplasm. Basophilic stippling of erythrocytes refers to numerous very small coarse or fine blue granules within the cytoplasm. When the stippled particles are due to iron granules (demonstrable by the Prussian blue stain), they are termed Pappenheimer bodies. Malaria parasites may appear as cytoplasmic inclusion bodies within erythrocytes. Platelets overlying erythrocytes may be mistaken for erythrocyte inclusions.
- Toxic granulation refers to small, dark blue-staining granules in neutrophils. Döhle bodies are light blue cytoplasmic inclusions, 1–2 μm in diameter.
- The Pelger-Huët anomaly, a disorder characterized by impaired nuclear segmentation of mature neutrophilic granulocytes, appears morphologically as cells with bilobed nuclei (dumbbell or eyeglass shapes) or with round or oval nuclei (Stodtmeister cells).
- Hypersegmented neutrophils are cells in which there are six or more nuclear lobes.
- Reactive lymphocytes are usually larger than small lymphocytes, may have cytoplasmic vacuolization, sometimes have deep blue staining of the periphery of the cytoplasm, and contain nuclei that may be kidney-bean or monocytoid in shape.
- Most platelets in the peripheral blood have diameters between 1 and 3 μm. Platelets greater than 3 μm in diameter are "large" (megathrombocytes). In a normal person, usually less than 5% of the platelets appear large.

32. Characteristic features of deferoxamine, deferiprone, and deferasirox. *Ref: Hoffbrand 7/e p46*

Variables	Deferoxamine	Deferiprone	Deferasirox
Structure	Hexadentate	Bidentate	Tridentate
Iron-chelator complex	1:1	1:3	1:2
Half-life	20 minutes	1–3 hours	10–16 hours
Iron excretion route	Urine + fecal	Urine	Fecal
Daily dose	40 mg/kg	75–100 mg/kg in three divided doses	20–30 mg/kg once daily
Side-effects	Ototoxicity, retinal toxicity, and cartilage and bone abnormalities	Agranulocytosis, arthropathy	Skin rashes, gastrointestinal disturbance, renal impairment
Reported efficacy	Efficient hepatic and cardiac iron removal	More effective in removing cardiac iron, less efficient in hepatic iron clearance	More efficient clearance of hepatic iron, also effective in cardiac iron removal

33. Antifungal agents.

Class	Drugs	Mechanism of action
Azole	Fluconazole, itraconazole, posaconazole, ravuconazole, tetraconazole, voriconazole	• Inhibition of sterol 14-alpha-demethylase • Erg11p, impairing ability of the fungal cell to produce ergosterol for the cell membrane
Polyene macrolides	Amphotericin B, Mepartricin	Binding of sterol component of fungal cell membrane and pore formation, leading to increased permeability
Echinocandins	Anidulafungin, caspofungin, micafungin	Interference with (1,3)-beta-glucan synthesis, leading to loss of fungal cell wall integrity

34. Direct oral anticoagulants (DOACs).

DOAC	Target	Peak level at (hour)	Half-life (hour)	Dose in VTE	Renal excretion
Dabigatran	Factor IIa	1–2	12–17	150 mg BD	80%
Rivaroxaban	Factor Xa	3–4	7–12	15 mg BD for 3 weeks then 20 mg OD	35%
Apixaban	Factor Xa	3–4	10–14	10 mg BD for 7 days, then 5 mg BD	25%
Edoxaban	Factor Xa	1–2	9–10	60 mg OD	35%

(BD: twice a day; OD: once a day; VTE: venous thromboembolism).

35. Lymphomas and genetic abnormalities.

Disease	Genetic abnormality	Gene involved
Follicular lymphoma	t(14;18)(q32;q21)	BCL2
Burkitt's lymphoma	t(8;14)(q24;q32) or t(2;8)(p12;q24) or t(8;22)(q24;q11.2)	MYC
Mantle cell lymphoma	t(11;14)(q13;q32)	CCND1
ALK positive- ALCL	t(2;5)(p23;q35)	NPM1–ALK
T-prolymphocytic leukemia	t(14;14)(q11;q32)	TCL1

(ALCL: anaplastic large cell lymphoma; ALK: anaplastic lymphoma kinase; BCL2: B-cell leukemia/lymphoma 2).

36. Novel drugs for various hematological diseases.

S. No.	Drugs	Mechanism of action	Comments
1	Voxelotor	Antisickling agent	Sickle cell disease
2	Acalabrutinib	Bruton's tyrosine kinase (BTK) inhibitor	Chronic lymphocytic leukemia
3	Givosiran	Aminolevulinic acid synthase 1 (ALAS1) inhibitor, decreases neurotoxic heme intermediates ALA and PBG	Acute hepatic porphyria
4	Crizanlizumab	Monoclonal antibody inhibiting interaction of P-selectin glycoprotein ligand 1 by binding to P-selectin	Sickle cell disease
5	Zanubrutinib	BTK inhibitor	Mantle cell lymphoma
6	Luspatercept	Smad2/3 signaling inhibitor	Transfusion dependent beta thalassemia, MDS
7	Daratumumab	IgG1k monoclonal antibody directed against CD38	Multiple myeloma
8	Fedratinib	JAK2-selective inhibitor	Myelofibrosis
9	Polatuzumab vedotin	CD79b-directed antibody-drug conjugate	Diffuse large B-cell lymphoma
10	Gilteritinib	FLT3 inhibitor	Refractory acute myeloid leukemia
11	Venetoclax	BCL-2 inhibitor	CLL, AML
12	Caplacizumab	Targets the A1 domain of the ultra-large von Willebrand factor (vWF), preventing the interaction between vWF and platelets	Acquired thrombotic thrombocytopenic purpura
13	Tagraxofusp	CD123-directed cytotoxin	Blastic plasmacytoid dendritic cell neoplasm
14	Ravulizumab	C5 inhibitor	Paroxysmal nocturnal hemoglobinuria
15	Calaspargase pegol	Depleting plasma L-asparagine	Acute lymphoblastic leukemia
16	Romiplostim	Thrombopoietin receptor agonist	Immune thrombocytopenia
17	Gilteritinib	FLT3 inhibitor	Refractory acute myeloid leukemia
18	Truxima	Biosimilar to rituximab	B-cell non-Hodgkin's lymphoma

(ALA: alpha-linolenic acid; AML: acute myeloid leukemia; BCL2: B-cell leukemia/lymphoma 2; CLL: chronic lymphocytic leukemia; FLT3: fms like tyrosine kinase 3; IgG1k: immunoglobulin G1 kappa; JAK2: Janus-associated kinase-2; MDS: myelodysplastic syndrome).

37. Novel drugs for various hematological diseases.

S. No.	Drugs	Mechanism of action	Comments
1	Moxetumomab pasudotox	CD22-directed cytotoxin	Refractory hairy cell leukemia
2	Mogamulizumab	CCR4 inhibitor	Refractory mycosis fungoides
3	Lusutrombopag	TPO agonist	Thrombocytopenia in adults with chronic liver disease
4	Pembrolizumab	PD 1 checkpoint inhibitor	Refractory primary mediastinal large B-cell lymphoma, refractory Hodgkin's lymphoma
5	Fulphila	Pegfilgrastim biosimilar	Febrile neutropenia
6	Avatrombopag	TPO agonist	Thrombocytopenia in adults with chronic liver disease
7	Tisagenlecleucel	CD19-directed genetically modified autologous T-cell immunotherapy	Refractory large B-cell lymphoma
8	Selinexor	Selective inhibitor of nuclear export (SINE) by blocking protein XPO1	Multiple myeloma
9	Vemurafenib	BRAF inhibitor	Hairy cell leukemia
10	Axicabtagene ciloleucel	CD19 CART cell therapy	Diffuse large B-cell lymphoma
11	Inotuzumab ozogamicin	Blocks CD22	Refractory B-cell precursor acute lymphoblastic leukemia
12	Ibrutinib	BTK inhibitor	Chronic graft-versus-host disease
13	L-glutamine oral powder	Antioxidant	Sickle cell disease
14	Miristen	MicroRNA inhibitors	Chronic myeloid leukemia
15	Midostaurin	FLT3-specific small molecule inhibitors	AML, mast cell leukemia
16	Glasdegib	Hedgehog *pathway* inhibitor	Acute myeloid leukemia
17	Emapalumab	Monoclonal antibody that binds and neutralizes interferon gamma	Primary hemophagocytic lymphohistiocytosis
18	Emicizumab	Bispecific monoclonal antibody binding both factor IX and to factor X	Hemophilia A

(CART: chimeric antigen receptor therapy; CCR4: CC chemokine receptor 4; PD 1: Programmed cell death protein 1; TPO: thyroid peroxidase).

38. Diagnostic criteria for Erdheim-Chester disease (ECD)

Ref: Goyal G, Heaney ML, Collin M, et al. Erdheim-Chester disease: consensus recommendations for evaluation, diagnosis, and treatment in the molecular era. Blood. 2020;135(22):1929-45.

Clinical and morphological
- Symmetric diaphyseal and metaphyseal osteosclerosis in the legs; best seen by PET scan
- Other typical ECD findings: perirenal infiltration or periaortic sheathing (CT), right atrial pseudotumor (MRI), or physical examination findings of xanthelasma, exophthalmos, or osteosclerosis of facial sinuses

Histopathological
- Foamy or lipid-laden histiocytes, fibrosis, and sometimes Touton giant cells
- Staining for CD68 or CD163 and negative for CD1a

Molecular
- BRAFV600E mutation
- Other activating mutations of the MAPK pathway: KRAS, NRAS, MaP2K1, ARAF, MAP3KI, and others
- Gene fusion activating the MAPK pathway or
- Activating mutation in CSF1R

39. T cell leukemias and lymphomas and their cell of origin.

Ref: Sharma SK. What a clinical hematologist should know about T cells? International Blood Research & Reviews, 2020;11(4):20-32 and WHO Book, 2017.

Type of T ALL/T cell lymphoma	Cell of origin	Organ of origin/ Localization
Early T precursor ALL	CD4-, CD8-, Double negative	Recent immigrants from the bone marrow to thymus
Cortical T ALL	CD4+, CD8+, Double positive	Thymic Cortex
Medullary T ALL	CD4-/CD8+ or CD4+/CD8- Single positive	Thymic Medulla
Peripheral T cell lymphoma (PTCL), NOS	CD4+ central memory T cell	Lymph node
Angioimmunoblastic T cell lymphoma	CD4+T follicular helper (TFH) cells	Lymph node
Anaplastic large cell lymphoma (ALCL)	CD4+ T cell	Lymph nodes and extranodal sites
Mycosis fungoides	A mature skin-homing CD4+ T cell	Skin
Sezary syndrome	Central memory CD4+ T cells	Lymph node, bone marrow, skin
Adult T cell leukemia/lymphoma (ATLL)	T-regs	Lymph node, peripheral blood
T cell large granular lymphocytic leukemia (T-LGL)	CD8+ T cell	Bone marrow, peripheral blood

40. FLT3 inhibitors.

Drug	Type	Active as monotherapy	Cellular potency	Selectivity	Half-life	Protein binding (%)	Clinical resistance mechanisms	FDA-approved	FDA approved for AML
Midostaurin	I	No	++	+	19 h	>99.8	One reported case of an acquired FLT KD mutation (N676K)	Yes, in combination with induction chemotherapy only	Yes
Sorafenib	II	Yes	++	++	25-48 h	99.5	FLT3 KD mutations (D835, F691L)	Yes	No
Quizartinib	II	Yes	+++	+++	~1.5 d	>99	FLT3 KD mutations (D835, F691L)	No	Development ongoing
Crenolanib	I	Yes	++	++	6-8 h	95.9	F691L, Ras pathway mutations	No	Development ongoing
Gilteritinib	I	Yes	++	++	113 h	~94	F691L, Ras pathway mutations	Yes	Yes

Index

A

ABO
 blood group 308, 315, 399
 hemolytic disease 308
Abortion
 recurrent 94
 threatened 78
Absolute neutrophil count 240
Acetazolamide 150
Acid
 fast bacilli 327, 328
 hemolysis 115
 phosphates stain 407
Activated partial thromboplastin time 118, 271
Activin receptor trap ligand 100
Adenocarcinoma 330
 metastatic 330
Adenosine diphosphate 47, 331
Adenovirus 330
Adipocytes, predominance of 327
Adriamycin 129
Adult T-cell
 leukemia 271
  cell of origin of 185
 lymphoma, cell of origin of 185
Aggregation 47
Agranulocytosis 358
Alanine aminotransferase 325
Alcohol abuse 328, 331, 340
Alemtuzumab 154, 390, 416
 therapy 153, 390
Alkaline phosphatase 325
Allogeneic stem cell transplantation 142, 162, 164, 176, 227, 235, 237, 238, 364, 379, 415
Alloimmune
 antibody 78
 thrombocytopenia, neonatal 422
Allophycocyanin 284
Allopurinol 229
Allosteric inhibitor 351
All-trans retinoic acid 376
Alpha-helical light-chains 214
Alpha-thalassemia 83, 327, 328, 337
 trait 84
Amoxicillin 39
Amyloid
 light-chain amyloidosis 205
  diagnosis of 204
 symptomatic cardiac 212
Amyloidosis 95, 203, 205
 cardiac 204
 causes of 204
Anaplastic lymphoma kinase 173
Anemia 32, 38, 60, 84, 182, 328, 329, 331, 397, 402, 403
 acquired aplastic 274, 287, 396
 autoimmune hemolytic 35, 63, 78, 154, 306, 311, 327, 328, 385, 415
 causes of 154

chronic
 hemolytic 60, 67
 hereditary nonspherocytic hemolytic 404
 neutrophilic 278
congenital dyserythropoietic 103, 288, 365, 411, 414
Coombs' positive hemolytic 115
development of 16
hemolytic 59, 75, 76, 329, 338, 385
hepatitis associated aplastic 274
hereditary nonspherocytic hemolytic 65
idiopathic aplastic 287
immune hemolytic 75
macrocytic 32, 38, 39, 327
megaloblastic 18, 38, 39, 278, 285, 327
microangiopathic hemolytic 44, 385
microcytic 327, 336
 hypochromic 31
myelophthisic 19
nonspherocytic hemolytic 60
pernicious 38, 39, 41, 77, 93, 328-330
refractory sideroblastic 400
severe
 aplastic 103, 381, 430
 hemolytic 65
 macrocytic 38
sideroblastic 32, 34, 224, 402
warm autoimmune hemolytic 326
Anfibatide 44
Angiogenesis 13
Angular cheilitis 40
Anisocytosis 34, 328
Anisopoikilocytosis 84
Ankyrin 61
Anlotinib inhibits 347
Ann Arbor staging system 427
Anthracyclines 125
Antibiotic therapy 327
Antibody 76, 77, 137, 390
 anticardiolipin 259
 monoclonal 100, 308
 screening 305
Anticoagulation, prophylactic 290
Antifungal effective against mucormycosis 416
Antigen presenting cells 319
Anti-intrinsic factor antibodies 41
Antimalarial prophylaxis 327
Antimetabolite 361
Antimicrobial antibody development 319
Antiphospholipid syndrome 53, 54, 260, 392, 428
Antithrombin deficiency 56, 331, 359
Antithymocyte globulin 319
 mechanism of action of 414
Anti-thyroid antibodies 40
Anti-tissue factor pathway inhibitor 100
Anti-tuberculous medications 80
Anxiety 307
Aplastic anemia 103, 105, 108, 284, 327, 329, 338, 379, 400, 414
 severity of 430

Apoptosis 3, 4
 sensors of 274
Arsenic
 therapy 381
 trioxide 376
Arterial thrombosis 53
Arthralgia 103
Arthritis 103
 worsening 328, 331
Arylsulfatase 110
Asciminib 346
Ascorbate 34
Asparaginase 125, 131
Aspartate aminotransferase 325
Aspergillus 146
Aspirin 56
Asthma 93
 bronchial 364
Ataxia 418
Atenolol 70
Atherosclerosis, accelerated 282
Atrial fibrillation, chronic 54
Auer rods 28, 275, 365
Autoantibody 305
 against red cells 395, 398
Autoimmune disease 43
Autologous stem cell transplant 115, 150, 172, 238, 379
Azacitidine 226
 plus venetoclax 146

B

Bacteria, antigens of 308, 316
Bacterial infection 109
Band 3 protein 282
Basket cell 25
Basophilia 277, 398, 399
Basophilic disorders 110
Basophilic stippling 16, 287, 407
Basophils 111, 143, 165, 222, 393
 granules of 290
B-cell 319
 acute lymphoblastic leukemia 383
 lymphocytosis 279
 lymphoma, high-grade 185, 330, 339
 maturation antigen 352
 prolymphocytic leukemia 182
 quantification 319
Belantamab mafodotin 205
Bence-Jones proteins 330, 366
Bendamustine 204, 357
Bernard-Soulier syndrome 42, 97, 285, 331, 398
Beta-galactosidase 6
Beta-glycoprotein 288
Beta-thalassemia 83, 85, 88, 327, 328, 331, 335
 cause of 83
Bevacizumab 345
Bing-Neel syndrome 184
Biopsy 251
Birbeck granules 329

Bispecific antibody 348, 384
Bite cells 68
Bleeding 95, 259, 369
　causes of 392
　diathesis 95
　disorder 420
　gastrointestinal 98, 410
　massive 260
　time 99
Bleomycin 178
Blinatumomab 127, 345
Blood
　banking 305
　cells 401
　components
　　irradiation of 414
　　leukodepletion of 306
　　therapy 397
　flow, stasis of 45
　group 213, 416
　　antibodies 307
　　system 305, 307
　loss, acute 40, 308
　sample 366
　sugar, high 372
　tests 105
　transfusion 38, 46, 83, 274, 305, 308
　　massive 307
Bombay blood group 308
Bone marrow 12, 33, 188, 221, 273, 274, 278
　aspiration 11, 407
　autologous 236
　biopsy 11, 103, 219, 329, 407
　blasts 280
　cells 14, 400
　examination 216, 367
　　indication of 276
　failure syndromes, inherited 103, 204
　flow cytometry 405
　frequency of 220
　involvement 153, 389
　iron stain 273
　karyotype 325
　normal component of 12
　plasma cells, assessment of 319, 321
　stem cells 8
　test 103
　treatment of 238
Bordetella pertussis 25
Bortezomib 205, 286, 357
　side effects of 204, 357
Brain 214
Breath, shortness of 66, 306, 326
Brentuximab vedotin 171, 172, 346, 384, 420
Bright-field microscopy 50
Bronchoalveolar lavage 89
Brucellosis 326
Bruton's agammaglobulinemia 81
Bruton's tyrosine kinase 159
Buffy coat 306
　collection 307
Bulky disease 171
Burkitt's lymphoma 183, 185, 229, 275, 325, 329, 420
Busulfan 236

C

Calcitriol 369
Cancer 55, 380

Caplacizumab 50, 345
Carbohydrates 417
Carboxyhemoglobin 19, 367
Carcinoma
　colon 44, 259
　prostate 16
Cardiomyopathy 85, 352
Carfilzomib 205
Caspases 4
Castleman disease, multicentric 278
Cat scratch disease 325
Cataract surgery 94
Cedazuridine 353
Celiac disease 413
Cell 3
　adhesion molecules 3
　biology 3
Cellulose acetate electrophoresis 275
Central nervous system 69, 126, 181, 189, 198, 211, 381, 399, 427
　lymphoma 182
　primary diffuse large B-cell lymphoma of 184
Centrifugation 312
Cephalohematoma 95
Cerebriform nucleus 182
Cerebrospinal fluid 366, 391
Cervical lymph node biopsy 80, 325, 326
Chemical meningitis 359
Chemoimmunotherapy 189
Chemokines 5, 10
Chemotherapy 132, 140
　consolidation 135
　intensive 227
Chest syndrome, acute 69, 306
Chimeric antigen receptor-T cells 127, 319
Chlorambucil 154
Chloramphenicol 78, 364
Cholecystectomy 54
Cholestasis 243
Cholesterol, serum 56
Chromosome 179, 292
　loss of 6
Cidofovir 248
C-kit mutations 276
Cladribine 216, 217
　plus rituximab 218
Clastogenic agent 103, 381
Clonal hematopoiesis 228, 271
　age-related 386
Clonal somatic mutations 224
Cobalamin
　deficiency 38, 39, 402, 406
　low serum 39
Cohesin complex genes 280
Cold
　agglutinin disease 61, 75, 76 182, 308, 315, 416
　antibodies 308
Competitive xanthine oxidase inhibitor 231
Complete blood count 16, 54, 60, 83, 260, 326, 396
Computed tomography scan 171, 367
Concizumab 96, 120
Coombs' test 259
　direct 56, 75, 76, 78, 305, 308, 326, 365, 399, 406, 408, 415
　indirect 306, 405
Copper deficiency 34, 36
Coronary artery disease 259
Corticosteroids 27, 306

COVID-19
　coagulopathy 419
　infection 368, 420
　pneumonia 275
Crizanlizumab 70, 345
　mechanism of action of 70
Crizotinib 345
Crow-Fukase syndrome 367
Cryoprotectant solutions 239
Cyanmethemoglobin 17, 21
　method 16, 18
　　principle of 17
Cyclophosphamide 129, 235, 236, 357
　post-transplant 237, 415
Cyclosporine 107, 243, 251, 367
　toxicity, chronic 104, 381
Cytarabine 126, 144, 148, 164, 359
　high-dose 383
　liposomal formulation of 386
Cytogenetic abnormalities 4, 136, 153, 380, 389, 392, 399
Cytokine, multilineage 12
Cytomegalovirus 192, 235, 245, 330, 381
　drugs effective against 381
　infection 305
　transmission 307
Cytopenia 223
　refractory 224, 228, 271
Cytosine 98

D

Dabigatran 54, 413
Daclizumab 308
Dacryocytes 23
Dactylitis 115
Daratumumab 205, 308, 315, 346, 394
　mechanism of action of 346
Dasatinib 163, 165, 279
Daunorubicin 151, 386
　side effects of 357
De novo purine synthesis 252
Decitabine 147
Deep vein thrombosis 44, 54, 358, 413
Deferiprone 86, 432
Deferoxamine 402, 432
Dehydration 70
Denintuzumab mafodotin 134
Denosumab, mechanism of action of 204
Deoxyhemoglobin polymerization 72
Deoxynucleotidyl transferase assay 328
Dephosphorylation 168
Dermal venous thrombosis 331
Desferrioxamine, side effects of 83
Desmopressin 96, 117
Dexamethasone 51, 129, 149
Diabetes
　insipidus 329
　mellitus 278, 327
Diarrhea 305
Diepoxybutane 400
Diffuse large B-cell lymphoma 181, 183, 184, 330, 351, 352
DiGeorge syndrome 80, 81
Digestive enzymes 25
Dilute Russell's viper venom time 99
Diphenhydramine 250
Direct antiglobulin test 306

Disease-modifying antirheumatic drug therapy 32
Disseminated intravascular coagulation 43, 95, 119, 415
Diverticulosis 326
Döhle bodies 28, 93, 373
Dolichos biflorus 307
Donath-Landsteiner syndrome 367
Donor lymphocyte infusion 162, 237, 383
Donor T cells 239
Double-hit lymphoma 184, 185, 199, 275
    treatment for 185
Down's syndrome 137, 293
    transient leukemia of 393
Downey cells 28
Dry cough 306
Dutcher bodies 401
Dyserythropoiesis 274
Dyskeratosis congenita 103, 104, 389
Dysplasia 135, 225, 227
    multilineage 223, 228

E

Ecchymoses 260
Ecchymotic spots 80
Eculizumab 114, 249, 358, 390, 401
Edema, pulmonary 328, 331
Ektacytometer 62
Elliptocytes 330
Elliptocytosis, hereditary 59, 328
Elotuzumab 394, 395
Eltrombopag 357, 368, 379
    mechanism of action of 357
Embolism, pulmonary 375
Emicizumab 96, 97, 345, 346, 376, 392
    mechanism of action of 96
Enasidenib 349, 376
Endothelial cells 47
Engraftment syndrome 238
Enzyme deficiency 60
Eosinophilia 89, 367
    cause of 89
    reactive 407
    severe 89
Eosinophilic disorders 89
Eosinophils 329
    maturation of 89
Epithelial cells 14, 15
Epsilon aminocaproic acid, usual dose of 390
Epstein-Barr virus 24, 330, 340
    infection 281, 327, 328, 410
Erdheim-Chester disease 418, 434
Erythroblasts 37
Erythrocyte 287
    overcentrifugation of 308
    sedimentation rate 366
Erythrodontia 415
Erythroferrone true statement 33
Erythroid 11, 275, 393
    dysplasia 278
    hyperplasia 274
    precursors 366
Erythroleukemia 329, 372
Erythropoietin 11, 17, 32, 143, 166, 272, 306, 416
    elevated serum 365
    serum 329, 338
    therapy 104
Escherichia coli asparaginase, half-life of 125
Esterases 110
Ethanolamine 421
Ethylenediaminetetraacetic acid 19
Extracorporeal photopheresis 244

F

Facial
    bones, frontal prominence of 274
    skin 329
Factor V Leiden mutation 53, 55, 57
Fanconi's anemia 103, 104, 239, 326, 381, 389, 400
Fasciotomy 422
Fatigue 260, 327, 329
Febrile nonhemolytic transfusion reaction 305, 306
Fedratinib 415
Ferric gluconate 36
Ferritin
    aggregates of 291
    elevated serum 31
    serum 34
Fetal hemoglobin 70
    hereditary persistence of 369
Fetal warfarin syndrome 358
Fever 306
    cause of 423
    high-grade 43, 105
    low-grade 325
    sudden onset of 327, 331
Fibrin degradation product 406
Fibrinogen 305, 372
    deficiency 307, 313
Fibrosis, degree of 221
Fludarabine 154, 159
Fluorescein-labeled proaerolysin 271
Folate
    deficiency 36, 38, 39, 41, 399
    treatment 39
Folic acid 38, 39, 368
Follicular lymphoma 182-184, 326 427
    international prognostic index 181, 183, 427
    relapsed 182
Fondaparinux 54, 57
Fontolizumab 319, 321
Foscarnet 248
Fostamatinib 345
Fragmentation 328
Fragmented red cells 17
Franklin disease 421
Fresh frozen plasma 236, 307, 390, 390
    volume of 413

G

Gallstones 63, 67
Gamma interferon 13
Gammopathy, monoclonal 203, 280, 328
Ganciclovir 240, 248, 381
Gangliosides, cerebral 3
Gastrectomy 402
Gastritis, atrophic 326
Gaucher disease 329
Gemtuzumab ozogamicin 137
Gene expression profile 133
Genetic defect 104, 406
Germinotropic lymphoproliferative disorder 278
Glanzmann thrombasthenia 331, 340
Globulin 206
Glucarpidase 384
Glucocorticoids 104
Glucose-6-phosphate dehydrogenase deficiency 63, 65, 66, 327, 328, 336
Glutathione 22
Glycolytic pathway 19
Glycoprotein 6
Glycosylphosphatidylinositol 271, 401
Gonadal mosaicism 4
Graft-versus-host disease 251, 319, 379, 381, 399
    acute 379
    Glucksberg staging of 428
    risk of 235
    transfusion-associated 305
Graft-versus-host reaction 235
Granules, azurophilic 91, 393
Granulocyte 305, 330
    colony stimulating factor 12, 92, 126, 245, 399
    development, stage of 91
    transfusions 280
Granulomas 327
Granulomatous disease, chronic 59, 80, 91
Granulopoiesis 400
Gray-zone lymphomas 394
Groin pain, triad of 96
Growth factors, transduction pathway of 3
Gum 94
    bleeding 43
    hypertrophy 34

H

Haemophilus influenzae pneumonia 79
Hair loss 168, 179
Hairy cell 218
    leukemia 216, 329, 338, 416
        diagnosis of 216
        feature of 403
Ham's test 114
    sensitivity of 104
Haploidentical stem cell transplant 237
Haptoglobin 367, 404
Hasenclever index 171, 428
Hasford system 162, 383
Headache 142, 148, 182, 235, 329, 403
    worsening 330
Hearing loss 278
Heart disease
    cyanotic congenital 260, 413
    rheumatic 54, 259
Heinz body 68, 327, 365
Hemangioma
    hepatic 259
    surgery of 264
Hemarthrosis 94
Hematemesis 18, 262
Hematocrit 13, 18
Hematologic disorders 328
Hematology, benign 29
Hematoma, splenic 330
Hematopathology 271
Hematopoiesis 11, 393, 406 411
    extramedullary 12, 219
Hematopoietic stem cell 11, 93, 251, 393
    cryopreservation of 239
    transplantation 233, 415
Hematuria 43
Heme oxygenase deficiency 67
Hemochromatosis 33, 34, 83, 326
    hereditary 328, 331, 337, 341
    primary 365

Hemoglobin 16, 17, 70, 260, 280, 404
  abnormal 73
  concentration 16
  E disease 328, 396
  solubility test 404
  types of 17
Hemoglobinuria 16, 76, 330
  hemolytic paroxysmal nocturnal 358
Hemolysis
  chronic extravascular 65, 385
  degree of 61
  drug-induced 66
  extravascular 65, 405
  severity of 76
Hemolytic
  disease 305, 306, 308
  transfusion reaction 306
  uremic syndrome 53, 307
Hemopexin 367
Hemophagocytosis 279
Hemophilia 94, 97, 100, 347, 368, 388, 390
  A 96, 100, 307, 329, 331, 428
    incidence of 388
    treatment of 95, 346
  acquired 118
  autosomal 379
  B, Leyden phenotype of 388
  C 96
  frequency of 96
  severe 94, 388
  symptomatic 388
Hemopoietic proliferation 137
Hemorrhage 20
  acute 12
  cerebral 43, 351
  intracranial 260
  small petechial 45
Hemorrhagic disease 99, 370
Hemosiderin 8, 35
Hemostatic disorder 42, 99
Henoch-Schönlein purpura 48, 368
Heparin 46, 55
  unfractionated 44, 53
Hepatic sinusoidal obstruction syndrome 242
Hepatitis
  A 64
  B 305
    virus 187
  C
    antibody 305
    infection 326, 330
    virus 107, 305, 309, 330
Hepatosplenic T-cell lymphoma 184, 185, 200
Hepatosplenomegaly 18, 38, 329, 330
Hepcidin 274, 401
Hexose monophosphate shunt pathway 60
High apoptotic tumor cell death 399
Highly active antiretroviral therapy 49
High-performance liquid chromatograph 25, 396
High-pressure liquid chromatography 83
Hip flexure 96
Histone deacetylase inhibitor 349
Hodgkin's disease 403
Hodgkin's lymphoma 76, 171, 172, 325, 326, 328-330, 332, 370, 384, 420
  classical 173, 384
  nodular lymphocyte predominant 171, 173
Howell-Jolly bodies 21, 60, 274, 325, 328, 333

Human bone marrow 44
Human immunodeficiency virus
  associated
    immune thrombocytopenia 412
    lymphoma, treatment of 183
  disease 412
  infection 326
Human leukocyte antigen 24, 272, 306, 405, 416
Human T-lymphotropic virus 329
Hunter disease 3
Hydration 231
Hydronephrosis 80
Hydroxide 32
Hydroxycarbamide 69, 163
Hydroxycobalamin 40
Hydroxyurea 69, 70, 385, 416
Hyperbilirubinemia 76
Hypercalcemia 206, 230
  treatment of 365
Hypereosinophilic syndrome 89
  diagnosis of 89
Hypergammaglobulinemia 47, 279, 374
Hyperhemolysis, features of 415
Hyperimmunoglobulin E syndrome 404
Hyperimmunoglobulin M syndrome 319, 331, 340
Hyperkalemia 229
Hyperphosphatemia 229, 231
Hyperplasia
  megakaryocytic 327
  reactive 326
Hypersplenism 12, 105
  cause of 12
Hypertension 70
  portal 326
  pulmonary 71
Hyperviscosity 203, 385
  syndrome, manifestation of 365
Hypochromasia 328, 337
Hypochromia 16
Hypofibrinogenemia, congenital 405
Hypogammaglobulinemia, transient 331
Hypohomocysteinemia 55
Hypothalamic infarcts 51
Hypothermia 51
Hypoxia 8
  discovery of 352

I

Ibrutinib 155
  induced bleeding 155
  side effects of 154
Ibuprofen 93
Idarucizumab 350, 413
Idelalisib 345
Idiopathic pneumonia syndrome 239
Idiopathic thrombocytopenic purpura 95, 326, 328, 336
Iduronate sulfatase 6
Imatinib 89, 90, 163, 383
  dose of 398
  inhibits 162
  therapy, side effects of 163, 383
Imerslund-Gräsbeck disease 39
Immune thrombocytopenia 42, 45, 46, 260, 348, 380, 397
Immunity, innate 278
Immunodeficiency diseases, primary 79

Immunoglobulins, cytoplasmic 130
Immunohematology 317, 319
Immunosuppressive therapy 265
Impetigo 80
Indeterminate cell histiocytosis 279
Indirect antiglobulin test 306, 307
Infertility 57
Inflammatory cytokines 319
Infliximab 308
Inosine monophosphate dehydrogenase 244
Interferon 164, 166
Interleukin 15
International prognostic
  index 383, 426
  Scoring System 223
International Society on Thrombosis and
  Haemostasis Score 415
International Staging System for Multiple
  Myeloma 430
Intravascular hemolysis 60, 65, 305, 385, 410
  cause of 60, 65
Intravascular large cell lymphoma 181
Intravenous immunoglobulin 154, 305
  mechanism of action of 357
Intravenous iron formulations 402
Invasive aspergillosis, risk of 91
Inversion 7, 409
Ipilimumab 351
Iron 62
  absorption of 31, 34
  deficiency 31-33, 105, 396
    anemia 9, 19, 31, 33 36, 61, 329, 402
  metabolism 32
  overload 401
  serum 31, 32, 329, 408
  stores 18
Isochromosome 4, 6
Isocitrate dehydrogenase 376
Ivosidenib 376

J

Janus-associated kinase-2 397
Jaundice 60, 63, 67, 76, 259, 305, 407
Joint hematoma 94

K

Keratinocyte growth factor 418
Keratoconjunctivitis sicca 253
Ketonuria 325, 332
Khorana score 380, 421
Kills intracellular bacteria 289
Knee joints, swelling of 407
Kostmann syndrome 288, 411

L

Lactate dehydrogenase 65, 76, 306
Lactoferrin 92
Lambda light chain 278
Langerhans cell histiocytosis 329, 338, 368
Lap score 264
Large cell lymphoma, nucleus of 275
Lead poisoning 36, 331, 413
Leflunomide 248
Leg ulcers 72
Lenalidomide 204, 357, 395

Leptomeninges 198
Letermovir 381
Leucocyte alkaline phosphatase score 367
Leucovorin administration 384
Leukemia 126, 136, 366, 399, 417
    acute 260, 280, 365, 405, 406, 409
        basophilic 423
        erythroblastic 280
        lymphoblastic 99, 125, 126, 271, 319, 326, 328, 329, 337, 366, 379, 410, 428
        megakaryoblastic 280, 281, 292
        monoblastic 281
        monocytic 291
        myelogenous 326, 333
        myeloid 135-137, 224, 235, 237, 276, 277, 306, 328, 349, 382, 386, 391, 400, 417, 430
        myelomonocytic 280, 281
        promyelocytic 136, 148, 275, 276, 305, 376, 381-383, 386
        undifferentiated 280, 281
    atypical chronic myeloid 162
    chronic
        eosinophilic 374
        lymphocytic 75, 143, 153-155, 182, 271, 276, 306, 326, 329, 331, 334, 418, 429, 430
        myelogenous 326, 328
        myeloid 92, 161-163, 167, 231, 357, 373, 404, 416, 418, 428
        myelomonocytic 223, 395, 431
        neutrophilic 162, 276, 404
    congenital 399
    cutis 135, 146
    inherited 136
    juvenile myelomonocytic 162, 396
    lymphoblastic 326
    mature B-cell 127
    megakaryoblastic 135
    prolymphocytic 154
    spontaneous remission of 136, 399
Leukemic lineage switch 319
Leukemoid reaction 326
Leukocyte 25, 149
    adhesion deficiency 80, 113
    alkaline phosphatase 104, 407
        score 325
Leukocytosis 27, 114, 278
Leukodepletion 306, 307
Leukoerythroblastosis 326, 408
Leukopenia 280, 325
Leukostasis 409
L-glutamine therapy 345
Light-chains 373
    deposition disease 393
Liposomal cytarabine 386
Lithium 367, 373
Liver 12, 13
    cirrhosis of 413
    disease 274
        active 41
        alcoholic 260
        dysfunction 412
        function tests 103
Low fibrinogen levels 99
Low mean cell volume 62
Low molecular weight heparin 44, 53, 358
Low reticulocyte count 39

Lung
    disease, chronic obstructive 259
    injury, transfusion-associated 306, 312
Luspatercept, mechanism of action of 96
Lymph node 177, 279
Lymphadenopathy 38, 105, 156, 327, 329, 330
    diffuse 260
    generalized 24, 329
        cervical 325
    inguinal 79, 325
    multiple suppurative 80
    supraclavicular 325
Lymphoblasts 365
Lymphocyte 24 28, 153, 171, 328, 329, 330
    atypical 325
    intraepithelial 279
    monomorphic 326
    predominant cells 173
    small mature 325
    syndrome 413
Lymphocytosis 24, 292, 395, 411
    monoclonal B-cell 395, 398
Lymphohistiocytosis, hemophagocytic 350, 380, 382, 428
Lymphoid 319
    infiltrates, atypical cutaneous 373
    neoplasms 367
    organ, primary 24
    tissue lymphoma, mucosa-associated 383
Lymphoma 181, 186, 271, 330, 386, 397, 399, 403, 407, 433
    anaplastic large cell 183, 201, 349
    angioimmunoblastic 183, 350
    B-lymphoblastic 275
    cells 279
    classification 185
    lymphoblastic 125
    lymphocytic 326
    lymphoplasmacytic 182, 191, 273, 198, 403
    marginal zone 193, 375
    pediatric
        follicular 182
        T cell 183
    plasmablastic 185, 275
    primary cutaneous 373
    small lymphocytic 153, 389
Lymphoproliferative disorder 237, 420
    post-transplant 237, 238
Lysozyme 92, 110

M

M protein 376
Macrocephaly 108
Macrocytes 66
Macrocytosis 402
Macroophthalmia 364
Macro-ovalocytes 330
Macrophage
    activation syndrome 413
    disorders 112
Macrothrombocytopenia 43
Macular rash, erythematous 330
Magnesium 108
Magrolimab 346
Major histocompatibility complex 16
Major orthopedic surgery 47
Malabsorption syndrome 51
Malaise 39, 325, 326
    generalized 325

Malaria 305, 327
Malignant cells 179
Malmö protocol 97
Mantle cell lymphoma 185, 191, 193, 198, 201, 275
Manual reticulocyte count 11
Maribavir 248
Marrow 12
    cells 15
    failure, post-hepatitis 381
    fibrosis 397
    gelatinous transformation of 367
Mass
    abdominal 259
    anterior mediastinal 127
    lesion 330
Mast cell 110, 112
    cytoplasmic granules 110
    disease 405
Mastocytosis
    cutaneous 110, 279
    systemic 278
McLeod phenotype 61, 416
Mean corpuscular
    hemoglobin concentration 19, 62, 76
    volume 38, 83, 325
Mean platelet volume 412
Megakaryoblasts 276
Megakaryocyte 50
    cytoplasm of 49
Megaloblastic anemia 18, 38, 39, 278, 285, 327
    syndrome 402
    treatment of 38
Megaloblastosis 402
Melphalan 208
Memory B-cells 156
Menarche 94
Menorrhagia 94
Mental
    confusion 326
    retardation 403
Mercaptopurine 358
Mesenchymal stem cells 252
    surface antigen expression of 252
Mesenteric vein thrombosis 331
Metamyelocyte 28, 92
Metarubricyte 12
Methemalbumin 367, 373
Methemoglobinemia 73
    acquired causes of 73
    clinical manifestations of 73
Methotrexate 40, 243, 358
    high dose 193, 384
    intrathecal injection of 357
Methylene blue 13, 74
    reticulum 17
Methylprednisolone 244, 252
Microangiopathy 47
Microcytic hypochromic cells 84, 409
Microcytosis 407
Micromegakaryocyte 169, 280
Microscope lens 366
Microtubules 6
Midostaurin 137, 386
Minimal bone marrow toxicity 133
Minimal residual disease 126, 205
Miracle mouth wash 239
Mitomycin C 400
Mitosis 91

Molecular defects 135
Molecules, antiapoptotic 274
Monoblast 371
Monocyte 111-113, 328-330
Monocytosis 279, 397, 407
Mononine 351
Mononucleosis 24
    infectious 77, 326, 327
Monosomal karyotype 391
Moxetumomab pasudotox 347
Mucoproteins 28
Multi-nucleate giant cells 279
Multiple myeloma 167, 203-205, 215, 283, 325, 330, 352, 358, 401, 420
    staging of 203, 385
    symptomatic 428
Mycophenolate mofetil 236, 256
Mycosis fungoides 186, 190, 325, 329, 338
Myeloblasts 137, 371
Myelocyte 92
Myelodysplasia 327, 329, 336
Myelodysplastic syndrome 103, 135, 223, 224, 271, 280, 347, 388, 430
    high-risk 223
    pathophysiology of 223
    primary 223
    secondary 223
Myelofibrosis 13, 166, 219, 326, 334, 347
    causes of 408
    nonmalignant cause of 162, 383
    percentage of 404
    prefibrotic 219
    primary 219
Myeloid 275, 319, 367
    cells
        immature 327, 335
        mature 327, 335
    development, stage of 393
    leukemia 133
    leukemic blasts 146
    marker 399
    neoplasms 224, 228
    reconstitution syndrome 395
    sarcoma, treatment for 135
Myelokathexis 92
Myeloma 27, 205, 430
    cells 203
Myeloperoxidase 91
    stains 137, 275
Myeloproliferative disorder 327-329, 336, 387
Myocardial infarction 71, 107
Myoglobinuria 16
Myopathy 210

N

Natural killer cells 272, 280
Nausea 327, 331
Neisseria gonorrhoeae 27
Neoplasms, myeloproliferative 219
Neoplastic cells 280
Neural tube defect 41
Neurofibromatosis 279, 397, 398
Neuropathy, peripheral 384, 418
Neutropenia 91, 92, 103, 112, 375
    absolute neutrophil count 174
    benign ethnic 401
    chronic idiopathic 91
    febrile 126

    persistent severe 278
    severe congenital 228
Neutrophil 93, 225, 226, 260, 328, 329, 393
    alkaline phosphatase activity 91
    hypersegmented 91, 92, 224, 328, 336
    macrocytic 92
Neutrophilia 92, 418
Neutrophilic disorders 91
Night sweats 325
Nivolumab, mechanism of action of 173
Non-Hodgkin's lymphoma 13, 181, 182, 330, 339, 403, 427
    development of 182
    pathogenesis of 181
Noonan syndrome 279
Nuclear hypersegmentation 40
Nucleic acid test 415
Nucleus 22, 275
    loss of 22
Numerous plasma cells 325, 332
Nutritional deficiency 413

O

Oligoclonal 422
Omalizumab 358
Opthalmoplegia 418
Oral anticoagulants, direct 433
Oral iron 20
    therapy 32, 402
Oral penicillin 371
Oral swab culture 325
Orthochromatic normoblast 15
Osmotic fragility test 59, 60, 62, 85, 329, 412
Osteoblasts 112
Osteopenia 107
Otitis media 79, 80, 91
Oxygen tension 327

P

Packed red blood cell 305
    volume of 21
Pacritinib 353
Pain, abdominal 18, 327, 330, 331
Palifermin, dose of 248
Pallor 260
Pancytopenia 56, 103, 259, 305, 309, 412
Papilledema 142
Pappenheimer bodies 21, 60, 287
Paragonimiasis 89
Parasitic infection 266
Paroxysmal cold hemoglobinuria 76
Paroxysmal nocturnal hemoglobinuria 104, 114, 115, 271, 347, 363, 374, 401
    feature of 104
Partial thromboplastin time 326, 327, 331
Parvovirus infection 105, 327, 331, 341
Paterson-Kelly syndrome, features of 32
Pearson marrow-pancreas syndrome 36
Pedal edema, bilateral 331
Pelger-Huet anomaly 93
Pembrolizumab 384
Peptic ulcer disease 331
Periodic acid Schiff staining 25, 128, 137
Peripheral blood
    counts 14
    film 60
    lymphocyte 25, 329
    smear 25, 39, 43, 59, 274, 326-331, 367, 431
    stem cells 236
Phagocytic disorder 80

Phagocytosis 25, 319
Pharyngitis 325
Phenytoin 367
Philadelphia chromosome 366, 379
Phlebotomy 369, 387
Phophoethanolamine 421
Phosphatases 110
Phosphate 32
Phosphoglycerate kinase deficiency 66
Pink test 398
Plasma 306
    cell 28
        leukemia 203, 385
        sheets of 327
    exchange 44, 49
        therapy 48
    hemoglobin 67
    homocysteine levels 409
    volume 35
Plasmablasts 278, 401
Plasmacytoid dendritic cell 272
    neoplasm 276
Plasmacytoma 330, 373
    extramedullary 204
Plasmic score 44
Plasminogen 98
Plasmodium
    falciparum 305
        malaria 409
    vivax 305, 310, 365
        infection 329
Platelet 42, 44, 71, 305, 306, 309, 311
    aggregation 408
    average life span of 379
    count 18, 38, 43, 44, 51, 95, 149, 260
    fraction, immature 415
    immune destruction of 43
    life span 407
    microparticles 392
    poor plasma 273, 395
    strongest activator of 43
    transfusion 48, 306, 307
Plerixafor 346
Plummer-Vinson syndrome 367
    features of 32
Pneumonia 72
    episode of 81
    recurrent 91
Poikilocyte 21
Poikilocytosis 328, 331
Polychromasia 330
Polycythemia vera 14, 18, 107, 162, 219, 220, 275, 278, 328, 331, 383, 387, 397, 408, 409, 431
    diagnosis of 409
Polyethylene glycol 306
Polyneuropathy, organomegaly, endocrinopathy, monoclonal gammopathy, and skin changes syndrome 204, 418
Polysaccharides 28
Polyspecific direct agglutinin test 422
Ponatinib 163, 360
Popcorn appearance 171
Porphyrin ring 20
Positron emission tomography scan 171
Posterior reversible encephalopathy syndrome 241
Post-haploidentical transplant 237

Postremission therapy 135
Postsplenectomy 59, 287
Postsplenectomy infection 365
Post-transfusion purpura 42, 305, 307
Potassium
    cyanide 21
    ferricyanide 21
Prilocaine hydrochloride 73
Primidone 367
Proerythroblasts 280
Progenitor cells, hypersensitivity of 143
Promyelocyte 93, 280
Pronormoblast, atypical 280
Prosthetic valve replacement surgery 54
Protamine neutralizes 379
Proteasome 9
    inhibition 351, 360
Proteins
    antiapoptotic 3
    C deficiency 54, 55
    proapoptotic 3
Proteinuria 325, 332
    subnephrotic range 38
Prussian blue 22
P-selectin inhibitor 72
Pseudolymphoma 367, 373
Pseudo-Pelger-Huët anomaly 223
Pseudothrombocytopenia 42, 379
Pseudotumor cerebri 390
Pure red cell aplasia 405
Pure white cell aplasia 112
Pyknotic nuclei 91
Pyridoxine responsive anemia 402
Pyrimethamine 66
Pyrimidine 5' nucleotidase-1 deficiency 66
Pyropoikilocytosis 59
Pyruvate kinase deficiency 66

Q

Quinacrine 327, 331

R

Radiation therapy 157
Radiotherapy 171, 189
Raised mean corpuscular hemoglobin
    concentration 416
Rasburicase 229
Ravulizumab 114, 345
Real-time quantitative polymerase chain
    reaction 416
Rectosigmoid region 253
Red blood cell 16, 36, 305, 308, 325, 333, 372, 399
    distribution 404
    exchange 422
    mature 16
    membrane 60
        disorders 59
    urea transporter 305
Red cell
    acanthocytosis 59
    adenosine deaminase 65
    antibodies 308
    aplasia 103
    distribution width 62
    enzyme
        defects 65
        disorders of 65
    indices 18
    maturation nucleus 12
    membrane 3, 417
        disorder, congenital 405
    protoporphyrin level 33
Reed-Sternberg cell 172, 178, 325, 382
Remission induction
    chemotherapy 135
    therapy 136
Renal dysfunction 167
Renal failure 209, 363
    causes of 229
    chronic 34
Respiratory failure 230
Respiratory infections, recurrent 79
Respiratory syncytial virus infection 51
Reticulocyte 16, 17
    count 11, 19, 31, 32, 60, 72, 109, 330, 411
    high 105
Reticulocytopenia 103
Reticulocytosis 36, 65, 66
Reticuloendothelial cell 112
Retinoblastoma 129
Retinoid acid syndrome 136
Reverse transcription-polymerase
    chain reaction 139
Rhesus incompatibility 63
Rheumatoid arthritis 32, 156, 197, 422
Ribavirin 385
Ribbon sign 252
Ribosome 20
    biogenesis, disorders of 274
Richter's syndrome 395
Richter's transformation 155
Ring sideroblasts 224, 282
Ristocetin-induced platelet aggregation 117,
    120, 272
Rituximab 46, 158, 195, 254, 308, 386
    addition of 181
    dose of 416
Rivaroxaban 364
Romiplostim 52, 394
Rough endoplasmic reticulum 25, 92
Ruxolitinib 219, 345

S

Saline, varying concentrations of 63
Sanger sequencing 417
Schilling test 39
Schistocyte 21, 328
Schnitzler syndrome 215
Schumm test 367
Scleroderma 330
Seborrheic eruption over scalp 329
Seizures 360
Seligmann disease 203, 385
Selinexor 347
Sensorineural hearing loss, progressive 278
Sensory loss, cutaneous 96
Serum amyloid P scintigraphy 211
Serum protein electrophoresis 208
Sevuparin 286
Sézary cell count 202
Sézary syndrome 185, 186, 420
    diagnosis of 186
Short stature 260
Shwachman-Diamond syndrome 104, 105, 389
Sickle cell
    anemia 69, 260, 273, 326-329, 348, 398, 409
    disease 69, 70, 72, 306, 349, 375, 416
    hemoglobin C 403
    trait 69
        complications of 70
Sickle hepatopathy 385
Sickling test 69
Sideroblast 18
Siderocyte 18
Siderotic granules 18
Silicone breast implants 185
Siltuximab 319
Sinusitis 91
Sinusoidal obstruction syndrome 238
Siplizumab 346
Sirolimus 252
Skin 279, 280
    biopsy 253
    lesions 280
    rash 305
Skull, computed tomography scan of 367
Smoldering myeloma 416
Smudge cell 28
Sodium metabisulfite test 72
Solitary plasmacytoma, diagnosis of 203
Soluble transferrin receptor levels 404
Somatic hypermutation 26, 319, 320
Somatocytosis 64
South-East Asian ovalocytosis 59, 387
Spectrophotometry 21
Spherocytes 60, 385, 404, 407, 410
Spherocytosis 328
    degree of 76
    hereditary 59, 60, 63, 327, 329-331, 387, 404,
        413, 414
Spleen 375
    function of 25
Splenectomy 24, 60, 405, 411, 414
    indications of 403
Splenic marginal zone lymphoma 155, 183
Splenomegaly 108, 242, 405
Spliceosome 8
Squamous cell carcinoma 108
Stem cell 9, 14
    donation 237
    markers 8
    mobilization 12
    transplantation 235, 237, 267, 280
        indications of 114
Stereotactic brain biopsy 330
Steroid 319
    therapy 89
Stomach 188
    alkaline pH of 34
Stomatocyte 21
Streptococcus
    infection 326, 333
    pneumonia 325
Stress, psychological 307
Stroke 267
Submandibular nodes 374
Sulfhemoglobin 21
Sunitinib 375
Supravital stain 20
Surrogacy 331
Systemic lupus erythematosus 76, 326, 330, 333,
    339

T

Tachycardia 327, 331
Tafasitamab 346
Target cells 59, 62, 72, 330, 387

Tartrate-resistant acid phosphatase 329, 330
Tazemetostat 346
T-cell 28, 253
- anaplastic large-cell lymphoma 417
- histiocyte-rich large B-cell lymphoma 185
- inhibition 179
- large granular lymphocytic leukemia 271
- leukemias 435
- lymphoblastic
  - leukemia 196
  - lymphoma 196
- lymphocytosis 279
- lymphoma, peripheral 185
- T-cell lymphoma 184

Tear drop cells 162, 330, 383, 385
Telangiectasia, hereditary hemorrhagic 95, 273
Telomerase 109
- inhibitor 346
Telomeropathies 105
Tempi syndrome 367
Testicular lymphoma 181
Tetralogy of Fallot 260
Thalassemia 33, 83, 87, 236, 396, 403, 411
- intermedia 403
- major 83, 406
- minor 330
- mutations 402
- syndromes 83
- trait 396
Thalidomide 204, 286
Threonine 170
Thrombin 47, 100, 421
- time 260
Thrombocythemia, essential 143, 219, 220, 278, 387, 404, 409, 431
Thrombocytopenia 43, 44, 94, 108, 224, 225, 260, 325, 347, 374, 380, 395, 406
- autoimmune 43
- cause of 42, 410
- drug induced 331, 341
- gestational 380
- heparin-induced 42, 307, 379, 411
- severe 305, 309
Thrombocytosis
- essential 166, 167, 397
- reactive 162, 383, 418
Thromboelastography 95
Thromboembolism
- pulmonary 54
- venous 394
Thrombophilia, evaluation of 53
Thrombopoietin 143
- receptors agonist 45
Thrombosis 53, 159, 210, 259, 411
- causes of 114
- high-risk of 120
- history of 222
- venous 53

Thrombotic thrombocytopenic purpura 307, 326, 334, 347, 379, 385
- post-transplant 238
Thymoma 367
Thymus 26
Tissue
- factor pathway inhibitor 117
- macrophage 112
- plasminogen activator 98
T-large granular lymphocytosis 422
T-lymphocytes 24
Tocilizumab 319, 345
Tonic clonic seizure 44
Tonsillectomy 95
Total hip replacement therapy 44
Total iron binding capacity 326
Total leukocyte count 18, 38, 141
Transferrin 402
- bound iron 36, 287
- deficiency 8
Transfusion
- medicine 303
- prophylactic 266
- therapy 12, 327, 331, 335
Trousseau syndrome 326
Tumor lysis syndrome 229, 383
- management of 229
Tympanic membrane 329
Typhoid 305, 310
Tyrosine kinase
- activity 358
- inhibitors 418, 429

U

Umbilical cord stem cells 8
Upper respiratory tract infection 79
Upshaw Schulman syndrome 51, 280, 416
Urea clot
- lysis test 98
- solubility test 266
Urticaria pigmentosa 110, 279
Urticarial, chronic 205

V

Valganciclovir 248
Vascular injury 42
Vaso-occlusive crisis 69
Vemurafenib 218
Venereal disease research laboratory 305
Venetoclax 147, 154, 155
Veno-occlusive
- disease 145
- syndrome 379
Villalta scoring system 394
Vincristine 129, 357, 359

Viral infection 237
Visceral leishmaniasis 90, 411
Vision, blurring of 148, 235
Vitamin
- B12 38
  - absorption 39
  - deficiency of 330, 368
  - levels 38, 413
    - serum 325, 367
- K
  - antagonists 358
  - deficiency 95, 274
Vomiting 148
von Willebrand
- disease 100, 117, 118, 307, 331, 373, 395
- factor 42, 117, 305
- syndrome, acquired 117
Vonicog alfa 118
Voriconazole prophylaxis 146
Vorinostat 345
Voxelotor 70
- mechanism of action of 70, 345

W

Waldenström macroglobulinemia 184, 198, 203, 380, 385, 411
Waldeyer's ring 367
Warfarin, teratogenic effect of 358
Warm antibody 76
White blood
- cell 306
  - count 260, 307, 325
  - types of 25
  - transfusion 308
Williams trait 395
Wiskott-Aldrich syndrome 47, 82, 285, 327

X

Xanthochromia 366
Xerocytosis, hereditary 61, 64
X-linked agammaglobulinemia 331
X-linked chronic granulomatous disease 79

Y

Y chromosome, loss of 282, 404
Yersinia enterocolitica 57, 85

Z

Zieve syndrome 414
Zoledronate 358
Zoledronic acid 204

www.ingramcontent.com/pod-product-compliance
Ingram Content Group UK Ltd.
Pitfield, Milton Keynes, MK11 3LW, UK
UKHW010821220425
457743UK00015B/118